RATE-CONTROLLED SEPARATIONS

RATE-CONTROLLED SEPARATIONS

PHILLIP C. WANKAT

School of Chemical Engineering, Purdue University,
West Lafayette, Indiana, USA

ELSEVIER APPLIED SCIENCE
LONDON and NEW YORK

ELSEVIER SCIENCE PUBLISHERS LTD
Crown House, Linton Road, Barking, Essex IG11 8JU, England

Sole Distributor in the USA and Canada
ELSEVIER SCIENCE PUBLISHING CO., INC.
655 Avenue of the Americas, New York, NY 10010, USA

WITH 28 TABLES AND 189 ILLUSTRATIONS

© 1990 ELSEVIER SCIENCE PUBLISHERS LTD

British Library Cataloguing in Publication Data

Wankat, Phillip C. *1944–*
Rate-controlled separations.
1. Chemical engineering. Separation
I. Title
660.2842

ISBN 1-85166-521-8 (casebound)
ISBN 1-85166-570-6 (paperback—USA only)

Library of Congress Cataloging-in-Publication Data

Wankat, Phillip C., 1944–
Rate-controlled separations / Phillip C. Wankat.
p. cm.
Includes bibliographical references and index.
ISBN 1-85166-521-8 (casebound)
ISBN 1-85166-570-6 (paperback—USA only)
1. Separation (Technology) I. Title.
TP156.S45W364   1990
660'.2842—dc20   90-38314

Printed in Great Britain by Galliard (Printers) Ltd, Great Yarmouth

PREFACE

Separations have always been very important in chemical engineering. This importance has recently escalated with the imminent emergence of new industries in biotechnology and high-performance materials. Separations will continue to remain important in bulk chemical manufacturing, petroleum processing, and the other standard areas of chemical engineering interest.

The development of new industries requiring the expertise of chemical engineers leads to problems and opportunities for chemical engineering education. Chemical engineering students need to be prepared for both the "known future" and the "unknown future." The known future includes the use of standard chemical engineering separation methods such as distillation and absorption which will remain important for many years. The unknown future involves the use of many relatively new separation methods such as adsorption, chromatography, electrophoresis, membrane separations.

A major question for chemical engineering education is what to teach. In the area of separations my personal answer has been to require undergraduates to study classical separations including distillation, adsorption and extraction. Then an elective course on newer methods which require a mass transfer analysis should be made available to seniors and graduate students. I would not mind if this second course were required of graduate students; certainly, that would be preferable to an additional distillation course.

My first book, *Equilibrium-Staged Separations*, was my response for the required undergraduate course. This book is my response to both the proposed second course, and to practicing chemical engineers who missed this material when they were in school.

v

This book, *Rate-Controlled Separations*, includes separation processes which require a rate analysis for complete understanding. This includes most of the newer separation methods. The style of this book is similar to the style of *Equilibrium-Staged Separations* and problem solving is emphasized throughout. However, a higher level of mathematical analysis is required, and an understanding of mass transfer is assumed.

The plan for this book is to start with crystallization which is essentially equilibrium based. Sorption separations which can be (but seldom are) operated as equilibrium staged systems are discussed next. Then membrane separations which are inherently rate processes are discussed. Finally, a progress report on selection and sequencing of separations is presented.

This book has been used in an elective course for seniors and graduate students at Purdue over a period of several years. My experience has been that the students have no great difficulty with crystallization even though this is their first exposure to population balances. The students find that the chapters on sorption separations are more difficult; possibly because of the inherent batch nature of these processes. The average and better seniors and all of the graduate students have been able to work their way through these difficulties. The membrane methods seem to pose no unusual difficulty for the students.

Many people have helped me with the writing of this book. My students have been most helpful in helping me develop clear methods to explain the separation methods. My teaching assistants (when I had this luxury), Sung-Sup Suh and Narasimhan Sundaram, have been very helpful in solving problems and finding errors. Professors Linda Wang and David Graves used parts of this book in their courses. Their comments were very helpful and have been incorporated into the text. Mr. Steve Leeper was very helpful in providing references on membrane separations. Dr. Scott Rudge did a very thorough review of Chapter 11, and he helped me appear to be reasonably knowledgeable in the area of electrophoresis. Professors Lowell B. Koppel and William R. Schowalter taught me my undergraduate and graduate courses in separations and awakened my interest in the field. Professor C. Judson King's book convinced me there were interesting research problems in separations. Professor L.B. Rogers who was in Chemistry at Purdue gave me my introduction to chromatography when I audited his course. My interest in problem solving was sparked by Professors Richard Noble and Donald Woods.

The keyboarding of this book was done by Mrs. Karen Parsons and Ms. Jan Gray. Their cheerfulness in the face of endless revisions is appreciated. Ms. Barbara Hildebrandt patiently drew and redrew the figures.

Finally, my wife Dot has supported me when I thought I would never finish, and my children Charles and Jennifer have provided light to my life.

Phillip C. Wankat

CONTENTS

PART II. SORPTION AND CHROMATOGRAPHY

PART III. MEMBRANES

PART IV. SELECTION AND SEQUENCING

Chapter 1

INTRODUCTION

This textbook considers separation processes where mass transfer rates need to be included for a complete analysis. Included in the book are crystallization, adsorption, chromatography, ion exchange, electrophoresis and membrane separations. We will start with equilibrium-based separation processes and gradually switch to rate processes. This will be done by starting with crystallization and finishing with membrane separations.

1.1. PART I: CRYSTALLIZATION

Crystallization is a complex, multifaceted subject. On one level of sophistication, crystallization can be considered entirely as an equilibrium stage separation process. This is done in Chapter 2 which could be included in a book on equilibrium staged separations. The coverage in Chapter 2 is concerned with crystallization from solution. Crystallization is done from a solution containing a solvent such as water or alcohol. This is the most common type of industrial crystallization. It is used for production of a large variety of inorganic salts and organic compounds. Usually, only a single equilibrium stage is required. The equilibrium diagrams discussed in Chapter 2 are similar to the enthalpy-composition diagrams used for distillation and the triangular diagrams used for extraction. Thus the principles will often be familiar although the diagrams may be more complex. In ternary systems such as two salts plus water, a single equilibrium stage operating at one temperature can produce a single pure salt plus a solution containing both salts. Fractional crystallization can be used to produce both salts as pure products. Fractional crystallization usually uses two equilibrium stages operating at different temperatures. These cycles are explained using triangular equilibrium diagrams.

1

When temperature has a large effect, a large amount of crystals can be obtained by *cooling* the solution. When temperature has a small effect cooling will have little effect. Crystallization then requires removal of solvent by *evaporation* or changing the solubility by adding another component (salting out). When there is a moderate temperature effect, both cooling and evaporation are used in a *vacuum* crystallizer. The equipment types used for these processes will be explained in Chapters 2 and 4.

The product from a crystallization is often sold as a solid (e.g. table salt or sugar). The size distribution and the shape of the crystals is very important in customer acceptance of the product. (It is annoying to buy a bag of sugar which is a single solid lump). The *crystal size distribution (CSD)* and the crystal shapes are *not* determined by equilibrium. Thus, if we stop at Chapter 2 we will miss a very important part of crystallization. To determine crystal size distributions, nucleation and growth rates are studied in Chapter 3.

Chapter 4 develops *population balances* (a count of the number of crystals in a given size range) and from this crystal size distributions are generated. The population balance is used first to develop the crystal size distribution for a simple case. From this several other distributions are calculated. Use of experimentally determined crystal size distributions to determine nucleation and growth rates is explored, and the effects of equipment variations on CSD are determined.

The second major type of crystallization is *melt crystallization*. In melt crystallization no solvent is present. Instead, the solid is melted and then slowly crystallized to purify it. This method is used for purification of organic chemicals, pharmaceuticals, and in the semi-conductor industry. Although many of the principles of melt crystallization are similar to crystallization from solution using cooling, the equipment is often very different. Some of the methods which will be discussed in Chapter 5 are normal freezing, zone melting, and counter-current column crystallizers.

The chapters on crystallization assume familiarity with equilibrium stage concepts and mass transfer. No prior knowledge of crystallization is required. The structure of the information is shown in Figure 1-1. This figure shows the

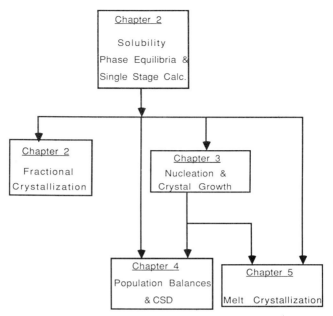

Figure 1-1.   Structure of knowledge for Part I. Crystallization.

path required to reach a particular topic. Chapter 2 is the basic chapter required for all other chapters. Note that some topics, such as fractional crystallization, although very interesting, are not prerequisites for later material.

1.2. PART II. SORPTION AND CHROMATOGRAPHY

In Chapters 6 to 10 we will switch gears and look at separation processes such as adsorption, chromatography, and ion exchange which separate based on the sorption of solutes onto a solid. These sorption separations all involve interaction with a solid but the mechanism of the interaction can be different. The separation is usually done in packed columns in a cyclic fashion. These separation techniques are thus usually quite different than equilibrium staged separations. The classical sorption separations use a column packed with small porous particles. The particles remove solutes from the fluid by adsorption or ion exchange. Since the solid is usually not moved, the solid will eventually become saturated. A separate desorption or regeneration step is required to remove and recover the desired solute. Operation is inherently time-dependent, and is not steady-state as are the equilibrium staged processes.

In Chapter 6 we will first look at a physical picture of what happens in adsorption and chromatography. Equilibrium expressions will then be considered. A simple theory of solute movement in the column will be developed for linear and then for non-linear equilibrium. This will allow us to determine when the column will be saturated. Then the rigorous mass and energy balances will be presented, and the solute movement results will be rigorously derived.

Chapter 7 discusses linear theories for chromatography and adsorption. The solute movement theory developed in Chapter 6 is used to explain chromatographic operations. The mass transfer equations are solved for systems with linear isotherms. Several linear chromatographic theories are compared.

In Chapter 8 several commercially significant packed bed adsorption processes are explored. The solute movement theory is used to delineate the basic principles of the process. The empirical mass transfer zone (MTZ) approach based on experimental data and theoretical constant pattern solutions are developed. Applications such as drying and pressure swing adsorption are discussed.

The topic of Chapter 9 is ion exchange. Electroneutrality and equilibrium will be discussed first. The properties of ion exchange resins are explored. Then the solute movement theory will be adapted to ion exchange. Several applications such as water softening and demineralization are discussed.

In Chapter 10 the development of counter-current and simulated counter-current processes for adsorption, ion exchange and chromatography will be discussed. These methods make the operation steady-state and the separations become analogous to equilibrium separations.

Figure 1-2 shows the structure of knowledge for Chapters 6 to 10. Chapter 6 is the key chapter required for all other chapters. Chapters 7 to 10

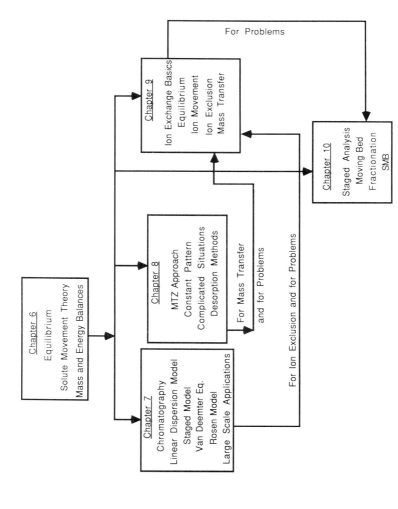

Figure 1-2.   Structure of knowledge for Chapters 6 to 10. Sorption separations.

are essentially independent of each other except that some problems will use analysis methods developed in previous chapters. These chapters assume familiarity with mass transfer concepts, but no previous knowledge of adsorption, chromatography or ion exchange. Chapters 2 to 5 are *not* prerequisites for Chapters 6 to 10.

Chapter 11 is an introduction to electrophoretic separations. These methods use migration of charged species in an electrical field to achieve separation. These methods have some similiarity to chromatographic separation methods; thus, Chapters 6 and particularly 7 are prerequisites for Chapter 11. Since electrophoretic methods are not currently used for large-scale separations, this chapter is a progress report.

1.3. PART III. MEMBRANES

Chapters 12 and 13 consider membrane separation methods such as gas permeation, reverse osmosis, ultrafiltration, dialysis, electrodialysis, prevaporation, and liquid membranes. The membrane separators, except dialysis and liquid membranes, can not operate as equilibrium separators. The separation is based on different rates of mass transfer through the membrane. These chapters assume familiarity with mass transfer concepts, but no previous knowledge of the membrane separators is required. Chapters 2 to 11 are *not* prerequisites for these two chapters.

Chapter 12 is an introduction to all of the membrane separators. First the basic concepts of membrane separators including membrane structure, flux, and geometry are discussed. Then each type of membrane separation is considered separately. First the method is defined and then the process is explained theoretically, but at a fairly simple level. This explanation includes permeability for gas permeators, osmotic pressure and concentration polarization for reverse osmosis, gel layer theory for ultrafiltration, electrochemical reactions and energy consumption in electrodialysis and diffusion in prevaporation.

Chapter 13 treats some of the theories for membrane separation in more detail. Chapter 12 is a prerequisite for this chapter. The theories of concentration polarization, gel formation and fouling in reverse osmosis and ultrafiltration are explained in detail. The effects of bulk flow patterns in the membrane module are modeled. Finally, irreversible thermodynamics is used to analyze transfer of solute inside the membrane.

1.4. PART IV: SELECTION AND SEQUENCING

Chapter 14 discusses selection and sequencing of separation methods. There are two very distinct problem categories. First, for new chemicals the problem may be finding *any* method or combination of methods which will do the desired separation. Second, if several separation methods will work the problem is determining the best method or sequence of methods to do the separation.

Three categories of methods have been developed for selection and sequencing. *Heuristics* are *rules-of-thumb* used to get one started. *Evolutionary* methods are techniques to move towards an optimum solution from the base case. *Algorithmic* approaches involve complete design of all alternatives. These three approaches are often used sequentially in the order listed. Unfortunately, these methods have been developed in detail for distillation, and to a lesser extent for extractive and azeotropic distillation, absorption, and extraction. Since very little research has been done on selection and sequencing of the separation methods covered in this book, Chapter 14 represents an unproven trial.

1.5. PROBLEM SOLVING

Engineers are problem solvers. Thus the ability to solve separation problems is critically important. To help you develop this ability example problems are solved in the text and homework problems are given at the end of each chapter.

An explicit problem solving strategy is often useful. The modification of the strategy developed at McMaster University (Woods *et al.*, 1975) is used for many of the examples. The discussion of this procedure closely follows that in Wankat (1988). The steps in problem solving are:

0. I want to and I can

1. Define the problem

2. Explore or think about it

3. Plan

4. Do it

5. Check

6. Generalize

Step 0 is a motivation and confidence step. It is a reminder that you got this far in your education because you can solve problems. The more different problems you solve, the better problem solver you will become. Remind yourself that you *want* to learn how to solve separation problems and you *can* do it.

In step 1 define the problem. Make sure that you clearly understand all the words. Draw the system and label its parts. List all the known variables and constraints Describe what you are asked to do. If you cannot define the problem clearly, you will probably be unable to solve it.

In step 2 you *explore* and *think about* the problem. What are you *really* being asked to do? What basic principles should be applied? Can you find a simple limiting solution that gives you bounds to the actual solution? Is the problem over- or underspecified? Let your mind play with the problem. Then go back to the Define step to make sure that you are still looking at the problem in the same way. If not, revise the problem statement and continue. Experienced problem solvers always include an Explore step even if they don't explicitly state it.

In step 3 the problem solver *plans* how to subdivide the problem and decides what parts to attack first. The appropriate theory and principles must be selected, and mathematical methods chosen. The problem solver assembles required resources such as data, paper, and calculator. While doing this, new subproblems may arise; you may find there are not enough data to solve the problem. Recycle through the problem-solving sequence to solve these subproblems.

Step 4, *Do it,* is often the first step that inexperienced problem solvers try. In this step the mathematical manipulations are done, the numbers are plugged in, and an answer is generated. If your plan was incomplete, you may be unable to carry out this step. In that case, return to the Explore or Plan steps and recycle through the process.

In step 5, *check* your answer. Is it the right order of magnitude? Does the answer seem reasonable? Have you avoided blunders such as plugging in the wrong number or incorrectly punching the calculator? Is there an alternative solution method that can serve as an independent check on the answer? If you find errors or inconsistencies, recycle to the appropriate step and solve the problem again.

The last step, *Generalize,* is important but is usually neglected. In this step you try to learn as much as possible from the problem. What have you learned about the physical situation? Did including a particular phenomenon have an important effect, or could you have ignored it? Generalizing allows you to learn and become a better problem solver.

I strongly encourage you to use this or another organized strategy and write down each step as you do homework problems. In the long run the use of an organized strategy will improve your problem-solving ability.

To become proficient in solving problems you must work on the homework questions and problems. The Homework at the end of each chapter is organized into a series of sections as follows.

A. Discussion Problems. These are questions requesting an essay type answer. The last question in each chapter asks for development of a *key relations chart.* This is your one-page summary of *everything* (key facts, equations, diagrams. etc.) which you need to trigger your memory. The key relations chart is an excellent way for you to summarize and review the chapter.

B. Generation of Alternatives. These problems ask you to brainstorm and develop alternatives. There is no one correct solution to these problems.

C. Derivations. These problems ask you to derive equations in the text or equations that are not given.

D. Single-Answer Problems. These are typical homework problems with a single answer.

E. More Complex Single Answer Problems. These are more complex problems or derivations.

F. Problems Requiring Other Resources. Some of these questions ask for a critical review of a classical paper. Others are problems which would have been in category D except some of the required data must be obtained from other resources.

Some chapters do not have categories B or E or F.

1.6. SUMMARY - OBJECTIVES

At the end of this chapter you should be able to

1. Briefly discuss the separation methods covered in this book.

2. List and define the steps in the problem solving strategy.

Part I
CRYSTALLIZATION

NOMENCLATURE CHAPTERS 2 TO 5

a	interfacial area/volume
a,b	empirical constants in Eq. (2-1b), or Eq. (3-15)
a_1 ,a_2	linear width of metastable zone, Eq. (4-67)
A	preexponential constant, Eq. (3-2)
A	cumulative area/vol of crystals
A	crystal surface area
A	area of heat exchanger, m^2
A	cumulative area/vol of crystals
A_c	cross sectional area
A_T	total area/volume of crystals
b	drying up points
B(L)	birth function, Eq. (4-59)
B	rate of formation of nuclei
C	fulcrum point
C_1 , C_2	Constants of integration for size dependent growth, Eqs. (4-61) and Table 4-3.
c	concentration, kg anhydrous crystals/kg water
c^*	equilibrium concentration
c_s	salt concentration or amount
C	flow rate crystals
C	constant of integration, Eq. (4-46b)
D	column diameter, m
D(L)	death function, Eqs. (4-59)

14

D	diffusivity
e	entrainment, Eq. (5-15)
f	solidification rate, cm/min
F	feed rate, kg/hr
F	flow rates, kg/hr
g	fraction of change frozen
G	linear growth rate, Eq. (3-5), m/s
h	heat transfer coefficient
i	order of nucleation, Eq. (3-4)
k	Boltzmann's constant $= 2.3085 \times 10^{-23}$ J/K
k_A	area shape factor, Eq. (4-20)
k_f	film mass transfer coefficient
k_i	linear distribution coefficient, Eq. (5-1)
k_N	rate constant for nucleation
k_r	rate constant
k_s	solubility product, Eq. (2-3b)
k_v	volume shape factor
K	constant, Eq (2-12)
K_G	overall coefficient
l	length of solid melted to form zone, m
L	liquid flow rate or amount
L	characteristic dimension of crystal
L	cumulative length m/m^3

L_D	dominant size mass distribution = $3G\tau$, m
L_f	size of fines, m
L_p	size product crystals, m
L_s	size seed crystals, m
m	mass solid deposited
M	mixed stream flow rate or amount
M	melt flow rate, kg/min
M	cumulative mass of crystals/volume
M_F	cumulative mass of fines/volume
M_T	magma density
MW	molecular weight
n	moles water per mole hydrate
n	population density
n	overall growth rate order, Eq. (3-16)
n^o	population density of nuclei
n_L	population density large crystals, Eq. (4-56b)
n_r	"order" for growth
n_s	population density small crystals, Eq. (4-56a)
N	kg solvent/kg salt
N	cumulative number crystals/volume
N	stirrer speed, rpm
N_T	total number of particles/vol.
P	product flow rate, kg/s

Q	volumetric discharge rate m^3/s
r	radius of particle or crystal, m
R	ratio retention times, Eq. (4-44a)
R	gas constant
S	kg salt in solution/hr
S	$c/c^* = $ supersaturation ratio
S_c	kg/hr crystals (hydrate form)
t	time
t_{col}	period of collection of magma, s
T	temperature °C or K
T_o	melting point temperature
T^*	temperature at equilibium
T_{cold}	coolant temperature
T_M	magma temperature
T_s	solid temperature
U	overall heat transfer coefficient
V	volume of magma, m^3
V	kg/hr vapor evaporated
V_M	molar volume of crystal
V_s	volume magma sieved, m^3
W	water flow rate, kg/hr
W_i	weight of crystals in sieve fraction i, kg
W_p	flow rate of product crystals, kg/hr

W_s	flow rate of seed crystals, kg/hr
x	mass fraction in solid
X	kg moles soluble salt/kg total salts
y	mass function impurity in the melt
y	mass or mole fraction salt in solution
y_{solute}	mass or mole fraction solute in vapor
Y	kg soluble salt/kg total salts
z	distance in zone melting, cm
z	increased fractional rate of removal of product

Greek

α	exponent in birth and death functions, Eqs. (4-59)
β	exponent in birth and death functions, Eqs. (4-59)
β	fraction of nuclei surviving point fines trap
β	constant in Eq. (2-12)
γ	constant for size dependent growth, Eqs. (3-15) and (4-60b)
δ	film thickness
Δ	delta or difference point
Δc	concentration supersaturation
Δc_{max}	maximum allowed supersaturation
ΔE	activation energy in Arrhenius Eq. (3-17)
Δg	fraction crystals melted.
ΔG	free energy change for formation of nuclei
ΔL_{growth}	$L_p - L_s$

ΔL_i size range sieve fraction i,m

ΔT supercooling temperature

λ molar heat of fusion

ρ_F feed density, kg/m^3

ρ_s solid density, kg/m^3

σ interfacial tension

τ V/Q, drawdown or retention time, s

τ_f retention time fines, s

τ_L retention time large crystals, s

τ_p retention time product, s

τ_s retention time small crystals, s

Chapter 2

CRYSTALLIZATION AND PRECIPITATION FROM SOLUTION-EQUILIBRIUM ANALYSIS

In the process of crystallization from solution the desired solute is dissolved in a solvent along with some impurities. The solution is made supersaturated by cooling and/or evaporation of solvent. Crystallization occurs usually on added seed crystals or on very small crystals (nucleii) broken off of other crystals. The crystals will grow and become larger until they are removed (harvested) from the crystallizer. Often the crystals will be pure and contain almost no impurity. This large separation factor is one of the reasons which makes crystallization a desirable separation method. After harvesting, the crystals are separated from the adhering solvent (mother liquor), and the crystals are prepared as a final product. A second reason why crystallization is often the separation method of choice is it can produce uniform crystals of the desired shape. This is important when a solid product is desired (e.g. with common salt or sugar).

Precipitation is a related process since solutes dissolved in a solvent precipitate out. However, the precipitate is usually amorphous and will have a poorly defined shape and size. Precipitates are often aggregates of several species and may include salts or occluded solvent. The precipitate is not pure and has a significantly lower separation factor than crystallization. Thus precipitation serves as a "rough cut" to either remove impurities or to concentrate and partially purify the desired product. Precipitation is an important separation method in production of many biochemicals and in mineral processing. Since many of the basic concepts of solubility and equilibrium are the same for crystallization and precipitation, these methods are considered together.

In this chapter we will explore solid solubility and phase equilibria for crystallization systems. The solubility diagrams will be used to explain and classify the different ways of doing crystallization commercially. Equilibrium methods for crystallization calculations will be developed, and fractional crystallization will be discussed. Finally, precipitation processes will be explored.

Equilibrium and equilibrium calculations are very important in crystallization design. However, equilibrium methods alone are not sufficient in crystallizer design as they can be for other equilibrium staged separations. Equilibrium calculations can tell the total mass of crystals produced, but equilibrium calculations cannot tell the size and number of crystals produced. For example, a mixture of one million particles each one mm in diameter has the same mass as 100 million particles each 0.1 mm in diameter. These two mixtures will be two very different products. To include the crystal size distribution in the design calculations, crystallization and nucleation rates and population balances must be included. These topics are the subject of Chapters 3 and 4.

2.1. SOLUBILITY

Solids have widely different solubilities in solvents. Since water is by far the most common solvent in crystallization, we will focus on the solubility of compounds in water. The effect of temperature on the solubility of different compounds is shown in Figures 2-1a and b and in Table 2-1 (Mullin, 1972). It is common to list concentration in mass ratio units such as kg of the anhydrous salt per 100 kg of water as shown in Figures 2-1a and b. Figure 2-1a shows the solubility of systems where only one crystalline phase is deposited over the range indicated. The materials with water attached such as $CuSO_4 \cdot 5H_2O$ are *hydrates*. The crystal is formed from a compound which consists of one molecule of $CuSO_4$ and 5 molecules of H_2O. This is the stable form of the solid from 0 to 100°C. Crystals with no water are called *anhydrous* (e.g. NaCl). Note that this type of diagram is slightly misleading since concentrations are plotted in terms of the anhydrous salt, but the stable form may be a hydrate. Obviously it is easy to calculate the kg of $CuSO_4 \cdot 5H_2O$ which are soluble from the kg of anhydrous salt which are soluble. Crystals can also change phase from one hydrate form to another or to the anhydrate. The phase transitions are illustrated in Figure 2-1b. A similiar figure for biochemicals is shown by Belter *et al* (1988).

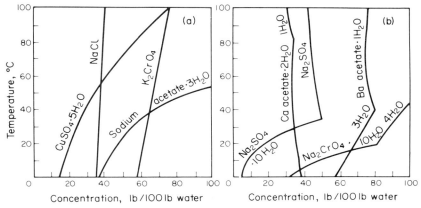

Figure 2-1.   Solubility diagrams. a. Systems without phase change. b. Systems with crystal phase changes. (Mullin, 1972). Reprinted with permission of Butterworths. Copyright 1972.

For ideal mixtures the solubility can be predicted with reasonable accuracy using the Vant'Hoff equation.

$$\ln y = \frac{\lambda}{R} \left(\frac{1}{T_o} - \frac{1}{T} \right) \qquad (2\text{-}1a)$$

where y is the mole fraction of non-solvated solute in solution, λ is the molar heat of fusion of the solute at it's melting point T_o, and R is the gas constant. Although Eq. (2-1a) does not work for non-ideal systems, an empirical modification will often fit the data

$$\ln y = \frac{a}{T} + b \qquad (2\text{-}1b)$$

Remember to use the absolute temperature in these equations. For many systems such as $CuSO_4 \cdot 5H_2O$ a plot of $1/T$ versus $\ln y$ will give a straight line. If a phase transition occurs, there will be two straight lines intersecting at the transition point. Some highly soluble salts such as sodium acetate do not satisfy Eq. (2-1b) and do not give straight lines on the $1/T$ vs $\ln y$ plot. Temperature increases can cause either marked increases in solubility as shown for sodium acetate or even a decrease in solubility (calcium acetate). This

22

decrease in solubility is called an *inverted solubility*. The temperature coefficient of solubility controls the type of crystallizer which can be used. This is discussed in the next section.

A considerable amount of solubility data has been collected in the literature. Standard references are Seidell (edited by Linke) (1958, 1965) and Stephen and Stephen (1963). Mullin (1972) also has fairly extensive solubility tables. A limited amount of solubility data is presented in Table 2-1. Thermodynamic methods for estimating solubility are discussed by Walas (1985).

Figures 2-1a and b show the saturation curves for the salts. For example, at 30°C twenty-five kg of anhydrous copper sulfate can be dissolved in 100 kg of water (see Table 2-1). This solution is stable and can be held indefinitely without crystallization. If a crystal of $CuSO_4 \cdot 5H_2O$ (the stable form of the solid at 30°C) is added, the crystal and the solution will be in equilibrium. Regions to the left of the saturation curves are *unsaturated* while regions to the right are *supersaturated*.

If the copper sulfate solution (with no crystals present) is either cooled or water is removed, the solution will become supersaturated. These processes are illustrated in Figure 2-2. Even though the solution is supersaturated no crystals may form. If a crystal were present it would grow, but crystals do not form spontaneously in this *metastable region*. If the cooling or water removal are continued until the system passes from the metastable into the *labile*

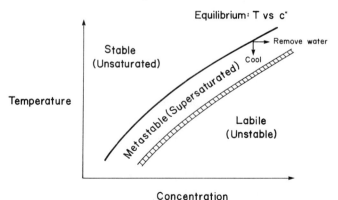

Figure 2-2.   Miers diagram showing metastable region.

(unstable) region then spontaneous formation of crystals does occur. Once crystals are present, the concentration of salt in solution will decrease as the crystals grow and the concentration will reapproach the equilibrium curve. The transition from the metastable region to the labile region is shown as a band since it depends on experimental conditions such as the degree of mixing. This is a kinetic transition, *not* an equilibrium transition. The plot shown in Figure 2-2 is often called a *Miers diagram*. Tavare (1987) summarizes studies on the metastable region.

Similar metastable regions can occur in vapor-liquid and liquid-liquid systems; however, there is a considerable difference in the size of the meta-stable regions. In crystallization and precipitation the metastable region is much larger. For instance, Miers found that a 53% solution of sodium nitrate in water could be supercooled by 14°C before spontaneous crystallization occurred.

Supersaturation is the driving force for crystallization and precipitation. Supersaturation can be defined as the concentration driving force

$$\Delta c = c - c^* \tag{2-2a}$$

or the supersaturation ratio

$$S = \frac{c}{c^*} \tag{2-2b}$$

Supersaturation can also be measured in terms of the supercooling.

$$\Delta T = T^* - T \tag{2-2c}$$

The solvent used, the addition of co-solvent and impurities can have a major effect on the solubility. The impurity may:

1. have no effect (this is unusual),

2. react with the solute,

3. cause the solute to precipitate (called *salting out*), or

4. cause the solution to become unsaturated (*salting in*).

Table 2-1. Solubilities of Selected Compounds (Mullin, 1972). grams anhydrous compuound per 100 g water.

Compound	Formula	Solubility °C								Stable Hydrate 0–25°C
		0	10	20	30	40	60	80	100	
Ammonium bicarbonate	$(NH_4)_2SO_4$	71	73	75.4	78	81	88	95.3	103.3	–
barium hydroxide	$Ba(OH)_2$	1.6	2.5	3.9	5.6	8.2	21	101		8
boric acid	H_3BO_3	2.7	3.6	5.0	6.6	8.7	14.8	23.8	40.3	--
calcium acetate	$Ca(C_2H_3O_2)_2$	37.4	36.0	34.7	33.8	33.2	32.7		29.7	2
copper chloride	$CuCl_2$	69	71	74	76	81			98	2
copper sulphate	$CuSO_4$	14.3	17.4	20.7	25.0	28.5	40.0	55.0	75.4	5
ferric chloride	$FeCl_3$	74.4	81.9	91.8				526	540	6
ferrous chloride	$FeCl_2$	61	64	68	73	77	89	100	106	6,4
lead chloride	$PbCl_2$	0.67	0.81	1.0	1.2	1.5	2.0	2.6	3.3	--
lead nitrate	$Pb(NO_3)_2$	39	48	57	66	75	95	115	139	--
lithium carbonate	$LiCO_3$	1.54	1.43	1.33	1.25	1.17	1.01	0.85	0.72	--
magnesium chloride	$MgCl_2$	52.8	53.5	54.5	56.0	57.5	61.0	66.0	73.0	6
potassium chloride	KCl	27.6	31.0	34.0	37.0	40.0	45.5	51.1	56.7	--

potassium chromate	K$_2$CrO$_4$	58.2	60.0	61.7	63.4	65.2	68.6	72.1	75.6	--
potassium nitrate	KNO$_3$	13.3	20.9	31.6	45.8	63.9	110	169	247	-
potassium sulphate	K$_2$SO$_4$	7.4	9.2	10.9	13.0	14.8	18.2	21.4	24.2	-
silver acetate	AgC$_2$H$_3$O$_2$	0.72	0.88	1.04	1.21	1.41	1.89	2.52	--	--
silver nitrate	AgNO$_3$	122	170	222	300	376	525	669	952	--
sodium acetate	NaC$_2$H$_3$O$_2$	36.3	40.8	46.5	54.5	65.5	139	153	170	3
sodium bicarbonate	NaHCO$_3$	6.9	8.2	9.6	11.1	12.7	16.4	decomp	--	--
sodium chloride	NaCl	35.7	35.8	36.0	36.3	36.6	37.3	38.4	39.8	--
sodium hydroxide	NaOH	42.0	51.5	109	119	129	174		340	4,3½
sodium nitrate	NaNO$_3$	73	80	88	96	104	124	148	180	--
sodium sulphate	Na$_2$SO$_4$	4.8	9.0	19.4	40.8	48.8	45.3	43.7	42.5	10
Acetamide	CH$_3$CONH$_2$	138	175	230	310	440	850			
Alanine (D)	CH$_3$CHNH$_2$COOH	12.7	14.2	15.8	17.6	19.6	24.3	30.0	37.3	
Alanine (DL)	CH$_3$CHNH$_2$COOH	12.1	13.8	15.7	17.9	20.3	26.3	33.9	44.0	
Benzoic Acid	C$_6$H$_5$COOH	0.17	0.20	0.29	0.40	0.56	1.16	2.72	5.88	
Citric Acid	C$_3$H$_4$OH(COOH)$_3$	96	118	146	183	215	277	372	526	1
Fructose	C$_6$H$_{12}$O$_6$	75	80	85	90					
Glucose	C$_6$H$_{12}$O$_6$	46	70	92	120	160	280	440		1
Lactose	C$_{12}$H$_{22}$O$_{11}$	12.2	15.0	19.5	25.2	33.3	57.5	102	153	1
Sucrose	C$_{12}$H$_{22}$O$_{22}$	179	190	204	219	238	287	362	487	1

In many cases it is difficult to predict if an impurity will cause salting out or salting in. However, if the added impurity has a common ion with the original solute, salting out will almost always occur. For example, if KCl is added to a saturated solution of NaCl, then NaCl will precipitate out.

The behavior of common ions can be predicted from the solubility product (Belter *et al*, 1988; Mullin, 1972). Consider the dissociation of a salt

$$P_m N_n = m\ P^+ + n\ N^- \tag{2-3a}$$

For a sparingly soluble salt where dissociation is complete and the activity coefficient is unity, the solubility product is

$$k_s = (c_{P^+})^m\ (c_{N^-})^n \tag{2-3b}$$

where c_{P^+} and c_{N^-} are ionic concentrations in any consistent set of units. The solubility product k_s usually follows an Arrhenius temperature dependance. In the example with KCl and NaCl, Cl^- is the common ion. Adding KCl increases c_{Cl^-}. Since k_{NaCl} is constant, increasing c_{Cl^-} requires that c_{Na^+} decrease which can occur only by precipitation of NaCl. Salting out can also be explained using ternary diagrams (see Example 2-3).

The solubility diagrams, Figures 2-1, and Table 2-1, are for systems with a single solute. When a second component is added or present in considerable amount, these simple diagrams are no longer adequate. More detailed phase diagrams are discussed in Section 2.4.

Figure 2-3. Cooling crystallizers. a. Indirect cooling with external circulation. b. Indirect cooling with internal circulation. c. Double-pipe scraped surface. (Garrett, 1961), Reprinted with permission from *Ind. Eng. Chem., 53*, 623 (1961), Copyright 1961, American Chemical Society. d. Direct cooling (Bennett, 1988). Reprinted with permission from *Chem. Eng., 95*(8) 118 (1988). Copyright 1988, McGraw-Hill Book Co.

27

a

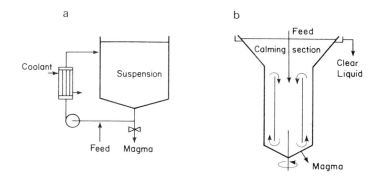

Coolant

Suspension

Feed   Magma

b

Feed

Calming section

Clear
Liquid

Magma

c

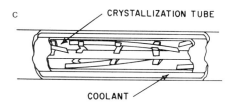

CRYSTALLIZATION TUBE

COOLANT

d

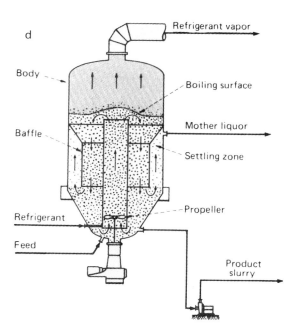

Refrigerant vapor

Body

Boiling surface

Baffle

Mother liquor

Settling zone

Refrigerant

Propeller

Feed

Product
slurry

2.2. EQUIPMENT TYPES

The solubility behavior of the system controls the type of equipment which can be used for commercial crystallization. This choice can be explored using the solubility diagrams discussed in the previous section. Most crystallization operations can be classified into one of five categories based on how the supersaturation is obtained. More details on the equipment are in Chapter 4 and in several reviews (Bennett, 1984, 1988; Mullin, 1972; Nyvlt, 1982; Moyers and Rousseau, 1987; Singh, 1979).

Cooling crystallizers obtain supersaturation by cooling the hot saturated solution. This method is applicable to systems where temperature has a large effect on solubility (for example, ammonium alum and sal soda, $Na_2CO_3 \cdot 10H_2O$). The method is not useful for systems like NaCl where temperature has little effect on solubility. A typical cooling crystallizer with an external heat exchanger is shown in Figure 2-3a while a jacketed tank, cooling crystallizer is shown in Figure 2-3b. A variety of trough type cooling crystallizers are also available with a variety of mixers. Scraped surface, double pipe heat exchangers (Votators) are used particularly for producing seed crystals (Figure 2-3c) Garrett (1961) and for viscous solutions such as crystallizing petroleum wax. Cooling can also be done by direct contact with an immiscible refrigerant. One method of doing this is shown in Figure 2-3d (Bennett, 1988). Cooling crystallizers are very desirable when they work since they have a high yield and low energy consumption.

Evaporative crystallizers supersaturate the solution by removing solvent through evaporation. These crystallizers are used when temperature has little effect on solubility (e.g. NaCl) or with inverted solubilities (e.g. calcium acetate). The crystallizer may be as simple as a shallow open pan heated by an open fire. This ancient technology is still in use for making maple syrup and fishery salt. For manufacture of common salt an evaporative crystallizer containing calandria (steam chest) is often used (see Figure 2-4a (Mullin, 1972)). The magma (mixture of crystals and solution) circulates by dropping through the central downcomer and then rises as it is heated in the calandria. At the top some of the solution evaporates increasing the supersaturation causing crystal growth. Forced circulation evaporative crystallizers are also commonly used.

One type is shown in Figure 2-4b (Bennett, 1988). These systems are obviously very similar to evaporators without crystallization (e.g., McCabe *et al.*, 1985; Mehra, 1986; Perry and Green, 1984). Spray evaporative crystallizers shown in Figure 2-4c (Bennett, 1988) are often useful when contact with air will not cause contamination problems. This cycle is very similiar to the forced circulation system.

The evaporators are often connected together to make a *multi-effect* evaporator as shown in Figure 2-4d. Here the vapor from the first unit is used as the steam to heat the second unit. This reduces the steam requirements per kg of product. The pressure must be varied as shown in the figure so that V will be at a temperature greater than the boiling temperature in the second stage. A variety of ways of connecting the different stages have been developed.

Any method for selectively removing the solvent could be used to supersaturate the solution. For example, Azoury *et al* (1987) used reverse osmosis to supersaturate aqueous calcium oxalate.

Vaccum crystallizers utilize evaporation to both concentrate the solution and to cool the mixture. Thus both of the methods used to cause supersaturation in evaporative and cooling crystallizers are used. The operating principles can be understood by referring to Figure 2-5a (Bennett, 1988). The hot liquid feed is at a higher pressure and temperature than the crystallizer. When this feed enters the crystallizer, it flashes and part of the feed evaporates. This flashing causes adiabatic cooling of the liquid (this is very similar to flash distillation). Crystals and mother liquor, containing any non-volatile impurities, exit the bottom of the crystallizer. Other variants of vacuum crystallizers have been developed. One example is the draft-tube baffled type shown in Figure 2-5b (Bennett and Van Buren, 1969). Because of the vacuum equipment required to operate at pressures from 5 to 15 mm Hg, the vacuum crystallizers are considerably more complex than the other types of crystallizers. Vacuum crystallizers are most common in large systems (more than 100,000 gal/day).

Salting-out processes add either a liquid diluent (anti-solvent) or a salt with a common ion pair to cause precipitation. For example, the effect of adding methanol on the solubility of common salts is shown in Figure 2-6 (Lozano, 1976). Addition of methanol to a saturated aqueous solution will

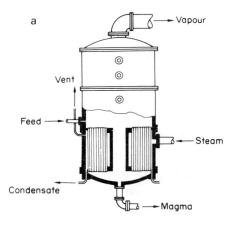

a

Vapour

Vent

Feed

Steam

Condensate

Magma

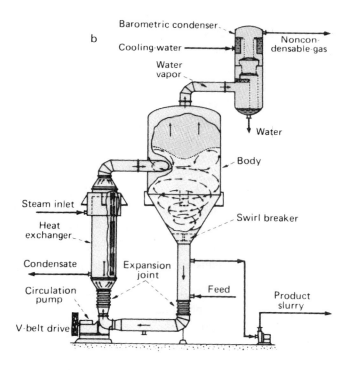

b

Barometric condenser

Cooling-water

Noncondensable gas

Water vapor

Water

Body

Steam inlet

Heat exchanger

Swirl breaker

Condensate

Expansion joint

Circulation pump

Feed

Product slurry

V-belt drive

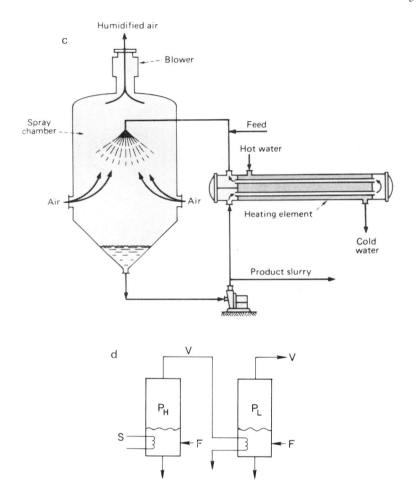

Figure 2-4.   Evaporative Crystallizers. a. Natural circulation with calandria (Mullin, 1972). With permission of Butterworths. Copyright 1972. b. Forced circulation, Swenson type. (Bennett, 1988). c. Spray evaporative crystallizer (Bennett, 1988), Parts c and b reprinted with permission from *Chem. Eng., 95*(8), 118 (1988), Copyright 1988, McGraw-Hill Book Co. d. Multi-effect system.

32

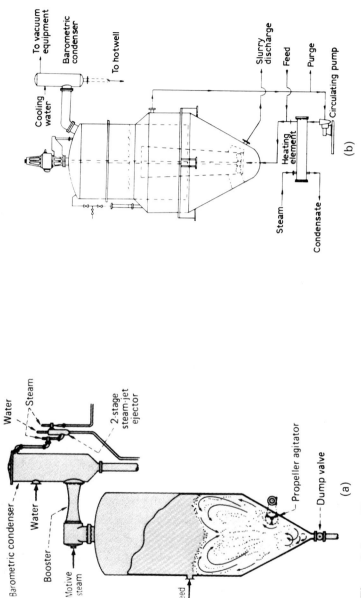

Figure 2-5. Vacuum crystallizers a. Batch (Bennett, 1988). Reprinted with permission from *Chem. Eng.*, 95(8), 118 (1988). Copyright 1988, McGraw-Hill Book Co. b. Swenson draft-tube baffled (Bennett and Van Buren, 1969). Reprinted with permission from *Chem. Eng. Prog. Symp. Ser.* 65 (95) 44 (1969). Copyright 1969, American Institute of Chemical Engineers.

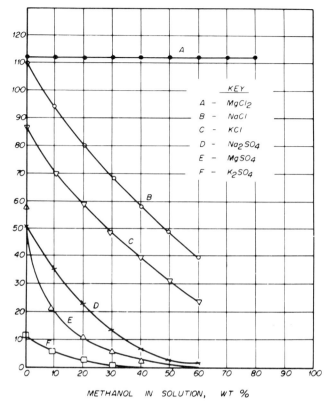

Figure 2-6.   Effect of methanol on solubility of common salts at 30°C
(Lozano, 1976). Reprinted with permission from *Ind. Eng.
Chem. Proc. Des. Develop., 15,* 445 (1976). Copyright 1976,
American Chemical Society.

often cause precipitation of the salt. Addition of alcohol has been used to salt
out $Al_2(SO_4)_3$ and to decrease the viscosity of the slurry. The crystallizer can
be a simple stirred tank, but additional equipment is required to recover the
methanol. A common use of salting out is the addition of $(NH_4)_2 SO_4$ to protein solutions to selectively precipitate different proteins. Sodium chloride has
been used commercially to salt out NH_4Cl. More details of salting-out methods
used in precipitation operations are in Section 2.6.

In *reaction crystallization* a solid product results from the reaction of gases and/or liquids. This process is commonly used in coke oven plants, the pharmaceutical industry, and in the production of some fertilizers. For example, ammonium sulfate is produced by reacting ammonia and sulfuric acid in a crystallizer. Reaction systems may produce a precipitate instead of well-defined crystals.

Both batch and continuous crystallizers are used. Generally, a production rate greater than about 50 ton/day is required to justify continuous operation (Bennett, 1988). The continuous operations tend to have higher yield and require less energy than batch, but batch is more versatile.

2.3. YIELD CALCULATIONS BASED ON SOLUBILITY DIAGRAM

When relatively pure solutions are crystallized or precipitated, the yield calculations can be done using the solubility diagram. A single stage process is almost always sufficient and can be done either batch or continuously. This is easiest to illustrate with two short examples.

Example 2-1A. Yield Calculation for Cooling Crystallizer.

A cooling crystallizer is used to crystallize sodium acetate, $NaC_2H_3O_2$, from a saturated aqueous solution. The feed is initially saturated at 40°C while the crystallizer is cooled to 0°C. If we initially dissolved the anhydrous salt in 100 kg of water/hr, how many kg of crystals/hr are collected?

Solution

In a cooling crystallizer there is essentially no loss of solvent. From Table 2-1 the feed solubility is 65.5 kg/100 kg water while the product solubility at 0°C is 36.3 kg/100 kg water. However, the amount of water available is reduced since the stable form of the crystals at 0°C is a hydrate with 3 moles of water (see Figure 2-1b or Table 2-1). A mass balance on the anhydrous sodium acetate is,

$$S_c \text{ (kg crystals/hr)}(\frac{MW_{anhydrous}}{MW_{hydrate}}) + c_{out}W_{out} = c_{in}W_{in} \qquad (2\text{-}4a)$$

where S_c is the kg of crystals/hr (hydrate form); c_{out} and c_{in} are concentrations of anhydrous $Na_2C_2H_3O_2$ per kg water, and W_{out} and W_{in} are the kg of liquid water/hour. A water balance is

$$W_{out} + S_c(\frac{n\, MW_{water}}{MW_{hydrate}}) = W_{in} \qquad (2\text{-}4b)$$

where n is the moles of water per mole of hydrate (3 in this example). Since c_{in}, c_{out}, W_{in} and the molecular weights are known, this represents two equations in the two unknowns S_c and W_{out}. Solving for S_c (see Problem 2-C1),

$$S_c = \frac{(\dfrac{MW_{hydrate}}{MW_{anhydrous}})(c_{in} - c_{out})W_{in}}{1 - c_{out}(\dfrac{MW_{hydrate}}{MW_{anhydrous}} - 1)} \qquad (2\text{-}5a)$$

For this example $MW_{anhydrous} = 82.04$, $MW_{hydrate} = 136.09$, $c_{in} = 0.655$ kg anhydrous/kg water, $c_{out} = 0.363$ kg anhydrous/kg water and $W_{in} = 100$ k/hr. Thus,

$$S_c = \frac{(1.66)(0.655 - 0.363)100}{1 - 0.363(1.66 - 1)} = 63.708 \text{ kg crystals/hour}$$

These crystals are $NaC_2H_3O_2 \cdot 3H_2O$. The mass of anhydrous material recovered is,

$$\text{Recovery, Anhydrous} = S_c\, \frac{MW_{anhydrous}}{MW_{hydrate}} = 38.405 \text{ kg/hour}$$

If the crystals were recovered directly as anhydrous material (e.g. with boric acid or lead chloride), Eq. (2-5a) can still be used. Now the ratio of molecular weights is unity and the equation simplifies considerably to,

$$S_c = (c_{in} - c_{out}) \, W_{in} \tag{2-5b}$$

Equations should never be used blindly. There may not be enough water available to form enough hydrate to crystallize all the material. Equation (2-5a) will predict incorrect results in this case (see Problem 2-D12).

Example 2-1B. Evaporative or Vacuum Crystallizers.

In evaporative and vacuum crystallizers some of the solvent is removed. This solvent removal must be included in the yield calculations. 1000 kg/hour of water is mixed with 280 kg/hour of copper sulphate at 40°C. The solution is cooled to 10°C and 38 kg/hour of water are evaporated in the process. How many kg/hour of crystals were collected?

Solution

From Figure 2-1A or Table 2-1 we notice that the stable crystal form at 10°C is $CuSO_4 \cdot 5H_2O$. A copper sulphate mass balance is,

$$(S_c, \text{kg crystals/hr})(\frac{MW_{anhydrous}}{MW_{hydrate}}) + c_{out} W_{out} + V y_{solute} = c_{in} W_{in}$$

Usually $y_{solute} = 0$. The water balance is

$$W_{out} + V + S_c(\frac{n \, MW_{water}}{MW_{hydrate}}) = W_{in}$$

where V is the kg/hour of vapor evaporated, $n = 5$, and the vapor is assumed to be pure water. Solving for S_c,

$$S_c = \frac{W_{in} \dfrac{MW_{hydrate}}{MW_{anhydrous}} [c_{in} - c_{out}(1 - V/W_{in})]}{1 - c_{out}(\dfrac{MW_{hydrate}}{MW_{anhydrous}} - 1)} \qquad (2\text{-}6a)$$

Note that Eq. (2-6a) reduces to Eq. (2-5a) when $V = 0$. For a salt such as NaCl which crystallizes in the anhydrous form Eq. (2-6a) reduces to

$$S_c = W_{in}[c_{in} - c_{out}(1 - V/W_{in})] \qquad (2\text{-}6b)$$

For this example, $MW_{anhydrous} = 159.61$, $MW_{hydrate} = 249.69$, $c_{in} = 0.280$ kg anhydrous/kg water, $c_{out} = 0.174$ kg anhydrous/kg water, $V = 38$ kg/hour, and $W_{in} = 1000$ kg/hr. Thus from Eq. (2-6a) we obtain,

$$S_c = \frac{1000(1.564)[0.280 - 0.174(1 - \dfrac{38}{1000})]}{1 - 0.174(1.564 - 1)} = 195.3 \text{ kg/hr crystals}$$

These crystals are $CuSO_4 \cdot 5H_2O$. Thus the mass of anhydrous crystals is,

$$\text{Anhydrous mass} = S_c(\frac{MW_{anhydrous}}{MW_{hydrate}}) = 124.88 \text{ kg/hr}$$

If this operation had been done in a cooling crystallizer (with $V = 0$) then $S_c = 183.84$ kg/hr.

The value of V (which was given in this problem statement) for a vacuum crystallizer can be determined from an energy balance. This is considered later. The vapor flow rate controls the diameter of the crystallizer. This calculation is essentially the same as for a vertical flash drum (e.g. see Wankat, 1988, Chapter 3).

Note in this example that the initial solution was not saturated. This did not change the calculation procedure. The final solutions are assumed to be in equilibrium, and thus are saturated.

The % recovery in this example is 124.88/280 x 100 = 44.6% which is low. The recovery can be increased by starting with a saturated solution at a higher temperature, operating the crystallizer at a lower temperature, or adding a second crystallizer such as a scraped surface crystallizer at very low temperatures.

Remember that these calculations assume that impurity concentrations are very low and do not affect the solubilities. If there are other components present then the phase diagrams considered in the next section are needed. The equilibrium calculations also do not give any information about the crystal sizes produced. For this the methods of Chapters 3 and 4 are required.

2.4. PHASE EQUILIBRIA AND SINGLE STAGE SYSTEMS

Phase equilibria for two component systems can be illustrated on temperature-composition, enthalpy-composition, and x-y diagrams. These equilibrium diagrams for solid-liquid systems are similar to those for vapor-liquid systems, but are often more complex. The principles remain the same. After presentation of two-component equilibrium data, three-component systems will be discussed. Three component systems can be shown on triangular diagrams. These presentations are similar to those for liquid-liquid extraction, but again the liquid-solid systems tend to be more complex. Data for many systems is given by Purdon and Slater (1946) and Seidell (1958, 1965).

2.4.1. Binary Systems

For binary systems Gibbs phase rule gives

$$F = C - P + 2 = 2 - 2 + 2 = 2$$

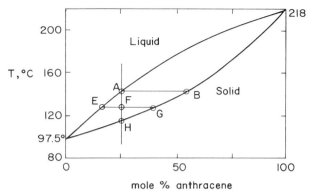

Figure 2-7.   Solid   solution   system: Phenanthrene   and   anthracene. Modified from figure in Walas (1985). Reprinted with permission of Butterworths, Copyright 1985.

degrees of freedom. In crystallization pressure is usually constant and there is one remaining degree of freedom. Graphically, temperature-composition and enthalpy-composition diagrams are convenient ways to represent the equilibrium data.

From the point of view of equilibrium diagrams the simplest binary systems are solid solutions. These systems are relatively common in melt crystallization. An example is the system phenanthrene-anthracene shown in Figure 2-7 (Walas, 1985). Cooling a liquid slowly to the liquidus line (point A) produces a solid (point B) in equilibrium with the solution. If the feed is cooled to a point in the two-phase region (point F) at equilibrium there will be a mixture of crystals (at pt. G) and solution (at pt. E). Further cooling to the solidus line (pt. H) will cause complete crystallization of a solid solution. The solid lines in Figure 2-7 are predictions made by UNIFAC (see Walas, 1985). For many solid-liquid systems excellent predictions can be made of the equilibrium data. This type of system requires a multi-stage contactor for purification and is discussed in more detail in Chapter 5.

A second type of phase diagram is the simple eutectic system illustrated in Figure 2-8 for the system naphthalene-phenol (Walas, 1985). This system could be considered as solution crystallization with phenol as the solvent or as

40

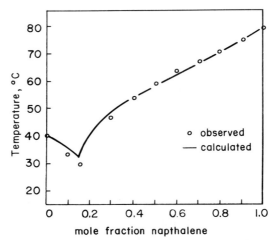

Figure 2-8.   Simple eutectic binary system: Phenol and naphthalene (Walas, 1985). Reprinted with Permission of Butterworths. Copyright 1985.

melt crystallization of a mixture of phenol and naphthalene. The *eutectic* is an equilibrium mixture which freezes at a constant composition. This is the point with the lowest freezing temperature (30°C). In the region from zero to the eutectic the crystals are pure phenol while in the region from the eutectic to 100% the crystals are pure naphthalene. For example, a mixture which is 60 mole % naphthalene would first form crystals of pure naphthalene at about 62°C. If this mixture was cooled to 40°C, then crystals of pure naphthalene would be in equilibrium with a solution containing about 21 mole % naphthalene. The relative amounts of the solution and the crystals can be found from mass balances or the lever-arm rule.

If the cooling is continued to the solidus line, the entire mass freezes. The solution remaining will freeze at the eutectic concentration which is approximately 17 mole % naphthalene. Thus the solid will contain crystals of pure naphthalene and crystals of the eutectic composition. This final freezing occurs at the eutectic temperature (~30°C). The eutectic is a physical mixture not a chemical compound. It can be considered as analogous to an azeotrope in distillation since it represents an equilibrium mixture of constant composition.

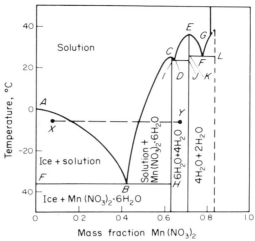

Figure 2-9.   Phase diagram for system Mn $(NO_3)_2$–water (Mullin, 1972).
With permission of Butterworths. Copyright 1972.

To obtain pure naphthalene crystals the feed concentration must be greater than
the eutectic composition; otherwise, pure phenol crystals will be obtained.
Note that a single stage system is capable of producing one pure product.
Methods to produce two pure products are discussed in Section 2.5.1.

Aqueous systems tend to be considerably more complex than solid solutions or simple eutectics. Figure 2-9 illustrates the system $Mn(NO_3)_2$ – water
(Mullin, 1972). Systems of a salt in water are complicated by the presence of
hydrates. From A to B the liquidus line separates solution from a mixture of
pure ice and solution. At point B the eutectic (or cryohydric point in aqueous
solutions) is reached. Then from B to C solution will crystallize to form pure
hexahydrate, $Mn(NO_3)_2 \cdot 6H_2O$. Point C represents the 25.8°C and 0.624 mass
fraction. Point C is congruent since solidification occurs with no change in
composition. Points D and F are additional eutectic points. Point E represents
the congruent melting point for $Mn(NO_3)_2 \cdot 4H_2O$ (37.1°C, 0.713 wt. frac).
Continuation of the equilibrium from F to G causes dihydrate to crystallize out.
Point G is a transition point where the dihydrate decomposes to form monohy-
drate and water. Thus this is an *incongruent* melting point since the composition changes. This diagram represents a rather simple example for salt solu-

42

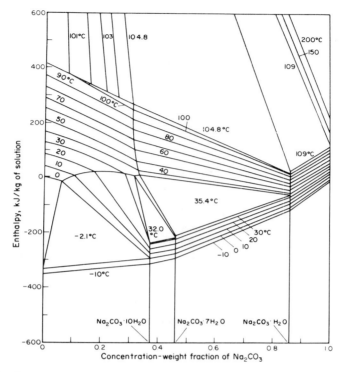

Figure 2-10. Enthalpy-concentration diagram for NA_2CO_3–water (Mullin, 1972). $p = 1$ atm. Reprinted with permission of Butterworths. Copyright 1972.

tions. Some compounds will form many hydrates, eutectics, congruent and incongruent melting points. A commonly cited example is $MgSO_4$ in water (Bennett, 1984; McCabe et al. 1985; Osburn, 1963).

Enthalpy-composition diagrams are complex, but contain all the information needed for energy balance and equilibrium calculations. *When available*, enthalpy-composition diagrams are extremely useful for calculations. Unfortunately, the diagrams are only available for a few systems (e.g. see Mullin, 1972), are difficult to prepare, and are not computer-friendly. One example of enthalpy-composition diagrams will be given to explain their use.

Figure 2-10 (Mullin, 1972) shows the enthalpy-composition diagram for Na_2CO_3-water. The zero point for enthalpy is arbitrarily set as pure, liquid water at $0°C$. The regions are marked on the diagram. The plateaus with three phases in equilibrium have

$$F = C - P + 2 = 2 - 3 + 2 = 1$$

degree of freedom which is used to set the pressure. (One atmosphere in Figure 2-10.) There are no additional degrees of freedom. Thus temperature is constant, and the compositions of the two solid phases and the solution (eutectic) in equilibrium are constant in these three phase regions. When two phases are in equilibrium, there remains one degree of freedom after setting the pressure. Thus, isotherms are shown in these regions.

Mass and energy balances can be done either using the data from the diagram, or directly on the diagram itself. The procedure is similar to that used for distillation on Ponchon-Savarait diagrams. This procedure is illustrated in Example 2-2.

Example 2-2. Crystallization Calculation with Enthalpy-Composition Diagram

100 kg of an aqueous solution which is 0.2 wt. fraction Na_2CO_3 at $60°C$ is cooled to $10°C$. What products result? How much of each product results? How much energy must be removed?

Solution.

The pertinent portion of Figure 2-10 is blown-up in Figure 2-11. The feed (point F) is cooled to $10°C$ (point M). This is assumed to happen without loss of water. Point M is in a two-phase region and will have crystals and solution in equilibrium. The crystals are $Na_2CO_3 \cdot 10H_2O$ (point C) which is 37.0% Na_3CO_3 while the liquid is at point L which is

44

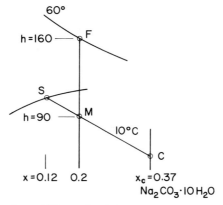

Figure 2-11. Expansion of Figure 2-10 for Example 2-2 (not to scale).

approximately 12% Na_2CO_3. The equilibrium is represented by the 10° isotherm. At equilibrium the mass balances are

$$100 = M = L + C$$

$$20 = Mx_M = Lx_L + Cx_C$$

This can also be written as the lever arm rule,

$$\frac{L}{C} = \frac{\overline{MC}}{\overline{LM}} = \frac{(x_C - x_M)}{(x_M - x_L)}$$

Solving for L and C we have C = 32 kg and L = 68 kg.

Energy removed is

$$(100 \text{ kg})(h_F - h_M)\frac{kJ}{kg} = 100(160-(-90)) = 25,000 \text{ kJ}$$

Note that the solution and the crystals have different enthalpies even though they are at the same temperature. Continuous calculations will be very similar to these batch calculations, but will be on a per unit time basis.

If some water is removed, point M will be more concentrated than the feed. If the amount of water removed is known, than point M can be determined and the calculation can be completed.

In a vacuum crystallizer pure water vapor is removed. The concentration of point M and the amount of cooling can be determined from mass and energy balances. The diagram shown in Figure 2-10 is at one atmosphere which does not correspond to the pressure of vacuum crystallizers. Thus, the vapor-liquid portion of Figure 2-10 will not be applicable. However, the liquid and solid parts will be affected only very slightly by changes in pressure, and Figure 2-10 can be used to closely approximate the liquid and solid equilibrium at reduced pressure. The vapor enthalpy can be determined from the steam tables. Thus the enthalpy-composition diagram can be used to estimate results for vacuum crystallizers. This calculation is explored in Problem 2-D4.

2.4.2. Ternary Systems

For ternary systems with two phases in equilibrium and constant pressure there are two remaining degrees of freedom. To represent the effect of temperature and composition a three-dimensional diagram would be required. (see Figure 2-13 as an example.) Since this is inconvenient, the equilibrium is often illustrated at constant temperature or with temperature as a parameter. To represent all three components we can use a triangular diagram similar to those used for extraction. Two representations for the system $KNO_3 - NaNO_3 - H_2O$ at 50°C are shown in Figures 2-12a and b (Mullin, 1972). Figure 2-12c shows the behavior at 25° and 100 °C.

On all three diagrams, points a and c represent the solubilities of pure KNO_3 and $NaNO_3$ in water, respectively. As $NaNO_3$ is added to a saturated solution of KNO_3, the solubility of KNO_3 decreases along line ab. This is the salting-out effect discussed earlier. In the region a-b-KNO_3 pure KNO_3 will be in equilibrium with solution. Thus equilibrium tie lines are straight lines through the KNO_3 vertex to the saturated liquid line ab. If KNO_3 is added to a saturated solution of $NaNO_3$, the solubility of $NaNO_3$ decreases along line cb and pure $NaNO_3$ will crystallize out. Region c-b-$NaNO_3$ represents mixtures

46

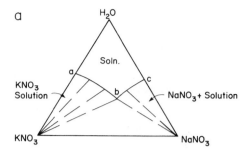

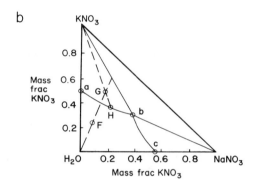

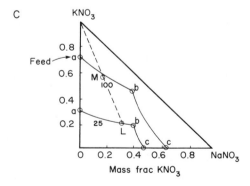

Figure 2-12.   Equilibrium data for System $KNO_3 - NaNO_3 - H_2O$. a. Equi-
lateral triangular diagram at 50°C. b. Right triangular diagram
at 50°C. c. Data at 25 and 100°C (M and L are for Example
2-3). Data replotted from Mullin (1972).

of pure $NaNO_3$ and solution. Tie lines are straight lines through the $NaNO_3$ vertex to line cb. KNO_3 and $NaNO_3$ crystallize as anhydrous salts. If one of the salts crystallized as a hydrate the tie lines would go from the composition of the hydrate to the saturated liquid line. This is illustrated later.

The effect of removing water is easily illustrated from any of these diagrams. For example, if we start with feed F shown in Figure 2-12b and remove pure water, we will follow the dilution line H_2O - F until the line intersects curve ab where pure KNO_3 starts to crystallize out. Further removal of water (say to pt. G) will produce a mixture which will separate into pure KNO_3 solid in equilibrium with solution of composition H. The dotted line to the KNO_3 vertex serves as a tie line in the a-b-KNO_3 region. When the line H_2O-F-G intersects the straight line KNO_3-b, the solid KNO_3 will be in equilibrium with solution of composition b. Removal of further water does not change the solution composition and b is known as the *drying up point*. The behavior of the system in the region b-c-$NaNO_3$ will be similar when water is removed, except pure $NaNO_3$ will be deposited.

In the region KNO_3–b–$NaNO_3$ both salts are in equilibrium with solution of composition b. Since temperature and pressure are fixed and 3 phases are in equilibrium, there are no remaining degrees of freedom. The relative amounts of each phase can change, but compositions and temperature are set in this region. By adding solvent (water), mixtures in this region can be moved into either the region a-b-KNO_3 or b-c-$NaNO_3$ allowing removal of pure KNO_3 or $NaNO_3$, respectively.

Temperature effects can be seen by comparing Figures 2-12b and 2-12c. Decreasing the temperature decreases the solubility of both salts and of mixtures of the salts. Thus in this system supersaturation can be caused by cooling, and/or by water removal and/or by salting out. Because of the variation of the saturation curves with temperature, fractionation of the two salts can be obtained using temperature cycles. This is explored in Section 2.5.1.

Mass balance and equilibrium calculations can be done directly on the triangular diagrams by a procedure similar to that used for extraction, or by extracting the equilibrium information from the diagram and doing the mass balances separately. These procedures are illustrated in Example 2-3.

Example 2-3. Crystallization of a Ternary System.

We wish to crystallize KNO_3 from a saturated solution of KNO_3 in water at 100°C by both cooling to 25°C and by salting out by adding $NaNO_3$. The feed is 100 kg/hr of saturated KNO_3 solution and 20 kg/hr of pure $NaNO_3$ are added. Find the yield of crystals and the final mother liquor concentration.

Solution

A. Define. The process is sketched in the figure.

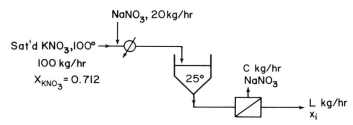

We wish to find C, L and the composition of the mother liquid x_i.

B. Explore. We can assume that the crystals and mother liquor are in equilibrium at 25°C. Thus Figure 2-12c can be used.

C. Plan. First add the $NaNO_3$ to the feed to find the mixing point M. This can be calculated graphically or analytically. Then this mixture separates into KNO_3 crystals and mother liquor. The concentration of the liquor can be read from Figure 2-12c while mass balances (graphical or analytical) can be used to calculate C and L.

D. Do It. Adding F plus $NaNO_3$ gives M = 120 kg/hr,

$$x_{M,KNO_3} = \frac{71.2}{120} = 0.5933 \, , \quad x_{M,NaNO_3} = \frac{20}{120} = 0.167$$

This is shown on Figure 2-12c. Then the tie line is from the KNO_3 vertex through M to ab at 25°C. Mother liquor is

$x_{NaNO_3} \sim 0.32$, $x_{KNO_3} \sim 0.22$ (see Figure 21-12c). To find C and L use mass balances

$$\text{Overall:} \quad C + L = M = 120$$

$$NaNO_3 : \quad (C)(0.0) + (L)(0.32) = (120)(0.167)$$

Solving for L, we have $\qquad L = \dfrac{0.167}{0.32} \, 120 = 62.63 \text{ kg/hr}$

and thus $\quad C = 57.37$ kg/hr.

E. Check. The KNO_3 mass balance can serve as a check:

$$C(1.0) + L(0.22) = M(0.593)$$

which is, $\quad 71.15 = 71.2 \quad$ which is OK.

This check is really closer than can be expected considering the size of the figure. Larger figures will in general be more accurate.

F. Generalization. The mass balances and equilibrium calculations can be conveniently done on triangular diagrams for single stage contact. This example showed first a mixing operation to find M followed by an equilibrium tie line to find x_i and mass balances to find C and L. The calculations are essentially the same as for single-stage extraction calculations on a triangular diagram. Only the form of the equilibrium data differs. This example also illustrated salting out when a common ion is present.

Note in this example that the mother liquor and crystals exit together. There will always be some mother liquor exiting with the crystals. Some crystallizers also remove an overflow mother liquor which is free of crystals. As shown in the example, the crystals must be separated from the mother liquor. This can be done in a centrifuge or filter and the crystals are usually washed to remove any adhering mother liquor which will contaminate the pure crystals.

50

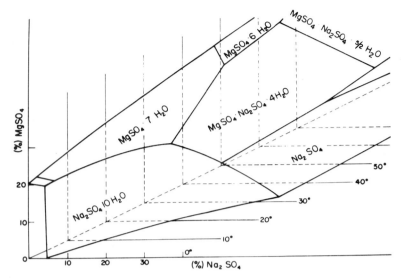

Figure 2-13.   Three-dimensional plot for equilibrium for the system Na_2SO_4–$MgSO_4$–water (Fitch, 1970). Reprinted with permission from *Ind. Eng. Chem.*, *62*, (12), 6 (1970). Copyright 1970, American Chemical Society.

Double salts can also occur in ternary systems. When a variety of hydrates and double salts are formed the equilibrium data becomes complex. An example for $MgSO_4$–Na_2SO_4-water is shown in Figure 2-13 (Fitch, 1970). Figure 2-13 shows a three dimensional plot for this system with temperature as the third axis. Note that three different hydrates and two double salts are shown.

Three-dimensional plots are not convenient for calculations. Projections at different temperatures are shown in Figures 2-14 a and b (Fitch, 1970). At 50°C (Figure 2-14a) the hexa-hydrate, $MgSO_4 \cdot 6H_2O$, the double salt astrakanite, $Na_2SO_4 \cdot MgSO_4 \cdot 4H_2O$, and anhydrous Na_2SO_4 will be the solid phases. At 20°C (Figure 2-14b) the hydrate is $MgSO_4$–$7H_2O$ while Na_2SO_4–$10H_2O$ precipitates instead of Na_2SO_4. At 20°C astrakanite still precipitates while at 10° and 0°C no astrakanite forms. The tie lines are shown in Figures 2-14. By

(a)

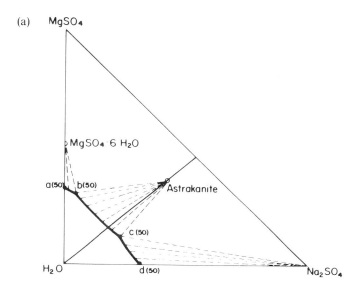

(b)

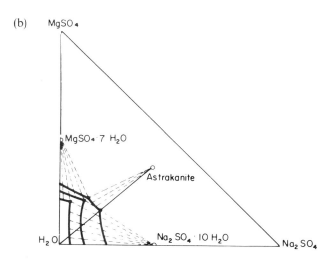

Figure 2-14.   Projections for system $Na_2SO_4-MgSO_4-$water. (Fitch 1970).
a. 50°C isotherm b. 20°, 10° and 0° isotherms. Reprinted with
permission from *Ind. Eng. Chem.*, *62*, (12), 6 (1970). Copyright 1970, American Chemical Society.

changing temperatures, cycles to fractionate the Na_2SO_4 and $MgSO_4$ are developed in the next section.

Solid solutions also occur in three component systems. The solid solution may cover the entire range of salt concentrations as does the system Pb $(NO_3)_2$ - $Ba(NO_3)_2$ - water. This system is discussed later (see Figure 2-21). The solid solution may also be discontinuous as is the system KBr - KCl - water. Systems which form solid solutions cannot be purified in a single equilibrium stage; thus, countercurrent cascades are used.

Note that the 3 component salt systems all have a common ion such as Cl^- or NO_3^-. A system such as KCl–$NaNO_3$-water is really a four component system. In water the double decomposition reaction

$$KCl + NaNO_3 = NaCl + KNO_3$$

occurs rapidly. Thus all four salts can be present. Since the composition can be expressed as the composition of three of the salts plus water, this is a four component system from the point of view of the phase rule. Alternately, it can be considered a 5 component system with one independent reaction. Then $F = C - P + 2 - N_{RX}$. This will give the same degrees of freedom. These *reciprocal salt pair* systems are important in commercial applications. Equilibrium data can be extremely complex and is discussed by Mullin (1972), Purdon and Slater (1946), and Fitch (1970).

This completes the discussion of phase equilibrium and equilibrium calculations for simple, single stage solution crystallizers. Most crystallization from solution is done in crystallizers which approximate a single equilibrium stage. Fractional crystallization requires more complex processes or countercurrent equipment and is discussed next.

2.5. FRACTIONAL CRYSTALLIZATION

For systems with two or more salts it is usually desirable to recover both salts as pure compounds. For instance, in Example 2-3 a method for producing pure

$NaNO_3$ was illustrated, but no mention was made of what to do with the saturated solution containing $NaNO_3$, KNO_3 and water. Processes which separate the solutes into two or more pure products are *fractional crystallization* systems.

When solid solutions are not formed, processes using single equilibrium stage crystallizers with various temperature cycles can be used. When solid solutions are formed, fractional crystallization schemes require counter-current cascades. Fractional crystallization can also be done by selective seeding (see Section 4.5.).

2.5.1. Fractional Crystallization Processes with Temperature Swings

Fractionation cycles for systems without double salts are easily developed (Fitch, 1970). The basic idea for a batch system is to operate at one temperature to produce pure crystals and solution at the drying-up point. Then add (or remove) water and change the temperature to produce pure crystals of the other component and solution at the second drying-up point. Then remove (or add) water and readjust the temperature to harvest the first component as pure crystals and return to the first drying-up point. This procedure is illustrated in Figure 2-15. Start at the drying-up point at temperature T_1, $b(T_1)$ on Figure 2-15a.

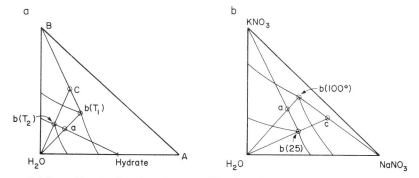

Figure 2-15.   Batch fractional crystallization for ternary systems without double salts. a. Schematic of basic process b. Application to system $KNO_3 - NaNO_3 -$water

54

Then add water (following line $b(T_1) - H_2O$) to point a. Change the temperature to T_2 and harvest product which is a hydrate of component A in equilibrium with solution $b(T_2)$. After removing the hydrate, remove water from solution $b(T_2)$ to point c. Change the temperature to T_1 and harvest crystals B in equilibrium with solution $b(T_1)$. This returns us to our starting point having harvested pure hydrate and pure B.

This basic scheme with minor modifications can be used for any ternary system which does not form double salts or solid solutions. A simple modification is illustrated in Figure 2-15b for the KNO_3-NaNO_3 - water system. Starting at $b(100°)$, water is added to reach point a and the system is cooled to 25°C. Pure KNO_3 crystals are harvested in equilibrium with $b(25°)$. Water is then removed to reach point c, and the mixture is heated to 100°C. Pure $NaNO_3$ crystals are harvested in equilibrium with the solution $b(100°)$. Now the process can be repeated.

The process can be made continuous by adding a feed stream. The feed can be added to either solution $b(T_1)$ or $b(T_2)$. Both approaches should be investigated. The continuous process is illustrated in Example 2-4.

Example 2-4. Continuous Fractional Crystallization of $NaCO_3-NaCl-$water.

A feed of 100 kg/hr which is 30 wt % Na_2CO_3 and 45 wt % NaCl is to be fractionally crystallized by alternating the temperature between 0° and 30°C. The drying-up points are (Fitch, 1970),

$b(0°)$: $= 0.028 \, Na_2CO_3$ and $0.242 \, NaCl$

$b(30°)$: $= 0.177 \, Na_2CO_3$ and $0.150 \, NaCl$

Anhydrous NaCl and $Na_2CO_3 \cdot 10H_2O$ hydrate are desired products. Find the yields of each product and the amounts of water added and evaporated when the feed is added to solution $b(30°)$.

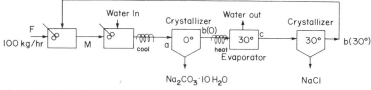

Figure 2-16.   Fractional crystallization system for Example 2-4.

Solution

A. Define. The process is sketched in Figure 2-16. In practice, several of the steps such as mixing solution b(30), F, and water will be done simultaneously, and the evaporation will probably be done in a vacuum crystallizer. We wish to find the flow rates of $Na_2CO_3 \cdot 10H_2O$, NaCl, water added and removed, and the recycle flow rate b(30°).

B and C. Explore and Plan. Required equilibrium data are given in the problem statement. External mass balances can be used to find product flow rates. The equilibrium diagram can be sketched (see Figure 2-17) and used as a guide. First find fulcrum point c at the intersection of lines H_2O - b(0) and NaCl - b(30). Since the flow rate of NaCl can be calculated and point c serves as a fulcrum, the flow rate of stream b(30), $F_{b(30)}$, can be calculated.

$$\frac{F_{b(30)}}{F_{NaCl}} = \frac{\overline{NaCl \cdot c}}{\overline{c \cdot b(30)}}$$

With $F_{b(30)}$ and the feed rate known, point M can be found.

$$\frac{F_{b(30)}}{F} = \frac{\overline{FM}}{\overline{M \cdot b(30)}}$$

and $F_M = F_{b(30)} + F$. Point a is found by the construction shown. Then water addition to get from M to point a can be found from the lever-arm rule.

$$\frac{F_{H_2O,in}}{F_M} = \frac{\overline{M \cdot a}}{\overline{H_2O \cdot a}}$$

or mass balances. Then $F_a = F_{H_2O} + F_M$. Flow rate of $b(0°)$ can be found from a mass balance

$$F_{b(0)} = F_a - F_{hydrate}$$

Finally, the water removal to go from $b(0°)$ to point c can be found from the lever arm rule.

$$\frac{F_{H_2O,out}}{F_{b(0)}} = \frac{b(0)·\overline{c}}{H_2O·c}$$

or from a mass balance (see Figure 2-16): $F_{H_2O,out} = F_{b(0)} - F_{NaCl} - F_{b(30)}$

D. Do It. Start with external balances,

$$F + F_{H_2O,in} = F_{H_2O,out} + F_{Na_2CO_3·10H_2O} + F_{NaCl}$$

Since the water flow rates are unknown, we need external balances for Na Cl and Na_2CO_3. All NaCl goes out in NaCl product,

$$F_{NaCl} = 0.45F = 45 \text{ kg/hr}$$

While Na_2CO_3 exits in the Na_2CO_3 product,

$$Na_2CO_3 {}_{out} = 0.3F = 30 \text{ kg/hr}$$

However, this product is a hydrate.

$$F_{Na_2CO_3·10H_2O} = (\frac{MW_{hydrate}}{MW_{anhydrous}})(F_{anhydrous})$$

$$= (\frac{285.99}{105.83})(30) = 81.07 \text{ kg/hr}$$

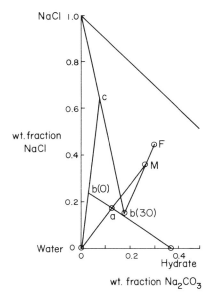

Figure 2-17. Solution to Example 2-4.

Plot points b(0) and b(30) which are the drying up points. Then plot NaCl = 1.00 and the hydrate, $x_{Na_2CO_3 \cdot 10H_2O} = 0.370$. Draw line H_2O - b(0°) and extend to extension with line NaCl - b(30°). Intersection is point c. See Figure 2-17. From the lever arm rule,

$$F_{b(30)} = F_{NaCl} \frac{\overline{NaCl \cdot c}}{\overline{c \cdot b(30)}} = (45) \frac{(9.25)}{(12.75)} = 32.6$$

To find M.

$$F_M = F + F_{b(30)} = 100 + 32.6 = 132.6$$

and the lever-arm rule is,

$$\frac{F_{b(30)}}{F} = \frac{32.6}{100} = \frac{\overline{F \cdot M}}{\overline{M \cdot b(30)}} \qquad \text{(see Figure 2–17)}$$

Draw lines b(0)-Hydrate and M-Water. Intersection is point a. Then water addition flow rate is,

$$F_{H_2O,in} = F_M \frac{\overline{M \cdot 1}}{H_2O \cdot 1} = (132.6)\frac{6.4}{5.4} = 157.2 \text{ kg/hr}$$

Then, $\quad\quad\quad F_a = F_{H_2O} + F_M = 289.8 \text{kg/hr}$

and $\quad F_{b(0)} = F_a - F_{hydrate} = 289.3 - 81.1 = 208.2 \text{ kg/hr}$

Finally, water out from the mass balance is,

$$F_{H_2O,out} = F_{b(0)} - F_{NaCl} - F_{b(30)}$$

$$= 208.2 - 45 - 32.6 = 130.6 \text{ kg/hr}$$

E. Check. The external water balance can be used as one check.

$$Fx_{F,H_2O} + F_{H_2O,in} = F_{H_2O,out} + F_{Na_2CO_3 \cdot 10H_2O}(\frac{10MW_{H_2O}}{MW_{hydrate}})$$

$$100(0.25) + 157.7 = 130.6 + 81.07(\frac{180.16}{285.99})$$

which is 182.2 compared to 181.7. This is OK since it is within the accuracy of the graph. A second check is to solve everything analytically. This is done in Problem 2-E1. Results agree within the accuracy of the graphical method.

F. Generalization. Although the details of the process will differ, the method employed here can be used for other systems which do not form double salts or solid solutions. Note that the calculation started with the drying-up solution, b(0°), which was *not* recycled. This allowed calculation of fulcrum point c and then the recycle stream flow rate $F_{b(30)}$. Then straight-forward mixing calculations could be used. This somewhat round-about approach is required whenever the flow rate of the recycle stream is unknown. Again the *idea* of this procedure can be applied to other systems.

An alternate method of doing this fractional crystallization is to add the feed to solution b(0°) instead of b(30°). This alternate process is explored in Problem 2-D7, and is probably preferable.

The fractional crystallization problems can also be set up for analytical solution instead of graphical solution. This requires quite a bit of algebra, but is computer friendly. For example, for Example 2-4 one would do the mass balances in the same order after solving the external mass balances. The equation for removal of water from solution b(0°) and for the separation of mixture c into pure crystals and solution b(30°) must be solved simultaneously. This gives 6 equations and 6 unknowns. Once the flow rate $F_{b(30)}$ is known, F_M and the coordinates of point M are easily found from mass balances for the mixing operation. Then F_a and $F_{H_2O,in}$ can be found from the mass balances for mixing in water and the mass balances for the separation of stream a. If the flow sheet is known, this procedure is straight-forward but a bit tedious. However, once the general equations have been developed, it is extremely convenient to study the effect of changing variables such as the feed composition. The analytical solution methods are explored in Problems 2-E1 and 2-E2. The graphical approach remains very useful for developing workable processes and for guiding the analytical calculations.

Note that the fractional crystallization process shown in Figure 2-16 is much more complicated than a simple crystallization. However, the fractional crystallization does produce two pure products and no saturated solutions which must be disposed of.

In the examples up to now the drying up points have been used as the saturated solutions. This will maximize the yield of the pure products, but is not always best choice. For the KCl - NaCl - water system shown in Figure 2-18 (Fitch, 1970) it is more economical to use an operating point (a) which

60

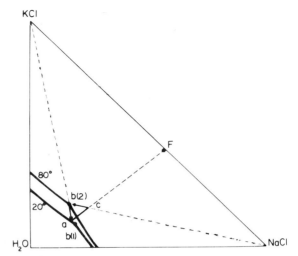

Figure 2-18.   Cycle for fractional crystallization of KCl and NaCl without evaporation or dilution. (Fitch, 1970). Reprinted with permission from *Ind. Eng. Chem.*, *62* (12), 6 (1970). Copyright 1972, American Chemical Society.

does not maximize yield instead of evaporating water to reach drying-up point b(1). The fractional crystallization cycle can be followed by starting at b(2). After cooling the solution to 20°C, a crop of KCl crystals can be removed. A saturated solution at 20°C (point a) results. The solution at point a is mixed with fresh feed and heated to 80°C to reach point c. KCl is leached from this mixture leaving NaCl and saturated solution b(2). This cycle is used commercially and avoids the need for evaporation or dilution.

The fractional crystallization of systems with double salts (e.g. $MgSO_4 - Na_2SO_4$-water shown in Figures 2-13 and 2-14) can be more complex. At 50°C (Figure 2-14a) the astrakanite is congruently soluble (adding water leads to a saturated solution in equilibrium with the astrakanite). It is possible to separate $MgSO_4 \cdot 6H_2O$ and astrakanite, or to separate Na_2SO_4 and astrakanite, but a complete separation is not possible at 50°. Isotherms where astrakanite either is not congruently soluble or where astrakanite ceases to exist must be found. Figure 2-14b shows that 0° and 10° the double salt

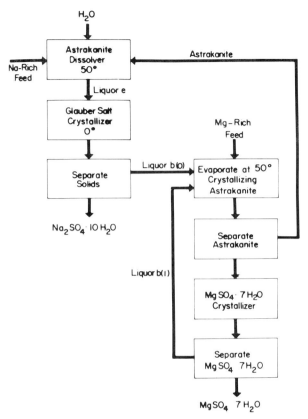

Figure 2-19. Process flowsheet for fractionation for Na_2CO_4 and $MgSO_4$. (Fitch, 1970). Reprinted with permission from *Ind. Eng. Chem., 62*, (12), 6 (1970). Copyright 1970, American Chemical Society.

astrakanite no longer forms. Thus one possibility is to develop a fractional crystallization cycle using these two temperatures. Several such cycles are possible (see Problem 2-B2) and will be similar to the cycles illustrated in Figures 2-15 to 2-18.

An alternative is to develop a process cycling between 50° and 0°C and using the astrakanite formed at 50°C as a recycle stream. A process flowsheet for this process is shown in Figure 2-19 (Fitch, 1970). This cycle requires three crystallizers; but will have lower evaporation costs than cycling between 0° and 10°C.

Trace components are usually present in the feeds to fractional crystallization processes. Unless these trace components are removed in a liquid purge stream, they will slowly build up in the liquid phase until it is saturated. Then the trace components are no longer traces and these components must be included in the phase equilibria. For simplicity, we will use purge streams to keep the concentration of trace components low.

More complex ternary, four-component and many-component systems are discussed by Fitch (1970). As the number of components increases the number of possible process configurations increases. The basic principles developed for ternary systems can still be used for these complex processes.

2.5.2. Processes Using Counter-Current Cascades

When solid solutions occur, a single equilibrium stage will not give either solute as a pure component. In this case counter-current cascades are required to obtain the desired fractionation. An example of a system which forms a solid solution throughout the entire range is $Pb(NO_3)_2 - Ba(NO_3)_2 -$ water. $Pb(NO_3)_2$ is the more soluble salt. A schematic of the counter current cascade for fractionation of these salts is shown in Figure 2-20. Each box is assumed to be an equilibrium stage. The more soluble $Pb(NO_3)_2$ tends to concentrate in

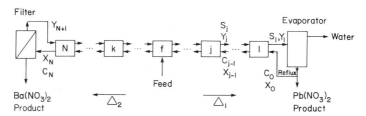

Figure 2-20.   Countercurrent cascade for fractional crystallization of solid solution.

the liquid. The less soluble $Ba(NO_3)_2$ tends to stay in the crystals. The net result is movement of $Pb(NO_3)_2$ to the right and $Ba(NO_3)_2$ to the left. The solution leaving the right end of the cascade is sent to an evaporator where water is removed. A portion of the crystals formed are taken as $Pb(NO_3)_2$ product while the remainder are refluxed. A portion of the crystals leaving the left end of the cascade are withdrawn as $Ba(NO_3)_2$ product. The remaining crystals are dissolved in water and refluxed (stream Y_{N+1}).

The counter-current cascade is very similar to fractional extraction columns (e.g., Wankat, 1988). The differences between overall and component flow rates of solid and liquid phases in each section of the cascade will be constant. Thus we can define difference points in the same way as for extraction. The resulting difference points can be plotted on triangular diagrams. Stages can now be stepped off on the triangular diagrams as done in extraction (e.g., Wankat, 1988). Unfortunately, this construction squeezes the difference points together near the solvent vertex.

An alternate construction is to plot the solvent to solute ratio, N, versus the fraction of salts which are the more soluble salt, $Pb(NO_3)_2$, in the solid and solution. This alternate is shown for crystallization in Mullin (1972). More detail is given in books and articles on extraction (Smith, 1963; Treybal, 1980; Wankat, 1982). Let N and Y be mass ratios in solution,

$$N = \frac{\text{kg solvent}}{\text{kg salts}} = \frac{\text{kg water}}{\text{kg Pb(NO}_3)_2 + \text{kg Ba(NO}_3)_2} \qquad (2\text{-}7a)$$

$$Y = \frac{\text{kg more soluble salt}}{\text{total salts}} = \frac{\text{kg Pb(NO}_3)_2}{\text{kg Pb(NO}_3)_2 + \text{kg Ba(NO}_3)_2} \qquad (2\text{-}7b)$$

and X is the mass ratio in the solid phase.

$$X = \frac{\text{kg more soluble salt}}{\text{total salts}} = \frac{\text{kg Pb(NO}_3)_2}{\text{kg Pb(NO}_3)_2 + \text{kg Ba(NO}_3)_2} \qquad (2\text{-}7c)$$

The equilibrium data (Mullin, 1972) are shown in these units in Figure 2-21 where both a McCabe-Thiele type diagram and a Ponchon-Savarit type diagram (similar to triangular diagrams) are shown. Equilibrium tie lines on

64

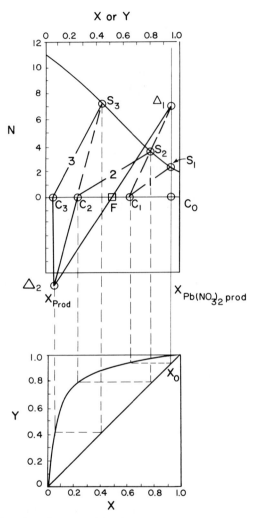

Figure 2-21. Fractional crystallization of solid solution Pb(NO₃)₂ − Ba(NO₃)₂ − water. Data from Mullin (1972).

the top diagrams can be obtained from the McCabe-Thiele diagram by the same methods used for enthalpy-composition or triangular diagrams (e.g., Wankat, 1988). The top diagram in Figure 2-21 is a transformation of the triangular diagram into the new set of variables.

These mass ratios are related to mass fractions,

$$N = \frac{y_W}{y_{Pb(NO_3)_2} + y_{Ba(NO_3)_2}} \qquad (2\text{-}8a)$$

$$Y = \frac{y_{Pb(NO_3)_2}}{y_{Pb(NO_3)_2} + y_{Ba(NO_3)_2}}, \qquad (2\text{-}8b)$$

$$X = \frac{x_{Pb(NO_3)_2}}{x_{Pb(NO_3)_2} + x_{Ba(NO_3)_2}}, \qquad (2\text{-}8c)$$

where x is mass fraction in the solid and y is mass fraction in the solution.

Since these mass ratio units are on a water-free basis, all flow rates must be converted to a water-free basis. Flow rate C is kg salt in the crystals per hour, and is already in this basis. Flow rate S is kg salt in solution/hr. S can be related to the total solution flow rate

$$S = (\text{Total solution flow rate}) \times (y_{Pb(NO_3)_2} + y_{Ba(NO_3)_2}) \qquad (2\text{-}9)$$

In these units the differences in passing streams to the right of the feed in Figure 2-21 are,

$$S_j - C_{j-1} = \Delta_1 = \text{constant} \qquad (2\text{-}10a)$$

where $P_{Pb(NO_3)_2}$ is the kg/hr of product. The $Pb(NO_3)_2$ and water balances are

$$S_j Y_j - C_{j-1} X_{j-1} = \Delta_1 X_{\Delta_1} = \text{constant} \qquad (2\text{-}10b)$$

$$S_j N_j - C_{j-1}(0) = \Delta_1 N_{\Delta_1} = \text{constant} \qquad (2\text{-}10c)$$

Similar equations are valid for Δ_2 on the left side of the feed in Figure 2-21. These equations allow calculations of the coordinates of Δ_1 and Δ_2. Since these equations are the same as mixing equations, they indicate that there is a straight line from the two passing streams (S_j and C_{j-1}) and the Δ point.

In the evaporator only water is removed. Since the ratios are on a water-free basis, $Y_1 = X_0$, and Δ_1 must be at this value of the abscissa. The location of Δ_1 can be determined from the external reflux ratio, $C_0/P_{Pb(NO_3)_2}$. From the lever-arm rule

$$\frac{C_0}{P_{Pb(NO_3)_2}} = \frac{\overline{\Delta_1 S_1}}{\overline{C_0 S_1}} \tag{2-11}$$

and the Δ_1 point can be found. The Δ_2 point can be found where the extension of the feed line $\Delta_1 F$ intersects the vertical line through $X_{Ba(NO_3)_2,product}$. This use of the feed line is the same use as in extraction and distillation. The Δ points are shown in Figure 2-21.

Stages can be stepped off on the Ponchon diagram using the same procedure used for triangular diagrams, or the McCabe-Thiele diagram can be used. In Figure 2-21 the McCabe-Thiele diagram is used to find tie lines and the Δ points are used for the operating lines. Figure 2-21 shows an example where the $Pb(NO_3)_2$ product is 93% $Pb(NO_3)_2$ while the $Ba(NO_3)_2$ product is 5% $Pb(NO_3)_2$. The feed is a 50 % mixture of both salts in crystal form, and a reflux ratio of 2.0 is used. A total of 3 equilibrium stages are required and the optimum feed is the second stage. If the McCabe-Thiele diagram is used to step off stages, curved operating lines must be generated from the Ponchon or triangular diagram (an example of this procedure is in Wankat, 1988).

Counter-current processes for fractional crystallization are *not* a common separation technique. There are only a few solid solutions which form a solid solution continuously over the entire range as $Pb(NO_3)_2 - Ba(NO_3)_2$ - water does. Other systems such as KBr - KCl - water form solid solutions over part of the range but there is a discontinuity in this range. A complete separation can be obtained only by operating two cascades at different temperatures and cycling between the temperatures (Fitch, 1976).

Another problem with counter-current fractional crystallization is mass transfer in crystallization is *not* analogous to distillation or extraction. There is essentially no mass transfer between the inside of a crystal and solution. To obtain equilibrium each stage in Figure 2-20 requires dissolution of the crystals followed by recrystallization. When solubility is temperature dependent, this can be done by heating crystals plus liquid to dissolve the crystals and then recooling. For other systems additional solvent may have to be added to dissolve the crystals. Then to cause crystallization the solvent has to be evaporated. These steps make the process more expensive. In addition, separation of the crystals from the mother liquor is usually not perfect. The entrained mother liquor reduces the stage efficiency. Fractional crystallization of solid solutions is probably applicable either when only a few stages are required or when the products are very valuable.

2.6. PRECIPITATION

Precipitation is an important industrial process which is closely related to crystallization from solution. In precipitation a solution is made supersaturated so that dissolved solutes precipitate out. Precipitation differs from crystallization since the precipitate is usually amorphous, has a poorly defined size and shape, is often an aggregate, and is usually not pure. Precipitation and crystallization are often complementary processes since precipitation is used for a "rough cut" while crystallization is used for final purification. Precipitation is commonly used in mineral processing and for the production of photographic chemicals, paints, polymers, pharmaceuticals, and will undoubtedly be an important unit operation in the emerging biotechnology industry.

Equipment for precipitation is often very similiar to that used for crystallization. Both batch and continuous operations are used, although batch is probably more common since many precipitations are done for relatively low volume products. Precipitation operations usually have a mixing operation where various reagents are added to make the solution supersaturated. This is followed by a holding period which allows for an induction period before nucleii form and a latent period before the supersaturation starts to decrease markedly. These periods are shown schematically in Figure 2-22 (Mullin, 1972). Once the precipitate starts to grow the desupersaturation often occurs at a constant rate as shown in Figure 2-22. Towards the end of the desupersaturation period the rate decreases as the concentration approaches equilibrium. During this period aging often occurs. During *aging* small crystals and precipitates redissolve and the solute is redeposited onto the larger precipitates. The result is a uniform crop of fairly large precipitate which is relatively easy to separate from the solution by centrifugation (Bell et al, 1983; Belter et al, 1988) or filtration (Belter et al, 1988). The kinetics of these steps are discussed in Chapter 3.

It is convenient to classify precipitation processes based on the method used to produce the supersaturation.

1. Cooling and solvent evaporation. Supersaturation can be caused by cooling and or evaporation of solvent. This is very similiar to crystallization and the equipment is very similiar.

2. Reaction. Some products are made by mixing reagents which react to form a precipitate. Examples are ammonium sulphate, sodium bicarbonate, and ammonium diuranate (Mullin, 1972).

3. Salting out. High salt concentrations often cause the precipitation of solute. This effect was explored for common ions in Eq. (2-3) and in Example 2-3. Salting out is also commonly used for protein precipitation (Bell et al, 1983; Belter et al, 1988). The Hofmeister series lists the effectiveness of anions as

citrate > phosphate > sulphate > acetate = chloride > nitrate > thiocynate

Cations follow the order
$$ammonium > potassium > sodium.$$

For the high salt concentrations required for salting out, the solubility of a protein usually follows the empirical Cohn equation,

$$\ln c^* = \beta - K\, c_s \qquad (2\text{-}12)$$

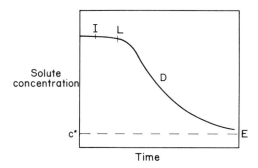

Figure 2-22.   Desupersaturation curve. I is induction, L is latent period, D is constant rate desupersaturation, and E is equilibrium.

where c_s is the salt concentration, and K and β are constants. Constant β depends on the protein, pH and temperature, but is usually independent of the salt. The slope of the salting out curve, K, depends on the salt and the protein. Note that Eq. (2-12) is valid only at high salt concentrations. At low salt concentrations the protein solubility becomes constant. Since relatively large amounts of salt are required, an inexpensive salt is desired. The combination of cheapness plus the Hofmeister series leads to $(NH_4)_2SO_4$ as the most common salt for protein precipitation. In fact, ammonium sulfate precipitation is so common that other salts may not be considered.

4. Antisolvents. Antisolvents or nonsolvents can be added to cause precipitation. This was illustrated in Figure 2-6. For proteins it is common to add ethanol, acetone or polyethylene glycol to cause precipitation. The precipitation is preferentially done at low temperature to prevent denaturation of the protein, and at ionic strengths in the range from 0.05 to 0.2 M (Belter et al, 1988). A major application of precipitation by addition of an antisolvent is the Cohn ethanol precipitation method used for the fractionation of blood plasma proteins. The Cohn fractionation procedure varies the mole fraction ethanol and pH in a strictly prescribed sequence to produce several (usually 6) fractions which contain different blood proteins (Bell et al, 1983).

5. pH. The solubility of many compounds will be effected by pH. Proteins

have a net charge of zero at a particular pH called the isoelectric point or pI. Each protein has a unique pI. Protein solubility goes through a minimum at the pI. For proteins precipitation is usually done by adjusting the pH to the isoelectric point, and then adding salt or an antisolvent. pH changes are also commonly used to precipitate metal ions from acidic sulphate solutions in the mining industry.

6. Temperature increases. Increasing the temperature usually increases the solubility; however, for proteins temperature increases may cause denaturation which can drastically decrease solubility. Details of this method are discussed by Belter et al (1988).

Precipitation can be carried out in one step to remove a large number of compounds in a single precipitate. This is the easiest application and is most common. Fractional precipitation requires a series of steps with each step optimized to precipitate one component. Since any solute left in solution during one step will probably precipitate in the next step, it is not possible to do extremely sharp purifications by fractional precipitation. In addition, in most cases any added salts or other chemicals have to be removed before the product can be used.

2.7. SUMMARY - OBJECTIVES

In this chapter equilibrium calculation methods for crystallization from solution have been explored. At the end of this chapter you should be able to do the following:

1. Explain and classify the types of crystallizers and precipitators used based on how supersaturation is achieved.

2. Plot solubility data and do yield calculations. Discuss the factors which effect solubility.

3. Use temperature-composition and enthalpy-composition diagrams for crystallizer calculations for binary systems.

4. Use ternary diagrams for crystallizer calculations.

5. Develop and do calculations for fractional crystallization processes for ternary systems without and with solid solutions.

REFERENCES

Azoury, R., W.G. Robertson, and J. Garside, "Generation of supersaturation using reverse osmosis," *Chemical Engr. Research Design, 65* (4), 342 (1987).

Bell, D.J., M. Hoare, and P. Dunnill, "The formation of protein precipitates and their centrifugal recovery," in A. Fiechter, (Ed.), *Advances in Biochemical Engineering/Biotechnology, 26, Downstream Processing,* Spring-Verlag, Berlin, 1983, 1-72.

Belter, P.A., E.L. Cussler, and W.-S. Hu, *Bioseparations. Downstream Processing for Biotechnology,* Wiley-Interscience, New York, 1988, Chapters 8 and 10.

Bennett, R.C., "Crystallization from solution", in R.H. Perry and D.W. Green (Eds.), *Perry's Chemical Engineer's Handbook,* 6th ed., McGraw-Hill, New York, 1984, p. 19-24.

Bennett, R.C., "Matching crystallizer to material," *Chem. Eng., 95* (8), 118 (May 23, 1988).

Bennett, R.C. and M. Van Buren, "Commercial urea crystallization," *Chem. Eng. Prog. Symp. Ser., 65* (95), 44 (1969).

Fitch, B., "How to design fractional crystallization processes," *Ind. Eng. Chem., 62* (12), 6 (Dec. 1970).

Fitch, B., "Design of fractional crystallization processes involving solid solutions," *AIChE Symp. Ser., 72* (153), 79 (1976).

Garrett, D.E., "Crystallization equipment applications," *Ind. Eng. Chem., 53,* 623 (1961).

72

Lozano, J.A.F., "Recovery of potassium magnesium sulfate double salt from seawater bittern," *Ind. Eng. Chem. Process Des. Develop., 15*, 445 (1976).

McCabe, W.L., J.C. Smith, and P. Harriott, *Unit Operations of Chemical Engineering*, 4th ed., McGraw-Hill, New York, 1985, Chapt. 28.

Mehra, D.K., "Selecting evaporators," *Chem. Eng.*, 93 (3), 56 (Feb. 3, 1986).

Moyers, C.G., Jr. and R.W. Rousseau, "Crystallization operations," in R.W. Rousseau (Ed.), *Handbook of Separation Process Technology*, Wiley, New York, 1987, Chapt. 11.

Mullin, J.W., *Crystallisation*, 2nd ed., Butterworths, London, 1972.

Nyvlt, J., *Industrial Crystallization*, 2nd Ed., Verlag Chemie, Weinheim, 1982.

Osburn, J.O., "Crystallization," in R.H. Perry, C.H. Chilton, S.D. Kirkpatrick (Eds.), *Chemical Engineer's Handbook*, 4th edition, McGraw-Hill, New York, 1963, 17-7.

Perry, R.H. and D.W. Green (Eds.), *Perry's Chemical Engineers' Handbook*, 6th ed., McGraw-Hill, New York, 1984.

Purdon, F.F. and V.W. Slater, *Aqueous Solution and the Phase Diagram*, Arnold, London, 1946.

Seidell, A., *Solubilities of Inorganic and Metal Organic Compounds*, 4th edition (W.F. Linke, Ed.), Vol. I, Van Nostrand, New York, 1958. Vol. II, American Chemical Society, Washington, D.C., 1965.

Singh, G., "Crystallization from solutions," in P.A. Schweitzer (Ed.), *Handbook of Separation Techniques for Chemical Engineers*, McGraw-Hill, New York, 1979, Section 2.4.

Smith, B.D., *Design of Equilibrium Stage Processes*, McGraw-Hill, New York, 1963.

Stephen, H. and T. Stephen, *Solubilities of Inorganic and Organic Compounds* (in 5 parts), Pergamon, London, 1963.

Tavare, N.S., "Batch crystallization: A review," *Chem. Eng. Commun., 61,* 259 (1987).

Treybal, R.E., *Mass Transfer Operations,* 3rd ed., McGraw-Hill, New York, 1980.

Wankat, P.C., "Advanced graphical extraction calculations," in J.M. Calo, and E.J. Henley, (eds.), *AIChE Modular Instruction,* Series B, *Stagewise and Mass Transfer Operations,* vol. 3, *Extraction and Leaching,* Module B 3.3, p. 17, AIChE, New York, 1982.

Wankat, P.C., *Equilibrium-Staged Separations,* Elsevier, New York, 1988.

HOMEWORK

A. *Discussion Problems*

A1. How does an evaporative crystallizer operated below one atmosphere pressure differ from a vacuum crystallizer?

A2. Sketch the entire process including methanol recovery if methanol were added to salt out KCl (see Figure 2-6).

A3. Crystallization processes which utilize only energy removal are usually preferred to those involving addition of a salt or antisolvent if all things are equal. Explain why. Give some examples of when the addition of a salt or antisolvent is desireable.

A4. A process for fractional crystallization of KCl and NaCl is shown in Figure 2-18. Sketch the flow-sheet for this process.

A5. Define the following terms.

    a. hydrate

    b. anhydrous

    c. Miers diagram

    d. metastable

    e. labile

    f. salting out

    g. eutectic

    h. congruent melting point

    i. incongruent melting point

    j. reciprocal salt pair

    k. double salt

A6. Why is it better to plot the concentration in Figures 2-1 as mass ratios in units, kg anhydrous salt/100 kg water, instead of in units kg hydrated salt/100 kg water? Focus on what happens at the phase change points.

A7. Explain how solubility data and temperature-composition diagrams correspond.

A8. Why are evaporation costs significantly higher at 10°C than at 50° C?

A9. Construct your key relations chart for this chapter. That is, on one page list all facts, equations, figures, etc. which you would want to help you solve problems on a test.

B. *Generation of Alternatives*

B1. In fractional crystallization many alternate processes are often available. For the fractionation for KCl from NaCl shown in Figure 2-18 several alternative processes using evaporation and addition of water can be used. Sketch the flow sheets for at least 3 such processes. Then sketch the processes on a triangular diagram.

B2. Develop at least two different cycles for fractionating $MgSO_4$ and Na_2SO_4 alternating between 0°C and 10°C (see Figure 2-14b). Sketch both the process flow sheet and the process on a triangular diagram.

C. *Derivations*

C1. Derive Eq. (2-5a). Note that
$MW_{hydrate} = MW_{anhydrous} + n\ MW_{water}$.

C2. Derive Eq. (2-6a).

C3. Show that Eq. (2-9) can also be written as

$$S = \frac{\text{(Total solution flow rate)}}{N+1}$$

C4. Write the Equations for Δ_2 for the cascade in Figure 2-21. Develop the coordinates of Δ_2.

C5. Prove that points $\Delta_1(X_{\Delta_1}, N_{\Delta_1})$, $S_j(Y_j, N_j)$ and $C_{j-1}(X_{j-1}, 0)$ are on a straight line in Figure 2-21.

D. *Problems*

D1. Determine if the following compounds in water satisfy Eq. (2-1b). If Eq. (2-1b) is satisfied determine the constants a and b. Data are in Table 2-1.

a. $CuSO_4 \cdot 5H_2O$

b. copper chloride

c. silver nitrate

d. sucrose

e. sodium sulphate

D2. Determine the yield of crystals deposited at equilibrium and the yield of anhydrous crystals for the following problems. Data are in Table 2-1.

    a. A saturated sugar solution (sucrose) is cooled from $80°$ to $20°C$. 100 kg of water are present.

    b. A saturated sucrose solution at $80°C$ has 1/2 of its water evaporated and the solution is then cooled to $20°C$. Initially 100 kg of water are present.

    c. A copper chloride solution initially saturated at $75°C$ is cooled to $10°C$. 100 kg of water are present. (See Problem 2-D1b for interpolation).

D3. 100 kg of a solution which is 0.60 wt. fraction Na_2CO_3 and 0.40 wt fraction water is cooled from an initial temperature of $80°C$. Data is in Figure 2-10.

    a. If the mixture is cooled to $35.4°C$ what three phases are present at equilibrium? If 20,000 kJ have been removed how many kg of each of these 3 phases are present.

    b. If the mixture is cooled to $0°C$, what two phases are in equilibrium? How much of each phase is present? How many kJ had to be removed to cool the original solution from $80°C$ to $0°C$?

D4. A vacuum crystallizer is operated so that the mixed magma has an overall concentration of 30 wt % Na_2CO_3 and 70 % water and is at $20°C$. The entering feed is a 25 wt % Na_2CO_3 solution and is under pressure so that it remains a liquid until it flashes in the crystallizer. Feed rate is 100 kg/hr. Data is in Figure 2-10.

    a. What crystals are formed? How many kg of steam are removed and how many kg of magma mixture are present?

    b. Data for the partial pressure of aqueous Na_2CO_3 at $20°C$ is (Perry & Green, 1984, p. 3-73).

wt. % Na$_2$CO$_3$	0	5	10	15
p, mm Hg	17.5	17.2	16.8	16.3

Estimate the pressure of the crystallizer.

c. From the steam tables saturated steam at 20°C has an enthalpy of ~ 2537 kJ/kg. (Perry & Green, 1984, p. 3-238). What is the required enthalpy of the feed? What temperature is it at? Is 1 atmosphere pressure high enough to prevent it from boiling?

d. How many kg of crystals are produced?

D5. We have a solid mixture of 80 % KNO$_3$ and 20 % NaNO$_3$ at 50°C (see Figures 2-12 a,b). What would you do to precipitate out pure KNO$_3$? If there is initially 100 kg of mixture, what is the maximum amount of KNO$_3$ which can be recovered. What is the concentration of solution in equilibrium with the pure KNO$_3$? Do this problem at 50°C. Do not use a fractional crystallization cycle.

D6. What happens if the feed to Example 2-4 also contains 0.02 wt % NaNO$_3$? Where would you add a purge stream? If we desire to keep the maximum concentration in the liquor below 1.0 wt % NaNO$_3$, what purge flow rate should be used?

D7. Redo Example 2-4, but with feed added to the solution b(0°) instead of solution b(30°). A flow chart of one way of doing this is shown below. Find crystal product flow rates, the water flow rates and recycle flow rate b(0°).

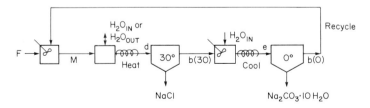

Note that you must determine whether water is added or removed from mixture M.

D8. Citric Acid (C_3H_4OH $(COOH)_3$) is dissolved in 10 kg water at 100°C to form a saturated solution. This solution is cooled to 20°C and simultaneously 0.8 kg of water are evaporated. Assuming the solution is saturated at 20°C, how many kg of hydrated crystals, C_3H_4OH $(COOH)_3 \cdot 1H_2O$ are formed? How many kg of anhydrous $C_3H_4OH(COOH)_3$ will result?

D9. We wish to separate $Pb(NO_3)_2$ from $Ba(NO_3)_2$. The feed is 55 wt % $Pb(NO_3)_2$ and 45 wt % $Ba(NO_3)_2$ on a water free basis, and enters stage N. The feed rate is 100 kg/hr of total salts in enough water so that the mixture is a saturated solution. A reflux ratio of 3.0 (lb crystals returned)/(lb crystals taken as $Pb(NO_3)_2$ product) is used. A crystal product which is 90 wt % $Pb(NO_3)_2$ is desired.
a. How many stages are needed?
b. How much water is required in the feed?
c. What is the composition of the $Ba(NO_3)_2$ crystals withdrawn from stage N?
Data are in Figure 2-21.

D10. We have 100 kg of a mixture which is 20 kg $MgSO_4$ (anhydrous), 10 kg Na_2SO_4 and 70 kg water. We evaporate 20 kg water. Operation is at 50°C. Data are in Figure 2-14a.

a. What are the composition of salt and of solution which result after crystallization is complete?

b. How many kg of each are obtained?

D11. At a particular pH bovine serum albumin (BSA) in $(NH_4)_2$ SO_4 has constants in the Cohn equation of approximately K = 7.65 and $\beta = 21.6$ where c_s is in moles/liter and c^* is protein solubility in g/liter (Belter et al, 1988). The initial charge is a saturated solution of BSA at c_s = 2.6M and we desire a 99.9% yield of BSA. What final salt concentration should be used?

D12. Repeat Example 2-1A, but for the case where the solution is initially at 100°C. Show that Eq. (2-5a) gives an impossible result. Explain why.

E.   *More Complex Problems*

E1.   Solve Example 2-4 with analytical equations instead of graphically. That is, solve the mass balances and find $F_{b(0)}$, F_c, $F_{b(30)}$, $F_{W,out}$, F_M, F_a, and $F_{W,in}$. Do this first in algebraic form without numbers. This would then be useful for a programmable calculator or computer solution. Then use the numbers of Example 2-4 and redo that example.

Hint: Read the paragraph following Example 2-4 which outlines the procedure.

E2.   Redo Problem 2-D7 but do it analytically instead of graphically. Follow the suggestions of Problem 2-E1.

Chapter 3

NUCLEATION AND CRYSTAL GROWTH

The crystal size distribution (CSD) and the shape of the crystals depends on kinetics and mass transfer in the crystallizer. Equilibrium data is needed to determine the driving forces for nucleation and crystal growth, but equilibrium data by itself is not sufficient to predict the CSD or crystal shape. In this chapter we will first look briefly at crystal shapes. Next, the imperfectly understood area of nucleation will be explored, and some empirical expressions for nucleation rates will be presented. Then theories of crystal growth and mass transfer will be developed. These theories will be used in Chapter 4 to predict crystal size distributions. While reading this chapter you should not think of this as the "truth". Instead, consider this as part way down the path to scientific knowledge.

This chapter continues to focus on crystallization and precipitation from solution. However, many of the fundamentals developed here are also applicable to melt crystallization.

3.1. CRYSTAL SHAPES

Every chemical compound has a unique crystal shape; however, the crystal shape depends enormously on the conditions in the crystallizer. This statement seems like a contradiction but is not. The unique aspect of the crystal is that the *angles* between adjacent faces are constant. The sizes of the faces can change, but the angles do not change and are characteristic of the substance. This is known as Haüy's law. These angles can be measured by an instrument

80

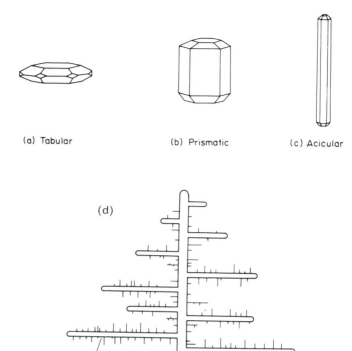

(a) Tabular   (b) Prismatic   (c) Acicular

(d)

Primary branch

Main stem   Secondary branch

Figure 3-1.   Shapes of a hexagonal crystal (a, b and c). a. Tabular. b. Prismatic. c. Needle or acicular. d. Dendrites. Mullin (1972). Reprinted by permission of Butterworths. Copyright 1972.

called a goniometer. With constant angles but different sizes of the faces, the shape of a crystal can vary enormously. This is illustrated in Figure 3-1 (Mullin, 1972) which shows three crystals which are all hexagonal. This variation in shape is called the crystal *habit*. The habit is affected by the rate of crystallization, impurities, agitation, solvent used, degree of supersaturation or supercooling and so forth. Note that some substances illustrate *polymorphism* which means the substance can crystallize into two or more unique forms. A good example is carbon which can crystallize into graphite or diamonds.

82

Crystallography (the study of crystals) is a well-developed science (Bunn, 1961; Mullin, 1972; Wyckoff, 1963-68). Most of the details of crystallography are beyond the scope of a book on separations. Thus, only a *very* brief account will be given here. A more detailed, but still brief, presentation is given by Mullin (1972).

There are 32 possible classes of crystals based on crystal symmetry. These 32 classes can be broken down into seven systems: regular (5 classes), tetragonal (7), orthorhombic (3), monoclinic (3), triclinic (2), trigonal (5) and hexagonal (7). The first six systems can be defined by referring to 3 axes while the hexagonal system requires 4 axes. The faces of the crystals can be numbered in terms of the Miller indices. More than 80% of the elements and sim-

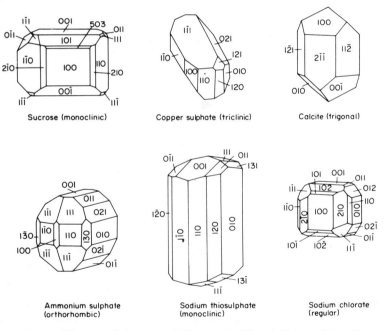

Figure 3-2.   Characteristic crystal forms. Miller indices of the faces are given. (Mullin, 1972). Reprinted with permission of Butterworths. Copyright 1972.

ple inorganic compounds belong to either the regular or hexagonal systems. Some characteristic crystal forms are shown in Figure 3-2 (Mullin, 1972).

Two or more substances which crystallize in almost identical forms are *isomorphous*. There will be small but measurable differences in the angles (Haüy's law says the angles are unique for each substance). Since the crystal shapes are so similar, these substances often form solid solutions. Isomorphs can also grow on top of crystals of the other substance.

Enantiomorphs are crystals of the same substance which are mirror images of each other. Compounds which are enantiomorphs are often optically active. These compounds are often of considerable interest in biological systems where one form may be biologically active while the other form is not.

Specific additives can be very useful in controlling both crystal morphology and purity (Davey, 1987; Randolph and Larson, 1988). Since impurities can be incorporated only through certain faces of the crystal, crystal purity is linked to crystal morphology. For example, optically active isomers will form pure D and pure L crystals, but separating the two types of crystals is very difficult. Suppose a small quantity of a resolved additive, say a D isomer, which inhibits crystallization is added. Then the D crystals will not grow and only the L crystals will form (Davey, 1987). Similiar separations based on the solid state chemistry can be developed.

In industrial crystallization the growth conditions are usually far from ideal. Thus, the individual crystals are also usually far from ideal. Only one-half or one-quarter of the maximum number of faces may develop. Combinations of different classes often occur. Crystals also often grow as composites formed by aggregation or intergrowth. Most crystals will have imperfections which may change the shape. Crystallization past phase transitions usually damages the crystals. Finally, when crystallization is very rapid dendrites (see Figure 3-1d) will often form. An example of dendrites is frost on windows. All of these variations from ideal conspire to make the shapes of industrially produced crystals considerably more complex than the ideal forms shown in Figure 3-2.

84

3.2. NUCLEATION

The steps in crystallization are:

1. Supersaturate or supercool.

2. Form crystal nuclei.

3. Grow crystals.

Nucleation is the least well understood of these. Part of the difficulty in understanding nucleation is there are several types of nucleation. In *primary* nucleation no crystals are involved in the nucleation. *Homogeneous* primary nucleation occurs in the bulk liquid phase with no solid surfaces present. *Heterogeneous* primary nucleation occurs on a solid such as a dust particle or the vessel wall. *Secondary* nucleation is heterogeneous nucleation induced by existing crystals.

3.2.1. Homogeneous Nucleation

Homogeneous nucleation occurs in the absence of crystals or any foreign particles. Since irregularities in the vessel wall or any crystals left over from previous crystallizations can serve as nucleation sites, the vessel must be meticulously cleaned and polished. In addition, the vessel must be closed since normal atmospheric dust will often cause heterogeneous nucleation.

The current picture of homogeneous nucleation is as follows: In a highly supersaturated solution a large number of solute units (atoms, molecules or ions) can aggregate together to form a cluster or embryo. Bringing together the solute units and expelling the solvent molecules requires work. This work or energy of nucleation serves as an energy barrier which controls the nucleation kinetics. If the cluster can reach a certain critical size, the free energy change upon further growth will be negative. Then the cluster is stable and serves as a nucleus for further growth. If the cluster cannot reach the critical size, it redissolves.

The solubility of small particles can be related to the equilibrium solubility by the Oswald-Freundlich or Kelvin equation

$$\ln \frac{c}{c^*} = \frac{2(MW)\sigma}{RT\rho_s r} \qquad (3\text{-}1)$$

where c is the solubility of the small particle, σ is the interfacial tension between solid and fluid, and r is the radius of the particle. Equation (3-1) predicts that $c > c^*$ for small particles and that solubility increases as the particle radius decreases. Thus, there is a tendency for the bigger particles to grow and the smallest ones to redissolve. This occurs because the system adjusts itself to a minimum total surface free energy. Since $c/c^* = S$, the supersaturation ratio, Eq. (3-1) indicates that very small particles require a certain degree of supersaturation or they will redissolve. This is one limit on the critical radius to form a nucleus.

Since there is an energy barrier to the formation of a nucleus, Arrhenius type kinetic equations for the rate of nucleation can be developed (Garside, 1985; McCabe and Smith, 1976; Mullin, 1972; Randolph and Larson, 1988). The rate of formation of nuclei, B°, defined as the number of nuclei formed/(time volume) is

$$B^\circ_{homogen} = \frac{dN}{dt} \Big|_{nuclei} = A \exp(-\Delta G/kT) \qquad (3\text{-}2)$$

where N is the cumulative number of crystals per unit volume which in this equation is the number of nuclei per unit volume, ΔG is the free energy change upon formation of nuclei, k is Boltzmann's constant = 1.3805×10^{-23} J/K, and the preexponential factor A is on the order of 10^{25}. Starting with Eq. (3-2), the eventual result is,

$$B^\circ = A \exp \left[-\frac{16\pi\sigma^3 V_M^2}{3k^3 T^3 (\ln S)^2} \right] \qquad (3\text{-}3)$$

where V_M is the molar volume of the crystal which is the reciprocal of the molar density. Equation (3-3) predicts an extremely rapid increase in the nucleation rate after some critical degree of supersaturation S is reached. At the critical supersaturation ΔG switches from a positive to a negative value and spontaneous nucleation can occur. Experiments agree with this initially, but then may show a maximum and a decrease in solubility. This equation is difficult to use since σ, the solid-liquid surface energy, is difficult to measure.

Homogeneous nucleation is well established as a real phenomena which will occur under well-controlled laboratory conditions. Equations (3-1) and (3-3) show that a considerable degree of supersatuation is required to have homogeneous nucleation. When homogeneous nucleation does occur, a very large number of nuclei may be produced, and the final product may consist of a very large number of small crystals. In properly operated commercial cooling, evaporative, and vacuum crystallizers homogeneous nucleation seldom if ever occurs. Homogeneous nucleation does occur in salting out and precipitation crystallizations.

3.2.2. Heterogeneous and Secondary Nucleation

In heterogeneous nucleation the crystal forms around a foreign object such a dust particle or a crack in the vessel wall. The foreign object lowers the surface energy because the solid is wetted by the solvent. The surface energy σ can drop from around 80 to 100 ergs/cm^2 to as low as 2 to 3 ergs/cm^2. Equation (3-3) is again applicable but with the absolute value of the argument of the exponential decreased by as much as 4 to 5 orders of magnitude. This obviously greatly increases the rate of nucleation at any supersaturation and decreases the critical supersaturation. The most effective particles will be in the range of 0.1 to 1.0 μm.

In industrial systems solutions are never completely free of suspended solids, cleaning of vessels is often less than perfect, and interior surfaces are often incompletely polished. Thus heterogeneous nucleation will occur at much lower supersaturations than homogeneous nucleation.

In secondary nucleation the object the crystal builds on is a very small crystal of the solute. This may be added on purpose as *seed crystals* to induce nucleation. The seed crystals can be the substance being crystallized or a substance which is isomorphous to the solid. Seeding is commonly used for production of borax from Trona ore, for crystallization of alumina, for production of sugar, and in citric acid crystallization. Citric acid is an example where nucleation is difficult if not seeded, but large crystals are easy to grow if seeded. Seed crystals may also be added accidentally as atmospheric dust or as crystals retained in tiny cracks from previous batches. When solutions are seeded, there is often a lag or induction period before secondary nucleation starts.

The presence of macroscopic growing crystals can also cause secondary nucleation by several different mechanisms (Nyvlt, 1982; Randolph and Larson, 1988; Strickland-Constable, 1972).

1. Initial breeding. Added seed crystals may have crystal dust on their surfaces. The crystal dust arises when the crystals are dried and retained mother liquor is dried onto the crystal forming a dust. When added to the crystallizer, the dust can wash off and serve as additional nuclei if the dust particles are larger than the critical radius. This can be an important nucleation mechanism in batch crystallizers.

2. Needle or dendrite breeding. Very rapid crystallization will cause the growth of needles and/or dendrites. Small crystals are easily broken off which will serve as nuclei.

3. Polymerization breeding. Crystals will often grow as agglomerates. These can break apart easily leading to nuclei.

4. Contact or collision breeding. The agitator or other parts of the vessel can knock off very small particles from a crystal. These small pieces serve as nuclei. Experiments show that different materials of construction (e.g. stainless steel versus polyethylene) will cause different nucleation rates. The rate with stainless steel is significantly higher. The required contact energy appears to be rather low, but repeated rapid contacts do not produce more nuclei. This is probably the most important

mechanism for secondary nucleation in continuous crystallizers (Garside, 1985; Rousseau, 1980).

5. Fluid shear breeding. Fluid shear by itself can apparently cause nucleation, but this does not appear to be an important mechanism.

In all cases the nuclei will grow only if they are larger than the critical radius. Thus secondary nucleation depends on the supersatuation. Since mixing is never perfect, the vessel will have higher supersaturation in some localities. Nucleation is most likely to occur in these places such as at cold walls or at the liquid surface when evaporation is used. Equation (3-3) is valid locally; although, for design it is often used for the entire volume. It is possible to have nuclei formed in one part of the vessel and then redissolve in other parts if the supersaturations are very different. This will not happen in a well-designed crystallizer.

Equation (3-3) can be derived from fundamental principles, but is only accurate within an order of magnitude. For design, empirical and semi-empirical equations are used. For heterogeneous and secondary nucleation the effective or apparent nucleation rate can often be correlated using the semi-empirical equation.

$$B^\circ = k_N((\Delta c)_{max})^i \qquad (3\text{-}4)$$

where $(\Delta c)_{max}$ is the maximum allowed supersatuation and i is the "order" of nucleation. Note that i is applied to a concentration difference and has no fundamental significance. For aqueous solutions the "order" lies between 2 and 9. Low molecular weight salts are at the lower end of this range. For secondary nucleation Eq. (3-4) again appears to be valid, but the order is significantly lower and is in the range from 0 to 3. Many commercial crystallizers appear to operate with orders in this range.

The nucleation rate is often correlated in terms of the linear growth rate of the crystal, G. This eliminates the need to know the system supersaturation which is often difficult to measure. G is defined as

$$G = \frac{dL}{dt} \qquad (3\text{-}5)$$

where L is a characteristic dimension of the crystal. Then $B°$ is

$$B° = \frac{dN}{dt} \Big|_{L=0} = \left[\frac{dN}{dL} \Big|_{L=0} \right] \frac{dL}{dt} = n°G \qquad (3\text{-}6)$$

In this equation N is the number of nuclei per unit volume and $n°$ (given by the term in parenthesis) is the population density of nuclei. Usually, the linear growth rate is proportional to the supersaturation, $G = k_G (\Delta c)$, while $B°$ is related by Eq. (3-4). Then equations

$$B° = k_N G^i, \quad \text{or} \quad n° = k_N G^{i-1} \qquad (3\text{-}7)$$

will correlate the data. A more general expression has been used by Garside and Shah (1980) in their review of experimental data on nucleation. This expression is

$$B° = K_R(T, \text{hydrodynamics, impurities}) (M_T)^j G^i \qquad (3\text{-}8a)$$

where M_T is the magma density in grams of crystals per liter and i,j are empirical constants. The dependence on magma density is expected when secondary nucleation occurs. The exponent i can range from -3.5 to +5 although most values are positive. The hydrodynamic term is sometimes separated out from K_R. Then

$$K_R = K'_R \ (T, \text{impurities}) N^k \qquad (3\text{-}8b)$$

where N is the stirrer speed in rpm and k is an empirical constant. The expressions and terms in this paragraph will be extensively used later when population balances and crystal size distributions are discussed. If this paragraph is not clear don't panic. Wait until after population balances and CSD have been covered.

Some of the correlations based on experimental data for nucleation are given in Table 3-1 (Garside and Shah, 1980). Note that the "constant" i for the same crystal often shows considerable variation between investigators. The negative i values are suspect since it is difficult to postulate a mechanism to

Table 3-1. Nucleation Kinetics from Aqueous Solution. Extracted from Garside and Shah (1980).

System	Temp. Range (°C)	Range M_T (g/l)	Range G (m/s × 10^8)	Range $(c-c^*)$ (g·hyd/gH$_2$O) × 10^3	Eq. for B° (#/L s)
Cooling and evaporation systems					
Ammonium sulphate	22	30-75	4.3-12.2	--	$2.09 \times 10^{12} M_T G^{1.5}$
Ammonium sulphate	34	--	--	--	$6.14 \times 10^{-11} N^{7.84} M_T^{0.98} G^{1.22}$
Potassium chloride	12-30	14-25	11.7-20.7	--	$2.86 \times 10^{21} G^{2.55}$ at 21°C
Potassium chloride	32	60-250	2-12	--	$7.17 \times 10^{39} M_T^{0.14} G^{4.99}$

Potassium sulphate	29	5-28	0.3-2.5	0.6-6.1	$4.07 \times 10^{-5} M_T^{0.4} G^{-1}$
Potassium sulphate	30	23-108	1.2-9.5	2.8-7.1	$1.67 \times 10^3 M_T G^0$
Potassium sulphate	~30	1-7	--	1.7-11.8	$2.62 \times 10^3 N^{2.5} M_T^{0.5} G^{0.54}$
Citric Acid	16-24	--	1.1-3.7	30-130	$1.09 \times 10^{10} M_T^{0.84} G^{0.84}$ at 20°C
Salting Out Systems					
Ammonium Sulphate/MeOH	27	110	1.4-3.3	--	$5.74 \times 10^{37} G^{4.0}$
Sodium chloride/	27	33	1.7-2.8	--	$2.02 \times 10^{75} G^{9.0}$
Ethanol	--	--	3.0-5.8	--	$4.54 \times 10^{14} G^{1.72}$
"	--	~13	2.3-3.9	32.5-53.5	$1.29 \times 10^{65} G^{7.9}$

give negative i. This variation in i and in the absolute value of B° (which can vary by several orders of magnitude) are an indication of the difficulty in reproducibly measuring nucleation rates. The values of i for salting out tend to be higher since nucleation is probably primary. The references for each system are given by Garside and Shah (1980). Nyvlt (1982) reports other values and Tavare (1987) reviews the literature.

At this point it may appear that the highest possible nucleation rate would be desired. This is not the case. If a huge number of nuclei are formed, then the crystals cannot grow very large. (Remember 10^9 particles 0.1 mm in diameter have the same mass as 10^6 particles 1 mm in diameter). Since relatively large crystals are usually desired, nucleation must often be supressed. For example, urea nucleates readily, but it is difficult to grow nice crystals. When seed crystals are added, it may be desirable to have a zero nucleation rate so that each seed crystal will become as large as possible.

3.3. CRYSTAL GROWTH

Crystal growth is a complex subject which like nucleation is not completely understood. On a microscopic level growth rates are irregular; however, averaged over a large number of crystals on a macroscopic scale growth rates are regular. Mass transfer rate limitations are usually used for design, but mass transfer theory cannot explain all phenomena. Thus, it will be useful to first explore another theory of crystal growth before discussing mass transfer.

3.3.1. Adsorption Theory

Adsorption layer or kinetic theories have proven to be quite fruitful in explaining crystal growth. (Garside, 1985; Ohara and Reid, 1973; Moyers and Rousseau, 1987; Mullin, 1972; Randolph and Larson, 1988; Tavare, 1987). These theories postulate that there is an "adsorbed" layer of units (atoms, ions or molecules) which is loosely held to the crystal face. These adsorbed units are free to move on the two-dimensional surface, but they have essentially lost one degree of freedom. If the surface is perfect and has no kinks, dislocations or crystallized units, the unit must crystallize at an edge or as a monolayer island nucleus. This two-dimensional nucleation requires a considerable supersaturation, but the energy required is considerably less than for a three-dimensional nucleation. The approximate ratio of energies is (Mullin, 1972)

$$\frac{\text{Energy two–dimensional nucleus}}{\text{Energy three–dimensional nucleus}} \sim \frac{1}{50}, \ S = 1.1$$

$$\sim \frac{1}{1.2}, \ S = 10$$

At lower supersaturations the energy required for this two-dimensional nucleation is considerably less than for normal nucleation. Thus, existing crystals can grow under conditions where three-dimensional nucleation will not occur. Once the initial two-dimensional nucleation has occurred, growth is easy since the units can fill in the face. Since each unit will fit with other units on at least two sides, the energy for growth is significantly less than that for two-dimensional nucleation.

Crystal growth will usually occur at supersaturation levels lower than can be explained by the two-dimensional nucleation theory. This happens because growth is much faster at any imperfection (kinks, pits, or dislocations) where the surface is not a perfect plane. Since crystals are usually not perfect, growth usually proceeds by a "filling-in" process. With linear imperfections the crystal will heal rapidly, and another two-dimensional nucleation would be required. Two-dimensional nucleation is not required if the crystal grows by a *screw-dislocation*. Crystal growth with a screw-dislocation mechanism is illustrated in Figure 3-3. Now the crystal can grow without healing the dislocation, and additional two-dimensional nucleations are not required. Equations resulting from this and similiar theories are discussed elsewhere (Garside, 1985; Moyers and Rousseau, 1987; Ohara and Reid, 1973; Randolph and Larson, 1988).

The adsorption theory helps to explain several experimental observations. First, rates of dissolution of crystals are invariably faster than rates of crystallization for equivalent differences from equilibrium saturation. Dissolution does not require two-dimensional nucleation. Since this is the slowest step

94

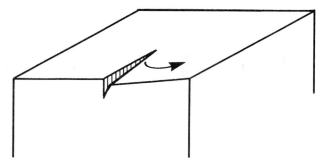

Figure 3-3.   Growth by screw dislocation.

in growth, dissolution would be expected to proceed at a higher rate. Second, small crystals often have linear growth rates, G in Eq. (3-5), which are significantly lower than large crystals. Small crystals are more likely to be perfect than large crystals. Thus the small crystals are much more likely to require two-dimensional nucleation. Large crystals are less likely to be perfect, and are more likely to be damaged by hitting the impeller or baffles. Thus, the large crystals can grow by healing kinks, pits and dislocations. Third, two crystals of the same size may have different growth rates although all conditions appear to be the same. This is called *growth rate dispersion* (Garside, 1985; Rousseau, 1980; Tavare, 1987). If one of the crystals happens to be more perfect than the other it will have a lower growth rate.

The adsorption theory is often incorporated into mass transfer theories. The adsorption theory explains the crystallization once a unit is at the surface. Mass transfer explains movement of the unit to the surface.

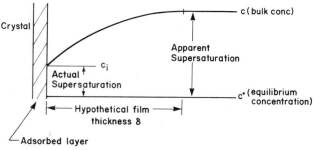

Figure 3-4.   Schematic of mass transfer process.

3.3.2. Mass Transfer Theory

Mass transfer or diffusion theory is similar to mass transfer theories for other processes. However, in crystallization the picture of the process is somewhat different and different empirical expressions are used. The mass transfer process is shown schematically in Figure 3-4. The steps in the process are

1. Bulk diffusion of solvated units through the film.

2. Diffusion of solvated units in the adsorbed layer.

3. Partial or total desolvation.

4. Surface diffusion of units to growth site.

5. Incorporation into lattice.

6. Counter diffusion of solvent through the adsorbed layer.

7. Counter diffusion of solvent through the film.

Since it is difficult to include all these steps in a theory, usually a simplified model is used which includes step 1, combines steps 2 to 5, and ignores steps 6 and 7.

The mass transfer across the film is,

$$\frac{dm}{dt} = k_f A(c - c_i) \tag{3-9}$$

where m is the mass of solute transferred across the film and thus m is also the mass of solid deposited. The film mass transfer coefficient is often written as $k_f = D/\delta$ where δ is the unknown film thickness. Next, steps 2 to 5 are combined as a single surface "reaction" or rearrangement of "order" n_r with rate constant k_r.

$$\frac{dm}{dt} = k_r A(c_i - c^*)^{n_r} \tag{3-10}$$

Realize that this is an empirical equation and does not correspond to steps 2 to 5 in detail.

In general, it is very difficult or impossible to determine the interfacial concentration c_i. *If* the surface reaction is of first order, $n_r = 1$, Eqs. (3-9) and (3-10) can be combined to remove c_i,

$$\frac{dm}{dt} = \frac{A(c - c^*)}{1/k_f + 1/k_r} = K_G A(c - c^*), \quad (n_r = 1) \tag{3-11}$$

For crystals where the faces are growing at the same rate, the mass and area of the crystal can be written as

$$m = k_v L^3 \rho_s, \quad A = k_A L^2 \tag{3-12}$$

where k_v and k_A are shape factors (see Eqs. (4-20)). Note that Eqs. (3-12) are not valid for crystals such as needles or plates where faces grow at different rates. Substituting Eqs. (3-12) into Eq. (3-11), we obtain

$$\frac{dL}{dt} = \left(\frac{k_A}{3\rho_s k_v}\right) \frac{(c - c^*)}{1/k_f + 1/k_r} \tag{3-13}$$

This simplifies to

$$G = \frac{dL}{dt} = k(c - c^*) = k\Delta c \tag{3-14a}$$

where G is the linear growth rate and k is a combined rate constant. For a constant supersaturation Δc, this is

$$\Delta L = G\Delta t \tag{3-14b}$$

where ΔL is the increase in linear size of the crystal. When Eq. (3-14b) is valid, the linear growth rate does *not* depend on crystal size. This is the McCabe ΔL *law* (McCabe, 1929; McCabe *et al.*, 1985; Mullin, 1972; Randolph and Larson, 1988).

The McCabe ΔL law is an important simplification which will be used in the next section. Because of the assumptions involved in the derivation (surface "reaction" is first order, all faces grow at same rate, constant coefficients, constant supersaturation in all parts of the crystallizer), it should not be surprising that many systems do not satisfy this law. Examples are the crystallization of potassium alum and of potassium sulfate. When the McCabe ΔL law is not valid, growth is size dependent. An empirical expression known as the Abegg-Stevens-Larson (ASL) equation (Abegg *et al.*, 1968)

$$G = G_{nuclei} (1 + \gamma L)^b \qquad (3\text{-}15)$$

is often used. In Eq. (3-15) b < 1 and γ are constants, and G_{nuclei} is the growth rate of the nuclei. This result can often be simplified by letting $\gamma = (G_{nuclei}\tau)^{-1}$. This reduces the number of parameters and simplifies determination of the crystal size distribution. Other models for size dependent growth are summarized by White *et al.*, (1976).

When n_r is not a simple integer, it is not possible to solve explicity for the growth rate. In these cases an empirical approach is to write the rate as

$$\frac{dm}{dt} = K_G A(c - c^*)^n \qquad (3\text{-}16)$$

where n is the "overall growth-rate order." For many inorganic salts n is in the range 1.5 to 2 (Mullin, 1972). Equation (3-16) allows for correlation of data, but it has no fundamental significance when n ≠ 1.

Temperature will affect both diffusion and the crystal rearrangement process. An Arrhenius type equation would be expected for both K_G and k_r. Thus plots of log K_G versus $1/T$ and log k_r versus $1/T$ will give straight lines. If either mass transfer or surface reaction controls, then the Arrhenius equation will be valid for the linear growth rate. In these cases

$$G = G(T_0)\exp[-\frac{\Delta E}{R}(\frac{1}{T} - \frac{1}{T_0})] \qquad (3\text{-}17)$$

When both mass transfer and surface reaction are important, Eq. (3-17) is not valid. Arrhenius plots for crystal growth data will thus usually give curved instead of straight lines.

Dissolution appears to be a much simpler process than crystallization. The overall dissolution rate is usually first order with respect to the concentration difference,

$$(\frac{1}{A} \frac{dm}{dt})_{\text{dissolution}} = k_d(c^* - c) \qquad (3\text{-}18)$$

Dissolution is usually significantly faster than crystallization (5 times quicker is not unusual). This probably occurs because two-dimensional nucleation and rearrangement to form the crystal lattice are not required.

Growth rates in the range of 10^{-6} to 10^{-7} m/s make it easy to grow crystals in the mm size range. Growth rates in the range of 10^{-9} m/s can take many days to reach this size range. According to Eq. (3-14a), G can be increased by increasing supersaturation. Unfortunately, nucleation is extremely sensitive to supersaturation, Eq. (3-4). If excessive nucleation occurs, large crystals cannot be grown unless the nuclei are destroyed (see the next chapter). In practice, it may be difficult to grow large crystals of materials with low growth rates with reasonable residence times.

3.4. SUMMARY-OBJECTIVES

This brief chapter covered crystal shapes, nucleation and crystal growth. At the end of this chapter you should be able to:

1. Discuss what is unique about crystal shape and define terms used.

2. Explain the types of nucleation, discuss when they are likely to occur, and calculate nucleation rates from empirical correlations.

3. Explain the adsorption layer theory of crystal growth.

4. Explain applications of mass transfer theory as applied to crystallization, and discuss the approximations used.

5. Be able to derive the McCabe ΔL law and explain the assumptions involved in this derivation.

REFERENCES

Abegg, C.F., J.D. Stevens, and M.A. Larson, "Crystal size distributions in continuous crytalizers when growth rate is size dependent," *AIChE Journal, 14*, 118 (1968).

Bunn, C.W., *Chemical Crystallography*, 2nd ed., Oxford, Clarendon Press, 1961.

Davey, R.J., "Looking into crystal chemistry," *The Chem. Engr.* (London), No. 443, 24 (Dec. 1987).

Garside, J. and M.B. Shah, "Crystallization kinetics from MSMPR crystallizers," *"Ind. Eng. Chem. Process Design Develop., 19,"* 509 (1980).

Garside, J., "Industrial crystallization from solution," *Chem. Eng. Sci., 40*, 3 (1985).

McCabe, W.L., "Crystal growth in aqueous solutions," *Ind. Eng. Chem., 21*, 30 (1929).

McCabe, W.L. and J.C. Smith, *Unit Operations of Chemical Engineering*, 3rd ed., McGraw-Hill, New York, 1976, Chapt. 28.

McCabe, W.L., J.C. Smith, and P. Harriott, *Unit Operations of Chemical Engineering*, 4th ed., McGraw-Hill, New York, 1985, Chapt. 28.

Moyers, C.G., Jr. and R.W., Rousseau, "Crystallization operations," in R.W. Rousseau (Ed.), *Handbook of Separation Process Technology*, Wiley-Interscience, New York, 1987, Chapter 11.

Mullin, J.W., *Crystallization*, 2nd ed., Butterworth, London, 1972.

Nyvlt, J., *Industrial Crystallization*, 2nd ed., Verlag Chemie, Weinheim, 1982.

Ohara, M., and R.C. Reid, *Modeling Crystal Growth Rates from Solution*, Prentice-Hall, Englewood Cliffs, NJ, 1973.

Randolph, A.D. and M.A. Larson, *Theory of Particulate Processes, Analysis and Techniques of Continuous Crystallization*, 2nd ed., Academic Press, New York, 1988.

Rousseau, R.W., "Crystallization: a review of recent developments," *Chem. Tech., 10, 566* (1980).

Strickland-Constable, R.F., "The breeding of crystal nuclei - a review of the subject," *AIChE Symp. Ser., 68,* (121), 1 (1972).

Tavare, N.S., "Batch crystallizers: A review," *Chem. Eng. Commun., 61* 259 (1987)

White, E.T., L.L. Bendig, and M.A. Larson, "The effect of size on the growth rate of potassium sulfate crystals," *AIChE Symp. Ser., 72,* (153) 41 (1976).

Wyckoff, R.W.G., *Crystal Structures,* (5 vols.), 2nd ed., Interscience, New York, 1963-1968.

HOMEWORK

A.   *Discussion Problems*

A1.   In any field it is important to understand the jargon. Define the following terms.

      a.   primary nucleation

      b.   homogeneous nucleation

      c.   heterogeneous nucleation

      d.   secondary nucleation

e.   two-dimensional nucleation

f.   isomorph

g.   G

h. $B°$

i.   screw-dislocation

j.   McCabe ΔL law

A2.   Why is empirical Eq. (3-15) often used instead of the usual mass transfer Eq. (3-9)?

A3.   Explain how different processes can cause secondary nucleation.

A4.   Explain why the Arrhenius relation is invalid for crystal growth rates when both mass transfer and surface rearrangement are important.

A5.   The "order" for secondary nucleation in Eq. (3-4) is usually less than the "order" for primary nucleation. What is the significance of this? Which will have higher Δc critical?

A6.   Explain why Eqs. (3-12) are not valid for plates, needles and dendrites.

A7.   Why do small crystals often grow slower than large crystals?

A8.   Construct your key relations chart for this chapter.

C.   *Derivations*

C1.   Derive Eq. (3-13) from Eqs. (3-11) and (3-12).

D.   *Problems*

D1.   Assuming that $G \propto \Delta c$, determine if the Arrhenius equation is valid for $(NH_4)_2SO_4$ crystallization. If it is valid, determine ΔE. Note: c^* depends on T.

Data (Mullin 1972): $30°C, S = 1.05, G = 5.0 \times 10^{-7}$ m/s
$60°C, S = 1.05, G = 8.0 \times 10^{-7}$ m/s
$90°C, S = 1.01, G = 6.0 \times 10^{-8}$ m/s

D2. Is $G \propto \Delta c$ for sucrose crystallization? If the relationship is linear, determine the proportionality constant.

Data (Mullin, 1972): $30°C, S = 1.13, G = 2.2 \times 10^{-8}$ m/s
$30°C, S = 1.27, G = 4.2 \times 10^{-8}$ m/s
$70°C, S = 1.09, G = 1.9 \times 10^{-8}$ m/s
$70°C, S = 1.15, G = 3.0 \times 10^{-7}$ m/s

D3. Estimate the nucleation rate for K_2SO_4 at $30°C$ at a supersaturation ratio $S = 1.07$. M_T is 25 g/l.

   a. Use the equations in Table 3-1.

   b. Assume homogeneous nucleation and use Eq. (3-3). Estimate σ as 80 ergs/cm^2. The density of K_2SO_4 crystals is 2.66 g/cm^3.

   c. Compare parts a and b.

Data: For $S = c/c^* = 1.07$, $G = 8.4 \times 10^{-8}$ m/s and growth was size dependent (Mullin, 1972).

F. *Problems Requiring Other Resources*

F1. Read the classical paper by McCabe (1929) where the McCabe ΔL law was first developed. Write a report on this short paper. Compare the development of the ΔL law in McCabe's paper to the development in this chapter.

Chapter 4

POPULATION BALANCES AND CRYSTAL SIZE DISTRIBUTIONS

Population balances will be introduced and will be used to derive crystal size distributions (CSD) for some simple growth kinetics. The crystal size distribution tells the number of crystals at each size range. This is important for product quality control and for ease of downstream processing. The CSD will be used to predict physically measurable quantities such as the sieve analysis. Methods for using an experimentally measured CSD to infer the nucleation and growth rates will be developed. The effect of equipment modifications on the CSD and more details of equipment for crystallization from solution will be discussed. Finally, the effect of the CSD on downstream processing will be briefly explored.

Population balances are the major theoretical tool used for predicting and analyzing crystal size distributions. The development of population balances in the 1960's was a major breakthrough which helped move crystallization from an art to more of a science. Population balances and CSD have been reviewed in many books and review papers (Garside, 1985; Larson and Randolph, 1969; McCabe et al., 1985; Mullin, 1972; Randolph and Larson, 1988; Rousseau, 1986). The most detailed source is Randolph and Larson (1988) while Garside (1985) has an extensive bibliography. Ramkrishna (1985) explores the general mathematical framework and other applications of population balances in considerable detail.

4.1. BASIC POPULATION BALANCE EQUATIONS

The population balance is a balance of the number of crystals within a given size range. The idea of the concept is easy to see from an analogy. Suppose we wish to determine the number of children in a school who are between 100 cm and 110 cm tall for a two month period. This number can be determined by a population balance on children in this height range. This balance can be written for the two month time period,

Initial No. children in range + No. children growing into range $\qquad$ (4-1)

+ No. children entering school in range = final No. children in range

+ No. children growing out of range + No. children in range leaving school

The population balance differs from a mass balance in that only the item balanced (children in this example) within a given size range (100 to 110 cm) are included. In addition, the item (children or crystals) can grow into or grow out of the size range.

The population balance for crystallization can be obtained by changing the words (No. of children) with (No. of crystals), and replacing "school" with "crystallizer." In addition, we will assume there is no crystal breakage. The size range is now for crystals within a range $L_2 - L_1 = \Delta L$. The size range is usually determined by a sieve or screen analysis.

Population balances for crystallizers are usually written in terms of the population density, n, instead of the number of crystals. This population density is defined as,

$$n = \frac{dN}{dL} = \lim_{\Delta L \to 0} \frac{\Delta N}{\Delta L} \qquad (4\text{-}2)$$

L is a measure of the linear size of the crystal, and N is the cumulative number of crystals per unit volume at the given size L. The units on n are number of crystals/m$-$m^3. The population density is shown schematically in Figure 4-1. The population density can be related to a count from a screen analysis, particle size analyzer, or count under a microscope by integrating,

$$\int_{L_1}^{L_2} n \, dL = \text{No. of crystals in sizes from } L_1 \text{ to } L_2/\text{volume} \qquad (4\text{-}3)$$

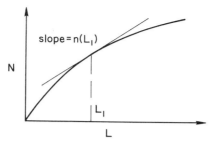

Figure 4-1.   Schematic representation of population density.

In terms of the population density, Eq. (4-1) for crystals can be written as (terms are in the same order)

$$V\overline{n}_{initial} \Delta L + V\, G_1 n_1\, \Delta t + Q_{in}\overline{n}_{in}\, \Delta L \Delta t$$

$$= V\overline{n}_{final} \Delta L + V\, G_2 n_2 \Delta t + Q_{out}\overline{n}_{out}\, \Delta L \Delta t \qquad (4\text{-}4)$$

Q_{in} is the volumetric feed rate while Q_{out} is the volumetric discharge rate, m^3/s. $\Delta L = L_2 - L_1$ is the size range. $\overline{n}$ is the average population density over the size range. n_1 and n_2 are shorthand for the average population densities over the range of sizes which will grow into and out of the range ΔL, respectively. G_1 and G_2 are the average growth rates of crystals growing into and out of the range ΔL. V = volume of *magma* (mixture of crystals and solution) which is assumed to be constant. The magma volume is assumed to be well-mixed so that n and Δc are constant throughout the volume.

Rearranging Eq. (4-4) gives

$$\frac{V(G_2 n_2 - G_1 n_1)}{\Delta L} + Q_{out}\overline{n}_{out} - Q_{in}\overline{n}_{in} + \frac{V(\overline{n}_{final} - \overline{n}_{initial})}{\Delta t} = 0 \qquad (4\text{-}5)$$

Taking the limit as $\Delta L \to 0$ and as $\Delta t \to 0$

$$V\frac{d(Gn)}{dL} + (Q_{out}\overline{n}_{out} - Q_{in}\overline{n}_{in}) + V\frac{d\overline{n}}{dt} = 0 \qquad (4\text{-}6)$$

This equation is the unsteady state population balance. In continuous operation the assumption of steady-state operation is usually made. Then the population balance simplifies to

$$V\frac{d(Gn)}{dL} + Q(\bar{n}_{out} - \bar{n}_{in}) = 0 \tag{4-7}$$

where we have also assumed that the volumetric feed and discharge rates are equal. This implies that the density (kg/m^3) is constant.

Solution of Eqs. (4-6) or (4-7) gives an equation for the population density distribution. From the population density distribution a variety of other distributions (number, length, area and mass) are easily generated. These crystal size distributions are developed in the next section.

4.2. DISTRIBUTIONS FOR SIZE INDEPENDENT GROWTH

In this section the CSD will be developed for steady-state crystallizers where the crystal growth rate does not depend on crystal size. This will be done for an idealized crystallizer known as the *Mixed Suspension, Mixed Product Removal (MSMPR)* crystallizer for the simplest possible case. The following assumptions will be made for the ideal MSMPR:

Steady-state

No product classification - crystals removed have same CSD as those in magma.

Constant magma volume.

Uniform supersaturation, Δc.

No crystal breakage.

Product crystals in equilibrium with mother liquor - no change in CSD after withdrawal and $\bar{n}_{out} = n$.

No crystals in feed, $\bar{n}_{in} = 0$.

Growth is independent of size. Thus G = constant since Δc is constant.

Many of these assumptions will be relaxed in later sections.

The steady-state population balance, Eq. (4-7) can now be simplified. The draw down or retention time is $\tau = V/Q$. Since the linear growth rate G is constant, Eq. (4-7) simplifies to

$$\frac{dn}{dL} + \frac{n}{G\tau} = 0 \qquad (4\text{-}8)$$

which upon integration is

$$n = n^\circ \exp(-\frac{L}{G\tau}) \qquad (4\text{-}9)$$

where n° is the population density of nuclei.

Equation (4-9) is *the result* we have been working towards. Taking the natural logarithm of both sides

$$\ln n = -\frac{L}{G\tau} + \ln n^\circ \qquad (4\text{-}10)$$

A plot of ln n versus L is a straight line with a slope of $-1/(G\tau)$ and an intercept of $\ln n^\circ$. This is illustrated in Figure 4-2. If n(L) is determined experimentally, n° and G can be determined from this plot. This will be illustrated in Example 4-2.

If G and n° are known, N and other distributions can be obtained starting with Eq. (4-9). The physical significance of these other distributions is easier to see than the physical significance of the population density. The first distribution is the cumulative number of particles at a given size L. From Eq. (4-2) and (4-9),

$$N = \int_0^L ndL = \int_0^L n^\circ \exp(-\frac{L}{G\tau})dL \qquad (4\text{-}11a)$$

which is

$$N = n^\circ G\tau[1 - \exp(-\frac{L}{G\tau})] \qquad (4\text{-}11b)$$

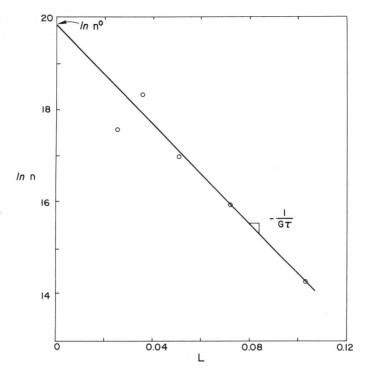

Figure 4-2.   Plot of population density following Eq. (4-10). Numerical values are for Example 4-2.

This distribution was illustrated in Figure 4-1. As $L \to \infty$, the exponential term becomes zero and

$$N_T = n^\circ G\tau \tag{4-12}$$

where N_T is the total number of particles per unit volume. Note that with the assumptions made for the ideal MSMPR each nucleus grows into one crystal in the product.

The cumulative length per unit volume is the length of crystals per unit volume if all crystals up to size L were laid end-to-end. Within a given size range, the end-to-end length per volume is LndL. Then the cumulative length per volume is

$$L = \int_0^L LndL = \int_0^L Ln^\circ \exp(-\frac{L}{G\tau})dL \qquad (4\text{-}13a)$$

which is

$$L = n^\circ G\tau \left\{ G\tau \left[1 - \exp(-\frac{L}{G\tau}) \right] - L \exp(-\frac{L}{G\tau}) \right\} \qquad (4\text{-}13b)$$

As L→∞ the total cumulative length per unit volume of all the crystals is

$$L_T = n^\circ (G\tau)^2 \qquad (4\text{-}14)$$

The cumulative area of crystals per unit volume, A, is of more interest. The cumulative area gives an idea of the area available for growth. The total area also gives an idea of the area on which mother liquor and impurities can adsorb. The cumulative area per unit volume can be calculated as

$$A = k_A \int_0^L L^2 ndL = k_A \int_0^L L^2 n^\circ \exp(-\frac{L}{G\tau})dL \qquad (4\text{-}15a)$$

where k_A is a shape factor [see Eq. (4-20b)]. This becomes,

$$A = 2k_A n^\circ G\tau \left\{ (G\tau)^2 - \left[(G\tau)^2 + (G\tau)L + \frac{1}{2}L^2 \right] \exp(-\frac{L}{G\tau}) \right\} \qquad (4\text{-}15b)$$

The total cumulative area per unit volume is found as L→∞.

$$A_T = 2k_A n^\circ (G\tau)^3 \qquad (4\text{-}16)$$

The cumulative mass of crystals per unit volume, M, is obviously of interest since it gives the weight of crystals up to a given size. The total mass per unit volume will give the concentration of crystals in the product. The cumulative mass per unit volume is

$$M = k_V \rho_c \int_0^L L^3 n dL = k_V \rho_c \int_0^L L^3 n^\circ \exp(-\frac{L}{G\tau}) dL \qquad (4\text{-}17a)$$

where k_V is the volumetric shape factor [Eq. (4-20a)] and ρ_c is the density of the crystals. This becomes

$$M = 6 k_V \rho_c n^\circ G\tau \left\{ (G\tau)^3 \right. \qquad (4\text{-}17b)$$

$$\left. - \left[(G\tau)^3 + (G\tau)^2 L + \frac{1}{2} G\tau L^2 + \frac{1}{6} L^3 \right] \exp(-\frac{L}{G\tau}) \right\}$$

The total mass of crystals per volume is determined as $L \rightarrow \infty$.

$$M_T = 6 k_V \rho_c n^\circ (G\tau)^4 \qquad (4\text{-}18)$$

This total cumulative mass of crystals per unit volume can also be determined from a mass balance. For a steady state process

$$M_T Q = S_c \qquad (4\text{-}19)$$

where S_c is the mass of crystals produced per time. S_c can be determined from steady-state equilibrium yield calculations such as Eqs. (2-5a) to (2-6b). Thus Eqs. (4-18) and (4-19) serve as a check on the population distribution or on the screen data. If n° is known, comparison of Eqs. (4-18) and the yield calculation allows determination of G.

The shape factors k_V and k_A are determined by comparing the volume or surface area of the crystals to the equations

$$\text{Volume} = k_V L^3 \qquad (4\text{-}20a)$$

$$\text{Surface Area} = k_A L^2 \qquad (4\text{-}20b)$$

where L is a length parameter. For cubes L = length of side, $k_V = 1.0$ and $k_A = 6.0$. For spheres L = diameter, $k_V = \pi/6$ and $k_A = \pi$. For octahedrons L = length of a side, $k_V = \sqrt{2}/3$ and $k_A = 2\sqrt{3}$. The shape factors are readily calculated for other regular geometric crystals. For platelets and needles the shape factors must be determined experimentally.

The distributions developed here are related to a mathematical method called *moment analysis*. The zeroth moment is

$$\frac{N}{N_T} = \frac{\int_0^L ndL}{\int_0^\infty ndL} = 1 - \exp(-\frac{L}{G\tau}) \qquad (4\text{-}21)$$

The first moment is

$$\frac{L}{L_T} = \frac{\int_0^L LndL}{\int_0^\infty LndL} = 1 - (1 + \frac{L}{G\tau})\exp(-\frac{L}{G\tau}) \qquad (4\text{-}22)$$

The second moment is

$$\frac{A}{A_T} = \frac{\int_0^L L^2 ndL}{\int_0^\infty L^2 ndL} = 1 - [1 + \frac{L}{G\tau} + \frac{1}{2}(\frac{L}{G\tau})^2]\exp(-\frac{L}{G\tau}) \qquad (4\text{-}23)$$

The third moment is

$$\frac{M}{M_T} = \frac{\int_0^L L^3 ndL}{\int_0^\infty L^3 ndL} \qquad (4\text{-}24)$$

$$= 1 - [1 + \frac{L}{G\tau} + \frac{1}{2}(\frac{L}{G\tau})^2 + \frac{1}{6}(\frac{L}{G\tau})^3]\exp(-\frac{L}{G\tau})$$

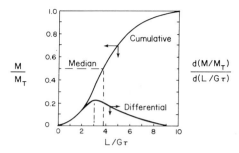

Figure 4-3.   Dimensionless cumulative and differential mass distributions from Eqs. (4-24) and (4-25b).

In Eqs. (4-21) to (4-24) the variable $L/(G\tau)$ is a dimensionless crystal size. $G\tau$ is the size of a crystal which has grown for a period equal to the residence time. Using the dimensionless crystal size, $L/(G\tau)$, the CSD can be analyzed without knowing the dependence of G on supersaturation. The ratio M/M_T is plotted in Figure 4-3. Table 4-1 is a short table of values for M/M_T. Complete tables of values of M/M_T are given by Randolph and Larson (1988) and Singh (1979). Obviously, values of M/M_T can be easily determined from Eq. (4-24) with a calculator.

Table 4-1. Values of Cumulative Mass Distribution [Eq. (4-24)]

$L/G\tau$	M/M_T	$L/G\tau$	M/M_T
0	0	5.00	0.735
1.00	0.019	5.51	0.799
1.74	0.099	6.00	0.849
2.00	0.143	6.68	0.900
2.29	0.199	7.00	0.918
2.76	0.299	7.74	0.950
3.00	0.353	8.00	0.958
3.21	0.400	8.50	0.970
3.67	0.500	9.00	0.979
4.00	0.567	9.50	0.985
4.17	0.599	9.99	0.990
4.76	0.700		

In a sieve analysis a series of sieves with different size openings are stacked together with the largest openings at the top. A charge of crystals is added to the top. After a period of shaking, the stack is opened and particles remaining between each pair of screens are collected. These particles will be in the size range from L_1 to L_2 where L_1 is the size of the screen opening for the lower screen and L_2 is the size of the opening in the upper screen. The easiest analysis of these fractions is to weigh each fraction. Thus the basic raw data is a differential mass distribution. The theoretical differential mass distribution is easily determined by differentiating the cumulative mass distribution. Differentiating Eq. (4-17b), we obtain

$$\frac{dM}{dL} = k_V \rho_c n^\circ L^3 \exp\left(-\frac{L}{G\tau}\right) \tag{4-25a}$$

In terms of the weight fraction, M/M_T, in this size range the differential mass distribution is,

$$\frac{d\left(\frac{M}{M_T}\right)}{dL} = \frac{L^3 \exp\left(-\frac{L}{G\tau}\right)}{6\,(G\tau)^4} \tag{4-25b}$$

The dimensionless differential mass distribution is shown in Figure 4-3.

Figure 4-3 shows that the maximum of the differential mass balance occurs at $L/(G\tau) = 3$. This is called the *dominant size*. The *median size* for the cumulative mass distribution is at $L/(G\tau) = 3.67$. Thus one half of the particles have a weight greater than the particles at this size.

Differential area, length and number distributions can also be defined. The dominant sizes for these distributions are $L/G\tau = 2$, 1 and 0, respectively. The median values for the cumulative distributions can be defined by setting A/A_T, L/L_T and N/N_T equal to 1/2. For example, the median of the cumulative number distribution is at $L/(G\tau) = 0.693$. Thus one half the particles are larger than $L = 0.693\ G\tau$.

Use of the distributions will be illustrated in Examples 4-1 and 4-2.

4.3. SIEVE ANALYSIS OF CSD

Experimental CSD's are usually determined by sieve analysis, particle size analyzer, or counting under a microscope. Since the principles to relate the theoretical CSD to the experimental CSD are similiar, we will discuss only the sieve analysis in detail. Mullin (1972) has an exhaustive analysis of sieving. We would like to convert M into a predicted sieve analysis. Usually standard sieves are used. An abbreviated table of sieve sizes is given in Table 4-2 (Perry and Green, 1984). We will first discuss the sieve analysis of experimental data and then prediction of sieve analysis from the weight distribution. For on-line measurements electronic zone-sieving devices (e.g. Coulter Counters) and laser-light-scattering instruments (e.g. from Leeds & Nothrup) are used.

Often G and n^o are not available in the literature. In this case laboratory

Table 4-2. Standard Sieve Sizes

Sieve Opening (mm)	Tyler mesh	Sieve Opening (microns)	Tyler mesh
8.0	2 1/2	841	20
5.66	3 1/2	707	24
4.76	4	595	28
4.00	5	500	32
3.36	6	420	35
2.83	7	354	42
2.38	8	297	48
2.00	9	250	60
1.68	10	210	65
1.41	12	177	80
1.19	14	125	115
1.00	16	88	170
		63	250
		44	325
		37	400

Source: Perry and Green (1984)

or larger scale experiments can be done to determine the kinetics of the process. This can be done by screening the crystals and experimentally determining a weight distribution. The data collected is:

W_i	= weight of crystals collected in sieve fraction i.
ΔL_i	= size range of sieve fraction i.
	= larger sieve opening – smaller sieve opening (see Table 4-2).
$\bar{L}$	= average size of sieve fraction i (Table 4-2).
	= 1/2 (larger sieve opening + smaller sieve opening).
t_{col}	= Period in which magma was sieved was collected.
or V_s	= Volume of magma sieved
τ	= $(V/Q)_{crystallizer}$ = crystallizer retention time.

From the sieve data M_T is easily determined from the total weight of crystals collected as

$$M_{T,exp} = (\sum_{\text{all sieve fractions}} W_i)/Qt_{col} = \frac{\sum W_i}{V_s} \qquad (4\text{-}26)$$

where Qt_{col} is equal to the volume of magma which was sieved.

The values of n° and G can now be found two different ways. One method is to generate an experimental cumulative mass distribution. The data of W_i versus $\bar{L}_i$ is a differential mass distribution. The experimental cumulative mass distribution is

$$M_{exp,i} = \sum_{\substack{\text{fraction under smallest size}}}^{\text{sieve frac.i}} (W_i)/V_s \qquad (4\text{-}27)$$

Then $M_{exp,i}$ or $M_{exp,i}/M_{T,exp}$ can be plotted versus $\bar{L}_i$.

The theoretical value of M/M_T versus $(L/G\tau)$ is known from Eq. (4-24), Figure 4-3 or Table 4-1. By comparing experimental and theoretical values, we can determine G and n°. For example, suppose one of the data points corresponds to $(M_{exp}/M_{T,exp})_i = 0.4$. Then from Table 4-1, $\bar{L}_i/G\tau = 3.21$. Since $\bar{L}_i$ and τ are known, this allows us to calculate G. If $(M_{exp}/M_{T,exp})_i$ is a number such as 0.442, the complete tabulations of M/M_T (Randolph and Larson, 1988; Singh 1979) can be used, or program Eq. (4-24) on your calculator. This procedure can be repeated for each sieve fraction. Then, average G according to the weight fraction of particles collected in each fraction.

$$\bar{G} = \frac{\Sigma\,(G_i\,W_i)}{\displaystyle\sum_{\text{all fractions}} W_i} \qquad (4\text{-}28)$$

Equation (4-28) assumes growth is size independent. This is not an additional assumption since it was already made to determine the population density function. The population density of nucleii can now be found from Eq. (4-18). Thus

$$n^\circ = \frac{M_T}{6k_V\rho_c(\bar{G}\tau)^4} \qquad (4\text{-}29)$$

The second approach is to calculate experimental values of the population density for each sieve fraction. G and n° can then be determined from Figure 4-2. To do this we first calculate $M_{T,exp}$ from Eq. (4-26). Then for each sieve fraction i

$$n_i = \frac{M_T W_i/\sum W_i}{\rho_c k_V \bar{L}_i^3 \Delta L_i} = \frac{W_i/V_s}{\rho_c k_v \bar{L}_i^3 \Delta L_i} \qquad (4\text{-}30)$$

To generate Figure 4-2, $\ln n_i$ is plotted versus $\bar{L}_i$ for each fraction. A regression analysis will then give the best values of n° and G.

Obviously, the two approaches should closely agree with each other.

Once n° and G are known the nucleation rate B° is readily calculated from Eq. (3-6), $B^\circ = n^\circ G$. To determine the functional dependence of B° as shown in Table 3-1 a series of experiments with different residence times and different stirrer speeds is done.

If G and equilibrium are known, the sieve analysis can be predicted. To predict the weight distribution from the theoretical mass distributions, we can first rearrange Eq. (4-26) to predict the total weight of crystals collected.

$$W_T = \sum_{\text{all fractions}} W_i = M_T V_s \qquad (4-31)$$

The weight W_i in a given sieve fraction is related to the differential mass balance, Eq. (4-25a) and (4-25b)

$$W_i = (\Delta L_i \frac{)(dM}{dL)_i} V_s = (\Delta L_i) \frac{V_s \bar{L}_i^3 M_T}{(G\tau)^4} \exp\left(-\frac{L}{G\tau}\right) \qquad (4-32)$$

The weight W_i can be calculated for each sieve fraction which will be collected. This is illustrated in Example 4-1. Note that we can calculate W_i without knowing the shape factor, k_V. This is useful since k_V will be unknown if the crystals are not ideal.

Example 4-1. CSD for Size Independent Growth.

Potassium chloride is being crystallized in a cooling crystallizer. The crystallizer approximates an MSMPR. Feed is initially saturated at 100°C and the crystallizer operates at 20°C. Feed is 10,000 kg/hr of total solution. The crystallizer has a volume of 2.0 m^3. Assume that the growth rate is 4.0×10^{-7} m/s. Predict the total mass distribution, M, as a function of crystal size L. If 0.1 m^3 of magma is sieved predict the weight of crystals collected between 24 and 28 mesh. Assume the system is operating in a high-yield mode where $\Delta c \sim 0$ (equilibrium) in the outlet liquid.

118

Solution

A. Define. The system is sketched in the figure.

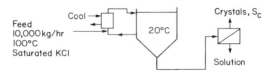

Plot M vs L and find W_i collected between 24 and 28 mesh.

B. Explore. Growth rate for this system is size independent (Mullin, 1972). The solution of the steady-state population balance Eq. (4-7) is Eq. (4-9), and the total mass distribution is given by Eq. (4-17b). Thus the theory developed in this section can be used.

C. Plan. External mass balances can be used to determine the crystal flow rate, S_c. Table 2-1 shows that KCl crystallizes as anhydrous material. Thus S_c can be found from Eq. (2-5b)

$$S_c = (c_{in} - c_{out})W_{in}$$

where W_{in} is the water flow rate entering the crystallizer, and c_{in} and c_{out} are given in Table 2-1 at 100 and 20°C, respectively. W_{in} can be determined from a balance on the inlet stream

$$F = c_{in}W_{in} + W_{in} \text{ or } W_{in} = \frac{F}{1 + c_{in}}$$

The volumetric feed rate $Q = F/\rho_f$ and $\tau = V/Q$. Then from Eq. (4-19), $M_T = S_c/Q$, and M can be calculated from Eq. (4-24) even though n^o and k_V are unknown.

To determine the weight collected between 24 and 28 mesh we will use Eq. (4-32)

D. Do It. From Table 2-1, c_{in} = 0.567 kg KCl/kg water, c_{out} = 0.340 kg KCl/kg water. Then

$$W_{in} = \frac{F}{1 + c_{in}} = \frac{10,000 \text{kg/hr}}{1 + 0.567} = 6382 \text{ kg water/hr}$$

and $S_c = (c_{in} - c_{out})W_{in} = (0.567 - 0.340) (6382) = 1449 \text{ kg/hr}$

The feed density is ~1208 kg/m^3 (extrapolated using data from Mullin (1972) or from Perry and Green, (1984)).

Then
$$Q = \frac{F}{\rho_F} = \frac{10,000 \text{ kg/hr}}{1208 \text{ kg/m}^3} = 8.278 \text{ m}^3/\text{hr}$$

$$\tau = \frac{V}{Q} = \frac{2.0}{8.278} = 0.2416 \text{ hr} = 870 \text{ sec}$$

and
$$M_T = \frac{S_c}{Q} = \frac{1449}{8.278} = 175.0 \text{ kg/m}^3$$

M can be determined from Table 4-1 or Figure 4-3 with M_T = 175.0 and $G\tau = (4.0 \times 10^{-7})(870) = 3.48 \times 10^{-4}$ m. To find M multiply M/M_T by 175. To find value of L (in meters) multiply $L/G\tau$ by 3.48×10^{-4}.

The dominant size of the mass distribution is

$$3G \tau = (3) (3.48 \times 10^{-4}) = 1.04 \times 10^{-3} \text{m} = 1.04 \text{ mm}$$

and the median size of the mass distribution is

$$3.67 G \tau = (3.67)(3.48 \times 10^{-4}) = 1.28 \times 10^{-3} \text{ m} = 1.28 \text{ mm} \qquad [1]$$

The median size for the number distribution is

$$(0.693) (G \tau) = 2.41 \times 10^{-4} \text{m} = 0.241 \text{ mm}$$

The differential mass distribution can also be obtained from Figure 4-3 using the same multipliers.

The mass of crystals collected in a sieve analysis can be predicted using Eq. (4-29). From Table 4-2 a 24 mesh screen has an opening of 0.707 mm while a 28 mesh screen has an opening of 0.595 mm. Then the average

$$\bar{L} = 0.5 \ (0.707 + 0.595) = 0.65 \ \text{mm} = 0.65 \times 10^{-3} \ \text{m}$$

For this $\bar{L}$, $\bar{L}/G\tau = 1.871$. Since $\Delta L = 0.707 - 0.595 = 0.112$ mm, Eq. (4-32) becomes

$$W_i = \frac{(\Delta L_i) V_s \bar{L}_i^3 M_T \exp(-\frac{L}{G\tau})}{(G\tau)^4}$$

$$= \frac{(0.112 \times 10^{-3} \text{m})(0.1 \text{m}^3)(0.65 \times 10^{-3} \text{m})^3 (175)(0.154)}{(3.48 \times 10^{-4})^4} = 5.65 \ \text{kg}$$

This is a fraction $\dfrac{W_i}{W_T} = \dfrac{5.65}{(175)(0.1)} = 0.32$ of all the crystals collected [W_T is calculated from Eq. (4-31)]. A complete sieve analysis can be predicted by calculating W_i for all pairs of sieves.

E. Check. Since n° is unknown and the external balances have already been used, a good check is difficult.

F. Generalization. When the linear growth rate is independent of size, the dimensionless solution for M shown in Figure 4-3 and Table 4-1 can be used. Then the engineer's job is to determine M_T and $G\tau$ so that the dimensional values can be determined. If M_T and $G\tau$ are constant, the distribution will be unchanged even when other variables are changed. For example, if F = 1000 kg/hr and V = 0.2 m^3, W_{in}, S_c and Q are all reduced by a factor of 10. However, G, τ, and M_T remain constant and the distribution is unchanged. This is helpful in scaling crystallizers to larger sizes. The growth rate for KCl crystals is rapid compared to that of many other crystals. Thus, the residence time used in this example is low compared to that required for other crystallizations.

Example 4-2. Kinetics from Experimental CSD

Urea was crystallized in a commercial Swenson DTB crystallizer. For one run the following data was obtained (Bennett and Van Buren, 1969)

			Tyler Screen Sizes				Magma
τ,hrs	14	20	28	35	48	65	Density, g/L
3.97	19.0	38.5	63.5	81.5	98.0	100	404

The screen numbers are cumulative weight %. Urea, NH_2CONH_2, has $\rho_c = 1.33$ g/cm^3. The crystals had $k_V \sim 1.0$. Determine G and n$^\circ$.

Solution

We will illustrate use of Eq. (4-30).

$n_i = \Delta N_i/\Delta L_i$ where $\Delta L_i = L_i - L_{i-1}$ is easily determined from Table 4-2. Then from Eq. (4-30)

$$\Delta N_i = \frac{(\text{Magma density})(\text{Weight fraction})}{\rho_c \, k_V \, \overline{L}_i^3}$$

where Weight fraction crystals in size fraction i $= \dfrac{W_i}{\Sigma W_i}$.

The weight fraction can be determined from the cumulative weight fraction as

$(\text{Weight fraction})_i = (\text{Cum. Wt. frac.})_i - (\text{Cum Wt. frac})_{i-1}$

Since Magma density, ρ_c and k_V are known,

$$\Delta N_i = \frac{303.8 \ \text{(Weight fraction)}}{\overline{L}_i^{-3}}$$

We can now generate the following Table.

Mesh	L	$\overline{L}$	ΔL	cum. frac.	wt. frac.	ΔN_i	n (in 1000)	ln n
14	.119			0.19	.19			
14/20	.0841	.10155	.0349	0.385	.195	56,562	1,621	14.3
20/28	.0595	.07180	.0246	0.635	.250	205,162	8,340	15.94
28/35	.0420	.05075	.0175	0.815	.180	418,306	23,903	16.99
35/48	.0297	.03585	.0123	0.980	.165	1,087,793	88,438	18.30
48/65	.0210	.02555	.0087	1.00	.020	372,929	42,865	17.57

Now plot ln n vs L. This result is shown in Figure 4-2.

$$G = \frac{-1}{(\text{slope}) \ \tau} = \frac{-1}{(-53.5)(3.97)} = 0.0047 \ \text{cm/hr}$$

Intercept $= 19.8 = \ln n^\circ$, which gives $n^\circ = 3.97 \times 10^8$

Notes: 1. Value of n° depends very much on how line is drawn.

2. The first mesh size (14) does not give a data point. Thus it is desireable if cumulative fraction for first screen is small. Use of a 12 mesh screen in addition to 14 mesh would have given another data point.

3. Obviously, data scatters with small screen openings.

4.4. EFFECT OF NUCLEATION AND GROWTH KINETICS ON CSD

Even when the McCabe ΔL law is valid, the kinetics of nucleation and growth can vary enormously. This was shown by Eq. (3-8) and the correlations in Table 3-1. In this section we will consider how nucleation and growth kinetics affect the CSD (Larson and Randolph, 1969; Randolph and Larson, 1988).

This section will illustrate how the equations can be manipulated to compare the effects of changing variables. The growth rate will be assumed to be independent of size. Size dependent growth is treated in Section 4.7.

Consider two cases where secondary nucleation does not occur. Equations (3-7) are valid and $n^\circ = k_N G^{i-1}$. First, compare two crystallizers where the suspension densities are equal, but the residence times $\tau_1 \neq \tau_2$. Setting $M_{T,1} = M_{T,2}$ and substituting in Eq. (4-18), we obtain

$$M_{T,1} = \tau_1^4 G_1^4 n_1^\circ (6k_V \rho_c) = \tau_2^4 G_2^4 n_2^\circ (6k_V \rho_c) = M_{T,2} \qquad (4\text{-}33a)$$

Canceling out the common terms and using $n^\circ = k_N G^{i-1}$ to remove n_1° and n_2°, this becomes

$$\tau_1^4 G_1^{3+i} = \tau_2^4 G_2^{3+i} \qquad (4\text{-}33b)$$

or

$$\frac{G_2}{G_1} = (\frac{\tau_1}{\tau_2})^{4/(3+i)} \qquad (4\text{-}34a)$$

Substituting $n^\circ = k_N G^{i-1}$ back into Eq. (4-34a), we have

$$\frac{n_2^\circ}{n_1^\circ} = (\frac{\tau_1}{\tau_2})^{\frac{4(i-1)}{3+i}} \qquad (4\text{-}34b)$$

Clearly, the exponent i has a major effect on the growth and nucleation rates in the two crystallizers. If $i=1$, $n_1^\circ = n_2^\circ$ and $G_2 = G_1(\tau_1/\tau_2)$. Thus growth rates depend inversely on the residence time and n° is independent of the residence time. Since G is proportional to Δc, the supersaturation difference Δc must also depend inversely on residence time. If residence time is halved, Δc doubles and G doubles.

If $i > 1.0$, G and n° increase as residence time increases. Then from Eq. (3-6), $B^\circ = n^\circ G$, the nucleation rate increases. When $i=2$, the exponents on Eqs. (4-34a and b) are equal. For $i > 2$ the exponent on Eq. (4-34b) is larger and n° grows faster than G. Thus as i becomes larger it is more and more difficult to grow large crystals since too many nuclei are formed. This tends to be the case for homogeneous and heterogeneous nucleation.

The nucleation rate $B°$ increases when the residence time is increased for $i > 1.0$. Then from Eqs. (3-6) and (3-4) the supersaturation Δc must increase. Increasing the residence time increases the supersaturation at constant magma density.

A second case without secondary nucleation compares two crystallizers with equal residence times, but different feed concentrations and hence different magma densities. Again we start with Eq. (4-18), $M_T = k_V \rho_c n° (G\tau)^4$. Set $\tau_1 = \tau_2$ equal for the two crystallizers, and cancel out common terms. Then,

$$\frac{M_{T,1}}{n_1° G_1^4} = \frac{M_{T,2}}{n_2° G_2^4} \tag{4-35}$$

Substitute in the expression $n° = k_N G^{i-1}$ and solve first for G_2/G_1,

$$\frac{G_2}{G_1} = (\frac{M_{T,2}}{M_{T,1}})^{\frac{1}{i+3}} \tag{4-36a}$$

and then solve for $n_2°/n_1°$.

$$\frac{n_2°}{n_1°} = (\frac{M_{T_2}}{M_{T_1}})^{\frac{i-1}{i+3}} \tag{4-36b}$$

Growth rates increase as magma density increases, and if $i > 1$ the nucleation population density, $n°$, increases as magma density increases even though secondary nucleation does not occur. If $i = 1$, $n°$ is constant while G and hence $B°$ both increase as magma density increases.

The dominant size of the mass distribution, $L_D = 3G\tau_1$, as easily determined from Eq. (4-36a).

$$\frac{L_{D,2}}{L_{D,1}} = (\frac{M_{T,2}}{M_{T,1}})^{1/(i+3)} \tag{4-36c}$$

Thus sizes are increased at higher magma density *if* secondary nucleation does not occur.

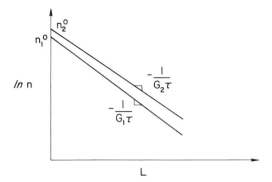

Figure 4-4.　Effect of magma density for size independent growth. $\tau_1 = \tau_2$, $M_{T,2} = 2M_{T1}$, $i = 3$. Calculated: $n_2^o/n_1^o = 1.2599$ and $G_2/G_1 = 1.1225$.

The population density distribution (and other distributions) can easily be determined for both cases since G and n^o have been calculated. Substituting the expressions for G and n^o into Eq. (4-9) or (4-10) will give the population density. The effect of changing M_T is illustrated in Figure 4-4.

Secondary nucleation is often important in commercial crystallizers. As a third case consider two crystallizers with equal residence times, but $M_{T,1} < M_{T,2}$. When secondary crystallization occurs, suspended solids are a source of nuclei. Then if the McCabe ΔL law, Eq. (3-14a), is valid $G = k\Delta c$. Equation (3-8) then becomes,

$$B^o = K_R \, k^i \, M_T^j (\Delta c)^i = K_R' \, M_T^j (\Delta c)^i \qquad (4\text{-}37a)$$

and Eq. (3-6) gives,

$$n^o = \frac{B^o}{G} = k_N \, M_T^j \, G^{i-1} = k_N' \, M_T^j (\Delta c)^{i-1} \qquad (4\text{-}37b)$$

With equal residence times Eq. (4-35) can again be derived. After substituting in Eq. (4-37b) for n^o, and solving for G_2/G_1, we obtain

$$\frac{G_2}{G_1} = (\frac{M_{T,2}}{M_{T,1}})^{\frac{1-j}{i+3}} \qquad (4\text{-}38)$$

126

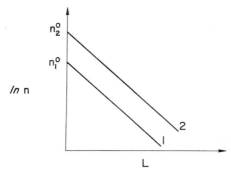

Figure 4-5.   Effect of magma density on population density when secondary nucleation occurs and $j = 1$. $M_{T2} > M_{T1}$

Experimental results often show $B^\circ \propto M_T$ (that is, $j = 1$). Then

$$G_2 = G_1 \,, \quad \frac{n_2^o}{n_1^o} = \frac{M_{T,2}}{M_{T,1}} \quad (j=1) \tag{4-39}$$

Equations (4-39) should be compared to Eqs. (4-36a) and (4-36b). When secondary nucleation occurs with $B^\circ \propto M_T$ ($j=1$), the growth rate does not depend on magma density and the nucleation population density depends linearly on the magma density. This is a greater dependence than shown in Eq. (4-33b). Neither n° nor G depend on i while in the absence of secondary nucleation they do. The population density graph with secondary nucleation is shown in Figure 4-5. Since $G_1 = G_2$, the slopes are equal. Since nucleation depends on magma density, it is difficult to obtain large crystals with high yield (which implies high M_T) when secondary nucleation occurs.

4.5. SEEDING

Problems can often be avoided by seeding the crystallizer. With added seeds the metastable region can be avoided. Thus the crystallizer can operate at lower supersaturations with no homogeneous nucleation and with small nucleation rates from other secondary nucleation processes. Sometimes seeding is the only practical way to grow crystals of the desired size range. If there is no additional nucleation, the weight of seeds required per hour, W_s is

$$W_s = W_p(\bar{L}_s^3 / \bar{L}_p^3) \tag{4-40}$$

where W_p = weight of product/hour, $\bar{L}_s$ and $\bar{L}_p$ are the mean particle sizes of seeds and products, respectively.

When there is no additional nucleation, the final product distribution can be determined from the CSD of the seed crystals. If growth is size independent, $\Delta L_{growth} = G\tau$ is the same for all crystals. Then for a crystal of a given initial size $L_{s,i}$, the final size is $L_{s,i} + \Delta L_{growth}$. The mass of the crystals is $\rho_c k_V (L_{s,i} + \Delta L_{growth})^3$. With no nucleation the number of crystals per volume is constant. Thus

$$\frac{dW_s}{\rho_c k_V L_{s,i}^3} = \frac{dW_p}{\rho_c k_V (L_{s,i} + \Delta L_{growth})^3}$$

or

$$dW_p = (\frac{L_{s,i} + \Delta L_{growth}}{L_{s,i}})^3 \, dW_s \qquad (4\text{-}41a)$$

In terms of sieve fractions

$$W_{p,i} = [\frac{L_{s,i} + \Delta L_{growth}}{\bar{L}_{s,i}}]^3 \, W_{s,i} \qquad (4\text{-}41b)$$

Equation (4-41a) or (4-41b) can be used to predict the differential weight distribution. The total weight is

$$W_{p,tot} = \int_0^{W_{s,tot}} (\frac{L_{s,i} + \Delta L_{growth}}{L_{s,i}})^3 \, dW_s \qquad (4\text{-}42a)$$

or in terms of sieve fractions

$$W_{p,tot} = \sum_{\text{all fracs}} (\frac{L_{s,i} + \Delta L_{growth}}{\bar{L}_{s,i}})^3 \, W_{s,i} \qquad (4\text{-}42b)$$

and the magma density is

$$M_T = \frac{W_{p,tot}}{V_s} \qquad (4\text{-}43a)$$

Since G and ΔL are unknown, the solution proceeds by first calculating

128

M_T from mass balances and equilibrium. Equation (4-19) can be used to calculate M_T except we should correct for the weight of seeds added. Then

$$M_T = (S_c + W_s)/Q \qquad (4\text{-}43b)$$

Usually, this correction will be small. Then Eq. (4-43a) gives $W_{p,tot}$. A trial-and-error procedure is used to find a ΔL_{growth} (and hence a G) which will give this value of $W_{p,tot}$ from Eq. (4-42). The shape of the product screen analysis will be different than the seed distribution since the relative increase in mass is greater for small particles than for large ones. A detailed example is given by Foust et al (1980). Experimental data may vary significantly from the distribution predicted since the McCabe ΔL law may not be valid.

Seeding can also be used to provide selective nucleation for fractional crystallization of a solution saturated in two or more solutes. (Rousseau and O'Dell, 1980). A modification of this procedure is used commercially for separation of racemic mixtures of amino acids. Assume we have a saturated mixture of the D and L isomers. If we cool the mixture but stay in the metastable region, neither isomer will crystallize. Selectively seeding with one of the isomers (e.g. the D isomer) will cause crystallization of that isomer. If contact nucleation occurs, a large number of nuclei will form. The mixture will approach saturation in the D isomer, but will remain supersaturated in the L isomer. After harvesting the D isomer crystals, removing any D isomer nucleii with a membrane or by heating followed by cooling to supersaturate the L isomer again; the L isomer can be crystallized out by seeding with the L isomer. Obviously, an operation such as this requires very careful control of conditions to prevent unwanted primary nucleation.

4.6. EQUIPMENT MODIFICATIONS

How does modifying the equipment affect the CSD? This is an important question for the design of crystallizers. In this section we will look at the removal of crystal fines, use of classified product removal and methods of suspending the solids. The analysis of CSD will again assume that growth rates are independent of crystal size.

4.6.1. Fines Removal

The purpose of fines removal is to remove excessive numbers of small particles so that a limited number can grow to larger sizes. The fines are removed by

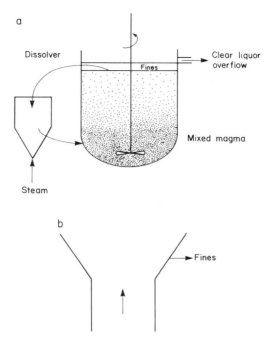

Figure 4-6.　　Methods for fines removal. a. partially mixed. b. fines trap.

some type of classification scheme. This is possible since the fine particles tend to move with the fluid while larger particles will settle out. Different classification methods are illustrated in Figure 4-6 (Mullin, 1972; Saeman, 1961). Figure 4-6a illustrates the situation where fines classification occurs because the crystallizer is not well mixed. Fines can be removed near the top of the crystallizer. By adjusting the level of the withdrawal tube the size of fines removed can be varied. The optimum size of fines to remove appears to be approximately 1/20 to 1/10 the mean product size. Once removed the fines are redissolved by heating and/or by adding solvent. This liquid is then recycled to the crystallizer. A different type of fines trap is shown in Figure 4-6b. Fines are collected at the level where particles larger than L_f have a settling velocity greater than the fluid velocity. The fines are then destroyed by heating the mixture. Fines dissolution can also occur in superheated regions inside the crystallizer since the small particles are more soluble than large particles.

The CSD can be analyzed using the population balances (Larson and Randolph, 1969; Randolph and Larson, 1988). Removal of fines decreases the residence time of most of the small particles. Some of the fines will escape the trap and grow to become product. Surprisingly, only 0.1 to 1.0% of the fines are allowed to grow to become product. If we let

$$R = \frac{\text{Product retention time}}{\text{Fines retention time}} \geq 1 \qquad \text{(4-44a)}$$

then if Q_{in} is the flow rate into the crystallizer, the withdrawal rate of fines by both destruction and in the product is RQ_{in}. The retention times for fines and product are,

$$\tau_f = \frac{V}{RQ_{in}}, \quad 0 \leq L \leq L_f \qquad \text{(4-44b)}$$

$$\tau_p = \frac{V}{Q_{in}} \quad L > L_f \qquad \text{(4-44c)}$$

where L_f is the maximum size of fines withdrawn.

The crystallizer with fines removal must have two population balances - one for fines and one for product. Equation (4-8) can be written twice.

$$\frac{dn}{dL} + \frac{n}{G\tau_f} = 0 \qquad \text{(4-45a)}$$

$$\frac{dn}{dL} + \frac{n}{G\tau_p} = 0 \qquad \text{(4-45b)}$$

Integrating these equations, the solutions are

$$n = n^\circ \exp(-\frac{L}{G\tau_f}) \quad L \leq L_f \qquad \text{(4-46a)}$$

$$n = C \exp(-\frac{L}{G\tau_p}) \quad L > L_f \qquad \text{(4-46b)}$$

where C is a constant of integration (see Example 4-3). Since the distribution is continuous, at $L = L_f$ the population densities are equal, $n_f = n_p$.

The distribution in Eqs. (4-46) can be compared to the distribution

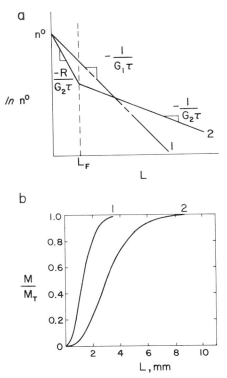

Figure 4-7.   Comparison of crystallizer with fines removal (2) to crystallizer without fines removal (1). a. Population density distribution. b. Dimensionless cumulative weight distribution. Case 1
is from Example 4-1 while Case 2 is from Example 4-3.

without fines removal. This is shown in Figure 4-7a for the population density,
and in Figure 4-7b for the dimensionless cumulative weight distribution. Since
the fines are of negligible mass, $M_{T,1} = M_{T,2}$. This condition forces

$$\frac{1}{G_2\tau} < \frac{1}{G_1\tau} < \frac{R}{G_2\tau}$$ (4-47a)

Thus the crystallizers have different growth rates and

$$G_{\text{with fines removal}} > G_{\text{w/o fines removal}}$$ (4-47b)

The same production ($M_{T,1} = M_{T,2}$) occurs with fines removal but on a much smaller number of larger particles. Since the total surface area is less for the large particles, the growth rate must be higher. Figure 4-7b shows that a significant increase in the mean particle size also occurs. The dominant particle size for the mass distribution will also increase significantly.

With higher growth rates with fines removal, the supersaturation must be higher. This will normally cause more nucleation and one would expect $n_2^o > n_1^o$. In this case fines removal is analyzed for an idealization called a *point fines trap*. A point fines trap destroys only nuclei.

We will compare crystallizer 1 to crystallizer 2 which has a point fines trap. The analysis is similar to the analyses of the previous section. The two crystallizers have the same V and Q. Hence, $\tau_1 = \tau_2$. Since nuclei represent an insignificant mass, the magma densities are equal, $M_{T_1} = M_{T_2}$. Then from Eq. (4-18)

$$M_{T,1} = 6k_V\rho_c n_1^o(G_1\tau)^4 = 6k_V\rho_c(\beta n_2^o)(G_2\tau)^4 = M_{T,2} \tag{4-48}$$

where β is the fraction of nuclei surviving the fines trap. Thus, βn_2^o is the population density of surviving nuclei. The value of β can be as low as 0.001 in practice. Next, the nucleation kinetics found by combining Eqs. (3-6) and (3-8),

$$n^o = k_N G^{i-1} M_T^j \tag{4-49}$$

are substituted into Eq. (4-48). After dividing out equal terms and rearranging, the result is

$$\frac{G_2}{G_1} = (\frac{1}{\beta})^{1/(3+i)} \tag{4-50a}$$

The dominant size of the mass distribution, $L_D = 3G\tau$, is

$$\frac{L_{D,2}}{L_{D,1}} = (\frac{1}{\beta})^{1/(3+i)} \tag{4-50b}$$

Since β is usually quite small, $1/\beta$ is large. Thus both the linear growth rate G_2 and the dominant size L_D are increased substantially. The degree of improvement is reduced as the order of nucleation i increases.

Both analysis procedures show that fines traps can significantly increase the median and dominant crystal sizes. Fines traps are often used on a variety of different crystallizers when large crystals are desired. Fines traps are relatively expensive to operate, but they are a universally valid method of controlling nucleation.

Example 4-3. CSD with Fines Destruction

Potassium chloride is crystallized in a cooling crystallizer with a fines trap. The feed is saturated at 100°C and has a total flow rate of 10,000 kg/hr. The crystallizer operates at 20°C and has a volume of 2.0 m³. The fines trap is operated to remove crystals where $L_f \leq 0.3$ mm. The product retention time is ten times the fines retention time. Determine the growth rate in this crystallizer. Predict the total mass distribution, M, as a function of crystal size L.

Solution

A. Define. This is the same system as in Example 4-1 except now there is a fines trap. We want to find G and plot M versus L.

B. Explore. Equations (4-46) give the population density function. The equilibrium and external mass balance calculations are the same as in Example 4-1. Thus $\tau_p = V/Q = \tau_{w/o\ fines\ removal} = 870$ sec from Example 4-1. The magma density is also the same as without fines destruction, and was obtained in Example 4-1 as $M_T = 175.0$ kg/m³. The growth rate will be higher and needs to be calculated.

C. Plan. The residence time for fines $\tau_p = V/(RQ_{in}) = \tau_f/R$ where R = 10. Thus $\tau_f = 87$ sec. The mass distribution M can be generated from the definition, Eq. (4-17a), and the population density functions, Eqs. (4-46). Thus some derivation is required. For small crystals,

$$M = k_V \rho_c \int_0^L L^3 n° \exp\left(-\frac{L}{G\tau_f}\right) dL , \quad L \leq L_f$$

Thus for $L \leq L_f$, M is the same as Eq. (4-17b). The cumulative mass of fines M_f at $L = L_f$ is,

$$M_f = k_V \rho_c \int_0^{L_f} L^3 n^\circ \exp(-\frac{L}{G\tau_f})dL$$

which from Eq. (4-17b) is

$$M_f = 6k_V\rho_c n^\circ G\tau_f \left\{ (G\tau_f)^3 \right.$$

(4-51)

$$\left. - \left[(G\tau_f)^3 + (G\tau_f)^2 L_f + \frac{1}{2}(G\tau_f)L_f^2 + \frac{1}{6}L_f^3 \right] \exp(-\frac{L_f}{G\tau_f}) \right\}$$

Since G is unknown this cannot be determined immediately.

For crystals where $L > L_f$, the cumulative population distribution is

$$M = M_f + k_V\rho_c \int_{L_f}^{L} C \exp(-\frac{L}{G\tau_p})dL \quad L > L_f$$

(4-52a)

which becomes

$$M = M_f + 6k_V\rho_c CG\tau_p \left\{ G\tau_p - \left[(G\tau_p)^3 \right. \right.$$

(4-52b)

$$\left. \left. + (G\tau_p)^2 L + \frac{1}{2}(G\tau_p)L^2 + \frac{1}{6}L^3 \right] \exp(-\frac{L}{G\tau_p}) \left. \right|_{L_f}^{L} \right\}$$

The total magma density M_T is obtained by letting $L \rightarrow \infty$ in Eq. (4-52b).

$$M_T = M_f + 6k_V\rho_c CG\tau_p \left[(G\tau_p)^3 \right. \tag{4-53a}$$

$$\left. + (G\tau_p)^2 L_f + \frac{1}{2}(G\tau_p)L_f^2 + \frac{1}{6}L_f^3 \right] \exp(-\frac{L_f}{G\tau_p})$$

Then, Eq. (4-52b) simplies to

$$M = M_T - 6k_V\rho_c CG\tau_p [(G\tau_p)^3 \tag{4-52c}$$

$$+ (G\tau_p)^2 L + \frac{1}{2}G\tau_p L^2 + \frac{1}{6}L^3] \exp(-\frac{L}{G\tau_p})$$

The value of $k_V n^\circ \rho_c$ can be estimated from the value of M_T found for the MSMPR without fines destruction (Example 4-1) and from Eq. (4-18).

$$M_T = 6k_V\rho_c n^\circ (G\tau)^4 = 175$$

Thus,

$$k_V\rho_c n^\circ = \frac{175}{6(G\tau)_{MSMPR}^4} = \frac{175}{6(3.48\times10^{-4})^4} = 1.9887\times10^{15}$$

Assume this is unchanged for the system with fines destruction.

For the system with fines destruction n is continuous at $L = L_f$. Setting Eq. (4-46a) equal to (4-46b) at $L = L_f$,

$$k_V\rho_c C = k_V\rho_c n^\circ \frac{\exp(-\dfrac{L_f}{G\tau_f})}{\exp(-\dfrac{L_f}{G\tau_p})} \tag{4-54}$$

Substituting M_f and $k_V \rho_c C$ into Eq. (4-53a)

$$M_T = (6k_V\rho_c n_o)\left\{\left[(G\tau_p)^4+(G\tau_p)^3 L_f + \frac{1}{2}(G\tau_p)^2 L_f^2\right.\right.$$

$$\left.+ \frac{1}{6}G\tau_p L_f^3\right]\exp(-\frac{L_f}{G\tau_f}) + (G\tau_f)^4 - [(G\tau_f)^4$$

$$+ (G\tau_f)^3 L_f + \frac{1}{2}(G\tau_f)^2 L_f^2 + \frac{1}{6}(G\tau_f)L_f^3]\exp(-\frac{L_f}{G\tau_f})\right\} \qquad (4\text{-}53b)$$

Since M_T is known, this represents one equation with G being the only unknown. Solve for G. Then can find M for $L \leq L_f$ from Eq. (4-17b), M_f from Eq. (4-51) and M for $L > L_f$ from Eq. (4-52c).

D. Do It. $\tau_p = 870$, $\tau_f = 87$, $L_f = 3 \times 10^{-4}$ m

$$\frac{M_T}{6k_V\rho_c n_o} = \frac{175}{(6)(1.9887\times 10^{15})} = 1.4666 \times 10^{-4} \text{m}^4$$

This is equal to the term in brackets in Eq. (4-53b). A trial and error solution is required. The result is

$$G = 9.251 \times 10^{-7} \text{ m/s}$$

This equation is very sensitive to the value of G used. It is best to do a problem like this on a programmable calculator or a computer.

The value of $k_V\rho_c C$ can now be calculated from Eq. (4-54).

$$k_V\rho_c C = 1.9887 \times 10^{15} \frac{\exp(-1.7275)}{\exp(-0.3727)} = 6.9444 \times 10^{13}$$

Calculate M_f from Eq. (4-51), $M_f = 0.2561$. Note that M_f is a small fraction of M_T. M can be calculated from Eq. (4-52c). This equation becomes

$$M = 175 - (4.1666{\times}10^{14})(8.048{\times}10^{-4})[5.2134{\times}10^{-10}$$

$$+ 6.4776{\times}10^{-7}L + 4.024{\times}10^{-4}L^2 + \frac{1}{6}L^3]\exp(\frac{-L}{8.0484{\times}10^{-4}})$$

This is valid for $L \geq L_f$. Programming this on a calculator we obtain:

L (m)	M	M/M_T
0.0003	0.2561	0.0015
0.001	6.728	0.038
0.002	41.985	0.24
0.002953	87.5 = Median	0.50
0.0003	89.595	
0.004	127.91	0.73
0.005	151.68	0.87
0.006	164.32	0.94
0.007	170.38	0.97
0.008	173.11	0.989
0.009	174.25	0.996
0.010	179.71	0.998
0.011	174.89	
0.012	174.96	
0.013	174.986	
0.02	174.9999	1.0

This distribution is plotted in Figure 4-7b. Values of M below L_f can be found from Eq. (4-17b).

E. Check. There are some consistency checks. As expected $G=9.251 \times 10^{-7} > G_{w/o} = 4.0 \times 10^{-7}$. Since fines have very little weight, the small value of M_f/M_T is expected. The median size is $L = 0.00295$ where $M = 0.5\, M_T$. This is at $L = 3.67\, G\tau_p$.

F. Generalization. This is a rather complex example. It illustrates the steps necessary to determine M_f, M and M_T for fines removal. Similar steps can also be used for determining the analogous quantities for classified product removal, or for other complex situations. The methods for determining the constant of integration and for determining G from M_T can also be used in other problems. Solution of the equation for G and generation of the cumulative mass distribution are straightforward on a programmable calculator or computer, but difficult without these tools.

If an experimental crystal size distribution is available, then G and $n°$ can be determined. First, calculate the experimental values of M_T and M_i from Eqs. (4-26) and (4-27). The theoretical values for M_T and M_i are given by Eqs. (4-53b) and (4-52c) with C from Eq. (4-54). Relating $(M_i/M_T)_{exper}$ to $(M/M_T)_{theory}$ gives an equation in G_i. The average G can be found from Eq. (4-28) and $n°$ can then be found from Eq. (4-53b).

Note that the median at $L = 3.67 \ G\tau_p$ is what would be expected for a simple distribution. This occurs since M_f is so small. Note that the median = 2.95 mm is significantly greater than the median = 1.28 mm found without fines removal (Example 4-1). Fines removal works!

It is interesting to compare this crystallizer to an equivalent MSMPR with the same growth rate and same magma density. This comparison (see Problem 4-D6) shows that the cumulative mass distributions are essentially the same. However, the equivalent MSMPR must have a nuclei population density significantly less than the crystallizer with fines destruction. Removal of fines is a practical way of controlling nucleation.

4.6.2. Classified Product Removal

Removal of crystals of the desired size by classifying the crystals and withdrawing these crystals at a higher rate is another possible equipment modification. This can be done in an elutriation leg where small crystals are fluidized by the upflowing liquid. Large crystals have higher settling velocities and thus can be concentrated. Product classification also often occurs inadvertently if mixing is inadequate to keep particles suspended.

If we could perfectly classify the product, then product classification would produce a product with larger crystals. However, in practice the smallest crystals are not separated, but occur in the product at approximately the same concentration as in the mixed magma. The concentration of large particles in the elutriation leg will be higher than in the mixed magma. Thus, a reasonable approximation is that classified product removal accelerates the removal of larger particles without affecting the removal of small particles.

All crystals with $L \geq L_p$ are removed at a rate zQ where $z \geq 1$. Crystals with $L < L_p$ are removed at a rate Q which is the volumetric flow rate through the crystallizer. Then the residence times are,

$$\tau_S = V/Q, \quad L < L_p \qquad (4\text{-}55a)$$

$$\tau_L = V/zQ, \quad L \geq L_p \qquad (4\text{-}55b)$$

The population balance Eq. (4-8) can be solved for each residence time.

$$n_S = n^{\circ} \exp(-\frac{L}{G_2 \tau_S}), \quad L < L_p \qquad (4\text{-}56a)$$

$$n_L = C \exp(-\frac{L}{G_2 \tau_L}), \quad L \geq L_p \qquad (4\text{-}56b)$$

where G_2 is the linear growth rate in the crystallizer with classified product removal. At $L = L_p$ the population densities are equal, $n_S = n_L$. This allows calculation of the constant of integration C.

The population densities are plotted in Figure 4-8 where they are also compared with an MSMPR. The MSMPR is assumed to have the same nucleation population density n° and the same production of crystals. With the same productivity, M_T,

$$M_T = k_V \rho_c \int_0^{\infty} L^3 n dL \qquad (4\text{-}57)$$

must be the same for the two crystallizers. This will require that the MSMPR have a slope intermediate between the two slopes of the classified product removal case. Thus $G_2 > G_1$ since $\tau_1 = \tau_{MSMPR}$. Since the classified product removal system has more small crystals (larger n for small L) and fewer large crystals, the MSMPR has a larger mean and dominant size for the weight distributions. Thus the MSMPR produces larger crystals! The classified product

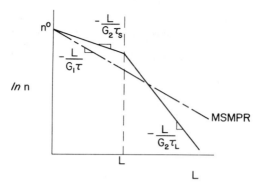

Figure 4-8.   Comparison of MSMPR and crystallizer with classified product removal.

withdrawal system does have a tighter distribution of product sizes. These results agree with experiments.

Sharper distributions with larger crystals can be obtained by using both a fines trap and classified product removal. In this case there will be three solutions to the population balance (see Problems 4-C7 and 4-D8 and Figure 4-13). Unfortunately, these modifications tend to increase the tendency towards instability (Garside, 1985; Randolph and Larson, 1988, Randolph *et al.*, 1977). Crystallization of KCl with classified product removal and fines destruction showed low order cycling of CSD. Such cycling causes undesirable variations in product quality and causes higher operating costs.

Another method of increasing magma density and average product size is called *clear-liquor advance*. A quiescent region of the settler is used to withdraw clear liquor. The product crystals are then drawn off at a much lower rate. This method effectively increases residence times, increases the average size, decreases the supersaturation, and increases M_T. The limit to using clear-liquor advance is the increase in secondary nucleation as M_T increases.

4.6.3. Methods of Suspending Solids

Crystallizers can be classified based on the method of suspending the growing crystals. One classification scheme for doing this is (Singh, 1979).

1. Circulating magma. Growing crystals are circulated through the zone

where supersaturation occurs. May also have fines removal and classified product withdrawal. This type of equipment can be an MSMPR. Examples were shown in Figures 2-3 a, b; 2-4 a, b; and 2-5 a. More examples of mixing methods are discussed below.

2. Circulating liquor. Some type of crystal settling or screen is used so that only clear liquor is recycled. The method is used in Krystal (or Oslo) type crystallizers. Some authors (e.g. Saeman, 1961) see no advantage to this method.

3. Scraped Surface. The wall of the heat exchanger is scraped with some type of blade. This was illustrated in Figure 2-3c and d. This method keeps the surface of the exchanger clean and gives high heat transfer rates. However, scraping the crystals off the walls breaks up the larger crystals. Thus only small crystals are produced. The effect of breakage of crystals causes "death" in one size range and "birth" in smaller size ranges (see the next section). These crystallizers are used to produce seed crystals, for viscous mixtures, and when very low temperatures are desired.

4. Tank Crystallizers. Both agitated or static tanks are used with cooling to the atmosphere or through a jacket. Static tanks will not be well mixed and a wide CSD will result. For example, ammonium alum crystals in the size range of +6 mesh to 2 inches are produced in tank crystallizers. Tank crystallizers are used for small throughputs of relatively easy to crystallize materials.

Mixing in crystallizers is very important, and is one of the major problems in scale-up. If the crystals and solvent have close to the same density, the crystals will be easy to suspend. Crystallizers equipped with mixers and baffles work well for these systems. If an external heat exchanger is used, an external pump is required. By returning the circulating liquid tangentially, much of the desired mixing can be achieved. The turn-over rate of the suspension must be high enough. This can be calculated by determining the sedimentation rate of crystals, and limiting the distance they can fall in the time required to mix the entire volume.

Draft tube or conduit mixing is commonly used if the crystals are difficult to suspend. This is illustrated in Figure 4-9 (Nyvlt, 1982; Saeman, 1961). The fast rise, slow fall requires the least energy, works very well with difficult to suspend crystals, and works well with fines traps. An air-lift can be used instead of the mixer (this is called a Pachuca type). The air lift also provides for some evaporation. Conduit mixing with fast rise can also be used

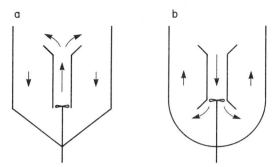

Figure 4-9.   Draft tube mixing methods. a. Fast rise-slow fall; b. Fast fall-slow rise.

with an external pump directing return liquor into the conduit. The fast fall, slow rise is used on the Oslo-Krystal design. It is also useful when a trap is used for fines removal, or when classification of product in the bottom of the crystallizer is desired. Examples of these crystallizers are shown by Mullin (1972), Nyvlt (1982), Rousseau (1986), and Singh (1979).

Scale-up of the mixing can be difficult. Unless growth is remarkably fast, all regions of the mixer should have about the same supersaturation. In a ten liter laboratory mixer a tracer bead may go through the entire mixing circuit in a few seconds. A commercial-scale crystallizer could easily be 10 feet tall and 15 feet in diameter. The time to traverse the mixing circuit must be longer if reasonable velocities are to be used. The half-life for supersaturation ranges from a few seconds to several minutes while circulation times can range from 0.2 seconds in a 0.2 m diameter tank to about 35 seconds in a 3 meter diameter tank (Garside, 1985). Thus, the two tanks can have significantly different supersaturations and hence different nucleation and growth kinetics. Generally, the large scale system is designed to be flexible so that its operation can be adjusted to give acceptable results.

4.7. CSD FOR COMPLEX CRYSTALLIZATION KINETICS

Crystallization can be much more complex than the situations discussed up to now. Two other commercially important cases will be briefly discussed here. The first is the inclusion of the birth and death of crystals in a given size range. The second is determination of CSD for size dependent growth.

In real crystallizers there is invariably some attrition of crystals. If the attrition results in contact nucleation, this effect can be accounted for in the nucleation kinetics used in the population balance (see Eqs. (4-37) to (4-39)). Since the pieces removed from the large crystal are tiny, no other adjustments in the population balance are required. In some crystallizers (e.g. scraped surface) and with some types of crystals large crystals are often fractured into two or more pieces. This results in the removal ("death") of crystals in one size range, and the simultaneous "birth" of two or more crystals in smaller size ranges. Including birth and death in the population balance is simple in a formal sense, but difficult to do in a form useful for calculation. Equation (4-8) is easily modified to include birth and death of crystals. The result is (Randolph and Larson, 1988).

$$G \frac{dn}{dL} + \frac{n}{\tau} = B(L) - D(L) \qquad (4\text{-}58)$$

where $B(L)$ and $D(L)$ are the birth and death functions which are obviously related to each other.

To solve Eq. (4-58) functions for $B(L)$ and $D(L)$ must be developed. Two-body death and birth effects are usually postulated. Experimentally, larger crystals are more likely to break. Thus a power-law death model is often assumed.

$$D(L) = k\, n\, L^{\beta} \qquad (4\text{-}59a)$$

where k is a rate constant and β represents the size selectivity. Since contact of crystals will be proportional to magma density, it would also be reasonable to include magma density in the death function.

$$D(L) = k\, n\, L^{\beta}\, M_T^{\alpha} \qquad (4\text{-}59b)$$

The birth function is obviously related to the death function since mass must be conserved. Depending on the assumptions made, various birth functions can be derived. If a power law is used for the death function, the birth function will also have a power law form.

The population balance Eq. (4-58) has been solved for the power law death function, Eq. (4-59a), with a related birth function (see Randolph and Larson, 1988). The results show a significant narrowing of the CSD with a

144

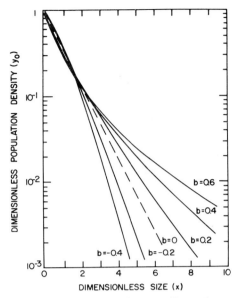

Figure 4-10.   Population density plot for size dependent growth (Abegg *et al*, 1968). Reprinted from *AIChE Journal 14*, 118 (1968) with permission. Copyright 1968, AIChE.

downward shift in the dominant size. The population density of the largest size crystals plummets. Thus, when large crystals are desired, breakage needs to be minimized. This can be done by using gentle mixing and by making impellers and baffles from a soft material such as polyethylene.

A second situation which commonly occurs is size dependent growth. In this case, the empirical model shown in Eq. (3-15) is often used. The solution of the population balance Eq. (4-7), along with Eq. (3-15) is (Abegg *et al.*, 1968).

$$n(L) = Kn^{\circ}(1 + \gamma L)^{-b} \exp\{-(1 - \gamma L)^{1-b}/[G_{nuclei}\tau\gamma(1-b)]\} \qquad (4\text{-}60a)$$

where

$$K = \exp\left[\frac{1}{G_{nuclei}\tau\gamma(1 - b)}\right] \qquad (4\text{-}60b)$$

Table 4-3.   Integration Constants for Size Dependent Growth Eqs. (4-61a, b).

b	C_1	C_2
0.9	5,841,000	1,681
0.8	6205	57.00
0.7	539.0	19.03
0.6	140.9	10.75
0.5	57.75	7.431
0.4	29.93	5.688
0.3	17.86	4.622
0.2	11.70	3.904
0.1	8.177	3.389
0.0	6.000	3.000
-0.1	4.569	2.696
-0.2	3.583	2.452
-0.4	2.356	2.084
-0.6	1.659	1.819
-0.8	1.221	1.618
-1.0	0.9341	1.461
-2.0	0.3438	1.000

Source: O'Dell and Rousseau (1978)

Equation (4-60a) agrees with Eq. (4-9) if b = 0 and $\gamma = 1/(G_{nuclei}\tau)$. This value for γ will be used in the following analysis.

When growth rate increases with size (this is the common case), b is positive. Examples are the growth of K_2SO_4 and $Na_2SO_4 \cdot 10H_2O$ crystals. Equation (4-60a) is plotted in Figure 4-10. Faster growth as size increases results in more crystals in this larger size range compared to size independent growth (b = 0). This is usually desirable. Note in Figure 4-10 that all the curves converge together for $L/(G\tau) < 2$. Thus size independent growth models give good results for small crystals. Abegg et al., (1968) obtained good fits with experimental data for both $Na_2SO_4 \cdot 10 H_2O$ and alum.

The weight distribution can be determined from Eq. (4-60a) or the parameters for the size dependent growth, Eq. (3-15) can be determined experimentally from weight distributions. The weight distributions are complicated functions involving definite integrals (O'Dell and Rousseau, 1978). The magma density and dominant size of the weight distributions can be calculated from

$$M_T = C_1 \rho_c k_V n^\circ (G_{nuclei} \tau)^4 \qquad \text{(4-61a)}$$

$$L_D = C_2 G_{nuclei} \tau \qquad \text{(4-61b)}$$

where C_1 and C_2 are calculated from definite integrals and are given in Table 4-3 (O'Dell and Rousseau, 1978). Equations (4-61) are valid when $\gamma = 1/(G_{nuclei} \tau)$ in Eq. (3-15).

4.8. BATCH CRYSTALLIZATION

Many crystallizations and precipitations are done as batch operations particularly for biochemicals. Batch processes will be the choice if the yearly production rate is fairly low or the equipment must be used to produce several different products. Unfortunately, batch processes usually produce a poorer quality product than continuous processes since the crystals are usually smaller. Better products can be obtained by controlling the cooling rate.

The population balance for unsteady state systems was derived in Eq. (4-6) while on the way to the continuous results. Equation (4-6) with birth and death functions added would be a logical starting point to develop CSDs for batch crystallizers. Unfortunately, although it has been tried (see Garside, 1985 and Tavare, 1987, for references) this approach has not proven to be extremely useful. Instead, an analysis incorporating the seeding analysis of Section 4.5 has been useful in predicting how to control the crystallizer temperature.

Batch crystallization usually starts with a hot, saturated solution which is seeded and then cooled and/or evaporated to cause supersaturation. The rate at which the solution is cooled will have a major impact on the CSD. The "normal" or "uncontrolled" method of cooling would start cooling the hot saturated solution with the cooling fluid at its usual temperature. From the heat transfer equation

$$Q = UA (T_M - T_{cold}) \qquad \text{(4-62)}$$

we can estimate the rate of cooling. This equation is more complicated than it

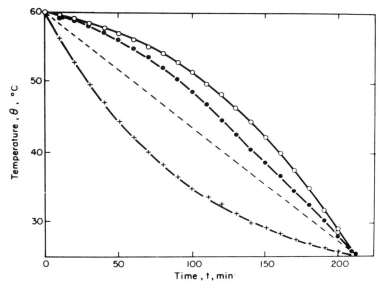

Figure 4-11.   Cooling curves determined for batch crystallization of potassium sulphate. From top down: Controlled cooling - theory, Eq. (4-72); Controlled cooling -- simplified theory, Eq. (4-74); Linear; Uncontrolled cooling. (Mullin and Nyvlt, 1971). Reprinted with permission from *Chem. Eng. Sci.*, 26, 369 (1971). Copyright 1971, Pergammon Press.

initially appears. The magma temperature, T_M, decreases during the crystallization and the overall heat transfer coefficient U is probably not constant because of fouling and the increase in viscosity of the magma. However, Eq. (4-62) can easily be used to estimate the initial rate of cooling when $T_M = T_F$ and the heat transfer surface is clean. Q will be large initially, and will decrease as both U and $(T_M - T_{cold})$ decrease. The cooling curve calculated for this case is curve d in Figure 4-11 (Mullin and Nyvlt, 1971). This rapid initial removal of heat will rapidly cool the magma temperature and supersaturate the solution. The result is likely to be the production of a large number of nucleii instead of sustained growth on the controlled number of seed crystals. This uncontrolled nucleation then causes a CSD with a very large number of rather small crystals. This is illustrated in Figure 4-12 (Jones and Mullin, 1974).

    Much better results can be obtained by controlled cooling (Mullin and

148

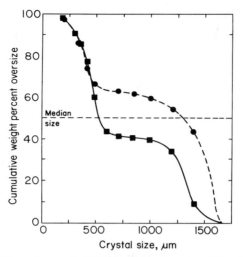

Figure 4-12. Experimental CSD for batch crystallization using different cooling methods. methods. ◆ Uncontrolled ● Following Eq. (4-74). (Jones and Mullin, 1974). Reprinted with permission from *Chem. Eng. Sci. 29*, 105 (1974). Copyright 1974, Pergamon Press.

Nyvlt, 1971; Mullin, 1972; Jones and Mullin, 1974; Belter et al, 1988). In controlled cooling the cooling rate will be slow at first to minimize excessive nucleation and will be fast after the growing crystals have reduced the supersaturation (see Figure 4-11). The improvement in CSD which can be obtained is illustrated in Figure 4-12.

To determine the temperature versus time or cooling curve desired for controlled cooling we start with a supersaturation balance (Mullin and Nyvlt,1971; Mullin, 1972).

$$-\frac{d(\Delta c)}{dt} = \frac{dc^*}{dt} + K_g \, A \, (\Delta c)^n + k_N \, (\Delta c)^i \qquad (4\text{-}63)$$

Δc is the supersaturation defined by Eq. (2-2a), A is the total area, K_g and k_N are the rate constants for growth and nucleation from Eqs. (3-16) and (3-4), respectively, and n and i are orders of growth and nucleation, respectively. The left hand side of this equation is the change in supersaturation with time. On the right hand side the first term represents the change in the saturation concentration with time. Since c^* is a function of temperature and we are cooling the solution, this corresponds to the creation of supersaturation according to

$$\frac{dc^*}{dt} = \frac{dc^*}{dT} \frac{dT}{dt} \qquad (4\text{-}64)$$

where $-dT/dt$ is the cooling rate. The term dc^*/dT can be determined from the solubility data such as Figure 2-1. The second and third terms in Eq. (4-63) correspond to the reduction of supersaturation caused by growth and nucleation, respectively.

Usually, we seed the batch and want to minimize other nucleation. To do this we operate within the metastable region illustrated in Figure 2-2. If we assume that we are successful in eliminating nucleation, the last term in Eq. (4-63) will be zero.

The left-hand-side of Eq. (4-63) can be written as

$$\frac{d(\Delta c)}{dt} = \frac{d(\Delta c)}{dT} \frac{dT}{dt} \qquad (4\text{-}65)$$

Now Eq. (4-63) becomes,

$$\frac{dT}{dt} = \frac{K_g A(\Delta c)^n}{\dfrac{dc^*}{dT} + \dfrac{d(\Delta c)}{dT}} \qquad (4\text{-}66)$$

The metastable zone width in Figure 2-2 probably depends upon temperature. Thus, the supersaturation Δc will depend upon temperature. If we assume a linear dependance, we have

$$\Delta c(T) = a_1 - a_2(T_o - T) \qquad (4\text{-}67)$$

Often the metastable zone width will not change ($a_2 = 0$), and $d(\Delta c)/dT = 0$.

We are now left with only the term $K_g A(\Delta c)^n$ to evaluate. From Eq. (3-16) this term equals dm/dt which can be related to the crystal size by Eq. (3-12).

$$K_G A(\Delta c)^n = 3L^2 k_V \rho_s \frac{dL}{dt} = 3L^2 k_V \rho_s G \qquad (4\text{-}68)$$

With no nucleation the seed crystals will grow to the final size.

$$L = L_{seed} + \sum_{i=0}^{t-1} G_i \qquad (4\text{-}69)$$

The summation over a series of growth rates occurs because G can be a function of both temperature and crystal size. Substituting Eqs. (4-69) and (4-68) into Eq. (4-66) we obtain

$$\frac{dT}{dt} = \frac{3k_V\rho_s G[L_{seed} + \sum_{i=0}^{t-1} G]^2}{\dfrac{dc^*}{dT} + \dfrac{d(\Delta c)}{dT}} \qquad (4\text{-}70)$$

The volumetric shape factor k_V can be difficult to predict. If the seeds grow without changing shape, we can use Eq. (3-12) to determine $k_V\rho_s$ from the known weight and size of the seed crystals.

$$k_V\rho_s = \frac{W_{seed}}{L_{seed}^3} \qquad (4\text{-}71)$$

Substitution of this result into Eq. (4-70) gives

$$\frac{dT}{dt} = \frac{3\,W_{seed}\,G\,[L_{seed} + \sum_{i=0}^{t-1} G]^2}{\left[\dfrac{dc^*}{dT} + \dfrac{d(\Delta c)}{dT}\right] L_{seed}^3} \qquad (4\text{-}72)$$

This equation gives the desired cooling rate as a function of time. Numerical integration of this equation gives the temperature versus time results shown in Figure 4-11.

Equation (4-72) is somewhat awkward to use. A considerably simpler form can be obtained by making additional assumptions, but the engineer must be aware that these assumptions may not be valid for a particular system. If the linear growth rate does not depend on temperature or crystal size, the summation in Eq. (4-72) becomes G. Often the supersaturation is constant and $d(\Delta c)/dT = 0$. Equation (4-72) then simplifies to

$$\frac{dT}{dt} = \frac{3\,W_{seed}\,G}{(dc^*/dT)\,L_{seed}^3}\,(L_{seed} + G)^2 \qquad (4\text{-}73)$$

If dc^*/dT can be assumed to be constant, this equation is easily integrated to obtain the required controlled temperature as a function of time.

$$T = T_o - \frac{3Gt}{L_{seed}} \frac{W_{seed}}{(dc^*/dt)} [1 + \frac{Gt}{L_{seed}} + \frac{1}{3} (\frac{Gt}{L_{seed}})^2] \qquad (4-74)$$

The cooling curve obtained using this simplified result is compared in Figure 4-11 to the result obtained by numerical integration of Eq. (4-72). The improvement in CSD when temperature is controlled following Eq. (4-74) instead of being uncontrolled is shown in Figure 4-12. An example of the use of Eq. (4-74) is given by Belter et al (1988).

4.9. DOWNSTREAM PROCESSING METHODS

The magma exiting from the crystallizer contains both crystals and mother liquor. Some downstream processing steps are required to recover the crystals. These steps are affected by the size and shape of the crystals as well as the properties of the liquor.

The most common downstream processing steps are filtration and centrifugation. To remove the mother liquor, which contains impurities, the crystals are often washed with solvent or water. However, the wash step depends on the size distribution and shape of the crystals. Regular shape prismatic crystals (Figure 3-1B) are much easier to filter without excessive pressure drops than either tabular (Figure 3-1A) or needle forms (Figure 3-1C). Washing of the prismatic crystals is also easier since the filter cake is more porous and the surface-to-volume ratio is lower. These steps are also simpler with larger crystals with tight CSD. Centrifugation is an alternative to filtration, and the same comments hold.

The crystals may require a final drying step to remove any remaining solvent or mother liquor. This is again easiest to do for large prismatic crystals with tight CSD.

Screening or sieving or other size classification methods may be required to produce a product within the desired size range. This step is reduced or eliminated if the crystallizer can produce a tight CSD of the desired median size. Screening and sieving separate based on the second largest dimension. Referring to Figure 3-1, both tabular and needle forms will bounce on the screen until the smallest cross-sectional area has a chance to slip through the screen opening. For example, needles which are much longer than the screen opening will readily pass through. If accurate sizing is required, it may be necessary to grow prismatic crystals.

Bulk storage, movement and packaging of crystals are all made easier when it is free flowing and not dusty. Large, prismatic crystals with a tight CSD are most likely to be free flowing. Crystals will produce less dust if mother liquor is removed before drying; otherwise, drying of the mother liquor often deposits a dust of solute on the crystals.

In summary, unless the product requires tabular or needle form crystals, prismatic shaped crystals are best for downstream processing.

4.10. SUMMARY-OBJECTIVES

This chapter has focused on the theoretical aspects of population balances and crystal size distributions. The objectives are:

1. Be able to derive the population balance.

2. Solve the population balance for size independent growth. Generate the number, area and weight distributions.

3. Use experimental weight distributions to determine crystallizer kinetics.

4. Determine the effect of changing residence time and magma density on crystallizer kinetics with and without secondary nucleation.

5. Explain the effect of and do calculations for fines destruction, classified product withdrawal, and different mixing procedures.

6. Utilize CSD for size dependent growth.

7. Determine the cooling curve for batch crystallization.

REFERENCES

Abegg, C.F., J.D. Stevens, and M.A. Larson, "Crystal size distributions in continuous crystallizers when growth rate is size dependent," *AIChE Journal, 14,* 118 (1968).

Bennett, R.C. and M. Van Buren, "Commercial urea crystallization," *Chem. Engr. Prog. Symp. Ser., 65* (95), 44 (1969).

Canning, T.F., "Interpreting population density data from crystallizers," *Chem. Eng. Prog. 66,* (7) 80 (1970).

Foust, A.S., L.A. Wenzel, C.W. Clump, L. Maus, and L.B. Andersen, *Principles of Unit Operations,* 2nd ed., Wiley, New York, 1980, 526-529.

Garside, J. and M.B. Shah, "Crystallization kinetics from MSMPR crystallizers," *Ind. Eng. Chem. Process Design Develop., 19,* 509 (1980).

Garside, J., "Industrial crystallization from solution," *Chem. Eng. Sci., 40,* 3 (1985).

Larson, M.A. and A.D. Randolph, "Size distribution analysis in continuous crystallization," *Chem. Eng. Prog. Symp. Ser., 65* (95), 1 (1969).

McCabe, W.L., J.C. Smith, and P. Harriott, *Unit Operations of Chemical Engineering,* 4th ed., McGraw-Hill, NY, 1985, Chapt. 28.

Moyers, C.G., Jr. and R. Rousseau, "Crystallization operations," in R. Rousseau, (Ed.), *Handbook of Separation Process Technology,* Wiley, New York, 1987, Chapt. 11.

Mullin, J.W., *Crystallization,* 2nd ed., Butterworth, London, 1972.

Nyvlt, J., *Industrial Crystallization,* 2nd ed., Verlag Chemie, Weinheim, 1982.

O'Dell, F.P. and R.W. Rousseau, "Magma density and dominant size for size dependent crystal growth," *AIChE Journal, 24,* 738 (1978).

Ramkrishna, D., "The status of population balances," *Rev. Chem. Engr.,* 3 (1), 49 (1985).

Randolph, A.D. and M.A. Larson, *Theory of Particulate Processes. Analysis and Techniques of Continuous Crystallization,* 2nd Ed., Academic Press, New York, 1988.

Randolph, A.D., J.R. Beckman, and Z.I. Kraljevich, "Crystal size distribution dynamics in a classified crystallizer," *AIChE Journal, 23,* 500 (1977).

Rousseau, R.W. and F. P. O'Dell, "Separation of multiple solutes by selective nucleation," *Ind. Eng. Chem. Process Des. Develop., 19,* 603 (1980).

154

Saeman, W.C., "Crystallization equipment design," *Ind. Eng. Chem.*, *53*, 612 (1961).

Singh, G., "Crystallization from solutions," in P.A. Schweitzer, (Ed.), *Handbook of Separation Techniques for Chemical Engineers*, McGraw-Hill, New York, 1979, Section 2.4.

Tavare, N.S., "Batch crystallization: A review," *Chem. Eng. Commun.*, *61*, 259 (1987).

HOMEWORK

A. *Discussion Problems.*

A1. Why is the median size for the dimensionless number distribution, $L/(G\tau) = 0.693$, less than that for the dimensionless weight distribution, $L/(G\tau) = 3.67$?

A2. Explain the concept of a population balance in your own words.

A3. Define the following terms.

  a. MSMPR

  b. population density

  c. moments

  d. τ

  e. $L/(G\tau)$

  f. dominant size

  g. point fines trap

  h. classified product removal

  i. clear liquor advance

  j. birth and death

A4. Sketch the expected plot of ln n vs L to compare a crystallizer 1 without a point fines trap to crystallizer 2 which has a point fines trap.

A5. Why is a weight average used to determine $\overline{G}$ in Eq. (4-28)?

A6. When secondary nucleation does not occur and $\tau_2 > \tau_1$ but $M_{T,1} = M_{T,2}$, Eqs. (4-34) relate growth rates and nucleation population densities. Sketch the graph of ln n versus L if,

   a. $i = 1$

   b. $i = 3$

   Comment on your graphs.

A7. Construct your key relations chart for this chapter.

C. *Derivations*

C1. Derive Eqs. (4-11b), (4-13b), (4-15b), and (4-17b).

C2. Derive Eqs. (4-25a and b).

C3. Prove that the dominant sizes for differential mass, area, length and number distributions are $L/(G\tau) = 3, 2, 1$ and 0, respectively.

C4. Prove that the median size for N/N_T is at $L/(G\tau) = 0.693$. Find the median of the cumulative area distribution, A/A_T.

C5. Show that Eq. (4-49c) follows from Eq. (4-49b).

C6. Complete the details of the derivation of Eqs. (4-47a and b) for a point fines trap.

C7. Combinations of fines destruction and classified product removal can be analyzed using the population balances. Solve the population balance, Eq. (4-8), for this combination. A population density plot for an industrial crystallizer (a Swenson DTB) producing KCl is shown in Figure 4-13 (Canning, 1970). Interpret this plot in terms of the population density function. What is happening in each zone? What are the values of $G\tau$, R and z?

156

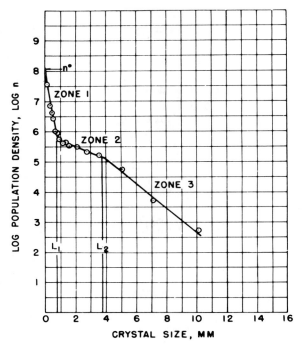

Figure 4-13.   Experimental population density results for KCl crystallizer with fines removal and classified product withdrawal (Canning, 1970). Reprinted with permission from *Chem. Eng. Prog.*, *66* (7), 80 (1970). Copyright 1970, AIChE.

D.   *Problems*

D1.   For the crystallization of urea in a large draft tube, baffled evaporative crystallizer the following data were obtained.

G = 0.0240 mm/hr, τ = 6.70 hours, and $\ln n^o$ = 11.45 where n^o is No./mm-L. See 4-D2 and 4-D5 for other data.

Predict the screen analysis if the following screens are used: 14, 20, 28, 35, 48, 65.

D2.   For Problem 4-D1 determine the distribution for n, N, *L*, A and M.   Plot these distribution. Assume $k_V = 1.0$ and $k_A = 6.0$. Do this for the continuous distributions.

D3. For Problem 4-D1 determine the sieve analysis distributions for n, N, L and A.

D4. A cooling crystallizer is used to crystallize KCl. At 60°C the following Tyler screen data are obtained.

Screen	14	16	20	24	28	32	42	60	80	115
Wt, kg	0.001	0.029	0.136	0.139	0.276	0.210	0.209	0.049	0.012	0.002

KCl forms cubic crystals with $\rho_c = 1.98$ g/ml. At 60°C the saturated fluid has a density of $\rho_F = 1.198$ g/ml. $V_s = 10$ liters. Residence time in crystallizer is 15 min. Find G and n°.

D5. An evaporative crystallizer is used to crystallize urea. The following data are obtained (Bennett and Van Buren, 1969)

τ, hrs			Tyler Screen Sizes				Crystallizer Density, g/L
	14	20	28	35	48	65	
a) 5.9	36.0	62.0	80.5	92.5	98.5	100	510
b) 3.12	26.2	51.5	76.2	94.0	99.5	100	317

where the screen numbers are cumulative weight % measured experimentally. Urea, NH_2CONH_2, has $\rho_c = 1.33$ g/cm^3. The crystals are "chunky", use $k_V = 1.0$. Find G and n° for parts a and b.

D6. A sodium acetate crystallizer receives a saturated solution at 60°C. This solution is seeded with 0.2 mm average size crystals and cooled to 10°C. What is the mean size of the product crystals $\bar{L}_p$? If the residence time is $\tau = 21$ hours, what linear growth rate G is required? Use a basis of 100 kg of entering water to which 0.25 kg of seeds are added. Data are in Figure 2-1 and Table 2-1. Why would this crystallizer be difficult to operate?

D7.   Example 4-3 showed that the crystallizer with a fines trap had a linear growth rate of G = 9.251 x 10^{-7} m/S.

  a.   Calculate the cumulative mass distribution M for an MSMPR operating with this G value, $\tau = \tau_p$ = 870s, and $M_T = M_{T,with\ trap}$ = 175 kg/m^3. Compare these results to the distribution found in Example 4-3.

  b.   What value of ($k_V \rho_c n^\circ$) will this MSMPR have?

D8.   When we crystallize potassium chloride without a fines trap, we find that M_T = 175 kg/m^3, τ = 870 sec, G = 4.0 x 10^{-7} m/s, and the order of nucleation i = 3.5. We desire the CSD to have a median size of 3 mm for the cumulative mass distribution when we use a point fines trap. Calculate the fraction of nucleii which can survive the point fines trap to achieve this median size. Residence times and magma densities for the crystallizers with and without the point fines trap are identical.

D9.   Glauber salt ($Na_2SO_4 \cdot 10H_2O$) demonstrates size dependent growth. Abegg *et al.*, (1968) found a good fit to data when

$$n^\circ = 8.0 \times 10^6 \text{ No./g cm--cm}^3$$

$$\gamma = \frac{1}{G_{nuclei}\tau} = \frac{1}{0.008}(\text{cm}^{-1}) , \quad b = 0.2$$

Predict the magma density M_T and the dominant size L_D. Crystal density ρ_c = 1.46 g/cm^3, k_V = 1/2.

E.   *More Complex Problems*

E1.   A classified product removal is used to remove crystals larger than 1.0 mm at a rate 4 times faster than removal of small crystals. Otherwise, the crystallizer is the same as the MSMPR explored in Example 4-1. Assume that the population density of nuclei and the magma densities are the same for the MSMPR and the classified product removal system. Determine G, the median size of the weight distribution, and the cumulative weight distribution for the classified product removal system. Compare your results to the MSMPR.

E2. The product from Problem 4-D4 (crystals + solution) will be fed to a second cooling crystallizer operating at 20°C. Assume that the feed to this crystallizer (at 60°) is a saturated mixture and that the product magma is in equilibrium at 20°C. Assume no nucleation occurs. Residence time is 15 min.

a. Predict M_T

b. Predict the crystal size distribution

c. Predict G.

Saturated KCl solution at 20°C has a density of 1.174 g/ml.

Chapter 5

CRYSTALLIZATION FROM THE MELT

In crystallization from the melt a liquid mixture is separated by crystallization. No solvent is present. For example, a mixture of impure xylenes can be purified by crystalization since the p-xylene crystallizes at a much higher temperature. Since both melt and solution crystallization are crystallization processes, there are many similarities. For example, many of the phase equilibrium behavior illustrated in Chapter 2 and nucleation and growth processes discussed in Chapter 3 are similar.

There are also significant differences between solution and melt crystallization which will be highlighted in this chapter. In solution crystallization a variety of methods of causing supersaturation are used to induce crystallization. In melt crystallization cooling is almost always used. Most industrial processes for solution crystallization use a single equilibrium stage while devices with the equivalent of many stages are often used in melt crystallization. Since there is no solvent in melt crystallization, there is no need for solvent removal and recovery, and there is no possibility of contamination by the solvent. However, there is also no way to reduce the viscosity, increase the diffusivity or remove energy by solvent evaporation. In addition, the chemicals being purified must be stable at the melting point - there is no way to significantly lower the operating temperature. For systems such as salts where the melting points are very high, crystallization from solution is less expensive. Lower operating temperatures usually make the separation easier. Distribution coefficients can be orders of magnitude more favorable at the lower temperatures possible in solution crystallization.

These comparisons show why crystalization from solution is much more common for bulk separations. Melt crystallization becomes advantageous when the presence of a solvent would be detrimental. This occurs in two situations: 1. When the melting point is at a convenient temperature and equilibrium is favorable for separation, melt crystallization is used for bulk separations. Examples are purification of p-xylene and separation of dichlorobenzenes. If crystallization from solution were used, a solvent other than water would be required and the solvent would have to be recovered. The solvent recovery costs make crystallization from solution more expensive than melt crystallization for these chemicals. 2. When an ultrapure product is desired, solvent would be an impurity which would have to be removed. Several different melt crystallization processes such as normal freezing and zone melting have been developed for ultrapurification. Ultrapure organics, metals and semiconductors are all purified this way.

In the first section of this chapter the fundamentals of melt crystallization will be briefly discussed. This section will build on Chapters 2 and 3. Then methods for doing melt crystallization will be explored. First, slurry crystallization method where the crystals are in a slurry of crystals and liquid melt will be discussed. Then, ultrapurification methods such as normal freezing and zone melting are discussed. In these processes the solid is continuous and is not in a slurry.

5.1. FUNDAMENTALS OF MELT CRYSTALLIZATION

5.1.1. Equilibrium

Phase diagrams for three melt systems were shown in Figures 2-7 and 2-8. Solid solution behavior for phenanthrene and anthracene was shown in Figure 2-7. Eutectic behavior for naphthalene, phenol and naphthalene, 1-naphthol was illustrated in Figure 2-8. Note in Figure 2-8 that quite good predictions can be made using activity coefficients predicted with computer routines (Walas, 1985). In ultrapurification only a small section of the diagram (up to a few percent impurity) is needed.

Equilibrium data for melt systems is available in a variety of sources. The Landolt-Börnstein (1956) tables summarize data for many binary and a

162

Table 5-1.   Selected distribution coefficients, Eq. (24-1), for inorganics (Shoemaker and Smith, 1967) and organics (Zief, 1967).

Compound	T, °C	Impurities (k_i)
Al	659.7	Co (0.14), Cr (0.8), Ca (0.06), Fe (0.29), Ga (<0.1), La (<0.1), Mn (1), Sc (0.17), Sm (0.67), W (0.32)
Fe	1535	C (0.29), O (0.022), P (0.17), S (0.04 to 0.06)
Ga As	1238	Cd (<0.2), Cu (<0.002), Fe (0.003), Ge (0.018)
H_2O	0	D_2O (1.021), HF (10^{-4}), NH_3 (0.17), NH_4F (0.02)
Sn	231.9	Ag (0.03), Bi (0.5), In (0.5), Sb (1.5), Zn (0.05)
Anthracene		Anthraquinone (0.005), carbazole (> 2.0), fluorene (0.1), phenanthrene (0.06), tetracene (0.06)
Naphthalene		2-naphthol (1.85 and 2.3)
2-Naphthol		Naphthalene (0.4)
Phenol		p-nitrophenol (0.22)
Pyrene		Anthracene (0.125), 1, 2-benzanthracene (1.95)
Cyclohexane		Methylcyclopentane (0.6)
Benzene		Cyclohexane (~ 0.15)
Hexadecanol		Octadecanol (0.75)

few ternary systems. Timmermans (1960) also has data on a large variety of binary systems. Phase diagrams for metals are available in Hanson (1958) and Rhines (1956). Data on oxides and ceramics are given by Alper (1970-78) and Levin *et al.* (1964,1969). Calculations are summarized by Walas (1985).

Since melt crystallization methods, particularly normal freezing and zone melting, often operate with only a percent or less impurity, equilibrium is often represented as a distribution coefficient. The distribution coefficient is usually defined as

$$k_i = \frac{\text{concentration of impurity i in solid}}{\text{concentration of impurity i in melt}} \qquad (5\text{-}1)$$

Any consistent set of units can be used for the concentration measurement. Distribution coefficients for a large number of inorganic materials (Shoemaker and Smith, 1967) and a few organic materials (Zief, 1967) have been tabulated. Selected values are given in Table 5-1. For most impurities k < 1.0 and the impurity is excluded from the crystal. In some cases such as eutectic systems k << 1.0 and exclusion is essentially complete for systems at equilibrium.

The distribution coefficient can be related to the complete phase diagrams. For a solid solution system, illustrated by Figure 2-7, k_i can be obtained at any temperature. For instance, if phenanthrene is considered to be the impurity, k_i at 200°C is

$$k_i \sim \frac{1-0.95 \text{ mole frac anthracene}}{1-0.72} = \frac{0.05}{0.28} = 0.18$$

If the liquidus and solidus lines are straight, k_i will be constant. Otherwise, k_i will depend on concentration. For a eutectic system such as Figure 2-8 the solid will be pure at equilibrium. Thus $k_i = 0$. The apparent distribution coefficient will be greater than zero because of inclusions, imperfect washing and other non-idealities. At low concentrations, the distribution coefficients of different impurities are often independent. However, this is not true for semiconductors where large interactions often occur (Wilcox and Estrin, 1982).

5.1.2. Heat and Mass Transfer

Heat and mass transfer processes are usually very important in melt crystallization. Heat transfer is usually much more important in melt crystallization than in solution crystallization. The temperature and composition profiles are shown schematically in Figure 5-1. The solid temperature is usually somewhat greater than the liquid temperature since the latent heat of solidification must be dissipated. The solid is usually assumed to be at its melting point. In very slow processes such as normal freezing and zone melting the amount of supercooling, $T_s - T_{bulk}$, may be only a few tenths of a degree.

If $k_i < 1$, impurity is rejected at the growing interface of the crystal. Thus there will be a tendency for impurity to build up at the interface unless either mixing is vigorous or diffusional mass transfer is rapid. Usually the

164

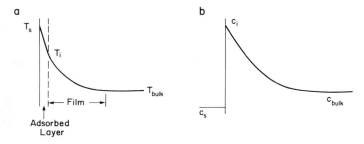

Figure 5-1.   Schematic of temperature and composition profiles in melt crystallization. a. Temperature. b. Concentration of impurity with $k_i < 1$.

interface can be assumed to be at equilibrium; thus, $k_i = c_s/c_i$ is the actual equilibrium constant. The apparent equilibrium constant $k_{app} = c_s/c_{bulk}$ will always be closer to unity than k_i.

The heat transfer analysis for a growing crystal can be treated formally in an approach similar to the mass transfer theory given in Eqs. (3-9) to (3-17). The heat transfer across the films is,

$$\frac{dq}{dt} = hA(T_i - T) \qquad (5\text{-}2a)$$

where A is the area of the crystal and h is the film heat transfer coefficient. This film coefficient can be written as $h = k_{cond}/\delta_T$ where k_{cond} is the thermal conductivity and δ_T is the hypothetical film thickness. Unfortunately, δ_T is not known and δ_T is not equal to the film thickness for mass transfer. It is often convenient to express the heat transfer in terms of an overall heat transfer coefficient U, since the interface temperature T_i is not required.

$$\frac{dq}{dt} = UA(T_s - T) \qquad (5\text{-}2b)$$

The solid temperature T_s will essentially be the melting point. Thus T_s is known while T_i is not.

The energy which must be dissipated is the latent heat of fusion, λ. Then,

$$\frac{dq}{dt} = \lambda \frac{dm}{dt} \qquad (5\text{-}3)$$

where m is the mass of solid deposited. The latent heats are readily available (Mullin, 1972; Nyvlt, 1982; Perry and Green (1984). The rate of mass transfer, dm/dt, was given by Eqs. (3-9) to (3-11) or Eq. (3-16) depending on the surface rearrangement.

If heat transfer controls the rate of growth of the crystal, then setting Eqs. (5-2b) and (5-3) equal we obtain

$$\frac{dm}{dt} = \frac{UA(T_s - T)}{\lambda} \qquad (5\text{-}4)$$

Heat transfer will often control in processes such as zone melting and normal freezing where there is very little impurity and the impurity has little effect on the kinetics of crystalilization. When large amounts of impurity are present, mass transfer will often be limiting and the analysis of Chapter 3 is valid. For in-between situations both heat and mass transfer need to be included (Meyer and Shen, 1970).

5.2. SLURRY PROCESSES

In slurry processes melt crystallization is operated with discontinuous crystals in a continuous liquid. The three methods of slurry operation are staged systems, end-feed columns and center feed columns. These systems are commonly used for bulk separations although they can be used for ultrapurification of eutectic systems.

The melt crystallizer must compete with other bulk separation processes such as distillation or crystallization from solution. The latent heat of fusion for organic compounds is approximately 1/3 the heat of vaporization. Thus, a crystallization process will require less energy than distillation all other things being equal. However, distillation has much higher mass and heat transfer rates; thus, distillation columns are much cheaper per equilibrium stage. Crystallization is favored over distillation for bulk separations only when distillation does not work well. Distillation may not be the separation of choice when: 1. The relative volatility is close to one. Separation factors for crystallization may be much higher. 2. Azeotropes are formed. Eutectics may not occur, or may be less of a problem. 3. Very high temperatures or thermal decomposition occur in distillation. Crystallization operates at lower temperatures. 4. The product is desired as a crystalline solid. A crystallizer may be able to do the required separation and produce the desired product in one step. 5. An existing crystallizer can be used. Capital expenses will be very low if existing equipment can be used. 6. A pure product is being further refined to higher purity. For example, distillation is usually very energy intensive when going from 99.9% to 99.99% purity.

5.2.1. Continuous Staged Processes

When equilibrium is favorable, a single equilibrium stage may be sufficient. For example, for both eutectic systems shown in Figure 2-8 pure naphthalene

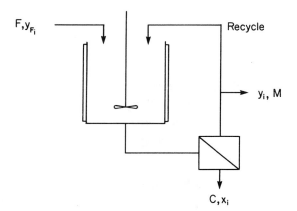

Figure 5-2.   Single stage continuous, steady-state crystallizer.

can be produced if the feed concentration is greater then the eutectic concentration. If the concentration of impurity (phenol or 1-naphthol in Figure 2-8) is quite small, a large amount of relatively pure naphthalene can be produced with a minimal amount of eutectic. The eutectic would then be separated by other methods (solution crystallization, distillation, extraction, etc.) and be recycled. For solid solution systems (see Figure 2-7) a single equilibrium stage will be sufficient only if the feed is already quite pure. The equilibrium calculations are essentially the same as those for solution crystallization (see Chapter 2).

If the distribution coefficient is constant, single stage calculations are straightforward. For the steady-state continuous well-mixed system shown in Figure 5-2 the mass balances are

$$F = M + C \qquad (5\text{-}5a)$$

$$Fy_{F,i} = Cx_i + My_i \qquad (5\text{-}5b)$$

where F is the feed flowrate, M is the melt flow rate, and C is the flow rate of crystals in any set of consistent units. To be specific we will treat flow rates F, M, and C in kg/hr. The weight fractions of impurity in the crystals and melt are x_i and y_i, respectively. Then the equilibrium expression is

$$k_i = x_i/y_i \qquad (5\text{-}5c)$$

where we assume that the impurities are independent. Combining Eqs. (5-6) to remove unknown M and y_i, the solution is

$$x_i = \frac{k_i y_{F,i}}{1 - \dfrac{C}{F}(1 - k_i)} \qquad (5\text{-}6)$$

This gives the concentration of the crystals. The adhering melt will contain more impurity. This can be removed either by partial melting and drainage or by reflux. These methods are discussed later.

168

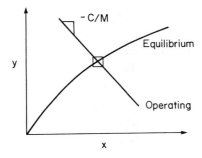

Figure 5-3.   McCabe-Thiele diagram for single stage crystallization. Either
continuous steady-state or batch crystallization with completely
mixed crystals.

An alternate analysis method for continuous crystallization is to use a
McCabe-Thiele diagram as shown in Figure 5-3. The mass balance Eq. (5-5b)
can be solved for y_i to develop the operating equation.

$$y_i = - \frac{C}{M} x_i + \left[1 + \frac{C}{M} \right] y_{F,i} \qquad (5-7)$$

The intersection of the operating line and equilibrum curve gives y_i and x_i.
This analysis is obviously applicable to nonlinear equilibria as long as the
solutes are independent.

If one equilibrium stage is not sufficient, crystallizers can be cascaded to
achieve additional separation. For solid solutions continuous operation will be
essentially the same as the counter-current cascade used for solid solutions for
solution crystallization (Figure 2-20). Between each stage the crystals and melt
must be separated from each other, and the crystals must be redissolved and
recrystallized. Thus, the process is expensive unless there are very few stages.
Equilibrium staged calculations can be done on an enthalpy-composition
diagram (Ponchon-Savarit diagram) which will look very similar to Figure 2-
21. Since this process will be rare in industrial practice, the development of
this analysis procedure is left as Problem 5C-1.

5.2.2. Batch Staged Crystallization

Batch crystallization calculations can be done several different ways. The simplest operation is to load the empty crystallizer with M_0 kg of feed mixture of weight fraction $y_{i,0}$. Then cool the charge and crystallize until the desired weight fraction, g, of the charge has frozen. The melt, $(1 - g)M_0$ kg, is then drained off and gM_0 kg of crystals remain. Assuming a homogeneous well-mixed crystal phase, equilibrium Eq. (5-6c) is valid at the end of the batch. The mass balance on impurity at the end of the batch is

$$gM_0 \; x_i + (1 - g) \; M_0 \; y_i = M_0 \; y_{i,0} \tag{5-8}$$

Assuming that the impurities are independent and combining Eq. (5-6c) and (5-8), we obtain

$$x_i = \frac{k_i \; y_{i,0}}{gk_i + (1-g)} \tag{5-9}$$

Note that if everything is frozen (g = 1) then $x_i = y_{i,0}$ and no separation is achieved.

A McCabe-Thiele analysis can be used for batch crystallization if the crystals are homogeneous and well mixed. Equation (5-7) is applicable if we interpret C and M as the kg of crystals and melt produced, and x_i and y_i are the weight fractions of the crystals and melt when the batch is done. With this interpretation, the McCabe-Thiele diagram is again shown by Figure 5-3.

Equation (5-9) or a McCabe-Thiele analysis are almost always oversimplifications. Crystals are usually *not* homogeneous. When the first layers of the crystal are formed, they will be in contact with solution of lower impurity concentration. As impurity is rejected its concentration in solution increases. Thus later layers will be less pure. To solve this problem we need a time dependent equation. Let dm/dt = rate of growth of crystals in kg/hr. dm/dt is set by the heat transfer rate and is assumed to be constant. Then the unsteady state mass balance is

$$-\left[\frac{dm}{dt}\right] x_i = \frac{d(My_i)}{dt} \tag{5-10}$$

where M is the kg of liquid melt in the crystallizer at time t. M can be related to the crystal growth rate by an overall mass balance.

$$M = M_0 - \left[\frac{dm}{dt}\right] t \qquad (5\text{-}11a)$$

Again defining g as the weight fraction of melt which has frozen

$$g = \frac{M_0 - M}{M_0} = 1 - \frac{M}{M_0} = \frac{(dm/dt)\, t}{M_0} \qquad (5\text{-}11b)$$

Equation (5-11a) was substituted in for M/M_0 to give the last equation in Eq. (5-11b). From Eq. (5-11b) we obtain both

$$M = M_0(1-g) \qquad (5\text{-}11c)$$

and

$$dt = \frac{M_0}{(dm/dt)}\, dg \qquad (5\text{-}11d)$$

These last two equations plus the equilibrium Eq. (5-6c) are substituted into Eq. (5-10). After rearrangement,

$$\frac{dx_i}{x_i} = (1 - k_i)\frac{dg}{(1-g)} \qquad (5\text{-}12a)$$

Integrating Eq. (5-12a) and applying the initial condition that the very first crystal is in equilibrium with the initial liquid,

$$x_i = k_i\, y_{i,0}, \quad \text{for} \quad g = 0 \qquad (5\text{-}12b)$$

we obtain

$$x_i = y_{i,0}\, k(1 - g)^{k_i - 1} \qquad (5\text{-}13)$$

This equation gives the instantaneous solid concentration as a function of y_0, k and g.

The average solids concentration can be obtained by integrating Eq. (5-13).

$$x_{i,avg} = \frac{\int_0^g x_i \, dg}{g} = \frac{y_{i,0} k_i \int_0^g (1-g)^{k_i-1} dg}{g} = \frac{y_{i,0}}{g}[1 - (1-g)^{k_i}] \tag{5-14}$$

Note that when the entire melt is frozen, (g = 1,) $x_{i,avg} = y_{i,0}$ which is the expected result. Comparison of Eqs. (5-14) and (5-9) shows that the progressive freezing calculation where the crystal is non-homogeneous results in a lower $x_{i,avg}$ that the completely mixed crystal. This analysis for a non-mixed crystal turns out to be the same analysis as for normal (or progressive) freezing (see Section 5.3.1).

The development leading to Eqs. (5-9) and (5-14) assumes equilibrium throughout the process. If the freezing rate is not very slow, then equilibrium is probably not reached. Equations (5-9) and (5-14) can still be used if an effective distribution coefficient k_{eff} is used. The effective distribution coefficient depends on all of the operating conditions. Equation (5-9) and (5-14) also assume that all of the contaminated melt can be removed from the crystals. This is often a problem when ultrapure product is required.

5.2.3. Partial Melting and Drainage

Additional purification can be obtained by partially melting the crystals and draining off the melt (this is also called *sweating*). Since the impurity lowers the freezing point, crystal layers with higher impurity concentration will melt first. Draining this melt washes the interstitial melt from the crystals, and can result in a considerable increase in purity. The freezing and melting can be done batch-wise in the same vessel. This "Proabd" process has been used commercially and is discussed later (see Section 5.3.1). An alternative is to do the freezing and thawing in separate vessels. This process has also been commercialized for purification of benzene, naphthalene and other organics (Molinari, 1967b).

The effect of partial melting and drainage can be seen by a simple addition to the equilibrium model for batch crystallization. When harvested, the crystals will entrain some weight fraction, e, of the melt even after the crystals are allowed to stand and drain.

$$e = \frac{\text{weight melt entrained}}{\text{weight of crystals}} \tag{5-15}$$

This entrained melt is assumed to be in equilibrium with the outer layer of the crystal.

$$y_i = x_i/k_i = y_{i,0}(1-g)^{k_i-1} \tag{5-16}$$

If this melt is not removed, the melt plus crystals have a total concentration of

$$y_{i,tot} = \frac{(ey_i + x_{i,avg})}{(e+1)} \tag{5-17}$$

which becomes

$$y_{i,tot} = \frac{ey_{i,0}(1-g)^{k_i-1} + \dfrac{y_{i,0}}{g}[1-(1-g)^{k_i}]}{e+1} \tag{5-18}$$

This is the product concentration which will be observed if the melt is not removed.

It is desirable to remove the entrained liquid since it is concentrated in impurity. This can be done by partially melting the crystals and allowing them to drain. Assume we crystallize a weight fraction g_1 of the initial charge. Then x_{avg} and y_{tot} are given by Eqs. (5-14) and (5-18) with $g = g_1$. Now melt a portion of the crystals Δg. Assume that the drainage occurs by displacing the old liquid with the new melt. If $\Delta g \geq eg_1$, with perfect displacement all of the old entrained liquid will be removed. The fraction of crystals collected is now

$$g_2 = g_1 - \Delta g \tag{5-19}$$

These crystals have an average composition of,

$$x_{i,avg2} = \frac{y_{i,0}}{g_2}[1 - (1 - g_2)^{k_i}] \tag{5-20}$$

This equation is obtained from the original crystallization since the interior of the crystals is unaffected by the partial melting.

The new melt entrained on the crystals can be a mixture of old melt plus the newly melted crystal layer. If all the old melt is removed, we can assume that the composition of the entrained material is the same as the melted crystal. Thus

$$y_{i,avg} = \frac{\int_{g_1}^{g_2} x_i dg}{\Delta g} = \frac{y_{i,0}k_i \int_{g_1}^{g_2} (1-g)^{k_i-1} dg}{\Delta g} = \frac{y_{i,0}[(1-g_2)^{k_i} - (1-g_1)^{k_i})]}{\Delta g} \tag{5-21}$$

The product composition will now be,

$$y_{i,prod} = \frac{(ey_{i,avg} + x_{i,avg2})}{(e + 1)} \tag{5-22}$$

where the fraction entrained is assumed to still be e. Excess liquid was drained off. This equation becomes

$$y_{i,prod} = \frac{y_{i,0}\left\{ \dfrac{e[(1-g_2)^{k_i}-(1-g_1)^{k_i}]}{\Delta g} + \dfrac{1-(1-g_2)^{k_i}}{g_2} \right\}}{(e + 1)} \tag{5-23}$$

Although less product is collected after partial melting and drainage, it is significantly purer. This is explored in Example 5-1.

Prediction of the entrainment e will be difficult. The entrainment will depend on the crystal shape, the crystal packing, viscosity, surface tension and the processing steps. Entrainment can be reduced by blowing an inert gas through the bed of crystals, by pulling a vacuum or by centrifuging the bed. To ensure removing all of the old entrained melt, a fraction of crystals significantly larger than eg_2 will often be melted. This reduces the yield, but gives a purer product. Partial melting and drainage can also be used with continuous processes (see Problem 5-C3).

Batch processes can be cascaded to increase the purity. After harvesting, the crystals are melted and then recrystallized. This reduces the initial concentration of impurity for the second crystallization, and will result in purer product crystals. The melt from this batch will be near the composition of the initial charge. Thus, this melt can be recrystallized to produce more crystals. These can then be recrystallized to form the final product. Methods for coupling batch processes to increase purity and yield are explored further in Problem 5-B1.

Example 5-1. Batch melt crystallization with partial melting.

Ten kilograms of a pyrene mixture containing 4 wt % anthracene is purified in a batch crystallizer. 60% of the original charge is frozen. After filtration, 0.08 weight fraction melt adheres to the crystals.

a. Find the product concentration.

b. If 1 kilogram of the crystals are melted and the melt is drained off, find the new product concentration.

Solution

a. The results of the initial freezing can be found from Eq. (5-14). $y_0 = 0.04$, $g = 0.6$, $k = 0.125$ (from Table 5-1). Then the anthracene concentration is

$$x_{avg} = \frac{y_0}{g}[1 - (1-g)^k] = \frac{0.04}{0.6}[1 - (0.4)^{0.125}] = 0.0072$$

The entrained melt is given by Eq. (5-16),

$$y = y_0(1-g)^{k-1} = (0.04)(0.4)^{-0.875} = 0.0892$$

Then the mix of entrained melt plus crystals is given by Eq. (5-17)

$$y_{tot} = \frac{ey + x_{avg}}{e + 1} = \frac{(0.08)(0.0892) + 0.0072}{1.08} = 0.0133$$

Note that the adhering melt causes a considerable increase in the impurity concentration of the product.

b. $\Delta g = 0.1$ since 1 of the original 10 kg is melted. Then g_2 is

$$g_2 = g_1 - \Delta g = 0.6 - 0.1 = 0.5$$

The remaining 5 kg of crystals have a composition given by Eq. (5-20).

$$x_{Avg,2} = \frac{0.04}{0.5} [1 - (0.5)^{0.125}] = 0.0066$$

Assuming that the old entrained melt is washed away by the newly melted material, the new adhering melt composition will be given approximately by Eq. (5-21).

$$y_{avg} = \frac{y_0[(1-g_2)^k - (1-g_1)^k]}{\Delta g}$$

$$= \frac{0.04 \, [(0.5)^{0.125} - (0.4)^{0.125}]}{0.1} = 0.0101$$

The product composition combining this melt with the crystals is given by Eq. (5-22).

$$y_{prod} = \frac{ey_{avg} + x_{avg,2}}{e + 1} = \frac{(0.08)(0.0101) + (0.0066)}{1.08} = 0.0069$$

This product is obviously much purer than the product obtained without drainage. In fact, this product is theoretically purer than the crystals before partial melting. This occurs because the most impure layers were melted off.

5.2.4. Column Crystallization

An alternate method for slurry melt crystallization when a single equilibrium contact is not sufficient is to have continuous contact between the solid and liquid in a column. Some method such as pulsed flow or a screw conveyor is used to move the crystals countercurrent to the liquid.

Two classes of column crystallizers have been developed. In the *end feed* system a slurry is fed to the column. The column operates as a stripping column to obtain further purification of the crystals. The largest application of end-feed columns has been in the Phillips process for purifying p-xylene by melt crystallization. This process is shown in Figure 5-4 (McKay, 1967). The first scraped surface crystallizer is operated at a low temperature to increase the recovery of the p-xylene. The crystals from the crystallizer are recovered in a rotary filter and then melted. This melt serves as the feed to the second scraped surface crystallizer which produces the slurry feed for the purification column. Note that this feed has already been through a two stage crystallizer. The crystal bed is moved downwards when the piston of the pulse unit retracts. Crystals are pulled into the melter. Some of the melt is removed as product while the remainder is refluxed. This reflux is warmer than the crystals and partially melts some of the crystals. The latent heat for melting is supplied by freezing some of the reflux. This partial melting of the most impure layers of the crystals (which have a lower melting point) and refreezing of the relatively pure reflux is one of the major reasons for the purification. The other major reason for purification is the contaminated melt is washed off by the countercurrent flow of much purer melt produced by the reflux. This washing is the main function of the countercurrent motion. The impure melt is removed through a filter or screen near the top of the column.

177

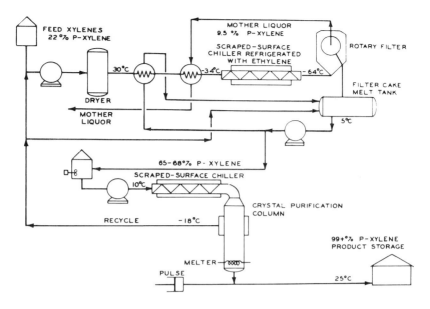

Figure 5-4. Phillips process for purifying p-xylene (McKay, 1967). Reprinted with permission from Zief, M. and Wilcox, W.R. (Eds.). *Fractional Solidification*, Marcel Dekker, NY, 1967. Copyright 1967, Marcel Dekker.

The xylene system is an extremely favorable system for melt crystallization. The melting points of ortho, meta and para xylenes are –46.9°C, –25.2°C and 15.3°C, respectively. The melting points are sufficiently far apart to make crystallization relatively simple, and the system does not form solid solutions. Thus the crystals are essentially pure p-xylene and the column removes entrained melt. Since the boiling points are very close, distillation is not feasible. Recently, adsorption using the Parex process (see Chapter 10) has been used for most new p-xylene purification plants. Existing crystallization plants continue to operate since their operating costs are low. Other products such as beer, fruit juices and other food products have been purified with end-feed column crystallizers. When the crystals are ice, the column is inverted and the solids move upward.

Several different designs for end feed crystallizers have been developed (Albertino *et al.*, 1967; Henry and Moyers, 1984; McKay, 1967; Moyers and Rousseau, 1987). Most of the large columns use the pulsed system shown in Figure 5-4. The pulses tend to prevent the formation of incrustations, and they sweep the screens free. Piston systems have also been used particularly for columns with ice. The piston systems use a piston to push the crystal bed through the column. The piston systems appear to be more difficult to scale up.

Center feed columns use a liquid melt as feed and form crystals inside the column. Schematically, the column can be arranged as shown in Figure 5-5a. The analogy to a distillation column is obvious. At the bottom, crystals are melted producing a product with the higher melting point. The reflux at the bottom of the column is equivalent to boilup. At the top of the crystallizer relatively pure lower melting product is withdrawn. Some of the melt is frozen and returned to the column as reflux. Conceptually, it should be easy to separate a binary mixture into two relatively pure products.

Unfortunately, the analogy between crystallization and distillation breaks down when one looks at hydrodynamics or mass transfer. For most systems the melt and the crystals have approximately the same density. This is another advantage of solution crystallization. Usually $\rho_c \gg \rho_f$ in solution crystallization while $\rho_c \sim \rho_f$ in melt crystallization. Thus gravity is usually insufficient to force rapid countercurrent flow of the melt and the crystals. Some positive means of forcing the crystals countercurrent to the melt is required. This can be done in a centrifuge, with a piston, in a pulsed column, or with a variety of mechanical conveyors. For center feed columns mechanical conveyors such as spirals are often used (Albertins, 1967; Henry and Moyers, 1984, Mullin, 1972; Moyers and Rousseau, 1987). A variety of specialized columns such as the Brodie or Schildknecht differ by the mechanical means used to move the crystals. A Brodie column is shown in Figure 5-5b. Exact design of the spiral and scale-up is difficult. Most commercial applications are relatively small systems. The size limit of a Brodie crystallizer is about 30 million pounds per year. Preliminary design calculations for a Brodie crystallizer are discussed by Moyers and Rousseau (1987). The 4C crystallizer (counter-current cooling crystallizer) developed by Tsukishima Kikai (TSK) in Japan and licensed by C.W. Nofs-

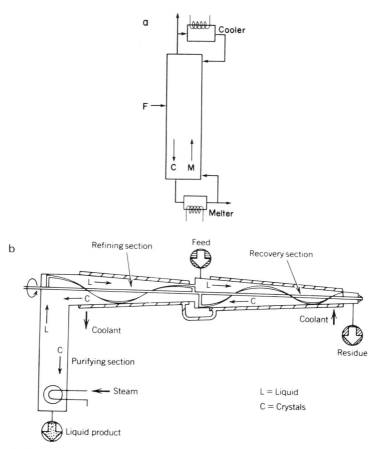

Figure 5-5.   Center feed melt crystallizer. a. Schematic b. Brodie type column.

inger in the U.S. is based on the Brodie crystallizer (Anon, 1988). It uses several tank-type scraped surface crystallizers and has a capacity about five times that of a Brodie crystallizer.

Mass transfer in a crystallizer differs from that in distillation. As has been mentioned before, molecules inside the crystal do *not* exchange mass with the melt. Thus an impurity can easily be carried to the melter where it may or may not be refluxed. The reflux does cause melting of the outer layers of the crystals and refreezing of the relatively pure reflux. The main function of the countercurrent motion seems to be to wash the interstitial melt from the crystals. Thus eutectic systems where the crystals are expected to be pure can be purified easily in a column crystallizer. Solid solutions which require a large number of contacts are much more difficult to purify. This is evident when one determines HETP or HTU values. These values are often large, and may not be constant when the column is made longer.

Both types of column crystallizers can be designed using either a staged analysis with an experimentally measured HETP or a mass transfer analysis. The staged analysis will be similar to that used in Chapter 2 for solution crystallization. The mass transfer analysis is preferred since it is closer to the actual process.

For eutectic systems the mass transfer analysis for end-feed crystallizers is straightforward if solid of eutectic composition is not present. Since equilibrium predicts that the crystals are pure (see Figure 2-8), the main purpose of the column is to wash impurities from the liquid adhering to the crystals. For a plug flow system the rate of mass transfer of the adhering liquid is

$$\frac{M}{A_c} \frac{dy}{dz} = ka(y_{ad} - y) \qquad (5\text{-}24a)$$

where M is the melt flow rate in kg/hr, A_c is the column cross sectional area, k is the mass transfer coefficient based on the interfacial area per volume, a, between crystals and liquid. The adhering melt has a weight fraction y_{ad}.

Rearranging this equation,

$$L = \int_0^L dz = \frac{M}{A_c ka} \int_{y_{in}}^{y_{out}} \frac{dy}{(y_{ad} - y)} \qquad (5\text{-}24b)$$

where we have assumed that $M/(A_c ka)$ is constant. This assumption and later assumptions in the mass balances can be approximately valid for end feed

181

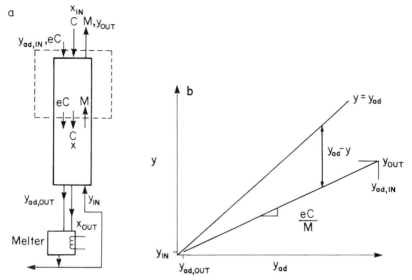

Figure 5-6.   End-feed column crystallizer. a. Schematic. b. Operating
                diagram.

columns which are adiabatic except at the melter. Equation (5-24b) can be
written as

$$L = (HTU)(NTU) \tag{5-24c}$$

where

$$HTU = \frac{M}{A_c ka} , \quad NTU = \int_{y_{in}}^{y_{out}} \frac{dy}{y_{ad} - y} \tag{5-24d}$$

To determine the NTU we must find $y-y_{ad}$ as a function of y. This can
be done with a mass balance for the end-feed column shown schematically in
Figure 5-6a. The adhering melt is entrained at a weight fraction e defined by
Eq. (5-15). The mass balance using the balance envelope shown in Figure 5-6a
is

$$eCy_{ad,in} + Cx_{in} + My = eCy_{ad} + Cx + My_{out} \tag{5-25a}$$

182

where we have assumed that crystal and melt flow rates, C and M, are constant. For eutectic systems $x_{in} = x = 0$. Solving for y

$$y = \frac{eC}{M} y_{ad} + y_{out} - \frac{eC}{M} y_{ad,in} \qquad (5\text{-}25b)$$

This is shown in Figure 5-6b where the difference $(y - y_{ad})$ is indicated. Solving Eq. (5-25b) for y_{ad} and substituting this into Eq. (5-24d), we obtain

$$NTU = \int_{y_{in}}^{y_{out}} \frac{dy}{[y_{ad,\,in} - \left(1 - \dfrac{M}{eC}\right) y - \dfrac{M}{eC} y_{out}]}$$

$$= \frac{1}{\left[\dfrac{M}{eC} - 1\right]} \ln \left[y_{ad,in} - \left(1 - \frac{M}{eC}\right) y - \frac{M}{eC} y_{out} \right] \Big|_{y_{in}}^{y_{out}} \qquad (5\text{-}26)$$

The usual specifications are $y_{ad,in}$ and $x_{product}$. Since the product is melted to produce reflux,

$$y_{in} = x_{product} \qquad (5\text{-}27a)$$

Since the crystals are pure, the product concentration is related to material leaving the crystallizer by

$$x_{product} = \frac{eC \, y_{ads,out}}{C \, (1 + e)} \qquad (5\text{-}27b)$$

From this equation we can determine $y_{ads,out}$. We can then determine y_{out} from an external balance around the crystallizer. With pure crystals this is

$$y_{out} = \frac{eC}{M} (y_{ad,in} - y_{ad,out}) + y_{in} \qquad (5\text{-}27c)$$

These calculations give us the limits needed to determine NTU.

Use of this analysis requires an estimate of the amount of melt adhering to the liquid. It also requires an estimate of HTU. In column crystallizers there is considerable mixing and dispersion which is not included in this analysis. More detailed analyses and comparison with experiments (Albertins *et al.*, 1967; Meyer and Shen, 1970) show that an effective dispersion coefficient should be included in the expression for HTU. Since the analysis is linear, this is mathematically valid. The analysis developed here can be used with the proviso that ka must be determined from experimental crystallization data, or that the HTU must be based on experimental data. In some small crystallizers purifying a eutectic a total HTU of 12.3 cm was measured while a solid solution had an HTU of 3.3 cm. (Albertins *et al.*, 1967).

The analysis of center feed columns is much more complex. Flow rates are not constant. The column is not adiabatic. Usually solid solutions are separated and the crystal composition plus the adhering melt must be considered. This analysis is beyond the scope of this book.

5.3. CONTINUOUS SOLID PHASE

Entrained melt can drastically decrease the purity when we desire to ultrapurify (see Example 5-1). Entrainment is a problem with slurry processes because of the very large surface area of the crystals. Entrainment can be drastically decreased by operating with a continuous solid phase (a single ingot) since there is very little surface area. Of course, reducing the surface area also decreases mass transfer rates. Thus the continuous solid phase systems are used only when ultrapurity (e.g. 99.9+%) is required.

A variety of clever methods for melt crystallization with a continuous solid phase have been developed (Henry and Moyers, 1984; Keller and Muhlbauer, 1981; Moyers and Rousseau, 1987; Pfann, 1966; Wilcox and Estrin, 1982; Zief and Wilcox, 1967; Zief, 1969). The two main variants, normal freezing and zone melting, will be discussed.

5.3.1. Normal Freezing

Normal or progressive freezing is a process in which a melt is slowly frozen in such a way that a single solid ingot is formed. It is desirable to form a flat

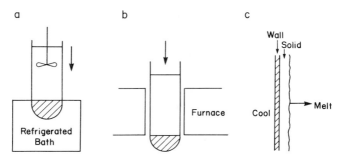

Figure 5-7.   Normal freezing. a. Refrigerated. b. Heated. c. On wall of heat exchanger.

interface since the entrainment of melt will be greatly reduced. Two ways to do this in the laboratory are shown in Figure 5-7 a and b. The melt is slowly lowered into a refrigerated bath or removed from a furnace so that a single solid ingot forms. The rate of movement is a few cm/hour or less. More rapid movement of the container causes the growth of crystals with facets or dendrites. These greatly increase the entrainment of melt and decrease the purity. Stirring of the melt will help remove impurity from the interface. The process can be done on the wall of a heat exchanger as shown in Figure 5-7c. The planar interface grows slowly into the melt. Laboratory equipment is discussed by Wilcox and Estrin (1982), Zief and Wilcox (1967), and Wynne and Zief (1967).

The geometry can be changed significantly. The freezing process can be done horizontally or from the walls of the container into the center. Further purification can be obtained by partial melting and draining of the ingot. For the system shown in Figure 5-7a the tube would be turned upside down and slowly warmed to achieve partial melting and drainage.

A variety of phenomena can reduce the separation (Wilcox, 1969). A completely planar interface is desired. If back diffusion of the impurity into the melt is slow, impurity will become concentrated at the interface. This change in impurity concentration causes a change in freezing point. At the interface the freezing point is lowest since impurity concentration is highest. Although the temperature increases as one moves into the melt (the melt is heated), the

185

increase in freezing point may be quicker. Then the melt will be supercooled a short distance from the interface. If this occurs, the interface can break down and structures such as grooved cells or dendrites will form which can trap melt. The result will be a large increase in the impurity level. The solutions to this problem are to freeze slowly and to stir the melt. Other phenomena which can adversely affect normal freezing are adsorption of impurity, variations in the freezing rate, and gas bubbles trapped at the interface.

A commercial progressive freezing process was developed by Proabd (Molinari, 1967a). Proabd observed that naphthalene in drums was always purer near the walls than in the center of the drum. This can be explained as a normal freezing process. The drum is filled with molten naphthalene. As it sets in the warehouse the drum slowly cools. The naphthalene freezes first along the walls and excluded impurities collect in the still molten center. Proabd used this observation to develop his process. The commercial equipment consists of a tank filled with finned tube heat exchangers. The charge is slowly cooled and most or all of it is frozen. The cooling rate is carefully controlled to prevent growth of dendrites and to maximize the segregation of impurity. The charge is slowly reheated and melt is drained from the vessel. The first melt is the most impure. As melting continues the melt becomes purer and purer. A variety of fractions can be collected. The Proabd process is available from BEFS Technologies (Mulhouse, France) and 31 plants have been installed mainly for purification of coal derived chemicals such as naphthalene and anthracene (Anon, 1988).

Another commercial process which is essentially a normal freezing process followed by partial melting and drainage is the MWB process developed by Sulzer Bros. Ltd. (Saxer and Papp, 1980). In this process the melt is slowly frozen on the inside of long vertical tubes. A thickness of product from 5 to 20 mm is built up during this normal freezing step. The system is then heated to slightly above the melting point to partially melt the crystals. The drainage which is high in impurity is stored. Then the entire crystal mass is melted and drained off. A new charge is then fed to the crystallizer and the process is repeated. The products from each step are stored separately and fed at different steps in the cycle to simulate a 3 to 5 stage countercurrent process. A variety of organics such as naphthalene, benzoic acid and fatty acids (with a solvent present) are commercially separated in 20 plants worldwide using this equipment (Anon, 1988).

The analysis for normal freezing is essentially the same as for the progressive freezing of crystals in a batch system, Eqs. (5-10) to (5-14). Melting and drainage are described by Eqs. (5-15) to (5-23). Since application of these equations to normal freezing is straight forward, no further amplification will be given. More detailed theories are discussed by Wilcox (1967).

5.3.2. Zone Melting

Zone melting is a technique for purification by melt crystallization. The method can be understood by referring to Figure 5-8a. An ingot of solid is heated locally so that a portion melts. As the heater is slowly moved along the bar, the molten zone also moves. At point m the solid melts while at f the crystal freezes. If impurity is excluded from the solid, $k_i < 1$, the impurity will concentrate in the molten zone. As this zone moves the impurity is swept to the ends of the bar. If any impurity has $k_i > 1$, it will concentrate at the other end of the bar. Thus the center of the bar may be the purest. Additional passes of the molten zone will sweep more and more impurity to the ends of the bar. The result is eventually an purification of most of the ingot.

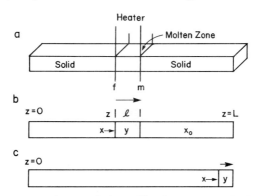

Figure 5-8.   Zone Melting. a. Schematic of apparatus, b. Bar when $z < L - l$, c. Bar when $z > L - l$.

This method has been extensively studied and used for ultrapurification of a wide variety of materials. Zone melting was invented by Pfann, and has since been extensively reviewed (Pfann, 1966; Wilcox and Estrin, 1982; Keller and Muhlbauer, 1981; Mullin, 1972; Zief, 1967, 1969; Zief and Wilcox, 1967; Shoemaker and Smith, 1967; Wynne, 1967; Moates and Kennedy, 1967). The method is easily automated in the laboratory for routine ultra purification. A home-made unit is sketched by Hudgins (1971), while more complicated units are discussed by Pfann (1966) and Wynne and Zief (1967). The process is routinely used for ultrapurification of materials particularly semiconductors. Between 100 and 200 metric tons of floating zone silicon single crystals are produced every year (Keller and Muhlbauer, 1981). Although the scale of operation is small compared to most other chemical engineering separations, the economic value is significant.

A large number of variations have been developed. For instance, it is easy to see that multiple zones can be used instead of the single zone shown in Figure 5-8a. Operation is often done vertically instead of horizontally. A wide variety of container materials and shapes are used. In fact, the container can be entirely removed in the floating zone method (Keller and Muhlbauer, 1981; Pfann, 1966; Wynne, 1967). This technique is almost necessary for materials melting above 1400°C. The ingot can be moved instead of the heaters. Continuous methods have also been developed (Pfann, 1966; Moates and Kennedy, 1967).

A variety of heating sources can be used. Below about 500°C electrical resistance heating is both convenient and inexpensive. For metals and semiconductors induction heating is useful since the container does not have to be heated. Induction heating also provides stirring of the molten zone which increases separation. Radio frequency (RF) induction heating is used for large-scale floating zone purification of silicon (Keller and Muhlbauer, 1981).

Since zone refining is used for ultrapurification, the initial charge is usually 99 wt % or more pure. The zone velocity can range from 0.1 to over 100 cm/hr. Typical values are 1 cm/hr for organics, 2.5 cm/hr for metals and 20 cm/hr for semiconductors (Henry and Moyers, 1984). Purification is higher at lower movement rates. Multiple zone passes are usually employed. Compounds purified by zone melting are surveyed by Shoemaker and Smith (1967) and Zief (1967).

The separation phenomena occurring in zone melting are very similar to those in normal freezing. Too rapid movement of the zone can cause the formation of dendrities or crystallite facets. This drastically decreases the separation. Dendrite growth is also a significant problem if impurity concentration is beyond one percent or so. Mixing helps to decrease these problems. Perhaps the major advantage of zone melting compared to normal freezing is the ease of using multiple zones. This allows many simultaneous passes of the molten zone and significantly increases the separation.

The molten zone should be stirred to mix the zone and increase mass transfer rates. For low temperature compounds a mechanical stirrer can be inserted in the zone. Care must be taken to avoid contamination. Induction stirring is convenient since it can be done as part of the heating. Electrical conductors can be stirred magnetically. Low melting point compounds can be stirred by pumping melt through an external heat exchanger.

The equilibrium analysis of batch zone melting is similar to that for normal freezing. The heater and hence the molten zone moves at a constant rate of f cm/min. We can relate f to the solidification rate dm/dt in kg/min as,

$$A_c \rho_c f = dm/dt \qquad (5\text{-}28a)$$

Note that dm/dt is also the rate at which the molten zone moves in kg/min. Since the linear zone movement rate f is kept constant, dm/dt is constant. Since tf = z, from Eq. (5-28a) and a mass balance

$$\frac{(dm/dt)t}{M_0} = \frac{z}{l} \qquad (5\text{-}28b)$$

where l is the length of solid melted to form the zone, and M_0 is the kg of melt in the molten zone (check the units on Eq. (5-28b) to understand it better). Differentiating Eq. (5-28b) we obtain

$$dt = \frac{M_0}{(dm/dt)l} \, dz \qquad (5\text{-}28c)$$

which will be useful to simplify the mass balance.

The solute mass balance must be done in two parts. First, consider Figure 5-8b where $z < L - l$. The mass balance is

$$\frac{dm}{dt}(x_0 - x) = M_0 \frac{dy}{dt} \qquad (5\text{-}29)$$

where x and y are the impurity weight fractions. If we assume that the zone is well mixed and that the freezing interface is in equilibrium with the melt, we can use the equilibrium expression $y = x/k$ in Eq. (5-29). Substituting in Eq. (5-28c) we obtain

$$\frac{k}{l}(x_0 - x) = \frac{dx}{dz}, \quad z < L - l \qquad (5\text{-}30a)$$

Before the start of the operation, $x = x_0$ for all z. When the first part is melted, $y = x_0$ (the melting interface is not in equilibrium with the melt). Then the first material refrozen is in equilibrium with y, or $x = ky = kx_0$. Thus the boundary condition is

$$x = kx_0, \quad z = 0 \qquad (5\text{-}30b)$$

The solution to Eqs. (5-30a,b) is

$$\frac{x}{x_0} = 1 - (1 - k)e^{-kz/l} \qquad (5\text{-}31)$$

During the end of the zone pass when $z > L - l$, the situation is shown in Figure 5-8c. Now the mass balance is

$$-\left[\frac{dm}{dt}\right]x = \frac{d(My)}{dt} \qquad (5\text{-}32)$$

since the size of the zone is shrinking. Note that Eqs. (5-32) and (5-10) are the same. The final step is essentially a normal freezing. Equations (5-11c) and (5-11d) can be used to write the equation in terms of g. Then Eq. (5-32) simplifies to Eq. (5-12a). The solution will be given by Eq. (5-13),

$$x = y_0 \, k(1-g)^{k-1}, \quad z \geq L - l \qquad (5\text{-}13)$$

190

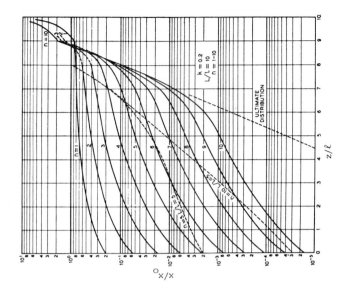

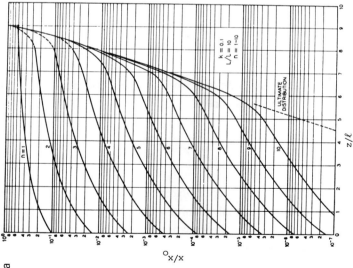

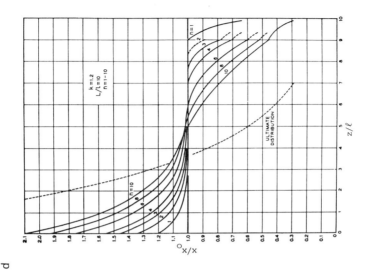

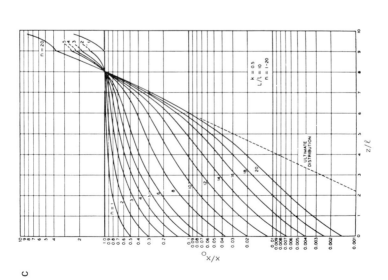

Figure 5-9. Relative solute concentration versus dimensionless zone length. n is the number of zone passes (Pfann, 1966). Reprinted with permission from Pfann, Zone Melting, 2nd ed., Wiley, N.Y., 1966. Copyright 1966, Wiley.

where y_0 is the concentration of the molten zone when the normal freezing starts. The value of y_0 can be found from Eq. (5-31) with $z = L - l$

$$y_0 = \frac{x}{k} = \frac{x_0}{k}[1 - (1 - k)e^{-k(L - l)/l}] \qquad (5\text{-}33)$$

When $z > L - l$, the parameter g is related to z by

$$g = \frac{z - (L - l)}{l} \qquad (5\text{-}34)$$

These results are for a single pass. For the next zone pass, x_0 in Eqs. (5-29) and (5-30a) is the x from the previous zone pass. Thus x_0 will be given by Eqs. (5-31) and (5-13). This makes Eqs. (5-29) and (5-30a) considerably more complicated. These equations have been solved numerically. This solution is shown in Figure 5-9 (Pfann, 1966) (see also Problem 5-E1).

Equation (5-31) and Figure 5-9 show that for $k < 1.0$ the purest material is at the starting end of the bar. Separation improves as k and zone length l decrease. As the number of passes n increases the separation becomes better. As $n \to \infty$ an "ultimate distribution" results. The ultimate distribution is approached when (Wilcox and Estrin, 1982)

$$n \geq 2(\frac{L}{l}) + 1 \qquad (5\text{-}35)$$

It appears that one would want to decrease l and do a lot of passes. Unfortunately, l is limited by heat transfer to a minimum of approximately the diameter of the rod. Usually, L/l is in the range from 4 to 10.

The purified ingot is usually harvested by cutting off the end of the bar. If some impurities have $k > 1$, both ends of the rod can be cut off. The resulting average composition is

$$x_{avg} = \frac{\displaystyle\int_{z_1}^{z_2} x \, dz}{(z_2 - z_1)} \qquad (5\text{-}36)$$

where z_1 and z_2 are the locations where the ends are cut off. If all $k_i < 1$ and the front end is not removed, then $z_1 = 0$. For a single pass x is given by Eqs. (5-31) and/or (5-13). If $z_2 < L - l$, the result for a single pass is

$$x_{avg} = x_0 \left[\frac{l\,(1-k)}{k\,(z_2 - z_1)} \left(e^{-z_2 k/l} - e^{-z_1 k/l} \right) + 1 \right] \tag{5-37}$$

For multiple passes the numerical solution for x (e.g. Figure 5-9) can be substituted into Eq. (5-36). The integration can then be done numerically. This is illustrated in Example 5-2.

This equilibrium analysis ignores mass transfer resistance and poor mixing in the molten zone. An effective distribution constant k_{eff} can be used instead of k to include mass transfer effects. When the film theory for mass transfer is solved, the value of k_{eff} is (Pfann, 1966),

$$k_{eff} = \frac{1}{1 + \left[\dfrac{1}{k} - 1 \right] e^{-f\delta/D}} \tag{5-38}$$

where δ is the film thickness, D is the diffusivity of impurity in the melt, and f is the linear freezing rate in cm/sec. δ/D is the mass transfer coefficient. Although δ is not known it can be measured by experiments. D can also be measured and usually lies in the range from 10^{-5} to 10^{-4} cm^2/sec. The value of δ was estimated as 0.1 cm in a horizontal zone of volume 1 cubic inch when mixing was caused by natural convection. With moderate stirring δ was estimated as 0.01 cm while with vigorous stirring δ was estimated as 0.001 cm (Pfann, 1966). These values can be used to estimate the actual separation. Wilcox (1967) lists experimental values of δ for both zone melting and normal freezing. More detailed theories are discussed by Wilcox (1967). Detailed analyses of the hydrodynamics and mass transfer during single crystal growth are reviewed by Brown (1988).

Example 5-2. Normal Freezing and Zone Melting

A bar of tin (Sn) contains 0.002 wt fraction indium (In).

a. If normal freezing is done and 75% of the tin is frozen, calculate the average crystal concentration.

b. Zone melting is done with one pass and $L/l = 10$. If the bar is cut at $z_2 = 0.75$ L, find the average product concentration.

c. Zone melting is done with ten passes and $L/l = 10$. If the bar is then cut at $z_2 = 0.75$ L, estimate the average product concentration.

Solution

A. Define. Three separate problems as delineated in the problem statement.

B. Explore. Part a is simple use of Eq. (5-14). Part b is use of Eq. (5-37) since $z_2 = 0.75$ L $< L - l = 0.9$L. Part c requires the numerical integration of Eq. (5-36).

C. Plan. Parts a and b were explained in the Explore step. For part c the numerical integration can be done in several ways. For example, with equal increments of size Δz,

$$x_{avg} = \frac{1}{z_2} \sum_{i=1}^{} x\left[z = \frac{i\Delta z}{2}\right]\Delta z$$

D. Do It. (a) For normal freezing Eq. (5-14) becomes

$$x_{avg} = \frac{y_0}{g}[1-(1-g)^k] = \frac{0.002}{0.75}[1-(0.25)^{0.5}] = 0.001333$$

(b) One pass zone melting. Eq. (5-37) becomes,

$$x_{avg} = x_0 [\frac{(1-k)l}{k(z_2-z_1)} (e^{-z_2 k/l} - e^{-z_1 k/l}) + 1]$$

Since $z_2 = 0.75L$, $z_1 = 0$, $L/l = 10$, $k = 0.5$, this is

$$x_{avg} = 0.002[\frac{(0.5)(0.1)}{(0.5)(0.75)} (e^{-0.75(10)(0.5)} - 1) + 1] = 0.00174$$

(c) Ten pass zone melting. If we do a numerical integration with $\Delta z_1 = \Delta z_2 = \Delta z_3 = .2$, and $\Delta z_4 = .15$, then the numerical calculation is,

$$x_{avg} = \frac{x_0}{0.75} \{0.2[x(\frac{z}{l}=1) + x(\frac{z}{l}=3) + x(\frac{z}{l}=5)] + 0.15x(\frac{z}{l}=6.75)\}$$

$$= \frac{(0.002}{0.75})[0.2(0.041 + 0.11 + 0.22) + 0.15(0.43)] = 0.00037$$

where the x values were determined from Figure 5-9.

E. Check. The normal freezing results can be checked by calculating x at $g = 0.75$. Then $y = x/k$ and the check is the mass balance

$$(0.75 \, x_{avg}) + 0.25 \, y = x_0 \ .$$

Unfortunately, the check is more work than the original calculation. The zone melting calculations are more difficult to check. The numerical integration can be checked by doing the integration with a different method. For example, using Simpson's rule (e.g. see Mickley *et al*, 1957)

$$x_{avg} = \frac{\frac{(z_2 - z_1)}{6} \left[x|_{z_1} + 4 \, x|_{(z_1 + z_2)/2} + x|_{z_2} \right]}{z_2 - z_1} \tag{5-39}$$

we obtain

$$x_{avg} = \frac{(0.75/6)(0.002)[0.0021 + 4(0.15) + 0.70]}{0.75} = 0.00044$$

where 0.0021 is x/x_0 at $z/l = 0$, 0.15 is x/x_0 at $z/l = 3.75$, and 0.70 is x/x_0 at $z/l = 7.5$. This disagrees with the other integration. The reason for this disagreement is the extreme sensitivity of the calculation to the amount of impurity near $z = 0.75$ L. Better agreement would be obtained by applying Simpson's rule in several steps.

F. Generalization. One perhaps surprising result is that normal freezing gives a better separation than one pass zone melting. This is generally true. The two methods become equal when $L/l = 1$. When the zone length equals the ingot length, zone melting becomes a normal freezing method. With additional passes zone melting produces a significantly better separation than normal freezing. Since the concentrated end of the bar has a major effect on the average purity level, particularly for small k_i, a small grid should be used for the numerical integration at this end.

5.4. SUMMARY-OBJECTIVES

This chapter has been a brief introduction to melt crystallization. At the end of this chapter you should be able to:

1. Discuss the effect of heat and mass transfer in melt crystallization.

2. Do equilibrium calculations for continuous and batch crystallizers including the effect of progressive freezing.

3. Do equilibrium calculations for partial melting and drainage.

4. Explain column crystallization systems and do mass transfer calculations for end feed columns.

5. Explain and do equilibrium calculations for normal freezing.

6. Explain and do equilibrium calculations for zone melting.

REFERENCES

Albertins, R., W.C. Gates, and J.E. Powers, "Column crystallization," in M. Zief and W.R. Wilcox, (Eds.), *Fractional Solidification,* Vol. I, Marcel Dekker, New York, 1967, 343-367.

Alper, A.M. (Ed.), *Phase Diagrams, Material Science and Technology,* Academic Press, New York, Vols. 1 to 5, 1970-78.

Anon., "CPI warms up to freeze concentration," *Chem. Engr., 95,* (6), 24 (April 25, 1988).

Brown, R.A., "Theory of transport processes in single crystal growth from the melt," *AIChE Journal, 34,* 881 (1984).

Hanson, M., *Constitution of Binary Alloys,* 2nd ed., McGraw-Hill, New York, 1958.

Henry, J.D. and C.G. Moyers, Jr., "Crystallization from the melt," in R.H. Perry, and D.W. Green, (Eds.), *Perry's Chemical Engineer's Handbook,* 6th ed., McGraw-Hill, New York, 1984, p. 17-3 to 17-12.

Hudgins, R.R., "Zone Refining. A student experiment," *Chem. Engr. Educ., 5,* 138, (Summer, 1971).

Keller, W. and A. Muhlbauer, *Floating-Zone Silicon,* Marcel Dekker, New York, 1981.

Landolt-Börnstein, *Zahlenwerte und Funktionen,* Vol. 2, Pts. a,b,c, Vol. 3, Springer, Berlin, 1956.

Levin, E.M., C.R. Robbins, and H.F. McMurdie, *Phase Diagrams for Ceramists,* American Ceramic Society, Columbus, Ohio, 1964 and 1969.

McKay, D.L., "Phillips fractional-solidification process," in M. Zief, and W.R.

198

Wilcox (Eds.), *Fractional Solidification*, Vol. I., Marcel Dekker, New York, 196?, 427-439.

Meyer, W. and P.K. Shen, "Design models for separation of eutectic systems by continuous countercurrent columnar crystallization," AIChE Meeting, Chicago, Nov. 29, 1970.

Moates, G.H. and J.K. Kennedy, "Continuous-zone melting," in M. Zief and W.R. Wilcox (Eds.), *Fractional Solidification*, Marcel Dekker, New York, 1967, 273-342.

Molinari, J.G.D., "The Proabd refiner," in M. Zief and W.R. Wilcox (Eds.), *Fractional Solidification*, Vol. I, Marcel Dekker, New York, 1967a, 393-400.

Moyers, C.G., Jr. and R.W. Rousseau, "Crystallization operations," in R.W. Rousseau (Ed.), *Handbook of Separation Process Technology*, Wiley, 1987, Chapt. 11.

Molinari, J.G.D., "Newton Chambers' process", in M. Zief and W.R. Wilcox (Eds.), *Fractional Solidification*, Vol. I., Marcel Dekker, New York, 1967b, 401-407.

Mullin, J.W., *Crystallization*, 2nd ed., CRC Press, Boca Raton, FL, 1972.

Pfann, W.F., *Zone Melting*, 2nd ed., Wiley, New York, 1966.

Rhines, N.F., *Phase Diagrams in Metallurgy*, McGraw-Hill, New York, 1956.

Saxer, K. and A. Papp, "The MWB crystallization process," *Chem. Eng. Prog.*, 76 (4), 64 (1980).

Shoemaker, C.E. and R.L. Smith, "Survey of inorganic materials," in M. Zief and W.R. Wilcox (Eds.), *Fractional Solidification*, Vol. I., Marcel Dekker, New York, 1967, 624-648.

Walas, S.M., *Phase Equilibria in Chemical Engineering*, Butterworth Pub., Boston, 1985, Chapt. 8.

199

Wilcox, W.R., "Mass transfer in fractional solidification", in M. Zief and W.R. Wilcox (Eds.), *Fractional Solidification*, Marcel Dekker, New York, 1967, 47-112.

Wilcox, W.R., "Fractional solidification phenomena," *Separ. Sci., 4,* 95 (1969).

Wilcox, W.R. and J. Estrin, "Crystallization and precipitation," in P.J. Elving, E. Grushka, and I.M. Kolthoff (Eds.), *Treatise on Analytical Chemistry,* Part I, Vol. 5, 2nd ed., Wiley-Interscience, New York, 1982, Chapt. 8, 281-370.

Wynne, E.A., "Batch zone melting," in M. Zief and W.R. Wilcox (Eds.), *Fractional Solidification,* Marcel Dekker, New York, 1967, 237-255.

Wynne, E.A. and M. Zief, "Laboratory scale apparatus," in M. Zief and W.R. Wilcox (Eds.), *Fractional Solidification,* Vol. 1, Marcel Dekker, New York, 1967, 191-236.

Zief, M. and W.R. Wilcox (Eds.), *Fractional Solidification,* Vol. I., Marcel Dekker, New York, 1967.

Zief, M., "Survey of organic materials," in M. Zief and W.R. Wilcox (Eds.) *Fractional Solidification,* Vol. I, Marcel Dekker, New York, 1967, 649-678.

Zief, M., (Ed.) *Purification of Inorganic and Organic Materials,* Marcel Dekker, New York, 1969.

HOMEWORK

A.	*Discussion Problems*

A1.	Construct a table contrasting and comparing solution and melt crystallization.

A2.   Suppose $k_i < 1$ in Eq. (5-7). What effect does the flow rate of melt, M, have on the purity of the crystals? What happens in the limit as $M = 0$? What happens if $k_i = 0$ and $M = 0$? Discuss this from both physical and mathematical viewpoints.

A3.   Explain the process of progressive freezing followed by partial melting and drainage in physical terms. Why is $x_{Avg,2}$ given by Eq. (5-20)? One could calculate y_{avg} as

$$y_{avg} = \frac{\int_{g_2+\delta g}^{g_2} x\, dg}{\delta g} \qquad (5\text{-}21a)$$

where $\delta g = eg_2$ instead of using Eq. (5-21). Explain Eq. (5-21a) physically. Does (Eq. (5-21) or Eq. (5-21a) predict a purer product?

A4.   Why do batch slurry crystallization and normal freezing give the same result for crystal composition? What are the advantages and disadvantages of each process?

A5.   What are the advantages of zone melting compared to normal freezing?

A6.   Construct your key relations chart for this chapter.

B.   *Generation of Alternatives*

B1.   A series of batch crystallizers can be cascaded to increase both yield and purity. Explore various ways to do this. Try not to produce any product streams of intermediate purity. (In other words, produce only a high purity product and a concentrated waste stream.)

B2.   We wish to purify pyrene which contains 0.8 wt % anthracene and 0.2 wt % 1,2-benzanthracene as impurities. A batch normal freezing apparatus is available. Develop a process to do this purification.

C.   *Derivations*

C1.   Develop the analysis procedure for a staged counter-current cascade for a binary melt crystallization system which forms a solid solution. The cascade will be similar to Figure 2-20. Plot enthalpy (both liquid and solid) as the ordinate versus mole fraction in both the liquid and solid phases. This is similar to Figure 2-21 with enthalpy replacing N. A plot of mole fraction in the liquid versus mole fraction in the solid (a McCabe-Thiele plot) is useful to obtain equilibrium tie lines. Develop the Δ points using two mass balances and the energy balance.

C2.   Single stage, batch crystallization can be treated in the same way as simple Rayleigh batch distillation. That is, assume that crystals are removed as soon as they are formed. Set up and solve the equation equivalent to the Rayleigh equation. Assume that $y = x/k$. Show that the results are the same as Eqs. (5-13) and (5-14).

C3.   The mass fraction impurity of the crystals for a single stage, steady state, continuous crystallizer is given by Eq. (5-6). a). If a weight fraction, e, of melt is entrained, find the average product concentration. b). If some fraction of the crystals are melted (fraction > e) and the excess liquid is drained, find the new product concentration.

C4.   Derive Eq. (5-28b). Explain why l is defined as the length of solid melted to form the zone instead of as the length of the heater.

C5.   Derive Eq. (5-37).

D.   *Problems*

D1.   A continuous single-stage, steady-state, equilibrium crystallizer is crystallizing 2-naphthol containing 0.007 wt frac naphthalene. Data in Table 5-1.

   a. If we crystallize 60% of the feed, calculate the concentration of the crystals and the concentration of the melt. Assume there is no entrainment.

b. If 9% by weight of melt is entrained with the crystals calculate the average product concentration.

D2. One hundred kilograms of a benzene mixture containing 0.45 wt % cyclohexane is purified in a batch crystallizer. We freeze 72% of the original charge and filter the crystals. Entrainment is 0.06 wt fraction. Data are in Table 5-1.

a. What is the product concentration?

b. If we melt 15% of the crystals and drain off the melt, find the new product concentration. Entrainment is unchanged.

D3. We are purifying naphthalene in a commercial batch crystallizer that functions as a normal freezer. The naphthalene charge is 1000 kg and is 99.87 wt % naphthalene. The impurity is unknown. If one half of the initial charge is frozen and the crystals are sampled (after centrifuging to remove melt), we find the average weight fraction is 99.93 wt % naphthalene. If we melt off and drain 125 kg of crystals, we find that the purity of the product (including entrained melt) increased to 99.932 wt % naphthalene. Find k_i and e.

D4. We wish to purify pyrene containing 0.005 wt fraction anthracene and 0.005 fraction 1,2-benzanthracene.

a. If we freeze 70% of the initial charge in a batch stirred tank, and collect the crystals plus entrained melt (assume e = 0.09), what is the product concentration?

b. If we freeze 70% of the initial charge, remove excess melt, and then melt and drain off another 15% ($\Delta g = 0.15$) of the melt, what is the concentration of the collected product (crystals plus entrained melt) for e = 0.09?

c. The product from part b is melted and then reprocessed by freezing 30% of the product and collecting crystals plus entrained melt (e = 0.09). What is the concentration of the non-entrained melt? What fraction of the original feed is collected as non-entrained melt?

Equilibrium data is in Table 5-1.

D5. We are purifying an unknown impurity from azobenzene in a screw-type, end-feed, counter-current column crystallizer. The azobenzene system is a eutectic system (crystals are pure azobenzene). The HTU was estimated as 12.3 cm and entrainment as e = 0.12. M/C = 0.13. The crystals enter after leaving a crystallizer where the melt contains 0.009 wt fraction impurity. The final product (crystals plus entrained melt) should contain 0.00002 wt fraction impurity. The final product is melted and some of this is refluxed. Find the crystallizer length required.

D6. Repeat Parts a and b of Example 5-2 except do not assume equilibrium. For the molten metal assume $D \sim 3 \times 10^{-5}$ cm^2/s. Calculate the separation for natural convection ($\delta \sim 0.1$ cm), moderate stirring ($\delta = .01$ cm) and vigorous stirring ($\delta = 0.001$ cm). The linear rate of movement of the zone is f = 2.5 cm/hr.

D7. We wish to use zone melting to purify 99.8% pure (wt. %) anthracene containing fluorene as it's only impurity. A zone melting system with the zone length 1/10 of the ingot length is used. Data are in Table 5-1.

a. After 6 passes, 20% of the ingot is cut off and discarded. Calculate the average composition of fluorene in the ingot.

b. Predict the weight fraction fluorene at z/L = 0.95 after one pass.

D8. Zone melting is done to purify an aluminum bar containing 0.003 wt frac scandium (Sc) as an impurity. The zone melting has $L/l = 10$. After n passes we cut off 20% of the rod. We desire an average impurity weight fraction of 0.00003 or less. How many passes are required? What is the actual average wt frac impurity in the bar? What are the highest and lowest impurity wt fracs in the bar? Assume equilibrium operation. Use Figure 5-9 to estimate the solutions. Data are in Table 5-1.

E. *More Complex Problems*

E1. Repeat Problem 5-D8 except solve Eqs. (5-28) to (5-34) and Eq. (5-36) by numerical integration for $L/l = 10$ and k = 0.17. Assume the molten zone is completely mixed. Note that the boundary condition equivalent to Eq. (5-30b) for passes 2 to n should include melting a length l of the bar, mixing the zone, and crystallizing a solid at $z = 0$. Thus boundary condition is

$$x_{j+1} = k\ x_{j,\text{avg from } z=0 \text{ to } z=l} \qquad\qquad z = 0$$

where j is the number of the pass.

F.   *Problems Requiring Other Resources*

F1.   A laboratory zone melting apparatus is being used to ultrapurify naphthalene. The apparatus is 1 cm wide and 1 cm deep. The heater moves at 1.1 cm/hr. The melt temperature is measured to be 84.55°C. Estimate the overall heat transfer coefficient U between the solid and the melt.

Part II

SORPTION AND CHROMATOGRAPHY

NOMENCLATURE CHAPTERS 6 TO 10

a, b	constants in Langmuir Eqs. (6-12) and (6-13) or constants in Eq. (6-15) or (6-18).
a_i	activities, Chapter 9.
a_p	external surface area/volume, m^2/m^3
A	van Deemter eddy dispersion term, Eq. (7-39)
A(T)	equilibrium parameter, Eq. (6-4) or (8-17b)
A_c	cross sectional area of column, m^2
A_{hole}	cross-sectional area of hole in sieve plate
A_o	preexponential constant, Eq. (6-4b)
A_w	wall area for heat transfer, m^2
b	equilibrium constant, Eq. (10-15)
b, b$'$	constants in quadratic Eqs. (9-22) and (9-24)
B	van Deemter molecular diffusion term, Eq. (7-40)
c	solute concentration of fluid, kg/m^3
c^*	equilibrium concentration
c_a	concentration after wave has passed
c_{change}	concentration changed by thermal wave, Eq. (6-39b)
c_E	equlibrium concentration
c_F	feed concentration
$c_{i,pore}$	concentration i in pore
c_i	normality, equivalents/m^3 in solution, Chapter 9
c_{max}	maximum concentration in peak

c_{R_i} concentration on resin, equivalents/m^3, in Chapter 9

c_T total equivalents/m^3 in solution, Chapter 9

C van Deemter mass transfer term, Eqs. (7-41)

$C_{P,f}$ heat capacity of fluid

$C_{P,s}$ heat capacity of solid

$C_{P,w}$ heat capacity of wall

d^* d_p/d_{ref}, Eq. (10-26b)

d_c coating thickness

d_p particle diameter, m

D column diameter, m

D_{eff} effective diffusivity, Eqs. (9-33) and (9-34)

D_m molecular diffusivity, cm^2/s

D_{mp} molecular diffusivity in pore

D_s surface diffusivity

D_T thermal diffusivity

e volume fraction particles in fluidized bed

erf   error function, Eqs. (7-11)

E_D eddy diffusivity, cm^2/s

E_{DT} thermal eddy diffusivity

F feed rate, L/min

F Faraday's constant, 96500 amp·sec/equiv

F_i moles of feed in pulse

g acceleration due to gravity

G	fluid flow rate, kg solute-free fluid/hr
G	mass velocity of gas
h	heat transfer coefficient across film, m/s
h	height of packing, m
h_p	lumped parameter particle heat transfer coefficient
h_w	wall heat transfer coefficient
H	height equivalent to a theoretical stage, m
HTU	height of transfer unit, Eq. (10-12c)
ΔH	heat of adsorption
j	stage number
J_i	total flux
$J_{i\,elec}$	flux due to electrical transference, Eq. (9-28)
$J_{i\,dif}$	diffusive flux
k'	relative retention or capacity factor, Eq. (7-32a)
k_1, k_{-1}	rate constants for adsorption and desorption in Langmuir expression, Eq. (6-5).
k_1, k_2	rate constants, Eq. (7-35)
k_2	constant, Eq. (6-5)
k_e	effective thermal diffusivity
k_f	film diffusion coefficient, m/s
k_m	lumped parameter mass transfer coefficient
k_s	surface diffusion coefficient
K	constant in pressure drop Eq. (8-23)

K	true equilibrium constant in Eqs. (9-8) and (9-13).
K	equilibrium constant in BET Eq. (6-10)
K_A	$= k_1/k_{-1}$ equilibrium constant in Langmuir expression, Eq. (6-6).
K_A^o	preexponential factor, Eq. (6-8)
K_{AB}	equilibrium constant or selectivity coefficient, Eqs. (9-10) and (9-11).
K_d	fraction of interparticle volume species can penetrate, Eq. (6-3).
K_{DB}	equilibrium constant for divalent-monovalent exchange, Eqs. (9-14) and (9-16b).
K_E	exclusion factor. Zero for excluded ions and 1.0 for non-excluded, Chapter 9.
K_i	Langmuir equilibrium constant for multicomponent system
l_p, l_{port}	length of travel of pulse, or packing height between ports, m
L	column length, m
L_{MTZ}	length of mass transfer zone in column, m
m	linear equilibrium constant
1/m	constant in LRC Eq. (6-11)
M_s	mass of stationary phase per stage
n	number of adsorbates
n	exponent in Eq. (10-32a)
n	constant in Eq. (7-44)
n	moles of gas
1/n	exponent in Freundlich isotherm, Eq. (6-14)
N	loading of molecular sieve, kg/kg adsorbent

N	number of stages
N_{max}	maximum loading
N_{Pe}	Peclet number based on d_p, Eq. (7-14b)
NTU	number of transfer units, Eq. (10-12c)
p	pressure, kPa.
$\bar{p}$	partial pressure of solute, kPa.
p_H	high pressure
p_L	low pressure
Pe_z	axial Peclet number, Eq. (7-12a)
P_1, P_2	product flow rates, m^3/min or kg/min
q	amount of solute adsorbed, kg/kg adsorbent
q_a	amount adsorbed after wave has passed
q^o	amount adsorbed from pure gas
q_s	$= q\,(R_p)$, surface adsorbate loading
$\bar{q}$	average amount adsorbed, Eq. (6-43b)
q^*	equilibrium amount adsorbed
q_{MAX}	monolayer coverage of adsorbent in Langmuir isotherm, Eq. (6-6), kg/kg adsorbent.
q_{mono}	amount adsorbed for monolayer coverage
q_{sat}	saturation capacity of adsorbent
Q	volumetric flow rate, m^3/min
r	radial direction
R	gas constant
R	resolution, Eq. (7-30)

R_N $(L/L_{MTZ})_{new}/(L(L_{MTZ})_{old}$

R_p $\Delta p_{new}/\Delta p_{old}$

R_p pore radius, m

R_T crossover ratio, Eq. (8-51)

Re   Reynold's number, $\varepsilon_e \, \rho_f \, vd_p/\mu$

S   solids flow rate, kg clean adsorbent plus fluid in pores/hr

Sc   Schmidt number, $\mu/\rho_f \, D_m$

Sh   Sherwood number, $k_f d_p/D_m$

t   time, min

$t_{A,band}$ bandwidth in displacement chromatography, min

t_{br} breakthrough time, Eq. (8-2)

t_{center} time center of breakthrough curve exits

t_F period of feed pulse, min

t_{MTZ} time for mass transfer zone to exit column, min

t_{NR} retention time of non-retained peak, min

t_p time between switching port locations, min

t_R retention time, min

T   temperature, °C or K

T^* equilibrium temperature

$\bar{T}, \bar{T}_s$ average temperatures, Eqs. (6-52)

T_a, T_b temperature after and before wave

T_C, T_H cold and hot temperatures

T_f, T_s temperature of fluid and solid

T_w, T_{ref}	temperature of wall and reference
u_A, u_B, u_s	solute wave velocity, m/min, Eqs. (6-23) or (6-24) .
u_{co-ion}	velocity of coion, Eq. (9-26b)
u_i	ionic mobility, Eq. (9-29)
u_{NC}	velocity of non-charged species, Eq. (9-26a)
u_p	pattern velocity
u_{pulse}	average pulse velocity, Eq. (10-10)
$u_{port,avg}$	average velocity port movement, Eq. (10-23)
$u_{s,cc}$	observed countercurrent solute velocity, Eq. (10-19)
u_{sh}	shock wave velocity m/min, Eq. (6-30).
u_{stm}	velocity of steam wave, Eq. (8-52)
u_{th}	thermal wave velocity m/min, Eq. (6-36).
$u_{total\ ion}$	ion wave velocity, Eq. (9-20).
v	interstitial fluid velocity, m/min
v^*	v/v_{ref}, Eq. (10-26b)
v_{hole}	velocity through hole in sieve plate
v_{mf}	minimum fluidization velocity, m/min
v_{solid}	superficial solid velocity, m/min
v_{super}	superficial fluid velocity, m/min
V	volume solution fed to column, m^3 or L.
$\overline{V}$	volume solution required to saturate column, Eqs. (7-12c) and (9-27b)
V_e	elution volume of non-adsorbed species, m^3 or L.
$V_{ec,feed}$	extracolumn volume on feed side, m^3, Eq. (8-32)

V_{Feed}	volume feed gas, m^3
V_F	volume feed pulse
V_i	internal void volume, m^3 or L
V_o	external void volume, m^3 or L
V_M	volume mobile phase/stage
V_{peak}	volume peak exits
V_{purge}	volume purge gas, m^3
V_R	volumetric flow rate resin, L/hr
V_S	volumetric flow rate solution, L/hr
Vp	vapor pressure
w_i	width of species i peak
W	weight of column wall per length, kg/m
x	see Eq. (7-47)
x	mole fraction in solid phase, Eq. (6-16),
x_E	equilibrium mass fraction in fluid
x_i	c_i/c_T, equivalent fraction ions in solution or c_A/c_{AF} in adsorption
X_A	general breakthrough solution
y	mole fraction in gas phase, Eq. (6-16)
y_E	equilibrium mass fraction on solid
y_i	$c_{R,i}/c_{R,tot}$, equivalent fraction ions on resin, Chapter 9.
y_{stm}	mole fraction water in steam
$y_{w,b}$	water mole fraction in vapor before steam wave
Y	mass ratio solute in fluid, kg solute/kg solute-free fluid

z	axial distance in column, m
z_i	valence of ion

Greek

α_{AB}	separation factor, Eq. (6-16)
α_{21}	A_2/A_1, selectivity
β_A	Eqs. (8-58)
β_i	empirical constant, Eq. (6-15)
γ	V_{purge}/V_{feed} in PSA
γ_i	activity coefficients, Eq. (9-9)
Δ	difference calculation
ε_e	external void fraction (between particles), Eq. (6-1a)
ε_p	intraparticle void fraction (within a particle), Eq. (6-1b)
ε_T	total porosity, Eq. (6-1c)
θ	fraction of surface covered by adsorbed solute
θ	$= t-z/v$, Eq. (7-47).
λ_W	latent heat of vaporization of water
μ	viscosity
v	see Eq. (7-53)
ρ_B	bulk particle density, kg/m^3, Eq. (6-2a)
ρ_f	fluid density, kg/m^3
ρ_p	particle density including fluid in pores, kg/m^3, Eq. (6-2b)
ρ_s	structural solid density, kg/m^3
σ	standard deviation, Eqs. (7-27).

σ_1,σ_2	Eqs. (7-37)
τ	tortuosity factor
τ	see Eq. (7-53)
τ	see Eq. (8-6)
ϕ	electrical potential
$\Phi_{i,j}$	parameter for calculation of mixture viscosity, Example 8-1
χ	see Eq. (7-53)
χ	volumetric fraction of swelled resin taken up by water

Chapter 6

BASICS OF SORPTION IN PACKED COLUMNS

What phenomena are involved in adsorptive and chromatographic separations? How do these phenomena combine to produce the desired separation? How can we simply predict the separation which will occur? In this chapter we will try to answer these and other questions.

Adsorption is a separation technique which uses a solid (the *adsorbent*) to adsorb a solute or *adsorbate* on its surface. Highly porous adsorbents with large surface areas are used. Usually, the adsorbent is held in a packed column as illustrated in Figure 6-1. This is a batch process consisting of a feed step followed by a desorption or regeneration step. The regeneration is done by increasing temperature, or dropping pressure, or using a chemical desorbent. Adsorption is used commercially for a wide variety of separations such as hydrogen purification, production of oxygen and nitrogen from air, drying gases and organic liquids, removal of pollutants from air and water, and purification of biochemicals. Various adsorption processes are discussed in detail in Chapter 8.

Chromatography is a similar separation process which is used for fractionating feeds into several components. A pulse of feed is injected into the column and the products are eluted with a carrier gas or solvent. The result is a series of separated peaks (for example, see Figure 7-1). Chromatography is most commonly used as an analytical method, but large scale chromatography is becoming a more common commercial method for sugar separations, in biotechnology and for purification of pharmaceuticals. Chromatographic separations are explored in detail in Chapter 7.

Ion exchange is a process where ions in solution are exchanged for ions held to a resin. The best known application is water softening where calcium

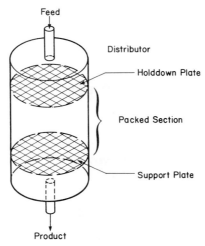

Figure 6-1.   Packed bed system.

and magnesium ions are removed and replaced with sodium ions. A variety of other ion exchange separations are also done commercially. The usual operation is done in fixed beds, and follows a cycle of load, regenerate and wash. Ion exchange is the subject of Chapter 9.

Adsorption, chromatography and ion exchange are also done commercially in moving beds, staged systems and simulated moving beds. These applications are explored in Chapter 10.

6.1. PACKING STRUCTURE

Commercially significant sorption operations (including adsorption, chromatography, ion exchange, ion exclusion, etc.) use solid particles (sorbents) which are highly porous and have large surface areas per gram of sorbent. The sorbent particles are commonly packed in a column as illustrated in Figure 6-1. In general the particles will be of different sizes and shapes. They will pack in the column and have an average interparticle (between different particles) porosity of ε_e. Since the particles are usually porous, each particle has an intraparticle (within the particle) porosity ε_p which is the fraction of the particle which is void space. The interparticle or extra particle porosity, ε_e, is defined as

$$\varepsilon_e = \frac{\text{volume between particles}}{\text{total volume of packed bed}} \tag{6-1a}$$

while the intraparticle or particle porosity, ε_p, is

$$\varepsilon_p = \frac{\text{volume of fluid inside all particles}}{\text{total volume of all particles (solid plus fluid)}} \tag{6-1b}$$

The total porosity, ε_T, of the bed is the sum of the voids within the particles and between particles.

$$\varepsilon_T = \varepsilon_e + (1 - \varepsilon_e)\,\varepsilon_p \tag{6-1c}$$

Note that all three porosities are dimensionless. The different porosities are shown in Figure 6-2.

In a poorly packed bed ε_e may vary considerably in different parts of the column. This can lead to poor flow distribution or channeling and will decrease the separation. If the solid particles are uniform, ε_p will be the same for all particles. Gel beads used for ion exchange have $\varepsilon_p = 0$ while 3 porosities can be defined for molecular sieves and some activated carbons.

Sorbents are provided in bulk. The bulk density ρ_B including the fluid in the pores and the fluid between particles is easy to determine. The bulk density

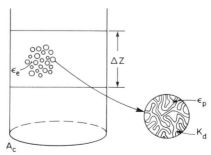

Figure 6-2.   Porosites in packed bed.

is related to the particle density ρ_P which includes the solid plus fluid in the pores.

$$\rho_B = (1-\varepsilon_e)\,\rho_P + \varepsilon_e\,\rho_f \qquad (6\text{-}2a)$$

The particle density can be estimated from the structural or crystalline density ρ_s which is the density of crushed and compressed solid containing no pores.

$$\rho_P = (1-\varepsilon_p)\rho_s + \varepsilon_p\,\rho_f \qquad (6\text{-}2b)$$

When supplied in bulk the fluid is usually air. Thus the fluid density, ρ_f, terms are often ignored in estimating ρ_P and ρ_s from ρ_B.

The pores are not of uniform size. Large molecules such as proteins or synthetic polymers may be sterically excluded from some of the pores. The fraction of volume of pores which a molecule can penetrate is called K_d. For a non-adsorbed species, K_d can be determined from

$$K_d = \frac{V_e - V_o}{V_i} \qquad (6\text{-}3)$$

where V_e is the elution volume, (that is the volume of fluid at which the species exits from the column), V_o is the external void volume between the particles, and V_i is the internal void volume. When the molecules are small and can penetrate the entire interparticle volume, $V_e = V_i + V_o$ and $K_d = 1.0$. When the molecules are large and can penetrate none of the interparticle volume, $V_e = V_o$ and $K_d = 0$. Exclusion phenomena are used commercially for separations. Examples are listed in Table 6-1. The zeolites are discussed in Section 6-2. Sephadex is a cross-linked dextran gel, Biogel P is a cross-linked polyacrylamide, Sepharose and Bio-gel A are cross-linked agarose gels. These are discussed in Chapter 7 and in more detail by Janson and Hedman (1982) for size exclusion chromatography (SEC). Styragel is a cross-linked polystyrene (Bidlingmeyer and Warren, 1988).

For the system shown in Figure 6-2, fluid containing solute flows in the void volume outside the particles. The processes which occur during a separation are as follows: (1) The solute diffuses through an external film to the particle. Here the solute may (2) sorb on the external surface or (3) (more likely)

Table 6-1. Separations using Steric Exclusion
(Collins, 1968; Janson and Hedman, 1982; Bidlingmeyer and Warren, 1988).

Packing	Molecules Included	Molecules Excluded	Typical Applications
3A Zeolite	H_2O, NH_3, He diameter <3 Å	CH_4, CO_2, C_2H_2, O_2, C_2H_5OH, H_2S diameter >3 Å	Drying cracked gas, ethylene, butadiene, and ethanol
4A Zeolite	H_2S, CO_2, C_3H_6, C_2H_5OH, C_4H_6 diameter <4 Å	C_3H_8, compressor oil diameter >4 Å	Drying natural gas, liquid paraffins, and solvents. CO_2 removal
5A Zeolite	n-Paraffins, n-olefins, n-C_4H_9OH diameter <5 Å	Iso-compounds, all 4 + carbon rings diameter >5 Å	n-Paraffin recovery from naphtha and kerosene
10X Zeolite	Iso-paraffins, iso-olefins diameter <8 Å	Di-n-butylamine and larger diameter >8 Å	Aromatic separation
13X Zeolite	Di-n-butylamine diameter <10 Å	$(C_4F_9)_3$-N diameter >10 Å	Desulfurization, simultaneous H_2O and CO_2 removal
Sephadex G-25	Salts, low MW compds <1000 to 5000	Proteins and compds >5000	Desalting-SEC
Bio-Gel P6	Salts, low MW compds <1000 to 6000	Proteins and compds >6000	Desalting-SEC
Sephadex G-50	<1500 to 30,000	>30,000	Insulin-SEC
Sephadex G-150	<5000 to 300,000	>300,000	Protein fractionation
Sephadex G-200	<5000 to 600,000	>600,000	Protein fractionation
Bio-Gel P-200	<30,000 to 200,000	>200,000	Protein fractionation
Bio-Gel P-300	<60,000 to 400,000	>400,000	Protein fractionation
Sepharose 2B	<7×10^4 to 4×10^7	>4×10^7	Protein fractionation
Sepharose 4B	<6×10^4 to 2×10^7	>2×10^7	Protein fractionation
Sepharose 6B	<10^4 to 4×10^6	>4×10^6	Protein fractionation
Bio-Gel A-1.5m	<10^4 to 1.5×10^6	>1.5×10^6	Protein fractionation
Styragel	<100 to 2000	>2000	SEC-Analytical

diffuse in the stagnant fluid in the pores. If the pores are tight for the solute this diffusion will be hindered. (4) The solute finds a vacant site and then sorbs by physical or electrical forces or by a chemical reaction. (5) While sorbed the solute may diffuse along the surface. This is called surface diffusion. (6) The solute desorbs, (7) diffuses through the pores, and (8) diffuses back across the external film and into the moving fluid. A given molecule may sorb and desorb many times during its stay inside a single particle.

While in the moving fluid the solute is carried along at the average interstitial fluid velocity, v, until the solute diffuses into another particle and the whole process is repeated. As far as migration down the column is concerned, the particle is either moving at the interstitial velocity, v, of the fluid or it has a velocity of zero when it is inside a particle. The average rate of movement of the solute depends on the relative amount of time the solute spends inside particles. Thus the solute movement depends on ε_e, ε_p, K_d, v, and the sorption equilibrium.

6.2. ADSORBENTS

The most commonly used adsorbents are activated carbon, zeolite molecular sieves, slica gel, organic polymers and activated aluminas. In chromatography a variety of specialized packing materials are used. These are discussed in Chapter 7. The polymeric resins used for ion exchange are discussed in Chapter 9.

Based on tonnage used and market value *activated carbon* is the most commonly used adsorbent. Activated carbon is made by first carbonizing a carbonaceous starting material such as wood, coal, petroleum coke, or coconut shells. The material is then partially gasified in a mild oxidizing gas such as CO_2 or steam. This activation process creates the desired porosity and surface area, and oxidizes the surface. Different grades of activated carbon for both gas and liquid separations are made (Bonsol *et al*, 1988). Activated carbon properties are listed in Table 6-2. Properties of a variety of commercially available carbons used for water treatment are tabulated by Faust and Aly

Table 6-2. Properties of Activated Carbon Adsorbents
(Keller *et al*, 1987; Lydersen, 1983; Ruthven, 1984,
Vermeulen *et al.*, 1984; Yang, 1987)

| Property | Liquid-Phase | | Vapor-Phase |
	Wood Base	Coal Base	Coal Base
Mesh Size (Tyler)	-100	-8 + 30	-6 + 14
Bulk density ρ_B (kg/m^3)	250-300	400-700	500-530
		500 (avg)	
Ash (%)	7	8	4-8
ε_p	~0.8	0.6-0.85	0.6-0.85
Pore vol. cm^3/g	0.15 to 0.50		
Surface area (km^7/kg)	0.8-1.8		0.9-1.2
Tortuosity, τ (Eq. 6-44b)		5-65	

Adsorption Capacity, Vapor-phase carbon:
CCl_4 0.4 to 0.7 kg adsorbate/kg
nC_4 (250 mm Hg, 25°)   25 wt %
water (250 mm Hg, 25°C)   5-7 wt %

(1987). Activated carbon is used for water and air purification, gas masks, solvent recovery, pollution control, decolorizing sugar, gold recovery, alcohol purification, adsorption of gasoline vapors from automobiles and a host of other applications.

Activated carbon has an essentially nonpolar surface. Thus, it does not strongly adsorb water. Because of this, activated carbon is commonly used for aqueous separations and activated carbon can be used to process humid gases. Water does adsorb, but it is by capillary condensation and is rather weak. Since activated carbon has a very large internal surface area, it usually has a higher capacity for nonpolar and weakly polar organics than other adsorbents. However, since the pores are small, $K_D < 1$ for relatively large molecules and the diffusion rates may be very low (it is not unusual to take 30 days for activated carbon to come to equilibrium). The maximum capacity of activated carbon for a variety of organics is listed in Table 8-3. Finally, since the heat of

224

Table 6-3. Commercially Available Zeolites
(Not all are used as adsorbents). (Vaughan, 1988).
Reprinted with permission from *Chem. Engr. Prog., 84* (2), 25 (Feb. 1988).
Copyright 1988, Amer. Inst. Chem. Engrs.

Zeolite	Pore Size	Si/Al	Cation	H_2O	nC_6H_{14}	C_6H_{12}	Vendors
Faujasite							
X	7.4Å	1-1.5	Na	28	14.5	16.6	GLPTU
Y	7.4	1.5-3	Na	26	18.1	19.5	GLPTU
US-Y	7.4	>3	H	11	15.8	18.3	GLPTU
A	3	1.0	K,Na	22	0	0	GLPTU
A	4	1.0	Na	23	0	0	GLPTU
A	4.5	1.0	Ca,Na	23	12.5	0	GLPTU
Chabazite	4	4	*N*	15	6.7	1	GU
Clinoptilolite	4×5	5.5	*N*	10	1.8	0	A
Erinoite	3.8	4	*N*	9	2.4	0	AM
Ferrierite	5.5×4.8	5-10	H	10	2.1	1.3	T
L type	6	3-3.5	K	12	8	7.4	LTU
Mazzite	5.8	3.4	Na,H	11	4.3	4.1	U
Mordenite	6×7	5.5	*N*	6	2.1	2.1	AU
Mordenite	6×7	5-6	Na	14	4.0	4.5	PTU
Mordenite	6×7	5-10	H	12	4.2	7.5	PTU
Offretite	5.8	4	K,H	13	5.7	2.0	U
Phillipsite	3	2	*N*	15	1.3	0	A
Silicalite	5.5	∞	H	1	10.1	0	U
ZSM-5	5.5	10-500	H	4	12.4	5.9	M

A = Anaconda Minerals, Letcher Minerals, Double Eagle mining, and others.
G = W.R. Grace & Co.; L = Laporte PLC; M = Mobil Oil Co.; P = PQ Corp.; T = Toyo Soda; U = Union Carbide Corp.
N = mineral zeolite; cations variable, and usually Na, K, Ca, Mg.
Note: Many small companies will mine and supply mineral zeolites on a custom basis as ground or sized rock, but they offer no process or fabrication services.

adsorption is modest, the energy requirements for regeneration are often modest. However, some adsorbates such as large organics are almost impossible to desorb and must be burned off.

A new type of carbon adsorbent is the *carbon sieve*. Carbon sieves differ from activated carbon since the pores are smaller and the pore distribution is more tightly controlled. Because of the tightly controlled pore size, gas molecules may have widely varying diffusion rates. Carbon sieves are used commercially for separating oxygen and nitrogen based on the different diffusion rates (see Ruthven, 1984; or Yang, 1987). This is of interest since it is apparently the only rate based adsorption separation being used commercially.

Zeolite molecular sieves can also separate molecules based on size although the most common applications are based on differences in adsorption. Zeolites are porous crystalline aluminosilicates of general formula.

$$C_{x/n} \left[(Al\ O_2)_x\ (SiO_2)_y \right] z\ H_2O$$

In this formula x, y, n, z are integers and $y \geq x$. n is the valence of cation C while z is the number of water molecules per unit cell. By changing x, y and the cation C a very large number of zeolites have been synthesized (Breck, 1974, Ruthven 1984,1988; Vaughan, 1988; Yang, 1987). A number of naturally occurring zeolites are also used commercially. These are listed in Table 6-3 (Vaughan, 1988) while other physical properties are listed in Table 6-4.

Zeolites are useful and in some ways unique since a rigid, three-dimensional cage structure with exact dimensions is formed. Molecules which are too large are excluded and do not adsorb. The most common separations which utilize steric effects are given in Table 6-1. The 3A zeolites are used for drying reactive gases since the reactive gas is excluded from the zeolite (Zeolites are also used as catalysts). The water is not excluded and is strongly adsorbed. The structural details of the zeolites are discussed in detail elsewhere (Breck, 1974; Ruthven 1984,1988; Yang, 1987).

Zeolites are also used for a variety of separations where the steric properties are not used. Examples would include the following:

Drying air to low dew points (see Table 8-2 and Figure 8-11)

Table 6-4. Physical Properties of Zeolite Adsorbents
(Keller *et al.*, 1987; Kovach, 1979; Ruthven, 1988;
Vermeulen *et. al.*, 1984; Yang, 1987)

Zeolite Type	Nominal Pore size (nm)	ρ_B, kg/m^3	ε_p	Equil. H$_2$O cap. (wt %)	Largest Molecule included
3A	0.3	670-740	0.30	20-23	H$_2$, H$_2$O
4A	0.4	610-720	0.32	22-28.5	C$_2$H$_6$, Xe
5A	0.5	600-720	0.34	21.5-28	CF$_4$, n-paraffins
10X	0.8	641		28-36	isoparaffins, benzene
13X	0.8-1.0	580-710	0.38	28.5-36	<10Å
Mordenite	0.3-0.8	720-800,880		12	
Chabazite	0.4-0.5	640-720		20	

Tortuosity, τ, Eq. (6-44b) varies from 1.7 to 4.5

Drying natural gas to low dew points
Drying liquids (see Figure 8-14)
CO$_2$ removal
H$_2$S removal
Separation of alcohol and water
Sugar separations
Separation of O$_2$ from N$_2$ in air
Separation of xylenes and ethylbenzene
Static desiccant in packaging and homes

The zeolite adsorbents can be fine-tuned for a particular separation by changing the structure and the cation.

Silica gel is an amorphous solid made up as spherical particles of colloidal silica, SiO$_2$. It is produced from the following reaction

$$Na_2SiO_3 + 2\ HCl + n\ H_2O \rightarrow 2\ NaCl + SiO_2 \cdot n\ H_2O + H_2O$$

Table 6-5. Physical Properties of Silica Gel.
(Keller *et al.*, 1987; Kovach, 1979;
Lydersen, 1983; Vermeulen *et al.*, 1984; Yang 1987)

Particle Size	0.1 to 3.0 mm
Bulk density	400 to 830 kg/m^3
	(700 to 820 common)
ε_p	0.38 to 0.55
Pore diameter (nm)	1-40 (depending on grade)
	2-5 and ~ 14 are common
Surface area m^2/g	400-830 (800 common)
Adsorption Capacity	0.3 to 0.6 kg H$_2$O/kg
Reactivation Temp	130-280°C
Tortuosity, τ, Eq. (6-44b)	2-6

The silica surface has a high affinity for water and the most common use of silica gel is for drying gases and liquids (see Table 8-2 and Figure 8-6). Silica gel is cheaper and easier to regenerate than zeolites (see Table 8-1), but cannot produce as dry a gas particularly at high temperatures. Since silica gel can be damaged by liquid water, it is important to avoid the presence of liquid water. The physical properties of silica gels are listed in Table 6-5. Other properties are shown in Figure 8-11 and are listed in Table 8-2.

Activated alumina, Al$_2$O$_3$, is made by dehydrating or activating aluminum trihydrate. The surface has a strong affinity for water, but the alumina is not harmed by immersion in liquid water. The most common application is drying both gases and liquids. The alumina surface can be modified to preferentially adsorb other compounds. At high water concentrations adsorbent loadings are higher than for zeolites. Physical properties are listed in Table 6-6 while other properties are given in Table 8-2 and Figure 8-11.

Organic polymer resins have been used for many years for ion exchange. More recently these resins in uncharged form have been used for adsorption of organics dissolved in water (Fox, 1985). In this application the organic polymers compete with activated carbon. Although more expensive, the polymers

Table 6-6. Physical Properties of Activated Aluminas
(Keller et al., 1987; Kovach, 1979;
Lydersen, 1983; Vermeulen et al., 1984; Yang, 1987)

Particle Size	14/28 mesh to 1/2 in spheres
Bulk Density	720-880 kg/m^3 (800 avg)
ε_p	0.50-0.57
Pore diameter (nm)	1-14 depending on grade
Surface area (m^2/g)	200-390 (320 avg.)
Adsorption Capacity	0.07 to 0.25 kg H$_2$O/kg
Regeneration Temp.	150-315°C
Tortuosity, τ, Eq. (6-44b)	2-6

appear to be economical for treating concentrated waste streams. Resin details are discussed in Chapter 9.

A variety of other adsorbents are used for special cases. These include clays for purification of vegetable oils, calcium silicate for fatty-acid removal, activated bauxite which is similar to activated alumina, Fuller's earth which has the same uses as clays and used to be the most commonly used adsorbent, and bone char which is used in sugar refining. There are also a variety of proprietary adsorbents which have been developed for very particular applications such as adsorbing traces of mercury vapor from air.

6.3. ADSORPTION EQUILIBRIUM

Since most adsorption processes are based on differences in the equilibrium adsorption of different chemicals, adsorption equilibrium is extremely important. Solute adsorbed on the solid surface is usually assumed to be in equilibrium with the solute in the fluid contained in the pores. At equilibrium the adsorbed solute concentration, q, is related to the solute concentration in the fluid, c. Usually q is determined in units such as moles/kg adsorbent or kg/kg adsorbent while c is in units such as moles/m^3 solution or kg/m^3 solution.

Equilibrium is strongly affected by temperature. Constant temperature equilibrium isotherms are usually measured.

Many forms of equilibrium isotherms have been developed. The simplest is the linear or Henry's law form

$$q = A(T)c \qquad (6\text{-}4a)$$

where $A(T)$ is the equilibrium constant which usually follows an Arrhenius function of temperature.

$$A(T) = A_o \exp(-\Delta H/RT) \qquad (6\text{-}4b)$$

The linear form is shown in Figure 6-3a. The linear form is often approximated at very low concentrations. This form is extremely convenient to use in theories and for this reason has been used where the data shows some curvature. Equation (6-4b) shows how adsorbents can be *thermally regenerated*. At higher temperatures less adsorbate is bound to the surface. The desorbed material must concentrate in the fluid and hence can be swept out of the bed.

A second isotherm form which is commonly used is the Langmuir isotherm. This isotherm is appealing because a simple physical picture can be used to develop the isotherm. Assume that a gas is being adsorbed on a solid surface and that a maximum of a monolayer of this gas can be adsorbed. The number of molecules striking the surface is proportional to the partial pressure of the solute, $\bar{p}$. Only the molecules striking a bare surface can adsorb and not all of these will adsorb. Thus the rate of adsorption is

$$\text{Adsorption rate} = k_1 (1 - \theta) \bar{p}$$

where θ is the fraction of surface covered by adsorbed solute and $(1 - \theta)$ is the fraction of surface which is bare. k_1 is an adsorption rate constant. The rate of desorption is assumed to depend on the amount adsorbed but not on the concentration in the gas phase.

$$\text{Desorption rate} = k_{-1} \theta$$

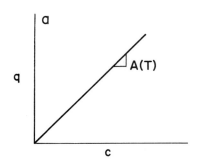

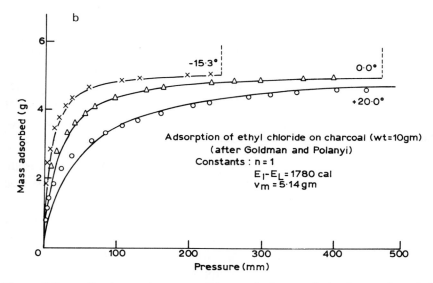

Figure 6-3. Isotherm shapes. a. Linear. b. Langmuir isotherms for ethyl chloride on charcoal (Brunauer *et al*, 1938). c. BET isotherms for nitrogen and argon (Brunauer *et al*, 1938). d. Freundlich. e. Exchange adsorption for ethylene-propylene on silica gel (Lewis *et al*, 1950b). f. Gas-liquid chromatography. Items b and c reprinted with permission from *J. Am. Chem. Soc., 60,* 309 (1938). Copyright 1938, American Chemical Society. Item e reprinted with permission from *Ind. Eng. Chem., 42,* 1319 (1950). Copyright1950, American Chemical Society.

c

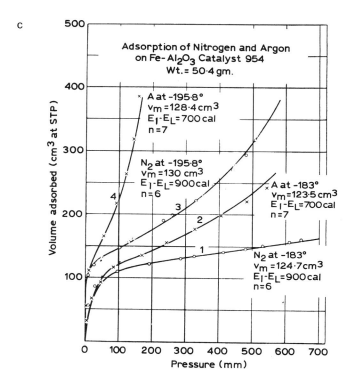

Adsorption of Nitrogen and Argon
on Fe- Al$_2$O$_3$ Catalyst 954
Wt. = 50·4 gm.

A at -195·8°
v$_m$ =128·4 cm^3
E$_I$-E$_L$ =700 cal
n =7

N$_2$ at -195·8°
v$_m$ =130 cm^3
E$_I$-E$_L$ =900 cal
n = 6

A at -183°
v$_m$ =123·5 cm^3
E$_I$-E$_L$ =700 cal
n =7

N$_2$ at -183°
v$_m$ =124·7 cm^3
E$_I$-E$_L$ =900 cal
n = 6

Volume adsorbed (cm^3 at STP)

Pressure (mm)

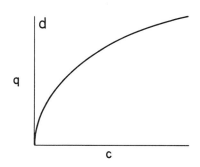

Figure 6-3.—*contd.*

232

e

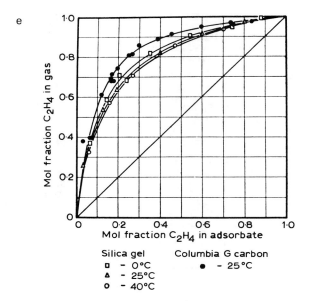

Silica gel Columbia G carbon
□ – 0°C   ● – 25°C
▲ – 25°C
○ – 40°C

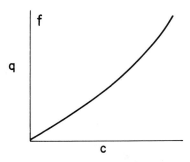

Figure 6-3.—*contd.*

where k_{-1} is the desorption rate constant. At equilibrium the desorption and adsorption rates are equal. Solving for θ at equilibrium we obtain,

$$\theta = \frac{k_1 \, \bar{p}}{k_{-1} + k_1 \, \bar{p}} = \frac{(k_1/k_{-1}) \, \bar{p}}{1 + (k_1/k_{-1}) \, \bar{p}}$$

Since the adsorbate concentrate on the solid, q, must be proportional to θ

$$q = k_2\,\theta = \frac{k_2\,(k_1/k_{-1})\,\bar{p}}{1 + (k_1/k_{-1})\,\bar{p}} \qquad (6\text{-}5)$$

When the surface is fully covered, $\theta = 1$, and $q = q_{MAX}$ which is the monolayer coverage. Thus Eq. (6-5) can be written

$$q = \frac{q_{MAX}K_A\,\bar{p}}{1 + K_A\,\bar{p}} \qquad (6\text{-}6a)$$

where $K_A = k_1/k_{-1}$ is the sorption equilibrium constant.

Equation (6-6a) is the Langmuir isotherm (Langmuir, 1918). The shape of Eq. (6-6a) is shown in Figure 6-3b (Brunauer *et al*, 1938). This is known as a *favorable* isotherm. The Langmuir isotherm is applicable for dilute, single component adsorption with an inert gas present or for pure gases at low pressures. In concentration units the Langmuir equation is,

$$q = \frac{q_{MAX}\,K_A\,c}{1 + K_A\,c} \qquad (6\text{-}6b)$$

At very low partial pressures the Langmuir equation is linear

$$q = K_A\,q_{MAX}\,\bar{p} \qquad (6\text{-}7a)$$

or at very low concentrations

$$q = K_A\,q_{MAX}\,c \qquad (6\text{-}7b)$$

If we plot q/q_F vs c/c_F where q_F is the amount adsorbed in equilibrium with fluid at the feed concentration, the equilibrium curve goes from 0 to 1.0. The shape is the same as vapor-liquid equilibrium with constant relative volatility. The term $(1 + K_A\,c_F)$ is equivalent to the relative volatility. Thus larger $(1 + K_A\,c_F)$ indicates a more *favorable* adsorption step.

Since K_A is a sorption equilibrium constant, we would expect its temperature dependence to follow an Arrhenius form.

$$K_A = K_A^\circ \exp\left(-\frac{\Delta H}{RT}\right)$$

(6-8)

where ΔH is the heat of adsorption. Since adsorption is exothermic, ΔH is negative. Thus, Eq. (6-8) correctly predicts that K_A and the amount adsorbed decrease as temperature is increased.

The Langmuir isotherm is often extended to multicomponent systems. The resulting isotherm equation is

$$q_i = \frac{q_{max} K_i \bar{p}_i}{1 + \sum_{j=1}^{n} (K_j \bar{p}_j)}$$

(6-9)

where n is the number of adsorbates. This equation shows competitive adsorption where less solute A is adsorbed when other solutes are present. Although very convenient, the multicomponent Langmuir isotherm often does not fit experimental data. Note that q_{max} must be the same for all solutes or the result is not thermodynamically consistent (LeVan and Vermeulen, 1981).

The Langmuir forms assume a maximum of a monolayer coverage. In some gas adsorption systems additional layers of adsorbate can form on top of the monolayer. Brunauer et al (1938) derived several isotherms which have become known as the BET isotherms. The simplest form of the BET isotherm for one adsorbate is

$$\frac{q}{q_{mono}} = \frac{K\bar{p}}{[(VP) + (K-1)\bar{p}]\,[1-\frac{\bar{p}}{(VP)}]}$$

(6-10)

where q_{mono} is the amount adsorbed for monolayer coverage and VP is the vapor pressure of pure adsorbate. The shape of this isotherm depends on the value of K and is shown in Figure 6-3c for adsorption of nitrogen or argon at different temperatures (Brunauer et al., 1938). Note that if $K \gg 1$ and $\bar{p} \ll$

(VP), Eq. (6-10) reduces to the Langmuir form. The BET isotherm is the basis of a method for determining the surface area of the packing (e.g. see Yang, 1987).

In zeolite molecular sieves the entire pores are filled with adsorbate. In this case adsorption is not by surface layers, but occurs by pore filling. The loading rate correlation (LRC) is a simple extension of the Langmuir equation where q_{max} is replaced by the maximum attainable loading N_{max}. For gas adsorption this equation is (Lee, 1972),

$$\frac{N}{N_{max}} = \frac{(k\overline{p})^{1/m}}{1 + (k\overline{p})^{1/m}} \tag{6-11}$$

a typical zeolite molecular sieve isotherm will be similar to a Langmiur isotherm except it is likely to be sharper. Other isotherm equations are also commonly used for zeolites (Lee, 1972; Ruthven, 1984; Yang, 1987).

For liquids it is common to generalize the Langmuir isotherm to,

$$q = \frac{a\,c}{1 + b\,c} \tag{6-12a}$$

where a and b do not have to be $q_{MAX}K_M$ and K_M, respectively. The constants a and b can be fit to experimental data. This is easiest to do if Eq. (6-12a) is rearranged to,

$$\frac{c}{q} = \frac{b}{a}\,c + \frac{1}{a} \tag{6-12b}$$

If the Langmuir isotherm is followed, a graph of c/q versus c will give a straight line with a slope of b/a and an intercept of $1/a$ (see Example 6-1). The multicomponent form of Eq. (6-12a) is

$$q_i = \frac{a_i\,c_i}{1 + \sum_{j=1}^{n}(b_j\,c_j)} \tag{6-13}$$

This is a convenient form to use but it may not fit experimental data.

A better fit to experimental data for liquids can often be obtained with the Freundlich equation,

$$q = A(T) \, c^{1/n} \quad n > 1 \tag{6-14}$$

The Freundlich isotherm is shown in Figure 6-3d. Unfortunately, the Freundlich equation does not approach a linear isotherm for very dilute solutions, and it does not approach a limiting asymptotic value observed for many systems. The Freundlich isotherm is commonly used to fit data for the adsorption of organic pollutants from aqueous solution unto activated carbon. Tabulations of A and n are given by Dobbs and Cohen (1980) and Faust and Aly (1987). An empirical combination of the Langmuir and Freundlich equations often gives a better fit to data (Fritz and Schluender, 1974).

$$q_i = \frac{a_{io} \, c_{io}^{b_*}}{\beta_i + \sum_{j=1}^{n} a_{ij} \, c_j^{b_{ij}}} \tag{6-15}$$

where a_{io}, b_{io}, β_i, a_{ij} and b_{ij} are empirical constants. Equation (6-15) is not thermodynamically consistent and needs to be used with caution.

In *exchange adsorption* two adsorbates are present and there is no carrier. The surface of the adsorbent is always saturated. The two adsorbates then exchange with each other for sites on the adsorbent. This is illustrated in Figure 6-3e for ethylene-propylene mixtures on silica gel at 25°C (Lewis *et al.*, 1950b). Note that this looks similar to vapor-liquid equilibrium data. For binary systems equilibrium can often be represented by a constant separation factor, α_{AB}.

$$\alpha_{AB} = \frac{y_A/x_A}{y_B/x_B} = \frac{y_A(1-x_A)}{x_A(1-y_A)} \tag{6-16}$$

where y and x are mole fractions in the gas and solid phases, respectively. This is analogous to a relative volatility. To predict the actual amount adsorbed, Eq.

(6-16) is solved simultaneously with the correlation (Lewis *et al*, 1950b),

$$\frac{q_A}{q_A^o} + \frac{q_B}{q_B^o} = 1 \qquad (6\text{-}17)$$

where q_A^o, q_B^o are the amount absorbed from a pure gas and q_A, q_B are the amount adsorbed from the mixture. Equation (6-17) is often valid even if the separation factor α_{AB} is not constant.

In gas-liquid chromatography the mechanism responsible for separation is essentially *absorption* of the solute into the stationary liquid phase not adsorption at a surface. At low concentrations the isotherms follow a Henry's law or linear relationship. Absorption is favored as more solute disolves in the stationary phase. The shape can be fit by an isotherm of the form.

$$N = \frac{a\,\overline{p}}{1 - b\,\overline{p}} \quad , \qquad b > 0 \qquad (6\text{-}18)$$

where N is the loading of solute on the packing. This shape isotherm is shown to Figure 6-3f. Absorption systems usually follow Henry's law for much higher ranges of $\overline{p}$ than adsorption systems.

More details of adsorption equilibrium are in Ruthven (1984) and Yang (1987). A review listing sources for gas adsorption data is available (Valenzuela and Myers, 1984). Valenzuela and Myers (1989) give references and show data for a very wide variety of pure gases, gas mixtures and liquids. Faust and Aly (1987) give data for removal of organics from water with activated carbon.

Example 6-1. Langmuir Isotherm

Tsou and Graham (1985) measured the sorption of the protein bovine serum albumin (BSA) on an ion exchanger, DEAE Sephadex A-50. The conditions were: T = 20 ± 1°C, pH = 6.9, 0.005 M phosphate

238

buffer. The results for c and q given below were read from a figure given by Tsou and Graham (1985).

c, mg protein per g solution	q, mg protein per g dry resin	c/q
0	0	0
0.05	5767	0.867×10^{-5}
0.10	6000	1.667×10^{-5}
0.20	6778	2.951×10^{-5}
0.30	7578	3.959×10^{-5}
0.50	7611	6.569×10^{-5}
0.50	7544	6.628×10^{-5}
0.70	8422	8.311×10^{-5}
0.90	7789	11.55×10^{-5}

Does this sorption follow a Langmuir isotherm? What are the values of a and b in Eq. (6-12a)?

Solution

Even though this is ion exchange and not adsorption, we can use the Langmuir isotherm. Equation (6-12b) shows that a plot of c/q versus c should be a straight line with a slope = b/a and an intercept of 1/a. Values of c/q are calculated in the table. The plot is shown in the figure. The line drawn is the best line from a linear regression routine on my calculator. The resulting parameter values are

$$b/a = 1.2111 \times 10^{-4} \qquad 1/a = 3.933 \times 10^{-6}$$

and the equilibrium expression is

$$q = \frac{254{,}259\,c}{1 + 30.79\,c}$$

Note that there is some scatter in the data; however, the duplicate data point is quite close.

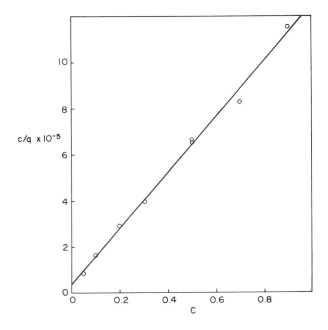

This example shows that unfamiliar systems (e.g. ion exchange of a protein) can easily be analyzed using the Langmuir isotherm. The values of q are very high compared to normal adsorption. This is possible since the gel swells in water and one gram of dry resin swells to fill 64.5 ml of column. The values of a and b differ slightly from those obtained by Tsou and Graham (1985) [268,925 and 32.7]. This probably occurs because of inaccuracy in reading the data points.

6.4. SOLUTE MOVEMENT

As solutes migrate through the bed they can be in the mobile fluid (external void volume, $\varepsilon_e\, A_c\, \Delta z$), in the stagnant fluid inside a particle (void volume $(1 - \varepsilon_e)\varepsilon_p\, A_c\, \Delta z$), or sorbed to the particle. (Refer to Figure 6-2.) The only solutes which are moving towards the column exit are those in the mobile fluid. Consider the movement of an incremental mass of solute added to a segment of the bed shown in Figure 6-2. Within this segment this incremental amount of solute must distribute to form a change in fluid concentration, Δc, and a change in the amount of solute adsorbed, Δq. The amount of this increment of solute in the mobile fluid compared to the total amount of the solute increment in this segment is,

$$\frac{\text{Amt. in mobile fluid}}{\text{Total amt. in segment}}$$

$$= \frac{\text{Amt. in mobile fluid}}{\text{Amt. in: (Mobile fluid + stationary fluid + sorbed)}} \qquad (6\text{-}19)$$

The individual terms on the right hand side of Eq. (6-19) can be determined. For instance,

$$\text{Amount solute increment in mobile fluid} = \qquad (6\text{-}20)$$

(Vol. column segment) (frac which is mobile fluid) (conc. moles/liter)

$$= (\Delta z\ A_c)\ (\varepsilon_e)\ (\Delta c)$$

After determining each term in Eq. (6-19), we obtain

$$\frac{\text{Amt. in mobile fluid}}{\text{Total amt. in segment}} = \qquad (6\text{-}21)$$

$$\frac{(\Delta z A_c)\ \varepsilon_e \Delta c}{(\Delta z A_c)\ \varepsilon_e \Delta c + (\Delta z A_c)\ (1-\varepsilon_e)\ \varepsilon_p \Delta c K_d + (\Delta z A_c)\ (1-\varepsilon_e)\ (1-\varepsilon_p)\ \rho_s \Delta q}$$

The K_d term is not included in the sorption term (last term in the denominator) since q is an experimentally measured quantity which will already include any steric exclusion effects. The solid density, ρ_s, is included in Eq. (6-21) to make the units balance. If q and c are in the same units the solid density is not included in Eq. (6-21). A_c is the cross sectional area, and z is the axial distance.

If the fluid has a constant interstitial velocity, v, then the average velocity of the solute in the bed u_s is,

$$u_s = v \times \text{(fraction solute in mobile phase)} \qquad \text{(6-22a)}$$

Assuming a random process of adsorption, desorption and diffusion in and out of the stagnant fluid, the solute wave velocity becomes

$$u_s = v \times \left[\frac{\text{amount solute in mobile phase}}{\text{total amount solute in column}} \right] \qquad \text{(6-22b)}$$

or, after rearrangement

$$u_s \ (T) = \frac{v}{1 + [(1-\varepsilon_e)/\varepsilon_e] \, \varepsilon_p K_d + [(1-\varepsilon_e)/\varepsilon_e] \, (1-\varepsilon_p) \rho_s \, (\Delta q/\Delta c)} \qquad \text{(6-23)}$$

Eq. (6-23) represents a crude, first order description of movement of solute in the column. It gives an "average" velocity, but because of the randomness of diffusion and equilibrium there will be spreading of zones. With a few additional assumptions Eq. (6-23) can be used to predict the separation in the system.

The most important assumption, and the assumption least likely to be valid, is that the solid and fluid are locally in equilibrium. Then Δq will be related to Δc by the equilibrium adsorption isotherm. This assumption allows us to ignore mass transfer effects. The second assumption is that dispersion and diffusion are negligible; thus, all of the solute will travel at the same average solute velocity. These assumptions greatly oversimplify the physical situation, but they do allow us to make simple predictions. As long as we don't believe these predictions must be exactly correct, the simple model which results can be extremely helpful in understanding these separation techniques.

With linear equilibrium, from Eq. (6-4a) $\Delta q/\Delta c = A(T)$, and Eq. (6-23) becomes

$$u_s \ (T) = \frac{v}{1 + [(1-\varepsilon_e)/\varepsilon_e]\varepsilon_p K_d + [(1-\varepsilon_e)/\varepsilon_e] \, (1-\varepsilon_p) \, \rho_s A(T)} \qquad \text{(6-24)}$$

For Eq. (6-24) the solute wave velocity is the same as the average solute velocity. Equation (6-24) allows us to explore the behavior of solute in the column for a variety of operating methods.

Several facts about the movement of solute can be deduced from Eq. (6-23) or Eq. (6-24). The highest possible solute velocity is v, the interstital fluid velocity. This will occur when the molecules are very large and $K_d = A(T) = 0.0$. For small molecules $K_d = 1.0$, and with porous packings small molecules always move slower than the interstitial velocity even when they are not adsorbed. If adsorption is very strong the solute will move very slowly. When the adsorption equilibrium is *linear*, Eq. (6-24) shows that the solute velocity does not depend on the solute concentration. This is important and greatly simplifies the analysis for linear equilibria. If the equilibrium is nonlinear, $\Delta q/\Delta c$ will depend on the fluid concentration and Eq. (6-23) shows that the solute velocity will depend on concentration. Since linear equilibrium is usually valid at very low concentrations, Eq. (6-24) is a limiting case which will be valid at low concentrations.

A convenient graphical representation of the solute movement is obtained on a plot of axial distance, z, versus time. Since the average solute molecule moves at a velocity of u_s (T), this movement is shown as a line with a slope u_s. This is illustrated for a simple chromatographic separation in Figure 6-4. Figure 6-4a shows the feed pulse while Figure 6-4b shows the solute movement in the column. The product concentrations predicted are shown in Figure 6-4c. Note that this simple model does not predict dispersion or zone spreading, but does predict when the peaks exit. *The solute movement diagrams will be used repeatedly; thus, you should study Figure 6-4 until you understand it.*

If desired, zone spreading can be included, but this will conceptually complicate the model. The advantage of this model is that it is simple and can be used to understand a variety of methods of operation. More detailed models including mass transfer effects are discussed in Chapters 7 and 8.

If the equilibrium isotherm is *nonlinear* the basic structure developed here is still applicable, but we must use Eq. (6-23) instead of (6-24). The solute velocity now depends on both temperature and concentration. Once a specific

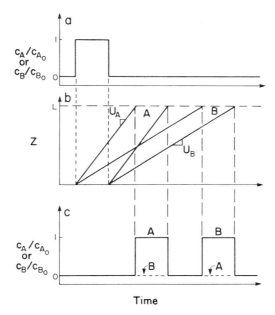

Figure 6-4.   Solute movement model for isothermal chromatography. a. Feed pulse. b. Trace of solute movement in column. c. Product concentrations.

isotherm is determined it can be substituted into Eq. (6-23). For example, if the Freundlich isotherm Eq. (6-14) is used, then

$$\lim_{\Delta c \to 0} \frac{\Delta q}{\Delta c} = \frac{\partial q}{\partial c} \Big|_T = \frac{A(T)}{n} c^{(\frac{1}{n}-1)} \tag{6-25}$$

and

$$u_s = \frac{v}{1 + [(1-\varepsilon_e)/\varepsilon_e]\, \varepsilon_p K_d + [(1-\varepsilon_e)/\varepsilon_e]\,(1-\varepsilon_p)\, \rho_s \dfrac{A(T)}{n} c^{(\frac{1}{n}-1)}} \tag{6-26}$$

The result for other isotherms such as the Langmuir isotherm is easily developed (see Problem 6-C4). Remember that $\partial q / \partial c$ is the slope of the equili-

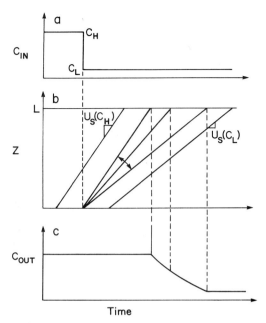

Figure 6-5.   Diffuse waves. a. Inlet concentration. b. Solute movement. c. Outlet concentration.

brium isotherm at c. Thus $\partial q/\partial c$ can be determined from data even if an equation is not known.

A diffuse wave (that is the solute is diffused or spread out) occurs when a concentrated solution is displaced by a dilute solution. This is illustrated in Figure 6-5 where the outlet wave concentrations are calculated. As long as the concentration is c_H, all solute waves move at the same velocity, u_s (c_H). When the concentration decreases, the solute wave velocity will decrease and a *diffuse wave* or *fan* is generated. This results in the zone spreading shown in Figure 6-5c. Note that this spreading is due to the *shape* of the isotherms and is proportional to the distance traveled. Thus this is called a *proportional pattern*. The diffuse wave shape can be determined by arbitrarily picking several concentrations between c_H and c_L. For each concentration u_s is calculated from Eq. (6-23) or the form written for a specific isothermal such as Eq. (6-26) for a

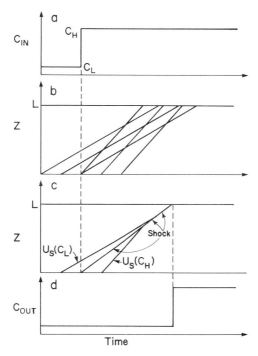

Figure 6-6.   Shock wave analysis. a. Inlet concentration. b. Physically impossible solute waves following Eq. (6-23). c. Shock wave following Eq. (6-30). d. Outlet concentration.

Freundlich isotherm. The solute movement line is drawn, and from this one point on the outlet concentration profile is determined (see Figure 6-5 and Example 6-2).

If we try the reverse (dilute solution displaced by a concentrated solution) then the limit in Eq. (6-25) does *not* exist since Δc has a finite value. A *shock* wave occurs. Another way of looking at this is Eq. (6-26) predicts a lower slope for dilute systems than for concentrated. When a concentrated solution displaces a dilute solution (Fig. 6-6a), the theory predicts that the solute lines overlap and two different concentrations occur simultaneously (Fig. 6-6b). This is physically impossible. To avoid this problem the mass balance must be done on a finite section of the column of length Δz. If the shock wave moves at a velocity u_{sh}, then the time required for the shock wave to move the distance Δz is

$$\Delta t = \Delta z/u_{sh} \qquad (6\text{-}27)$$

A mass balance for period Δt over segment Δz is,

$$IN - OUT - ACCUMULATION = 0 \qquad (6\text{-}28)$$

or

$$\varepsilon_e \, v \, \Delta t \, (c_2 - c_1) - [\varepsilon_e + K_d \, \varepsilon_p \, (1 - \varepsilon_e)](c_2 - c_1) \, \Delta z \qquad (6\text{-}29)$$

$$- (1 - \varepsilon_e) \, (1 - \varepsilon_p) \, \rho_s \, (q_2 - q_1) \, \Delta z = 0$$

where 1 refers to conditions before the shock wave and 2 to after the shock. Now we select the time interval $\Delta t = \Delta z/u_{sh}$ so that the shock has passed through the entire section. Solving for the shock wave velocity, we obtain

$$u_{sh} = \frac{v}{1 + [(1-\varepsilon_e)/\varepsilon_e]\varepsilon_p K_d + [(1-\varepsilon_e)/\varepsilon_e] \, (1-\varepsilon_p) \, \rho_s \, [(q_2-q_1)/(c_2-c_1)]} \qquad (6\text{-}30)$$

This is shown in Figure 6-6c and the outlet concentration is calculated in Figure 6-6d. Note that this result can also be obtained directly from Eq. (6-23) if we determine $\Delta q/\Delta c$ for the discrete step.

The shock wave velocity depends on q and c after and before the shock wave. Usually equilibrium between solid and fluid is assumed. Then q and c in Eq. (6-30) are related by the appropriate isotherm equation. For favorable isotherms (shapes shown in Figures 6-3b and 6-3c)

$$u_s \, (c_{high}) > u_{sh} > u_s \, (c_{low}) \qquad (6\text{-}31)$$

Because of Eq. (6-31) shock waves sharpen up and retain their shape. The more the curvature of the isotherm the stronger the tendency for the shock wave to sharpen. For the Langmuir isotherm $(1 + K_A c_F)$ is a measure of the tendency to sharpen. The larger $(1 + K_A c_F)$ the sharper the observed waves will be. In actual practice dispersion and finite rates of mass transfer smooth out the shock wave shown in Figure 6-6d. A balance is reached between the sharpening effect of the isotherm and the dispersive effects. A *constant pattern* S-shaped curve results. This shape does not change regardless of how long the column is. This concept will be discussed further in Chapter 8. Shock and diffuse waves can intercept each other and interact. This concept is discussed in Section 7.2.

The physical reasons for diffuse and shock waves can be clarified with a simple analogy. Suppose we have a line of cars moving on a one lane highway. If the cars are ordered in terms of speed with the fastest car in front and the slowest car last, the line will spread out as the cars move down the highway. This is a diffuse wave. If the slow cars are in front, all of the cars must move slowly. This result is similar to a shock wave.

Example 6-2. Solute Movement for Nonlinear Isotherms

The adsorption of acetic acid from aqueous solution onto activated carbon was extensively studied by Baker and Pigford (1971). The properties are:

$$\rho_s = 1.820 \text{ g/cm}^3, \quad K_d = 1.0, \quad C_{P,s} = 0.25 \text{ cal/g } °C$$
$$\varepsilon_e = 0.434 \quad\quad\quad\quad\quad\quad\quad C_{P,f} = 1.00 \text{ cal/g } °C$$
$$\varepsilon_p = 0.57 \quad\quad\quad\quad\quad\quad\quad \rho_f = 1.0 \text{ g/cm}^3$$

Adsorption follows a Freudlich isotherm, Eq. (6-14), with the following values:

Temperature	A(T)	n
4°C	3.646	3.277
60°C	3.019	2.428

where c is in gmoles/liter and q is gmoles/kg dry carbon.

a. An initially clean column ($c = 0$, $q = 0$) is fed with an acetic acid solution containing 0.25 gmoles/liter acetic acid. Superficial fluid velocity is 5 cm/min and the column is 2 meters long. Operation is at 60°C. Predict the shape of the solute wave and when it will exit the column.

b. After the column is saturated with $c = 0.25$ gmoles/liter, the acetic acid is removed with a solution with 0.05 gmoles/liter acetic acid at a superficial fluid velocity of 15 cm/min. Predict the shape and time the solute wave will leave the column.

Solution

A. Define. Sketches of the two parts are shown in the figure.

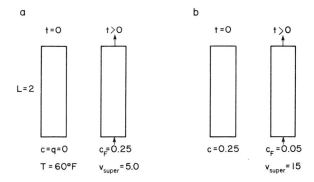

Find breakthrough profiles for each part.

B. Explore. The Freudlich isotherm is non-linear and has a favorable shape. Thus, we would expect a shock wave during part a and a diffuse wave during part b.

C. Plan. Use shock wave Eq. (6-30) for part a. Condition 1 before the shock wave is $c = 0$, $q = 0$. Condition 2 after the shock wave has $c_2 = c_F = 0.25$ and q_2 is in equilibrium with c_2. Plot this wave on a z vs t diagram.

For part b the diffuse wave velocity is determined from Eq. (6-26). The solute velocity is calculated for several concentrations from c = 0.25 to c = 0.05. The values are plotted on a z vs t diagram, and the outlet concentration profile is determined from this.

D. Do It. a. Shock Wave.

$$\text{Interstitial velocity} = v = \frac{v_{super}}{\varepsilon_e} = \frac{5.0}{0.434} = 11.52 \text{ cm/min}$$

$$q_2 = A(60)c_2^{\frac{1}{n(60)}} = 3.019(0.25)^{\frac{1}{2.428}} = 1.706$$

From Eq. (6-30)

$$u_{sh} = \frac{v}{1 + \frac{(1-\varepsilon_e)}{\varepsilon_e}\varepsilon_p K_d + (\frac{1-\varepsilon_e}{\varepsilon_e})(1-\varepsilon_p)\rho_s \frac{(q_2-q_1)}{(c_2-c_1)}}$$

$$= \frac{11.52}{1 + \frac{0.566}{0.434}(0.57)(1.0) + \frac{0.566}{0.434}(0.43)\frac{(1.82)(1.706-0)}{(0.25-0)}}$$

$$u_{sh} = 1.32 \text{ cm/min}$$

The shock wave exits at $t_{out} = L/u_{sh} = 200/1.32 = 151.5$ min. The outlet profile looks like Figure 6-6d with $c_{low} = 0$, $c_{high} = 0.25$ and $t_{out} = 151.5$ minutes.

b. Diffuse wave.

$$\text{Interstitial velocity } v = \frac{v_{super}}{\varepsilon_e} = \frac{15}{0.434} = 34.56 \text{ cm/min}$$

Diffuse wave velocity for Freundlich isotherm is given by Eq. (6-26).

$$u_s = \cfrac{v}{1 + (\cfrac{1-\varepsilon_e}{\varepsilon_e})\varepsilon_p K_d + (\cfrac{1-\varepsilon_e}{\varepsilon_e})(1-\varepsilon_p)\rho_s \cfrac{A(T)}{n} c^{(\frac{1}{n}-1)}}$$

$$= \cfrac{34.56}{1+(\cfrac{.566}{.434})(.57)(1.0)+(\cfrac{.566}{.434})(.43)(1.82)(\cfrac{3.019}{2.428})c(\cfrac{1}{2.428-1})}$$

We can determine u_s and t_{out} for several concentrations,

c	u_s, cm/min	$t_{out} = \dfrac{L}{u_s} = \dfrac{200cm}{u_s}$
0.25	7.53	26.9 min
0.20	6.93	28.9
0.15	6.18	32.4
0.10	5.22	38.3
0.05	3.81	52.5

Each one of these waves can be plotted starting from $t = 0$, $z = 0$ to $t = t_{out}$ at $z = L$. The result will look like Figure 6-5b. The outlet concentration profile can be plotted as shown in Figure 6-7.

E. Check. The outlet profiles have the shapes we expect. This is a visual check.

F. Generalization. For favorable isotherms we expect shock waves when feeding the column with a more concentrated feed, and diffuse waves when the column is eluted with a less concentrated stream. Note that the solute wave velocity decreases as concentration decreases and this is quite marked at the low velocities. In fact, the Freundlich isoth-

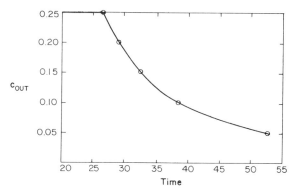

Figure 6-7.   Results from Example 6-2.

eïm predicts $u_s = 0$ when $c = 0$. This is usually not observed in experiments. Thus the Freundlich isotherm should not be used for diffuse wave calculations when $c = 0$. The reason for this incorrect prediction is the empirical Freundlich isotherm is not a good fit of experimental data for very low concentrations.

Note that plotting the solute movement diagram is not necessary for simple problems. For more complex problems the solute movement diagram is very useful to help understand the problem and to avoid errors. The solute movement diagram also provides a graphical representation which many people find useful.

6.5. EFFECTS OF CHANGING THERMODYNAMIC VARIABLES

Changes in temperature, pH, ionic strength or solvent concentration are often used to help desorb and elute the solute. Changes in these variables will change the equilibrium constants in the isotherm equations. For common adsorbents the amount of material adsorbed decreases as temperature is increased. Thus $A(T)$ and K_A are monotonically decreasing functions of temperature regardless of the validity of Eqs. (6-4b) and (6-8). One can either use a jacketed bed and change the temperature of the entire bed (called the direct mode) or one can change the temperature of the inlet stream and have a temperature wave propagate through the column (called the travelling wave mode). For most of the other elution methods (pH, ion strength, etc.) the travelling wave mode is used. Elution may be done either co-flow or counter-flow to the feed direction.

The velocity at which temperature moves in the column (the thermal wave velocity) can be obtained from an energy balance. If we can ignore the heat of adsorption and heat of mixing, and assume the column is adiabatic, then the average velocity of the thermal wave is

$$u_{th} = \left[\frac{\text{energy in mobile phase}}{\text{total energy in segment}} \right] v \qquad (6\text{-}32)$$

The fraction of energy stored in the mobile phase in a segment of the column is,

$$\frac{\text{Energy in mobile phase}}{\text{Total Energy in segment}}$$

$$= \frac{\text{Energy in mobile phase}}{(\text{Energy in: Mobile} + \text{Stagnant} + \text{Solid} + \text{Wall})} \qquad (6\text{-}33)$$

The numerator is

$$\text{Energy in mobile phase} = (\Delta z \, A_c) \, \varepsilon_e \, \rho_f \, C_{P,f} \, (T_f - T_{ref}) \qquad (6\text{-}34a)$$

while the denominator is

$$\text{Total energy} = \Delta z A_C \left[(\varepsilon_e + (1-\varepsilon_e)\varepsilon_p) \, \rho_f C_{P,f}(T_f - T_{ref}) \right]$$

$$\left[+ (1-\varepsilon_e)(1-\varepsilon_p)\rho_s C_{P,s} \, (T_s - T_{ref}) \right] + (\Delta z W)C_{P,w}(T_w - T_{ref}) \qquad (6\text{-}34b)$$

The C_P values are the heat capacities while W is the weight of column wall per length and T_w is the wall temperature. If we have local thermal equilibrium

$$T = T_f = T_s = T_w \qquad (6\text{-}35)$$

and the term $(T - T_{ref})$ divides out. Then combining Eqs. (6-32) and (6-34) we obtain the thermal wave velocity,

$$u_{th} = \frac{v}{1 + (1-\varepsilon_e)\varepsilon_p/\varepsilon_e + [(1-\varepsilon_e)(1-\varepsilon_p)C_{P,s}\rho_s + (W/A_c)C_{P,w}]/\varepsilon_e\rho_f C_{P,f}} \qquad (6\text{-}36)$$

Note that with the simplifying assumptions made here u_{th} is independent of temperature. Comparison of Eqs. (6-36) and (6-24) show they have a similar form but there is an additional term in Eq. (6-36) to account for thermal storage in the column wall, and effectively $K_d = 1.0$ for energy changes. Just as Eqs. (6-23) and (6-24) represented the movement of the average solute molecule, Eq. (6-36) represents the average rate of movement of the thermal wave. A more exact analysis is needed to include dispersion and heat transfer rate effects.

On a graph of axial distance z versus time t the thermal wave will be a straight line with a slope u_{th}. This is illustrated in Figure 6-8a. The outlet temperature profile is shown in Figure 6-8b. Note that this behavior is exactly the same as for a solute with a linear isotherm.

To complete the analysis we need to consider the change in solute concentration when the adsorbent temperature is changed. Since the following analysis is subtle, it needs to be followed closely. The effect of temperature changes on solute concentration can be determined by a mass balance on a differential section of column Δz over which the temperature changes during a time interval Δt. The appropriate differential section is shown in Figure 6-9a for a typical liquid system where

$$u_{th} > u_s (T_h, c_F) > u_s(T_c, c_F) \qquad (6\text{-}37a)$$

254

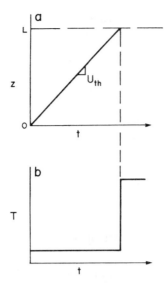

Figure 6-8.   Thermal wave. a. Trace of thermal wave in column. b. Product temperature.

Then the mass balance is

$$\varepsilon_e v \Delta t (c_2 - c_1) - [\varepsilon_e + K_d \varepsilon_p (1 - \varepsilon_e)](c_2 - c_1)\, \Delta z$$

$$- (1 - \varepsilon_e)(1 - \varepsilon_p)\, \rho_s (q_2 - q_1)\, \Delta z = 0 \qquad (6\text{-}38)$$

where 1 refers to conditions before the temperature shift and 2 to after the shift. Note that Eq. (6-38) is an application of Eq. (6-28) and is very similar to Eq. (6-29) used for shock waves.

To ensure that all material in the differential section undergoes a temperature change the control volume is selected so that $\Delta t = \Delta z / u_{th}$. The mass balance then becomes

$$\left[\varepsilon_e + \varepsilon_p (1 - \varepsilon_e)\, K_d - \frac{\varepsilon_e v}{u_{th}} \right] (c_2 - c_1)$$

$$+ (1 - \varepsilon_e)(1 - \varepsilon_p)\, \rho_s\, [q_2(c_2, T_2) - q_1(c_1, T_1)] = 0 \qquad (6\text{-}39a)$$

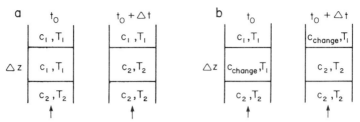

Figure 6-9.   Differential sections for mass balance when temperature changes. $\Delta t = \Delta z / u_{th}$. a. $u_{th} > u_s$ (T_2, c_2), $u_{th} > u_s$ (T_1, c_1). b. u_s $(T_h, c_F) > u_s$ $(T_C, c_F) > u_{th}$.

In this equation c_2 and q_2 are the unknowns. If we assume that solid and fluid are locally in equilibrium and that the equilibrium isotherm is *linear*, then Eq. (6-39a) reduces to

$$\frac{c(T_h)}{c(T_c)} = \left[\frac{1}{u_s(T_c)} - \frac{1}{u_{th}} \right] \Big/ \left[\frac{1}{u_s(T_h)} - \frac{1}{u_{th}} \right] \qquad (6\text{-}40)$$

In a typical liquid system where Eq. (6-37a) is satisfied, $c(T_h) > c(T_c)$. Thus, the solute is concentrated during elution. This concentration is calculated from Eq. (6-39a) or (6-40), and the solute movement diagram can be plotted as shown in Figure 6-10a. Concentrations are shown in Figure 6-10b. Note that the overall mass balance will be satisfied. The expected shape of the solute movement diagram for a particular example is shown in Example 6-3. If the equilibrium constant A does not change very much, $u_s(T_h) \approx u_s(T_c)$ and there will be little change in concentration during elution. Since A is not usually strongly dependent on temperature, large temperature changes are required. An alternative is to use a different elutant which has a major effect on the equilibrium constant. Eqs. (6-39) and (6-40) are still valid but with $u_{Elutant}$ replacing u_{th}.

In the direct mode the entire column is heated or cooled simultaneously through a jacket. In this case u_{th} is essentially infinite. Equation (6-40) for *linear* isotherms simplifies to

$$\frac{c(T_h)}{c(T_c)} = \frac{u_s(T_h)}{u_s(T_c)} \qquad (6\text{-}41)$$

256

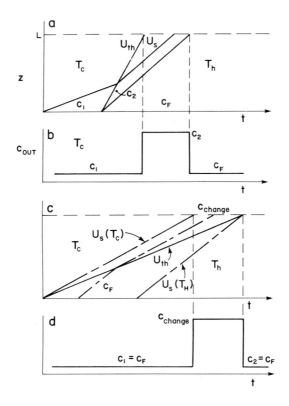

Figure 6-10. Effects of thermal waves for linear isotherms. a,b. Liquid systems where $u_{th} > u_s (T_2, c_2) > u_s (T_1, c_F)$. c,d. Dilute gas systems where $u_s (T_2, c_2) > (T_1, c_F) > u_{th}$.

For the usual adsorbent, $A(T)$ decreases (solute desorbs) as temperature increases. Thus u_s increases and, as expected, Eq. (6-41) predicts that the solute concentration increases as temperature increases.

Equations (6-39) and (6-40) were derived for a typical liquid system where Eq. (6-37a) is valid. In dilute gas systems it is common to have

$$u_s(T_h, c_F) > u_s(T_c, c_F) > u_{th} \qquad (6\text{-}37b)$$

A mass balance similar to Eq. (6-38) using the balance envelope shown in Figure 6-9b can again be developed. The result (see Problem 6-C6) is,

$$[\varepsilon_e + (1-\varepsilon_e)\varepsilon_p K_d - \frac{\varepsilon_e V}{u_{th}}](c_2 - c_{change})$$

$$+ (1-\varepsilon_e)(1-\varepsilon_p)\rho_s [q(c_2,T_2) - q(c_{change},T_1)] = 0 \qquad (6\text{-}39b)$$

where c_{change} is the concentration change caused by the temperature change. This concentration has now moved *ahead* of the thermal wave. In Eq. (6-39a) the unknowns are c_2 and $q_2(c_2,T_2)$ while in Eq. (6-39b) the unknowns are c_{change} and q (c_{change},T_1). Thus the differences in Eqs. (6-37a) and (6-37b) cause an important but subtle change. Equations equivalent to Eqs. (6-40) and (6-41) can also be derived for the case given in Eq. (6-37b) (see Problem 6-C6). This change is illustrated in Figures 6-10c and d. Note that with gas systems the changed (increased for a temperature increase) concentration wave comes out *ahead* of the thermal curve while in liquid systems (Figure 6-10b) the concentration waves comes out *after* the thermal wave.

A third case occurs when

$$u_s(T_h, c_F) > u_{th} > u_s(T_c, c_F) \qquad (6\text{-}37c)$$

and the temperature in the feed is increased. Now the solute waves for linear isotherms will intersect at the thermal wave as shown in Figure 6-11a. Since solute waves from both cold and hot sides intersect the thermal wave, the solute concentration must increase. Since the theory does not include zone broadening, this predicts an infinite concentration. To prevent this physically impossible result non-linear isotherms must be used. Now the concentration builds up *ahead* of the thermal wave so that

$$u_s(T_c, c_{change}) > u_{th}$$

Obviously, this can occur only with non-linear isotherms. The mass balance envelope will look like Figure 6-9b and the mass balance is given by Eq. (6-39b) (see problem 6-C7). This case is known as *focusing* (Wankat, 1986), and

258

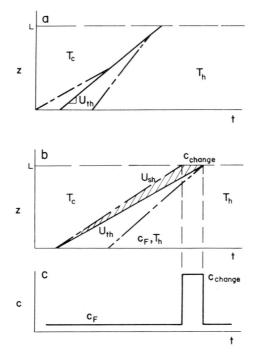

Figure 6-11.   Effect of thermal waves when focusing occurs, Eq. (6-37c). a. Physically impossible characteristic diagram for linear systems. b. Characteristic diagram for nonlinear systems. c. Concentration profile for nonlinear system.

is illustrated in Figures 6-11b and c. The concentration in the region moving ahead of the thermal wave can be calculated from Eq. (6-39b). Since this concentrated wave is displacing a dilute stream, there will be a shock wave which can be calculated from Eq. (6-30). Although rare, systems which focus can give large separation factors (see Problem 6-D10). Focusing is more likely to occur when thermodynamic variables other than temperature are changed. Separation methods can be devised which are based on focusing (see Wankat, 1986, and Section 7.10).

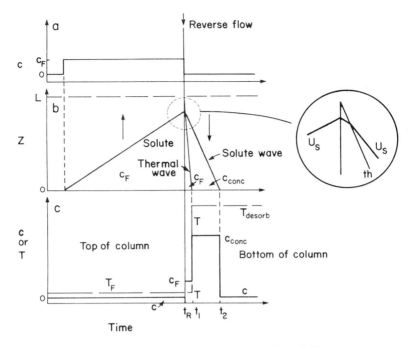

Figure 6-12.   Solute movement model for adsorption followed by counter-current elution with a hot fluid ($u_{th} > u_s$): a. Inlet concentration and temperatures. b. Trace of solute and temperature movement in bed. c. Product concentrations and temperatures.

Figure 6-12 illustrates elution using high temperatures for counter-flow desorption. In this case a single solute is adsorbed. The feed flow is continued until just before solute breakthrough (that is when solute appears in the outlet) occurs. Then counter-current flow of a hot fluid is used to remove solute. Upon reversing the flow the fluid first exits at the feed temperature and the feed concentration. When the thermal wave breaks through, the temperature and concentration both jump. Since the adsorption equilibrium constant is lower at high temperature, the solute velocity can be significantly greater at the higher temperature. In actual practice the outlet temperature and concentration waves will be S-shaped curves because of dispersion.

Example 6-3. Temperature Effects in Adsorption Columns.

A well insulated one meter long column containing activated carbon is saturated with an aqueous solution containing 0.4 g moles/liter acetic acid. Temperature is initially 4°C. The bed is eluted with a feed containing 0.04 gmoles/liter acetic acid at 60°C and a superficial velocity of 10 cm/min. Find the outlet temperature and composition profiles.

Solution

A. Define. The process is sketched in the figure.

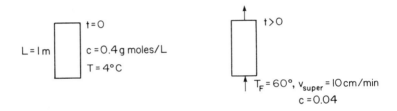

Find breakthrough profiles for temperature and composition.

B. Explore. Equilibrium, heat capacity, porosity and density data is available in Example 6-2. We expect a simple thermal wave in the column. This wave will cause an increase in acetic acid concentration since acetic acid will desorb at 60°C. The behavior of this more concentrated wave depends on the wave velocity compared to u_{th}. This will have to be calculated. The concentrated region is displaced by the hot dilute feed and a diffuse wave will result.

C. Plan. Calculate the thermal wave velocity from Eq. (6-36). Since no information is given on column diameter and wall effects, we will assume wall heat storage is negligible. This will be a good assumption for commercial systems, but not so good for laboratory columns. Next calculate c_2 (60°) from Eq. (6-38) assuming c_2 and q_2 are in equilibrium at 60°C. The equation is non-linear since equilibrium is represented by the Freundlich isotherm. Then determine u_s (c_2, 60°C) from Eq. (6-26). If u_s (c_2, 60°C) < u_{th}, the concentration at a point in the column will be 0.4 until the hot wave passes when it will jump to c_2. Finally, determine the diffuse wave from c_2 to 0.04 gmole/L.

D. Do It. With $\dfrac{W}{A_c} C_{P,w} = 0$, Eq. (6-36) is

$$u_{th} = \frac{v}{1 + \dfrac{1-\varepsilon_e}{\varepsilon_e}\varepsilon_p + \dfrac{(1-\varepsilon_e)(1-\varepsilon_p)\rho_s C_{P,s}}{\varepsilon_e \, \rho_f \, C_{P,f}}}$$

where $\quad v = \dfrac{v_{super}}{\varepsilon_e} = \dfrac{10}{0.434} = 23.04$ cm/min

thus,

$$u_{th} = \frac{23.04}{1 + \dfrac{0.566}{0.434}(0.57) + \dfrac{(0.566)(0.43)(1.82)(0.25)}{(0.434)(1.0)(1.0)}} = 11.53 \ \frac{cm}{min}$$

The thermal wave exits at $t_{th} = \dfrac{L}{u_{th}} = \dfrac{100}{11.53} = 8.67$ min.

To determine the effect of the temperature shift we need q_1 (4°C) in equilibrium with $c_1 = 0.4$. From the Freundlich isotherm

$$q_1 (4°) = A(4°)c_1^{1/n} = (3.646)(0.4)^{1/3.277} = 2.757 \ \text{gmoles/kg}$$

At 60°C, $q_2 = A(60)c_1^{1/n} = 3.019 \ c_2^{1/2.428}$

Substituting this into Eq. (6-38), we have

$$[\varepsilon_e + \varepsilon_p(1-\varepsilon_e)K_d - \frac{\varepsilon_e v}{u_{th}}](c_2 - c_1) + (1-\varepsilon_e)(1-\varepsilon_p)\rho_s[3.019c_2^{1/2.428} - q_1] = 0$$

Substituting in the values this equation becomes,

$$f(c_2) = 1.337\, c_2^{0.419} - 0.0732\, c_2 - 1.192 = 0$$

The second term will be small. If we ignore this term for the moment we have

$$c_2 = (\frac{1.192}{1.337})^{1/.4119} = 0.757$$

since the second term is subtracted, $f(0.757) = (-0.0732)(0.7511) = -0.055$. Thus try $c_2 = 0.80$ as first guess and calculate $f(.80) = -0.031$. This gives two guesses. Using some convergence procedure such as Newtonian or secant approach we find $c_2 = 0.857$. As expected $c_2 > c_1$.

Now we can calculate u_s $(c_2, 60°)$ from Eq. (6-26) which is,

$$u_s(60°, c_2) = \frac{v}{1 + \frac{1-\varepsilon_e}{\varepsilon_e}\varepsilon_p K_d + \frac{1-\varepsilon_e}{\varepsilon_e}(1-\varepsilon_p)\rho_s\, \frac{A(60)}{n}\, c_2^{(\frac{1}{n}-1)}}$$

$$= \frac{23.04}{1 + \frac{0.566}{0.434}(0.57)(1.0) + \frac{0.566}{0.434}(0.43)(1.82)\frac{3.019}{2.428}(0.857)^{(\frac{1}{2.428}-1)}}$$

$$= 7.354 \text{ cm/min}$$

Since u_s $(60°, c_2) < u_{th}$, we have the simple case outlined in the Plan.

For diffuse waves we use Eq. (6-26), but with varying concentrations.

These are easily calculated,

c	u_s (60°)	$t_{out} = L/u_s$
0.857	7.354	13.60
0.8	7.222	13.85
0.7	6.964	14.36
0.6	6.665	15.00
0.5	6.311	15.85
0.4	5.880	17.01
0.3	5.334	18.75
0.2	4.596	21.76
0.1	3.460	28.90
0.04	2.266	44.14

The total solute movement diagram and outlet concentration profile are shown in Figure 6-13.

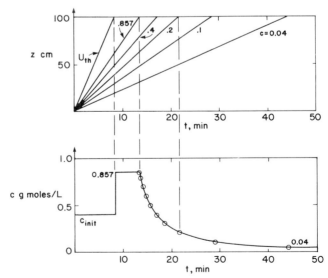

Figure 6-13.   Results of Example 6-3.

E. Check. The mass balance can be checked to see if IN-OUT = ACCUMULATION after the last wave has exited. This balance checks.

F. Generalization. Regeneration at high temperature is used because high concentrations and more rapid removal of the diffuse wave are achieved. The pattern achieved here with the thermal wave exiting with and causing the concentration wave is common for many liquid systems. However, if u_s $(T_h, c_2) > u_{th} > u_s$ (T_c, c_I) the pattern of the solute movement diagram and the outlet concentration profile will be quite different. This is illustrated in Example 6-4.

Example 6-4. Focusing.

Repeat Example 6-3, but for a special high heat capacity activated carbon with $C_{P,s} = 2.2$ cal/g°C.

Solution

Again assume $W C_{P,w}/A_c = 0$. Replace $C_{P,s} = 0.25$ with $C_{P,s} = 2.2$. Then, $u_{th} = 5.777$ cm/min and $t_{th} = 17.31$ min. Solute velocity at $c = 0.4$ is given by Eq. (6-26), which gives

u_s $(c = 0.4, 4°C) = 2.266$ cm/min

u_s $(c = 0.4, 60°C) = 5.88$ cm/min

Thus, Eq (6-37c) is satisfied and focusing occurs. Equation (6-39b) should be used to determine the effect of the temeprature change. For this balance $c_2 = 0.4$, $T_2 = 60°C$ and from the isotherm

$$q_2 = 3.019 \, c_2^{1/2.428} = 2.07$$

c_{ch} and q_{ch} (c_{ch}, $T = 4°C$) are unknown, but q is given by

$$q_{ch} = (3.646) \, c_{ch}^{1/3.277}$$

Then Eq. (6-39b) simplifies to

$$- 1.615 \, c_{ch}^{0.3052} + 0.9744 \, c_{ch} + 0.52715 = 0$$

Note that this nonlinear equation is significantly different than the nonlinear equation in Example 6-3. Since the unknown condition is now at $4°C$ instead of $60°C$ the exponent on c_{ch} has changed. This equation was solved by trial-and-error. The result is $c_{ch} = 1.22$

This high concentration displaces fluid with $c_1 = 0.4$ and $T = 4°C$. This gives a shock wave. Calculating

$$q_{ch} = 3.646 \, (1.22)^{1/3.277} = 3.874$$

we find,

$$\frac{\Delta q}{\Delta c} = \frac{3.8744 - 2.757}{1.22 - 0.4} = 1.362$$

$$u_{sh} = \frac{23.04}{1 + \dfrac{0.566}{0.434} (0.57) + \dfrac{0.566}{0.434} (0.43) (1.82) (1.362)} = 7.352 \text{ cm/min}$$

where the values of v, ε_e, ε_p and ρ_s are from Examples 8-1 and 8-3. This shock wave exits in

$$t_{sh} = L/u_{sh} = \frac{100}{7.352} = 13.60 \text{ min}$$

The results are shown in Figures 6-11b and c. Note that the concentration after the thermal wave immediately drops back to c_F since a solute wave at c_F and $T = 60°C$ exits at this point.

Obviously, the behavior illustrated in Examples 8-3 and 8-4 is very different (compare Figures 6-11 and 6-13). This occurred when only one variable, $C_{P,s,}$, was changed; however, this changed the system from a non-focusing to a focusing system.

6.6. THEORETICAL ASSUMPTIONS AND LIMITATIONS OF SOLUTE MOVEMENT THEORY

This completes the solute movement theory. As presented, this is not a rigorous mathematical model but was based on simple physical ideas. The equations developed here can be rigorously derived from the governing partial differential equations by making a group of assumptions called the local equilibrium assumptions and then using a mathematical method called the method of characteristics (see Section 6.9). Although some of the assumptions required for the rigorous development have been mentioned in passing, it is helpful to list them explicitly (Table 6-7).

If any of these assumptions are invalid the predictions can be way off. The most critical assumptions are the last three. Assumptions 14 and 15 cause the predicted outlet concentrations and temperatures to show sharp jumps instead of the experimentally observed S-shaped curves. Alternate mathematical models which are more realistic but much more complex are covered in Chapters 7 and 8. Assuming linear equilibrium can also cause physically impossible predictions, but fortunately this assumption is easily relaxed.

As we have seen, this model greatly oversimplifies the actual fluid flow and heat and mass transfer processes occurring in the column. Because of this the predicted separation is usually better than that obtained in practice. What is this model good for?

The solute movement model does include the reasons why separation occurs but not many of the phenomena which limit separation. The model is

Table 6-7. Common Assumptions to Simplify Mass and Energy Balances

	Assumption	Comments
1.	Homogeneous packing (no channeling)	Valid if careful-Poor packing can invalidate
2.	Negligible radial gradients	May not be valid if high heat loss
3.	Neglect thermal and pressure diffusion	Usually OK
4.	No chemical reactions except for sorption	Usually OK
5.	Neglect kinetic and potential energy terms	Usually OK
6.	No radiant heat transfer	Only absolutely true for isothermal Usually included with other heat transfer
7.	No electrical or magnetic fields	Usually OK
8.	No changes of phase except sorption	Usually OK
9.	Parameters are constant except for equilibrium	Never strictly true, but usually close enough
10a.	Velocity is constant across cross-section	OK if no channeling, no viscous fingering, no radial gradients
10b.	Velocity is not a function of z	OK for liquids, exchange adsorption, very dilute gases
11a.	Column is adiabatic, or	OK large columns with insulation
11b.	Column is at controlled constant temperature	OK small columns with jacket
12.	Heat of adsorption term is negligible	OK for liquids, exchange adsorption, dilute gases
13.	Solutes do not interact	OK for dilute systems
14.	Negligible thermal and mass axial dispersion and diffusion	Reasonable for liquids. Often lumped with mass transfer terms
15.	Heat and mass transfer rates are very high so that fluid and solid are locally in equilibrium	Never strictly true. Reasonable in diffuse waves. Obviously wrong in shock waves

simple and can thus be used to analyze rather complex processes. The model is a good guide for setting operating variables. Since this model predicts the best possible separation, the model can be used to determine if, at its best, a separation scheme is of interest. Since the predictions made are qualitatively correct, as long as the model predictions are interpreted in a qualitative or at best semi-quantitative sense the model is very useful. In addition, the prediction for diffuse waves is often good and can be used for design.

6.7. BASIC MASS TRANSFER EQUATIONS

The separation in adsorption, chromatography and ion exchange occurs because of differences in rates of solute or ion movement. However, as the experimental results of the previous section show the solute movement theory is far from the entire picture. The solute movement theory assumes that solid and fluid are locally in equilibrium. When equilibrium is the dominant phenomenon, the solute movement theory agrees with experimental data. Unfortunately, for shock waves resistance to mass transfer is always important. The result is a constant pattern, mass transfer zone which moves at the shock wave velocity. Mass transfer resistances will also spread out diffuse waves. However, equilibrium effects dominate except when mass transfer is very slow, and the solute movement theory results are often adequate for diffuse waves.

Mass transfer of solute in a packed bed can be thought of as occuring in several steps. First, the solute diffuses from the bulk fluid to the surface of the particles. This is often treated as occuring across a film. Next, the solute diffuses in the fluid through the pores. The solute then adsorbs and is held on the solid. Once on the solid the solute may diffuse along the solid or it may eventually desorb. Once desorbed, the solute may diffuse through the pores back into the bulk fluid, or the solute may diffuse to another site where it will adsorb. Since the pores in a particle are not straight (see Figure 6-2 for a schematic representation) the diffusing solutes must follow a torturous path. This picture is complex and all theories require experimental data to predict results.

A fundamental study of mass transfer can start with the differential solute mass balance for the packed bed. For the two porosity model this solute mass balance is,

$$\varepsilon_e \frac{\partial c_i}{\partial t} + K_{di}(1-\varepsilon_e)\varepsilon_p \frac{\partial \overline{c}_{i,pore}}{\partial t} + \rho_s(1-\varepsilon_e)(1-\varepsilon_p) \frac{\partial \overline{q}_i}{\partial t}$$

$$+ \varepsilon_e \frac{\partial(vc_i)}{\partial z} - \varepsilon_e(E_D + D_m) \frac{\partial^2 c_i}{\partial z^2} = 0 \qquad (6\text{-}42)$$

where D_m is the molecular diffusivity and E_D is the eddy diffusivity. Usually $E_D \gg D_m$. Equation (6-42) assumes the packing is homogeneous, there are no radial gradients, there are no chemical reactions other than adsorption or ion exchange, and there are no phase changes other than adsorption. The first term is the accumulation of solute in the mobile fluid, the second term is the accumulation in the stagnant fluid in the pores, and the third term is the accumulation of solute adsorbed to the solid. The terms $\overline{c}_{i,pore}$ and $\overline{q}_i$ are the volume average values inside the porous particles.

$$\overline{c}_{i,pore} = \frac{3}{R_p^3} \int_0^{R_p} c_{i,pore} \, r^2 \, dr \qquad (6\text{-}43a)$$

$$\overline{q}_{i,pore} = \frac{3}{R_p^3} \int_0^{R_p} q_i \, r^2 \, dr \qquad (6\text{-}43b)$$

The $3/R_p^3$ term comes from the volume of the spherical particle. Term 4 in Eq. (6-42) is the term for (out-in) due to bulk fluid movement, and the fifth term is the term for (out-in) due to axial dispersion and diffusion.

To use Eq. (6-42) we must relate the average amount adsorbed $\overline{q}_i$ to the fluid concentration c_i. Many ways of doing this have been proposed (e.g. Ruthven, 1984; Yang, 1987). Generally, fluid concentration in the pores $c_{i,pore}$ is calculated and q_i is assumed to be in equilibrium with the local pore concentration. Mass transfer inside the particles occurs due to some combination of normal (Fickian) diffusion in the pores, Knudsen diffusion in the pores, and surface diffusion. For spherical particles the equation for normal pore diffusion is

$$\frac{\partial c_{i,pore}}{\partial t} = D_{mp} \left[\frac{\partial^2 c_{i,pore}}{\partial r^2} + \frac{2}{r} \frac{\partial c_{i,} pore}{\partial r} \right] \qquad (6\text{-}44a)$$

where D_{mp} is the effective molecular diffusivity in the pore. The effective pore diffusivity is usually related to the molecular diffusivity,

$$D_{mp} = \frac{\varepsilon_p D_m}{\tau} \qquad (6\text{-}44b)$$

where τ is the tortuosity factor. The pellet porosity ε_p in the numerator takes into account the solid volume which is unavailable for diffusion. The tortuosity is the ratio of the actual distance of travel divided by the particle radius. Experimental ranges for τ are given in Tables 6-2, 6-4, 6-5 and 6-6. If there is drastically hindered diffusion or retardation of the solute, τ can be as high as 100 and D_{mp} can be two orders of magnitude lower than D_m. The safest approach is to use experimental data to determine D_{mp}, although expressions for estimating effective diffusivities are discussed by Ruthven (1984).

For gas systems with high loadings of adsorbate, surface diffusion is an important mechanism and can account for as much as 80% of the total flux (Yang, 1987). In surface diffusion the adsorbate does not desorb, but instead diffuses along the surface. We can define a surface diffusion coefficient, D_s, by analogy to Fick's law

$$\text{Flux} = -D_s \frac{dq}{dr} \qquad (6\text{-}45a)$$

Unfortunately, D_s shows a strong dependence on surface coverage, and Eq. (6-45a) is difficult to use in models. It is more common to write the surface diffusion effect as a lumped parameter expression,

$$\frac{d\overline{q}}{dt} = k_s(\overline{q} - q^*) \qquad (6\text{-}45b)$$

where k_s is the surface diffusion coefficient and q^* is the equilibrium value of surface concentration. For *linear* systems q = AC and Eq. (6-45b) can be written as

$$\frac{d\overline{q}}{dt} = k_s A(c - c^*) \qquad (6\text{-}45c)$$

Correlations for k_s are discussed in Section 8.3.

The pore fluid concentration at the wall $c_{i,pore}$ (R_p) can be related to the fluid concentration outside the pores, c_i, by the mass transfer equation across the surface film.

$$K_{d,i} \, \varepsilon_p (1 - \varepsilon_e) \frac{\partial \overline{c}_{i,pore}}{\partial t} + \rho_s (1 - \varepsilon_p)(1 - \varepsilon_e) \frac{\partial \overline{q}_i}{\partial t} = k_f a_p \left[c_i - c_{i,pore}(R_p) \right] \qquad (6\text{-}46)$$

In this equation k_f is the film mass transfer coefficient in units such as m/s and a_p is the external surface area per unit particle volume (m^2/m^3). For spherical particles $a_p = 3/R_p$. The left hand side of Eq. (6-46) is the accumulation of solute in the particle while the right hand side is the transfer rate across the surface film.

Equations (6-42) to (6-46) must be solved simultaneously with the appropriate equilibrium isotherm, initial and boundary conditions. This set of equations is difficult to solve. Although the Rosen solution does solve a similar set of equations for linear isotherms (see Section 7-8), it is common to drastically simplify the equations before solving. We will often assume that a lumped parameter expression similar to Eq. (6-46) is adequate.

$$\rho_s (1 - \varepsilon_p)(1 - \varepsilon_e) \frac{\partial \overline{q}_i}{\partial t} + K_{d,i} \, \varepsilon_p (1 - \varepsilon_e) \frac{\partial c_i^*}{\partial t} = (k_m \, a_p)(c_i - c_i^*) \qquad (6\text{-}47)$$

In this equation the entire particle is treated as having a constant amount adsorbed $\overline{q}_i$, and the stagnant fluid inside the pores is assumed to be in equilibrium with the solid. For gas systems the accumulation of adsorbate in the stagnant fluid is often ignored. Since the distributed concentrations c_i and q_i have been lumped, this is called a lumped parameter mass transfer equation.

Thus c_i^*, the fluid concentration in equilibrium with $\bar{q}_i$, replaces $\bar{c}_{i,pore}$. Equation (6-47) would be correct if mass transfer across the film were the controlling step. However, Eq. (6-47) is often used in other situations. Then k_m is the effective mass transfer coefficient. Correlations for k_m are discussed in Section 8.3.

Alternate forms of the mass transfer equation and the solute mass balance are used when a single porosity model is used. The solute mass balance is,

$$\varepsilon_e \frac{\partial c_i}{\partial t} + \rho_p(1-\varepsilon_e) \frac{\partial \bar{q}_i}{\partial t} + \varepsilon_e \frac{\partial(vc_i)}{\partial z} - \varepsilon_e(E_D + D_M)\frac{\partial^2 c_i}{\partial z^2} = 0 \qquad (6\text{-}48)$$

where ρ_p is the particle density of solid including the fluid in the pores and $\bar{q}_i$ now includes both adsorbed solute and solute in the stagnant fluid in the pores. Terms 1 and 2 are the accumulation terms while term 3 is the convection term and term 4 includes axial dispersion and diffusion. Equations (6-43) to (6-45) are unchanged. The coupling equation for mass transfer across the film becomes

$$\rho_p(1-\varepsilon_e)\frac{\partial \bar{q}_i}{\partial t} = k_f\, a_p \left[c_i - c_{i,pore}(r=R_p) \right] \qquad (6\text{-}49)$$

When the lumped parameter mass transfer expression is used, this equation is

$$\rho_p(1-\varepsilon_e)\frac{\partial \bar{q}_i}{\partial t} = k_m\, a_p(c_i - c_i^*) \qquad (6\text{-}50)$$

Equations (6-48) to (6-50) are the appropriate equations for non-porous solids and for gel-type ion exchange resins. These equations are somewhat simpler than Eqs. (6-42), (6-46) and (6-47), and thus the single porosity equations are often used when the two or three porosity models would be physically more realistic.

6.8. BASIC ENERGY BALANCES

For non-isothermal systems an energy balance for both phases and an energy transfer equation are required. We will assume that no electrical or magnetic fields are present, radiant heat transfer is negligible, viscous heating can be neglected, kinetic and potential energy changes are small, and density is constant. Then the energy balance for both phases is

$$\rho_f C_{P,f} \varepsilon_e \frac{\partial T}{\partial t} + \rho_f C_{P,f} \varepsilon_p (1-\varepsilon_e) \frac{\partial \overline{T}^*}{\partial t} + \rho_s C_{P,s} (1-\varepsilon_p)(1-\varepsilon_e) \frac{\partial \overline{T}_s}{\partial t} + \rho_f C_{P,f} \varepsilon_e \frac{\partial (vT)}{\partial z}$$

$$- (E_{DT} + D_T)\rho_f C_{P,f} \varepsilon_e \frac{\partial^2 T}{\partial z^2} = h_w A_w (T_{amb} - T_w) - C_{P,w} \frac{W}{A_c} \frac{\partial T_w}{\partial t} \qquad (6\text{-}51)$$

In Eq. (6-51) $\overline{T}^*$ and T_{amb} are the stagnant fluid and ambient temperatures, respectively, and h_w is the heat transfer coefficient for the column walls. Terms 1, 2, 3, and 7 represent accumulation in the mobile fluid, the stagnant fluid, the solid and the column walls, respectively. Term 4 is (out-in) with the flowing fluid while term 6 is (in-out) due to heat transfer through the column walls. Finally, term 5 represents the axial dispersive flow of energy.

The volume average values $\overline{T}^*$ and $\overline{T}_s$ are determined by equations analogous to Eqs. (6-43a,b)

$$\overline{T}^* = \frac{3}{R_p^3} \int_0^{R_p} T^* r^2 dr \quad , \quad \overline{T}_s = \frac{3}{R_p^3} \int_0^{R_p} T_s r^2 dr \qquad (6\text{-}52)$$

The temperatures inside the particles can be estimated from a diffusion equation

$$[(1-\varepsilon_p)\rho_s C_{P,s} + \rho_f C_{P,f} \varepsilon_p] \frac{\partial T}{\partial t} = \frac{k_e}{r^2} \frac{\partial}{\partial r} \left[r^2 \frac{\partial T_s}{\partial r} \right] + \Delta H_{ads} \frac{\partial q}{\partial t} \qquad (6\text{-}53)$$

where T^* and T_s are locally in equilibrium ($T^* = T_s$) and k_e is the effective thermal diffusivity including radiation effects. Equations (6-51) and (6-53) are coupled by film diffusion.

$$\rho_f C_{P,f} \varepsilon_p (1 - \varepsilon_e) \frac{\partial \overline{T}^*}{\partial t} + \rho_s C_{P,s} (1 - \varepsilon_p)(1 - \varepsilon_e) \frac{\partial \overline{T}_s}{\partial t} = ha_p [(T - T_s(R_p)] \tag{6-54}$$

where h is the heat transfer coefficient in units such as m/s. These equations are analogous to the mass transfer expressions. Equations (6-51) to (6-54) are a formidable set. Suprisingly, the equivalent single porosity set for heat transfer with no adsorption can be solved with a few simplifications (see Problem 7-E3 and Section 7.8.).

A relatively simple form of the energy transfer equation is obtained by assuming that an overall linear driving force model is adequate. Then the energy balance for the solid is,

$$\rho_s C_{P,s} (1-\varepsilon_p)(1-\varepsilon_e) \frac{\partial \overline{T}_s}{\partial t} + \rho_f C_{P,f} \varepsilon_p (1-\varepsilon_e) \frac{\partial \overline{T}^*}{\partial t}$$

$$= - h_p a_p (\overline{T}_s - T) + (1-\varepsilon_p)(1-\varepsilon_e)\rho_s \Delta H_{ads} \frac{\partial \overline{q}}{\partial t} \tag{6-55}$$

In this equation h_p is the particle heat transfer coefficient, a_p is the particle surface area per unit volume, and ΔH_{ads} is the heat of adsorption, kcal/gm adsorbate. Usually Eq. (6-55) is satisfactory.

The single porosity forms of Eqs. (6-51), (6-53), (6-54) and (6-55) are often used. These are easily obtained by setting $\varepsilon_p = 0$, replacing ρ_s with ρ_p, and replacing $C_{P,s}$ with $C_{P,p}$ which is the particle heat capacity including solid and fluid in the pores.

Complete solution of Eqs. (6-42), (6-47), (6-51) and (6-55) or of the corresponding single porosity equations is difficult. The equations are *coupled*. That is, the mass balances depend on the energy balance equations since equilibrium is temperature dependent. The energy balance is coupled to the mass balances through the last term in Eq. (6-52).

6.9. LOCAL EQUILIBRIUM THEORY

How do these mass transfer and energy equations relate to the solute movement theory? The solute movement theory can be derived from the mass transfer and energy transfer equations if a variety of additional assumptions are made. These assumptions are all the assumptions listed in Table 6-7. The results are drastically simplified partial differential equations. With local equilibrium (assumption # 15) the diffusion equation (6-44) and the mass transfer Eqs. (6-47) or (6-50) are not required. When the assumptions in Table 6-7 are used, the solute mass balance for a single solute, Eq. (6-42), becomes

$$[\varepsilon_e + K_d(1-\varepsilon_e)\varepsilon_p] \frac{\partial c}{\partial t} + \rho_s(1-\varepsilon_e)(1-\varepsilon_p) \frac{\partial q}{\partial t} + \varepsilon_e v \frac{\partial c}{\partial z} = 0 \qquad (6\text{-}56)$$

Note that with local equilibrium $q = \bar{q}$ and $c = c_{pore}$. From the chain rule,

$$\frac{\partial q}{\partial t} = \frac{\partial q}{\partial c} \frac{\partial c}{\partial t} + \frac{\partial q}{\partial T} \frac{\partial T}{\partial t} \qquad (6\text{-}57)$$

Substituting this into Eq. (6-56) and rearranging we obtain

$$\frac{\partial c}{\partial t} + u_s \frac{\partial c}{\partial z} = -\frac{u_s}{v}(\frac{1-\varepsilon_e}{\varepsilon_e})(1-\varepsilon_p)\rho_s \frac{\partial q}{\partial T} \frac{\partial T}{\partial t} \qquad (6\text{-}58)$$

where u_s is given by Eq. (6-23) with $\Delta q/\Delta c$ replaced by $\partial q/\partial c$.

Appropriate initial and boundary conditions are,

$$c = c_0(z) , \qquad t = 0 \qquad\qquad (6\text{-}59a)$$

$$c = c_F(t) , \qquad z = 0 \qquad\qquad (6\text{-}59b)$$

For isothermal systems or for square temperature waves, $\partial T/\partial t = 0$, and the right-hand-side of Eq. (6-58) is zero. Then, Eq. (6-58) is easily solved by the method of characteristics (Sherwood *et al.*, 1975; Wankat, 1981). A simple approach to the method of characteristics is to compare Eq. (6-58) to the total derivative of concentration with respect to time.

$$\frac{\partial c}{\partial t} + \frac{\partial c}{\partial z} \frac{dz}{dt} = \frac{dc}{dt} \tag{6-60}$$

If

$$\frac{dz}{dt} = u_s \tag{6-61}$$

then, the left hand side of Eq. (6-58) is the same as the left hand side of Eq. (6-60). This forces (when $\partial T/\partial t = 0$)

$$\frac{dc}{dt} = 0 \tag{6-62}$$

Thus concentration is constant along the lines represented by Eq. (6-61). This result is exactly the same as the solute movement theory developed earlier using a physical argument.

The local equilibrium or solute movement model is extremely simple compared to other adsorption models. This simple model includes the first and fourth terms in Eq. (6-42). The second and third terms are also included but with the assumption of local equilibrium. This assumption means that Eq. (6-47) is automatically satisfied. The fifth term in Eq. (6-42) is ignored. Any equilibrium form can be used. The model thus includes diffuse waves due to nonlinear equilibrium, but does not include mass transfer and dispersion which also broaden zones. Extensions of this model can be made to relax assumptions 10b to 14 in Table 6-7 (see Sections 7.4 and 8.5).

The mass transfer equations will be solved for systems with finite dispersion and mass transfer resistances in Chapters 7 and 8. Chapter 7 considers systems where the isotherm is linear and then applies the solutions to chromatography. Chapter 8 uses both the solute movement theory and non-linear solutions of the mass transfer equations to examine a variety of adsorption separations.

A simplified solution for the energy balance can be obtained by assuming local equilibrium $T = T^* = T_w = T_s = T_f$, assuming the heat of adsorption term is negligible, assuming h_w is zero, and ignoring axial dispersion and diffusion. These assumptions decouple the mass and energy balances, and make Eq. (6-55) automatically satisfied. The mathematical manipulations to solve Eq. (6-51) for this *local equilibrium* theory are essentially the same as those used to solve the mass balances (see Problem 6-C9). The results are exactly the same as those derived earlier for the solute movement theory by physical arguments.

6.10. SUMMARY - OBJECTIVES

At the end of this chapter you should be able to meet the following objectives:

1. Discuss which adsorbents are appropriate for a particular separation.

2. Use various equilibrium isotherm forms and determine the isotherm parameters from equilibrium data.

3. Use the solute movement theory for both linear and non-linear isotherms.

4. Explain the movement of energy waves and the effect of temperature on solute adsorption. Calculate thermal wave velocities and concentration changes.

5. Write and identify the terms in the mass and energy balances and the mass and energy transfer equations.

6. Show that the local equilibrium model is essentially the same as the solute movement theory.

REFERENCES

Baker, B. and R.L. Pigford, "Cycling zone adsorption: quantitative theory and experimental results," *Ind. Eng. Chem. Fundam., 10*, 283 (1971).

Bidlingmeyer, B.A., and Warren, F.V., Jr., "Column watch: Small-molecule gel permeation chromatography: A technique for everyone," *LC-GC*, *6*, 780 (1988).

Bonsal, R.C., J.-B. Donnet, and F. Stoeckli, *Active Carbon*, Marcel Dekker, New York, 1988.

Breck, D.W., *Zeolite Molecular Sieves*, Wiley, New York, 1974.

Brunauer, S., P.H. Emmett, and E. Teller, "Adsorption of gases in multimolecular layers", *J. Am. Chem. Soc.*, *60*, 309 (1938).

Collins, J., "Where to use molecular sieves," *Chem. Eng. Prog.*, *64* (8), 66 (1968).

Dobbs, R.A. and Cohen, J.A., "Carbon adsorption isotherms for toxic organics," EPA, Cincinnati, OH, 45268, EPA-600/8-80-023, April, 1980.

Faust, S.D. and D.M. Aly, *Adsorption Processes for Water Treatment*, Butterworths, Boston, 1987.

Fox, C.R., "Industrial wastewater control and recovery of organic chemicals by adsorption," in F.L. Slejko (Ed.), *Adsorption Technology*, Marcel Dekker, New York, 1985, 167.

Fritz, W. and E.V. Schluender, "Simultaneous adsorption equilibria of organic solutes in dilute aqueous solution on activated carbon," *Chem. Eng. Sci. 29*, 1279 (1974).

Janson, J.C. and P. Hedman, "Large-scale chromatography of proteins," in Fiechter, A. (Ed.), *Advances in Biochemical Engineering*, Vol. 25, Springer-Verlag, Berlin, 1982, 43-99.

Kovach, J.L., "Gas-phase adsorption," in P.A. Schweitzer (Ed.), *Handbook of Separation Techniques for Chemical Engineers*, McGraw-Hill, New York, 1979, Sect. 3.1.

Langmuir, I., "The adsorption of gases on plane surfaces of glass, mica and platinum," *J. Am. Chem. Soc., 40*, 1361 (1918).

Lee, M.N.Y., "Novel separations with molecular sieves adsorption," in N.N. Li (Ed.), *Recent Developments in Separation Science*, Vol. I, CRC Press, Boca Raton, FL, 1972, 75.

LeVan, M.D. and T. Vermeulen, "Binary Langmuir and Freundlich isotherms for ideal adsorbed solutions," *J. Phys. Chem., 85*, 3247 (1981).

Lewis, W.K., E.R. Gilliland, B. Chertow, and D. Bareis, "Vapor-adsorbate equilibrium. III." *J. Am. Chem. Soc. 72*, 1160 (1950a).

Lewis, W.K., E.R. Gilliland, B. Chertow, W.P. Cadogan, "Adsorption equilibria: hydrocarbon gas mixtures," *Ind. Eng. Chem., 42*, 1319 (1950b).

Lydersen, A.L., *Mass Transfer in Engineering Practice*, Wiley, New York, 1983, Chapt. 7.

Ruthven, D.M., *Principles of Adsorption and Adsorption Processes*, Wiley-Interscience, NY, 1984.

Ruthven, D.M., "Zeolites as selective adsorbents," *Chem. Eng. Prog., 84* (2), 42 (Feb. 1988).

Sherwood, T.K., R.L. Pigford, and C.R. Wilke, *Mass Transfer*, Chapt. 10, McGraw-Hill, N.Y., 1975.

Tsou, H.-S. and E.E. Graham, "Prediction of adsorption and desorption of protein on dextran based ion-exchange resin," *AIChE Journal, 31*, 1959 (1985).

Valenzuela, D. and A.L. Myers, "Gas adsorption equilibria," *Separ. Purific. Methods, 13*, 153 (1984).

Valenzuela, D.P. and A.L. Myers, *Adsorption Equilibrium Data Handbook*, Prentice-Hail, Englewood Cliffs, N.J., 1989.

Vaughan, D.E.W., "The synthesis and manufacture of zeolites," *Chem. Engr. Prog., 84* (2), 25 (Feb. 1988).

Vermeulen, T., M.D. LeVan, N.K. Hiester, and G. Klein, "Adsorption and ion exchange," in Perry, R.H. and D.W. Green (Eds.), *Perry's Chemical Engineers' Handbook*, 6th ed., Section 16, McGraw-Hill, N.Y., 1984.

Wankat, P.C., "Cyclic separation techniques," in Rodrigues, A.E. and Tondeur, D. *Percolation Processes, Theory and Application*, Sijthoff and Noordhoff, Alphen aan den Rijn, Netherlands, 1981, 443-516.

Yang, R.T., *Gas Separation by Adsorption Processes*, Butterworths, Boston, 1987.

HOMEWORK

A. *Discussion Problems*

A1. If V_{col} is the volume of an empty column, relate ε_e and ε_p to V_{col}, V_e, V_i, and V_o.

A2. You suspect that adsorption of a particular solute from a liquid satisfies the Freundlich isotherm. What would you plot to determine if the data does satisfy the Freundlich form? How could you determine A and n in Eq. (6-14)?

A3. Show that $(1 + K_A c_F)$ in the Langmuir isotherm is equivalent to the relative volatility.

A4. Explain each term in Eq. (6-21) in detail.

A5. For the isotherm shapes shown in Figures 6-3b or 6-3d show that Eq. (6-31) is valid. Do this based on slopes of the isotherm at a given concentration.

A6.   Explain in your own words the formation of shock and diffuse waves. When does each occur?

A7.   What conditions are required for Eqs. (6-6a), (6-6b), and (6-12a) to become linear?

A8.   Equations (6-42) and (6-48) are alternate expressions for the mass balance. Show how these equations are related. Compare the meaning of $\bar{q}$ for these two models. Which equation would be appropriate for:

   a. ion exchange

   b. size exclusion chromatography

   c. adsorption of a gas with a porous adsorbent

   d. adsorption of a liquid with a porous adsorbent

A9.   Why do liquid systems usually satisfy Eq. (6-37a) while dilute gas systems satisfy Eq. (6-37b)?

A10.   Workers entering adsorption columns containing zeolites always wear breathing apparatuses. Explain why.

A11.   Develop your key relations chart for this chapter. A key relations chart lists everything (equations, words, figures) you want to know on one page.

C.   *Derivations*

C1.   Show that Eq. (6-16) has the same form as the Langmuir equation (6-12a) except it is now in terms of mole fractions instead of q and c.

C2.   Many models use a single porosity, ε_e, and treat the packing material as a solid or gel without pores. This model is appropriate for ion exchange (see Chapter 9) since gel resins which do not have internal pores are often used. The model has also been used for adsorbents with porous particles because it is simpler. The equilibrium expression $q = f(c)$ must now include solute contained in the pore fluid if there are pores. Use the single porosity model to derive the solute wave velocity which is

$$u_s(T) = \frac{v}{1 + \dfrac{1-\varepsilon_e}{\varepsilon_e}\rho_p\left(\dfrac{\Delta q}{\Delta c}\right)}$$

(6-23a)

Note that when $\varepsilon_p = 0$, $\rho_p = \rho_s$.

C3.   Separation of fructose and glucose often uses a gel type ion exchange resin in the calcium form. Separation is based on different complexation equilibrium of the fructose and glucose with the calcium (this is not ion exchange). If $\varepsilon_p = 0$ and equilibrium is of the form $q_i = A_i\,c_i$ where q_i and c_i are both in the units g sugar/100 ml, derive the equation for solute velocity. HINT: Read problem 6-C2 first.

C4.   Derive the expression for the diffuse wave solute velocity for Langmuir equilibrium (Eq. 6-12a).

C5.   Derive Eq. (6-40) for linear isotherms starting with Eq. (6-39a).

C6.   Derive Eq. (6-39b) for the case shown in Figure 6-9b and in Eq. (6-37b). Also derive the equations for linear isotherms equivalent to Eqs. (6-40) and (6-41).

C7.   Derive the equation equivalent to Eq. (6-39b) when Eq. (6-37c) is valid. Show that the equation equivalent to Eq. (6-40) for linear isotherms predicts negative concentrations.

C8.   Making the assumptions listed in Table 6-7, derive Eq. (6-58).

C9.   Solve Eq. (6-51) for the local equilibrium model.

D.   *Single Answer Problems*

D1.   Data for the adsorption of propane on silica gel at 0, 40 and 100°C are given by Lewis *et al.* (1950a) and are repeated below. Over what pressure range is the Langmuir isotherm a good fit? Calculate the values of q_{max}, K_A and ΔH, (q is gram moles per kg adsorbent, p is mm Hg).

0°C		40°C		100°C	
p	q	p	q	p	q
16.6	0.2137	10.1	0.0418	96.4	0.0531
37.7	0.3960	27.9	0.0900	119.0	0.1471
64.4	0.5678	46.7	0.1407	406.5	0.2087
93.2	0.7307	92.2	0.2580	601.5	0.2781
129.3	0.9010	136.9	0.3352	753.7	0.3360
218.4	1.259	204.0	0.4470		
298.8	1.520	282.0	0.568		
429.4	1.881	373.0	0.6871		
587.1	2.241	462.6	0.7876		
762.6	2.582	554.9	0.904		
		643.0	0.9908		
		768.9	1.128		

D2. The adsorption of acetic acid from aqueous solution onto activated carbon was extensively studied by Baker and Pigford (1972). Their data is available in Example 6-2. We wish to do an experiment at a superficial velocity of 10 cm/min (superficial velocity = $\varepsilon_e v$). A column 100 cm long is packed with activated carbon at 4°C. The bed is saturated with a fluid containing 0.020 moles per liter. A feed of concentration 0.50 moles/liter at 4°C is introduced into the column for 10 minutes and is followed by fluid of concentration 0.020 moles/liter at 4°C. Predict the complete outlet concentration profile.

D3. Repeat Problem 6-D2, but with feed and following stream (concentrations 0.50 and 0.020) at 60°C instead of 4°C. Bed is initially at 4°C.

D4. Ching and Ruthven, *AIChE Symp. Ser.*, *81*, (242), 1, (1985) found that the equilibrium of fructose and glucose on ion exchange resin in the calcium form was linear for concentrations below 5 g/100 ml. Their equilibrium expressions are: $q_G = 0.51 c_G$, $q_F = 0.88 c_F$, at 30°C where both q and c are in g/100 ml. For this resin $\varepsilon_p = 0$ and $\varepsilon_e = 0.4$. A chromatographic column one meter long is operated with water flowing at a superficial velocity of 15 cm/min.

    a. If a very short feed pulse (~ 1 sec) is input, at what time will the fructose and glucose peaks exit the column?

    b. Assuming no zone spreading, what is the longest feed pulse (in minutes) which can be input which will just separate fructose and glucose in this column? At what time can the next feed pulse be introduced? What % of the time can feed be introduced to the column?

Note: See problem 6-C3 before doing this problem.

D5. We have a 60 cm long column packed with activated carbon. The column initially is filled with distilled water at 4°C. A feed at 4°C containing 0.25 moles acetic acid per liter is introduced at t = 0 minutes. This continues for 20 minutes. After 20 minutes, heating is used as specified in parts a and b. The same feed concentration is used but T = 60°C. Throughout the process the superficial velocity is 10 cm/min. Predict the outlet concentration profiles. Data is given in Example 6-2.

    a. The heating at 20 minutes is done through a jacket. Assume the entire column is heated instantaneously to 60°C.

    b. The column is insulated. Heating occurs because of the hot feed (at 60°C) only (a thermal wave is generated).

    c. Compare parts b and c.

D6. Estimate an average separation factor, $\alpha_{EP} = (y_E/x_E)/(y_P/x_P)$, for the ethylene-propylene equilibrium data shown in Figure 6-3e.

D7. A column packed with activated carbon is initially at 20°C. The column is 1 meter in diameter and 4 meters long. The carbon has the same properties as the carbon in Example 6-2. As part of the testing procedure the column is filled with water at 20°C. At 8:00 a.m. a water feed at 40°C is turned on and enters the bottom of the column. Superficial velocity is 20 cm/min. At 8:08 this water is turned off. Flow is reversed and water at 0°C enters the top of the column at a superficial velocity of 10 cm/min. At 8:20 this stream is shut off. Water again enters the column from the bottom. This water is at 60°C and has a superficial velocity of 20 cm/min. Predict the temperature profile in the bed at 8:25 a.m.

D8. The data listed below were obtained by Reich, Ziegler, and Rogers, *Ind. Eng. Chem. Process Des. Develop., 19*, 336 (1980) for the adsorption of methane on Type BPL activated carbon at 301.4 K. $\bar{p}$ is partial pressure in psia and q is mg moles/g carbon.

   a. Does this data satisfy the Langmuir equilibrium isotherm? If yes, what are good values of q_{max} and K_A? If no, can the Langmuir isotherm be used for some range of pressures? For what range of partial pressures is the Langmuir a good fit, and what values of q_{max} and K_A should be used?

   b. We have a column at 250 psia filled with hydrogen (which does not adsorb) and start adding a feed which is 20% methane in hydrogen at 250 psia. Predict at what time the shock wave will exit the column. The column is 2 meters long. Superficial velocity is 80 cm/min. Temperature is 301.4 K. Use the carbon properties listed in Example 6-2. Solve this problem using the data *and* using the appropriate Langmuir fit obtained in part a. Compare your results. Note: You must rederive Eq. (6-30) or change the equilibrium data to have the units work.

   c. Once the column is totally saturated with the 20% methane feed, the column is desorbed with pure hydrogen. Temperature, velocity, and pressure are the same as in part b. Predict the outlet concentration profile.

$\bar{p}$	q
19.1	0.765
39.8	1.304
67.8	1.825
98.3	2.256
129.8	2.604
168.6	2.953
209.4	3.256
249.3	3.501

D9. A column packed with alumina initially is saturated with pure cyclohexane. At $t = 0$ a stream containing $c = 0.01$ gmole/L anthracene in cyclohexane is input at a superficial velocity ($\varepsilon_e v$) of 30 cm/min. After 10 minutes a stream containing $c = 0.02$ gmole/L is input at the same velocity. Data are given in Example 7-1.

    a. If the column length is $L_1 = 75$ cm, predict the outlet concentration profile.

    b. If the column length is $L_2 = 150$ cm, predict the outlet concentration profile.

    c. It is often tempting to linearize the nonlinear isotherm. This can be done by using a linear isotherm calculated with $c = c_{Avg} = 0.01$ or $c = 0.02$. For example, if $c = 0.02$ then $q = 0.0512$. The linearized isotherm is set so that $q = 0.0512$ when $c = 0.02$. Thus, the linear equation is $q = 2.56 \, c$. Use the linear isotherm to redo Parts a and b. Compare your result with the solutions to Parts a and b.

D10. Fructose adsorption on a dihydroxyborylphenyl succinamyl derivative of aminoethyl cellulose is very pH dependent. Equilibrium isotherms at 25°C are (Busbice and Wankat, *J. Chromatogr.*, *114*, 369, 1975):

pH 8.0: $\quad q = \dfrac{0.0582 \, c}{1 + 1.52 \, c}$

pH 5:
$$q = \frac{0.000165\,c}{1 + 1.52\,c}$$

where q is g/g adsorbent and c is g/Liter. The pH wave velocity was measured as $u_{pH} = 0.40$ v. The feed concentration $c_f = 2$ g/L. $\varepsilon_p = 0.45$, $\varepsilon_e = 0.4$, $\rho_s = 1100$ g/L, $K_d = 1.0$. L = 50 cm, v = 20 cm/min

The column is initially saturated with feed solution (c = c_F) at pH 8.0. At t = 0 we input feed solution at pH 5.0. Predict the outlet concentration profile. Assume local equilibrium and use solute movement theory.

Chapter 7

LINEAR THEORIES OF SORPTION AND CHROMATOGRAPHY

In this chapter we will focus on linear theories for solving the mass transfer equations. These results are applicable for both adsorption and chromatography when the equilibrium is linear. Since chromatography is often operated at low concentrations where the equilibrium is linear, theories and applications for chromatography will be explored in this chapter.

The chapter starts with an introduction to a variety of types of analytical chromatography. Next, the application of solute movement theory to chromatography is briefly explored, followed by development of superposition principles in linear systems. Various linear solutions including a dispersion model, a staged model, Gaussian solutions, the Van Deemter equation, and the Rosen solution are discussed in Sections 7.4 to 7.8. After presenting programming and column switching, we then briefly discuss large scale applications of chromatography.

7.1. TYPES OF CHROMATOGRAPHY

Chromatography refers to a broad range of separation methods used to separate complex mixtures. Because of the very broad range of methods included in the general term, it is relatively easy to confuse methods. In this chapter chromatography will refer to a system with a fixed bed of particles which has a fluid (gas or liquid) flowing through it. This fluid is called the carrier gas or solvent. A feed pulse is input into the flowing fluid. The components of the feed pulse separate because they have different solute velocities. The solute movement theory of Chapter 6 can be used to explain the separation. In this section we will briefly discuss a variety of analytical chromatography methods.

Chromatography is an extremely powerful analytical tool for separating and analyzing complex mixtures. A schematic of an analytical chromatograph is shown in Figure 7-1. For liquid systems a pump is used to push the fluid through the column. A pulse of feed is injected into the system as was shown in Figure 6-3a. The column is often enclosed in an oven to control the temperature. After the column, the detector analyzes the stream for some parameter such as refractive index or ultra-violet (UV) absorbance which can be related to concentration. The purpose of the column is to separate the mixture into peaks which contain only one component in addition to the solvent. Then the detector response will be directly related to concentration. This is illustrated in Figure 7-1b where the chromatogram for separation of a protein sample by analytical ion exchange chromatography is shown. (Perkins *et al*, 1987). The ordinate in Figure 7-1b is the UV absorbance at 280 nm. For dilute samples this absorbance is directly proportional to the protein concentration. Note that the separation is quite sensitive to pH. In analytical systems the column is a small but critical part of the entire system. By changing the chemistry of the column, the separation can be vastly different. Analytical applications are usually at low concentrations where both the isotherm and the detector responses are linear.

In gas systems a carrier gas such as helium or hydrogen is used. The solvent tank and pump are then replaced with a gas cylinder under pressure. Injection is often done with a syringe into a small heater which vaporizes the liquid sample. The most common detectors are thermal conductivity detectors and flame ionization detectors (FID).

Two types of gas chromatographs with packed beds are used. In gas adsorption chromatography an adsorbent is used. This method is appropriate for separating mixtures which are normally gases. It has the disadvantage that the isotherms are often non-linear even at low concentrations (see Figure 6-3b). This causes the peaks to be skewed and makes analysis more difficult. Common adsorbents include zeolites, silica gel and activated alumina (Supina, 1985; Zweig and Sherma, 1972) which were discussed in Chapter 6.

The more common type of analytical gas chromatograph is *gas-liquid chromatography* (GLC). In gas-liquid chromatography an inert porous solid is

290

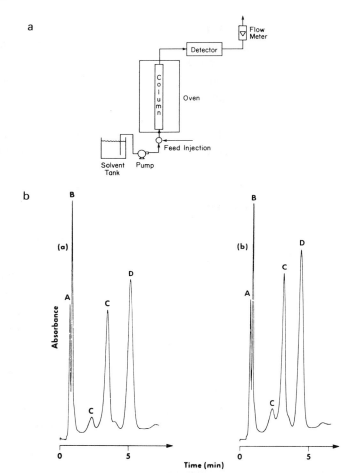

Figure 7-1.   Analytical Chromatograph. a. Equipment schematic. b. Isocratic ion exchange chromatography of 1 mg/mL protein standards at (a) pH 5.85 and (b) pH 6.5. Column: 10 cm × 4.6 mm
7-5μm WCX, 300-A pore size; mobile phase: 0.05 M phosphate with 0.2 M NaCl; flow rate: 1.5 mL/min; detection: UV
280 nm, 0.08 AUFS; injection: 10 μL. Peaks: A = ovalbumin,
B = conalbumin, C = cytochrome c, D = lysozyme. (Perkins *et
al*, 1987). Reprinted with permission from *LC-GC*, 5, 421
(1987). Copyright 1987, Aster Pub. Co.

coated with a viscous, high boiling liquid. This stationary liquid phase is what does the separation. An extensive list of GLC stationary phases is given by Zweig and Sherma (1972). The solid should be inert, have a high porosity and be inexpensive. Diatomaceous earth is most commonly used although a variety of other materials are available (Supina, 1985; Zweig and Sherma, 1972). The solutes in the feed can dissolve (or condense) in the stationary liquid phase and at a later time vaporize into the flowing gas. Separation is essentially based on relative volatility and is really an absorption-stripping operation. Equilibrium is often given by Eq. (6-18). At low concentrations the equilibrium reduces to Henry's law, Eq. (6-4a). Since the porous solid has a very thin coating of stationary liquid and the area for mass transfer is large, the rate of mass transfer is high. Thus the HETP will be low and the column has the equivalent of a large number of equilibrium stages. GLC was invented by James and Martin (1952) and revolutionized analytical chemistry. One major advantage of gas chromatographs in analytical systems is the detectors are very sensitive and work for any compound. Modern systems are covered by Grob (1985) and McNair and Bonelli (1969). GLC has been tried for large scale separations but has been significantly less successful. One problem is temperature stability since even slow vaporization of the stationary phase can, over time, significantly change the column characteristics. This loss of stationary phase also contaminates the product.

Capillary gas chromatography is a commonly used analytical method. A glass or fused silica capillary with a coating of adsorbent or high boiling solvent on the wall is used. Since the amount of stationary phase is small, the capacity is limited. However, the open capillary has little resistance to mass transfer and very sharp separation are observed. In addition, the open tube has a very low pressure drop and hence very long coiled columns (100 m or more) can be used. The result is a device which can rapidly separate complex mixtures. The capillary GC would be difficult to scale up for large-scale applications.

A variety of liquid chromatography systems have been developed. The oldest technique is liquid adsorption chromatography (see Johnson and Stevenson (1978) or Snyder and Kirkland (1979)). In this case an adsorbent is used. This is a common method for large scale applications and for separation of organic compounds. Silica gel and activated alumina are the most common adsorbents, and were discussed in Chapter 6. Details of chromatographic packings are given by Zweig and Sherma (1972). In large-scale applications liquid adsorption chromatography is often cheaper than other chromatography methods since the adsorbents are quite inexpensive.

In liquid-liquid chromatography (LLC) a stationary liquid phase is coated onto an inert, porous solid. The separation is thus essentially an extraction operation. LLC was invented by Martin and Synge (1941) for which they received the Nobel prize in chemistry in 1951. Modern applications are discussed by Johnson and Stevenson (1978) and Snyder and Kirkland (1979). This method is very useful for separating non-volatile compounds which cannot be separated by gas chromatography. The same porous solids are used as supports as in GLC. A large number of different stationary phases and modified mobile phases are used to take advantage of chemical interactions. *Bleeding* which is the slow loss of stationary phase into the mobile phase can be a problem and causes contamination of the product.

Modern liquid chromatography differs from LLC in two major ways. First, *bonded* phases are usually used. The stationary phase is now chemically attached to the inert solid. Very often silica is used as the solid. Great care has to be taken to cover all the active sites to prevent undesired adsorption. For large molecules special large-pore silicas with pores up to 300 nm in diameter are used. The coating still acts as a very thin liquid phase, but there is no loss of stationary phase by bleeding. The most common bonded phases use C_8 or C_{18} compounds attached to silica gel. Water is the most common solvent. For historical reasons this method is called *reverse phase chromatography*. The second major difference is that now short columns containing very small diameter packings are operated at high velocity and high pressure drops. The resulting *high performance liquid chromatography* (HPLC) has the equivalent of a huge number of equilibrium stages (100,000 is not uncommon). Modern analytical columns are often 10 to 25 cm long, 4 to 8 mm id, use packings from 3 to 10 μm (1 μm is 10^{-6} m) in diameter, and have pressure drops of several thousand psi. One advantage of liquid chromatography is that changing the solvent can have a major effect on the distribution coefficients and hence on the separation (Schoenmakers, 1986). See Johnson and Stevenson (1978) or

Snyder and Kirkland (1979) for details of analytical applications and details about bonded phase packings. Large scale applications are discussed later.

One particular type of liquid chromatography which has been extensively used for protein purification is *size exclusion chromatography*, SEC, (also called *gel filtration* or *gel permeation chromatography*). In this system there is no adsorption. Thus A(T) in Eq. (6-24) and ($\Delta q/\Delta c$) in Eq. (6-23) are zero. The only term which is different for different solutes is $K_{d,i}$ which depends on steric exclusion. Usually, the packing is a gel with a well defined distribution of pores. The method is particularly useful for separation of large molecules ($K_d = 0$) from small molecules ($K_d = 1.0$). The large molecules exit the column first. This is done commercially for purification of plasma proteins and as one step in purification of many other proteins, and analytically for protein separations and for analyzing polymer molecular weight distributions. A typical calibration curve for proteins is shown in Figure 7-2 (Andrews, 1964). Equation (6-3) can be used to determine K_d from V_e. Details of size exclusion chromatography are given by Determan (1969), Janson and Hedman (1982), and Yau *et al* (1979). Size exclusion chromatography of biological compounds often uses crosslinked polymer gels such as agarose, polydextrans (Sephadex) and polyacrylamides (Biogel) which are compressible. These gels can only operate at low pressure drops and hence low flow rates (from 10 to 200 cm/hr depending on the gel). Molecular weight cutoffs for these packings were given in Table 6-1. Extensive tables on the properties of SEC packings are given by Janson and Hedman (1982) and Zweig and Sherma (1972).

Supercritical fluid chromatography is a new method (Gere, 1983). The carrier fluid is a supercritical fluid. Compared to liquids, supercritical fluids have a solubility and density that are roughly half as large. The diffusivity is roughly an order of magnitude larger while the viscosity is over an order of magnitude lower. This gives significantly lower Δp and HETP. Carbon dioxide spiked with a modifier to enhance selectivity is the usual carrier. Applications of supercritical fluid chrometography in analytical chemistry are becoming common. Large-scale applications have not been announced yet.

The types of chromatography discussed up to now usually operate in a *migration mode*. In migration chromatography the solutes sorb and desorb

294

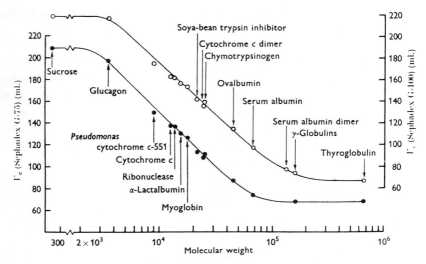

Figure 7-2.   Plots of elution volumes, V_e against log (molecular weight) for SEC of proteins on Sephadex G-75 (●) and G-100 (O) columns [2.4 cm. × 50 cm.; equilibrated with 0.05 M-tris hydrochloride buffer, pH 7-5, containing KCl (0.1 M)]. (Andrews, 1964). Reprinted with permission from *Biochem. J.*, *91*, 222 (1964). Copyright 1964.

many times and all solutes move at a finite solute velocity given by Eqs. (6-24) or (6-23). The solute movement diagram for migration chromatography was shown in Figure 6-4.

Ion exchange and affinity chromatography are usually operated with a rather different operating method called *on-off* chromatography (Wankat, 1986). In *affinity chromatography* the packing is modified by chemically attaching a compound which has a specific biochemical affinity for the desired molecules. The affinity matrix should be inert, readily accessible to the molecules being purified, rigid or close to rigid, easy to chemically modify and cheap. Agarose (a high molecular weight polysaccharide) has been most commonly used although it is not cheap. A variety of attachment procedures are used (Dechow, 1989; Gribnau et al, 1982). The resulting affinity chromatography packing can be very specific for the desired molecule. Thus, theoretically, one can pull out one molecule from a million undesired molecules. In actual practice, the presence of a large number of impurities can foul the packings. Thus affinity chromatography has been used as one of the last steps in commercial processing of biochemicals (Darbyshire, 1981; Dechow, 1989; Hill and Hirtenstein, 1983). Large scale applications are illustrated in Section 7.11. Ion exchange chromatography is also used for purification of biologicals and is usually used early in the process since ion exchange has high capacities and the resins are inexpensive. In the on-off mode of operation a molecule stays in the liquid phase until it finds an open site for sorption (either by specific affinity or electrical forces). Sorption is so strong that once sorbed the molecule does *not* come off. In order to remove the sorbates the conditions of the feed must be changed. Usually this means eluting with a solution of changed pH, ionic strength or high concentration of a compound with a specific attraction for the sorbate. This desorption can be done in several steps to remove one species at a time. The solute movement theory for on-off chromatography is developed in the next section. Ion exchange is discussed in Chapter 9.

There are also non-column chromatographic methods which are used for analysis. In *paper chromatography* the column is replaced by a sheet of paper. Solvent rises in the paper due to capillary forces. A spot of feed is placed on the paper. Separation occurs because of different migration rates of the solutes. One advantage of paper chromatography is a large number of feed spots can be analyzed simultaneously. This method was developed by Consden et al (1944) and modern applications are discussed by Smith (1969). *Thin-layer chromatography* was popularized by Stahl (1965). A glass or plastic plate is coated with a thin-layer of adsorbent such as silica gel or alumina. Operation is very similiar to paper chromatography. In *counter-current distribution* (*CCD*) (Craig and Craig, 1956) a series of extraction tubes is arranged so that only the top or only the bottom phase is transferred. A pulse of feed is input into one test tube and is eluted with additional solvent. Counter-current distribution is thus a liquid-liquid extraction that is operated in the same way as chromatography, and is very similiar to the staged model discussed in Section 7.5. A modern adaption of CCD called *countercurrent chromatography* was developed by Ito and his coworkers (e.g. to *et al*, 1974). The method winds a

296

helical coil in a centrifuge. Spinning the coil keeps the phases separate and the droplets of immiscible liquid will migrate through the coil. The result is essentially the same as CCD, but the apparatus is not as cumbersome. All of the types of chromatography discussed in this paragraph are commercially available as analytical instruments.

7.2. APPLICATION OF SOLUTE MOVEMENT THEORY TO CHROMATOGRAPHY

First, what does the solute movement theory tell us about migration chromatography? The solute velocity for linear systems was given by Eq. (6-24). The solute movement was shown graphically in Figure 6-4b. For a very small feed pulse the peak maximum exits at a retention time $t_{R,i}$ given as,

$$t_R = L/u_s \qquad (7\text{-}1)$$

For pulses which are fairly wide the retention time must be corrected. The center of the feed pulse will form the peak maximum. Thus

$$t_R = L/u_s + t_F/2 \qquad (7\text{-}2)$$

where t_F is the period of the feed pulse. For differential pulses Eq. (7-2) reduces to Eq. (7-1). In chromatography single porosity models are often used. An alternate expression for u_s is given later in Eq. (7-32b).

The solute movement theory (or a retention time argument) can be used to determine the linear equilibrium parameter from an experiment. Suppose a

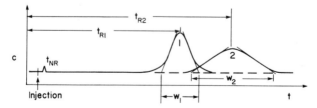

Figure 7-3.   Separation of two components in linear chromatography. Widths $w_1 = 4\sigma_1$ and $w_2 = 4\sigma_2$ where σ_1 and σ_2 are standard deviations of the peaks.

chromatograph is run in the laboratory with a very small pulse of feed and the result shown in Figure 7-3 is obtained. The non-retained peak which exits at time t_{NR} shows when a small, non-retained molecule will exit. Thus t_{NR} is a measure of the void volume between particles and inside the particles. An example is the air peak in gas-liquid chromatography. The retention time for solute 1, $t_{R,1}$, and solute 2, $t_{R,2}$, can be measured. Assume that 1 is a chemical which has a known equilibrium constant A_1. Then the equilibrium constant for solute 2 can be determined as,

$$\frac{t_{R,2} - t_{NR}}{t_{R,1} - t_{NR}} = \frac{A_2}{A_1} = \alpha_{21} \qquad (7\text{-}3)$$

Equation (7-3) is easily derived from the solute movement theory (see Problem 7-C1).

The selectivity, α_{21}, is the ratio of the equilibrium constants and is analogous to the relative volatility used for vapor-liquid equilibrium. Note that the

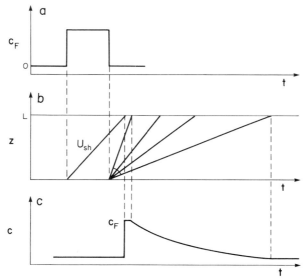

Figure 7-4.   Solute movement theory for one independent, non-linear solute with a wide feed pulse. Shock and diffuse waves are independent. a. Feed pulse. b. Solute movement diagram. c. Outlet concentration.

298

selectivity is easily determined from the experiment shown in Figure 7-3 even if neither A_1 nor A_2 are known.

For independent non-linear isotherms the solute movement theory can be used to predict the outlet concentration. Two situations can occur. When the input pulse is broad, the peak will exit at the feed concentration. This is illustrated in Figure 7-4. Note that the shock and diffuse waves do not interact; in effect, they are isolated by the plateau at $c = c_F$. Thus, the calculation of these waves and the outlet concentration profile is a straightforward application of the methods in Section 6.4.

For narrower pulses the shock and diffuse waves intersect before they

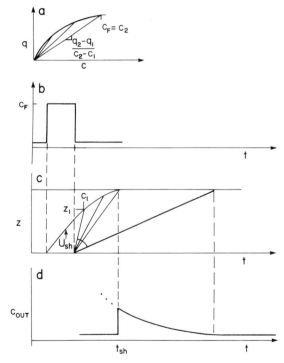

Figure 7-5.   Intersection of shock and diffuse waves for a narrow feed puse. Illustrated for Example 7-1. a. Chords on isotherm. b. Feed pulse. c. Solute movement diagram. d. Outlet concentration.

exist the column. Now c_2 and q_2 in Eq. (6-30) are decreased and the slope of the chord $(q_2 - q_1)/(c_2 - c_1)$ increases (see Figure 7-5a). The result is u_{sh} decreases and the shock wave is curved as shown in Figure 7-5c. The shock wave velocity needs to be calculated step-by-step or a mass balance over the cycle (IN = OUT) can be used to determine when the shock wave exists. This is illustrated in Example 7-1.

Figures 7-4 and 7-5 both assume that other solutes in the feed are independent. If the solutes interact such as with a multicomponent Langmuir isotherm, Eq. (6-9), then the relatively simple picutre shown in Figures 7-4 and 7-5 changes dramaticaly. This more complicated non-linear situation is discussed in Section 8.5.1.

For *on-off* or feed-elute chromatography systems the equilibrium isotherm can be approximated as the step function shown in Figure 7-6a (Wankat,

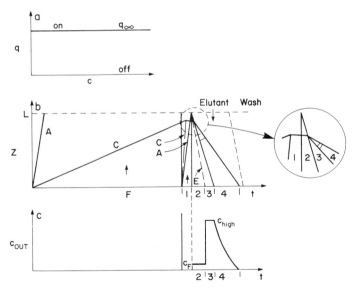

Figure 7-6.   On-off chromatography. a. Approximate equilibrium isotherm. b. Solute movement diagram. 1. Wash step. 2. C at feed concentration. 3. Concentrated C exiting after wave of elutant E. 4. Diffuse wave of C. c. Outlet concentration.

1986). The normal operating cycle consists of a feed step, a short wash step to remove non-adsorbed material, elution, and another wash step. During the feed the solute will move in a shock wave with the velocity given by Eq. (6-30). This is illustrated in Figure 7-6b (Wankat, 1986). In the wash step the adsorbed solute (C) quickly moves through the column until open sites are found. After sorption, no further movement occurs. Weakly or non-adsorbed solutes, A, are washed out of the column. Counter-flow elution is illustrated although co-flow elution is also commonly used. The elutant will move in a wave (E) in a fashion similar to a thermal wave. The solute first jumps to a high value when it is desorbed and then moves as a diffuse wave (for example, Eq. (6-26)). The outlet profile is shown in Figure 7-6c. If there are several adsorbed solutes, the elution can be done in steps with changes in elution concentration to remove different solutes. The final wash step is used to remove the elutant so that the column is ready for the next feed pulse. These systems can be analyzed in more detail using the non-linear approaches of Chapter 8.

Example 7-1. Solute Movement Theory for a Narrow Pulse

A 50 cm column is packed with activated alumina. The column is initially filled with pure cyclohexane solvent. At $t = 0$ a pulse of 0.009 gmole/L anthracene is input for 5 minutes. Superficial velocity is 15 cm/min.

Data $\varepsilon_e = 0.42$, $\varepsilon_p = 0$ (a single porosity model was used).

Equilibrium: $q = \dfrac{22\,c}{1 + 375\,c}$ where q = gmoles/kg and c = gmoles/L

The bulk density (measured in air) is $\rho_B = 0.85$ kg/L.

$K_D = 1.0$, ρ_f (cyclohexane) = 0.78 kg/L.

Solution

We need to determine the curved shock wave illustrated in Figure 7-5c. This will be illustrated first with a step-by-step calculation of u_{sh} and then by use of an overall mass balance.

A. Preliminary Calculations.

The particle density ρ_p can be determined from Eq. (6-2a)

$$\rho_p = \frac{\rho_B - \varepsilon_e \, \rho_{air}}{1 - \varepsilon_e} = \frac{0.85 - (0.42)\,(\sim 0.0)}{0.58} = 1.465$$

where the weight of the air is neglected.

From Eq. (6-2b) we see $\rho_s = \rho_p$ when $\varepsilon_p = 0$.

Velocity $v = \dfrac{V_{super}}{\varepsilon_e} = 35.71$ cm/min

Before the intersection of the shock and diffuse waves we can determine u_{sh} and u_s. For a single porosity model,

$$u_{sh} = \frac{v}{1 + \dfrac{1 - \varepsilon_e}{\varepsilon_e} \, \rho_p \, \dfrac{\Delta q}{\Delta c}}$$

The shock wave goes from $c_2 = 0.009$ to $c_1 = 0.0$.

Then $q_1 = 0$ and $q_2 = \dfrac{22\,(0.009)}{1 + (375\,(0.009)} = 0.04526$

$$u_{sh} = \frac{35.71}{1 + \dfrac{0.58}{0.42}\,(1.465)\,\dfrac{\Delta q}{\Delta c}} = \frac{35.71}{1 + 2.023\left[\dfrac{0.04526}{0.009}\right]} = 3.196 \, \frac{cm}{min}$$

Before the intersection with the shock wave the diffuse wave velocity is

$$u_s = \frac{v}{1 + \dfrac{1 - \varepsilon_e}{\varepsilon_e} \, \rho_p \, \dfrac{\partial q}{\partial c}} = \frac{v}{1 + \dfrac{1 - \varepsilon_e}{\varepsilon_e} \, \rho_p \, \dfrac{a}{(1 + bc)^2}}$$

where $a = 22$ and $b = 375$. Thus,

$$u_s = \frac{35.71}{1 + \dfrac{44.5}{(1 + 375\,c)^2}}$$

If there were no shock wave, the exit times are t_R (c) $= \dfrac{50}{u_s\ (c)}$.

The following table is easily generated.

Diffuse Wave if No Shock Wave Exits

c	u_s cm/min	$t_R = 50/u_s$,min	$t_F + t_R$
0.009	10.7415	4.655	9.655
0.008	9.446	5.294	10.294
0.007	8.141	6.142	11.142
0.006	6.851	7.298	12.298
0.005	5.594	8.938	13.938
0.004	4.395	11.377	16.377
0.003	3.290	15.196	20.196
0.002	2.300	21.744	26.744
0.001	1.456	34.350	39.350
0	0.785	63.698	68.698

B. Differential Analysis: Step-by-Step Changes in u_{sh}.

The shock wave and the solute wave at c = 0.009 intersect at z = z_1 when

$$u_{sh}\ (0.009\ \text{to}\ 0.0)\ t_1 = u_s\ (0.009)\ (t - t_F)$$

Then $t_1 = \dfrac{t_F\ u_s\ (0.009)}{u_s\ (0.009) - u_{sh}\ (0.009\ \text{to}\ 0.0)} = \dfrac{(5)\ (10.7415)}{10.7415 - 3.196}$

$t_1 = 7.118$ min and $z_1 = u_{sh}\ t = 22.75$ cm
This is shown in Figure 7-5c. The shock wave will now curve. From $c_2 = 0.009$ to $c_2 = 0.008$ the average $\bar{c}_2$ seen by the shock wave is $\bar{c}_2 = 0.0085$. Then

$$\bar{q}_2 = \dfrac{22\ (0.0085)}{1 + (375)\ (0.00851)} = 0.04466$$

and

$$u_{sh} \ (0.0085 \ \text{to} \ 0) = \cfrac{35.71}{1 + 2.023 \left[\cfrac{0.04466}{0.0085} \right]} = 3.071 \ \text{cm/min}$$

Note that the shock wave slows down. This shock will intersect the diffuse wave concentration $c = 0.008$ at t_2, z_2 where

$$z_1 + u_{sh} \ (t_2 - t_1) = u_s \ (0.008) \ (t_2 - t_F)$$

which gives

$$t_2 = \frac{z_1 + u_s \ (0.008) \ t_F - u_{sh} \ t_1}{u_s \ (0.008) - u_{sh}}$$

$$t_2 = \frac{22.75 + (9.446) \ (5) - (3.071) \ (7.118)}{(9.446 - 3.071)} = 7.548 \ \text{min}$$

Then, $\quad z_2 = u_s \ (0.008) \ (t_2 - t_F) = 24.07 \ \text{cm}$

From this point we can do another step. From $c_2 = 0.008$ to 0.007 the average concentration $\bar{c}_2 = 0.0075$. Then

$$\bar{q}_2 = \frac{(22) \ (0.0075)}{1 + 375 \ (0.0075)} = 0.0433$$

and

$$u_{sh} \ (0.0075 \ \text{to} \ 0) = \cfrac{35.71}{1 + 2.034 \left[\cfrac{0.0433}{0.0075} \right]} = 2.8176$$

Shock slows down more. This shock intersects $c = 0.007$ at t_3, z_3 calculated from

$$z_2 + u_{sh} (t_3 - t_2) = u_s (0.007) (t_3 - t_F)$$

Solving for t_3, we obtain

$$t_3 = \frac{z_2 + u_s (0.007) t_F - u_{sh} t_2}{u_s (0.007) - u_{sh}} = 8.173 \text{ min}$$

and $z_3 = u_s (0.007) (t_3 - t_F) = 25.83 \text{ cm}$

This tedious procedure can be continued until the shock wave exits at $z = L$. Note that relatively small steps must be used to have sufficient accuracy. Obviously, this approach is convenient to solve on the computer.

C. Integral Analysis: Overall Mass Balance

Fortunately, a less tedious integral analysis using a mass balance over an entire cycle can be used. From $t = 0$ to $t = \infty$ we must have In = Out since Accumulation = 0.

$$\text{In} = A_c v_{super} c_F t_F = (15) (0.009) 5 A_c = 0.675 A_c$$

$$\text{Out} = A_c v_{super} (\text{Area under diffuse wave from } t_{sh} \text{ to } t = \infty)$$

A trial-and-error integration of the area under the diffuse wave is required, but this is much easier than the previous calculation. The diffuse wave at $c = 0$ exits at $t_F + 63.698 = 68.698$ minutes. $c = 0$ from this time to $t = \infty$. Thus, we integrate backwards from $t = 68.698$ minutes to t_{sh}. This is trial-and-error to find a t_{sh} for which Area = $0.675 A_c/15 A_c = 0.045$. We set up the following table using the diffuse wave table for values

Interval	$\bar{c}$	Δt	$\bar{c}\,\Delta t$
c = 0 to 0.001	0.0005	68.698 − 39.35 = 29.348	0.01467
c = 0.001 to 0.002	0.0015	12.6	0.01891
Check #1			Area = 0.03358
c = 0.002 to 0.003	0.0025	6.548	0.01637
Check # 2			Area = 0.04995

This is too far (t_{sh} = 20.196 at c = 0.003). We could take smaller intervals to get Area exactly equal 0.045. Instead, will obtain an approximate answer with linear interpolation.

$$t_{sh} = 20.196 + \left[\frac{0.04995 - 0.045}{0.04995 - 0.0361}\right](26.744 - 20.196) = 22.54 \text{ min}$$

This procedure gives the outlet concentration profile shown in Figure 7-5d and it gives t_{sh}. The method can be expanded to give the shape of the shock wave shown in Figure 7-5c. (see Problem 7-D13). The dotted line shown in Figure 7-5d is the shape of the diffuse wave if the diffuse wave had not intersected the shock wave. For a Langmuir isotherm the integration of the diffuse wave can also be done analytically.

Notes

The results shown in Figures 7-4c and 7-5d oversimplify what is actually observed. Instead of a shock wave a constant pattern wave results (see Sections 8.1 and 8.2). The center of the constant pattern wave is at the shock wave. The diffuse wave results are often quite accurate. Thus the extensive tailing shown in Figures 7-4c and 7-5d due to the non-linearity is often the controlling effect. Profiles with similar shapes are commonly encountered in practice. The two procedures illustrated here can be applied to other situations (e.g. Problem 7-E4).

7.3. SUPERPOSITION IN LINEAR SYSTEMS

Systems with linear equilibrium are favorites to study theoretically. There are several reasons for this. At low enough concentrations adsorption and chromatography systems approach the linear isotherm, Eq. (6-4a). Analytical chromatography and removal of trace impurities by adsorption are almost always operated in the concentration region where isotherms are linear. Finally, the mathematical manipulations are greatly simplified for linear isotherms. Unfortunately, most commercial applications of adsorption, large-scale chromatography, and ion exchange are not operated in the linear concentration range. However, the linear theories are still useful as a limiting case valid at low concentrations.

When the isotherm is linear, the solute mass balances, Eqs. (6-42) or (6-48) and the mass transfer Eqs. (6-44), (6-47) or (6-50) will be linear. An extremely useful property of linear equations is *superposition*. If we have a solution for some simple operations, the results for more complex operations can be obtained by adding the solutions. For example, suppose that Eqs. (6-48), (6-50) and (6-4a) are simplified with some of the assumptions listed in Table 6-7. These equations are then solved for the breakthrough curve when an initially clean column has a step input of feed added. This resulting breakthrough solution is of the form,

$$x_{A,breakthrough} = \frac{c_A}{c_{A,F}} = X_A(z,t) \tag{7-4}$$

The function $X_A(z,t)$ can be any of the solutions for linear equilibrium which we will discuss later.

Now we wish to use this solution to determine the elution from an uniformly loaded column where $c_A/c_{A,F} = 1$ at $t = 0$. Subtracting the breakthrough solution from the uniformly loaded column solution, we obtain the solution for elution

$$x_{A,elution} = 1 - X_A(z,t) \tag{7-5}$$

Superposition can also be used to find the solution for a pulse input of feed. If the column is initially clean we have first a breakthrough solution, and then after time t_F a step down. The result is

$$x_{A,pulse} = X_A(z,t) - X_A(z,t-t_F) \tag{7-6}$$

In chromatography the pulse is often very small. Eq. (7-6) can be written as

$$x_{A,Pulse} = t_F \frac{\left\{ X(z,t) - X(z,t-t_F) \right\}}{t_F}$$

Taking the limit as $t_F \to 0$

$$x_{A,differential\ pulse} = t_F \frac{\partial X(z,t)}{\partial t} \tag{7-7}$$

is the solution for a differential pulse. Many other situations can be solved by superposition once the basic breakthrough curve X_A (z,t) is known. The use of superposition will be clarified by studying Example 7-2.

For linear systems superposition can also be used when several solutes are separated if the solutes do not interact with each other. Solve for each solute independently and superimpose the results. This was done in Figure 6-4 for the solute movement theory solution for linear chromatography. The super-position principle is valid for more complex theories which include mass transfer and dispersion effects.

The idea of superposition may seem trivial to you. However, superposition is *not* valid for non-linear systems. For example, the solute movement theory solution for breakthrough when the isotherm has a Langmuir shape is a shock wave. Thus X_A in Eq. (7-4) is a shock. The diffuse wave for elution of the loaded column is *not* given by Eq. (7-5).

One other result of superposition for linear systems is that variances (standard deviations squared) add. Thus the effect of any phenomena which increases the zone spreading can be added into the solution by adding variances. Unfortunately, once zone spreading has been observed it is not possible

308

to determine which of several possible phenomena caused it. This property of linear systems will be used in some of the linear theories.

Example 7-2. Superposition.

Determine the outlet concentration in terms of the breakthrough solution for the following input.

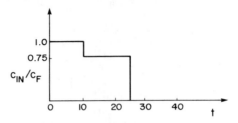

Solution

We have an initially uniformly loaded column followed by a step down to $0.75\ c_F$ followed by another step down to $0\ c_F$. From superposition solution is,

$$c_{out} = c_F - (1 - 0.75)c_F\ X(z,t - 10) - (0.75 - 0)c_F\ X(z,t - 25)$$

The first term on the right hand side is the initially loaded column. The second term is the step down to a value of $0.75\ c_F$ and the third term is the step down from $0.75\ c_F$ to zero. The solution $X(z, t)$ could be the error function solution given in Eq. (7-10), or it could be any other solution for a step input.

7.4. LINEAR DISPERSION MODEL

Lapidus and Amundson (1952) started with Eqs. (6-4a), (6-48) and (6-50) and considered two cases. In the first case they assumed very rapid mass transfer so that solid and fluid were in equilibrium. Then Eq. (6-50) is not needed. Equation (6-4a) was substituted into the single porosity mass balance, Eq. (6-48). After rearrangement, the resulting equation is,

$$[1 + \frac{1-\varepsilon_e}{\varepsilon_e} \rho_p A(T)] \frac{\partial x}{\partial t} + v \frac{\partial x}{\partial z} - (E_D + D_m) \frac{\partial^2 x}{\partial z^2} = 0 \qquad (7\text{-}8)$$

where $x = c/c_F$. For a step input the boundary conditions used were

$x = 1$ for $z = 0$, $t > 0$

$x = 0$ for $t = 0$, $z > 0$

$x = 0$ for $z \rightarrow \infty$, $t > 0$ $\qquad (7\text{-}9)$

For sufficiently long times the solution is (Lapidus and Amundson, 1952; Lightfoot et al., 1962)

$$x_A = \frac{c_A}{c_{A,F}} = \frac{1}{2} \left\{ 1 - \mathrm{erf} \left[\frac{z - \dfrac{vt}{1 + \dfrac{1-\varepsilon_e}{\varepsilon_e}\rho_p A(T)}}{\left[\dfrac{4(D_m + E_D)t}{1 + \dfrac{1-\varepsilon_e}{\varepsilon_e}\rho_p A(T)} \right]^{1/2}} \right] \right\} \qquad (7\text{-}10)$$

The error function, erf, is the definite integral

$$\mathrm{erf}(a) = -\,\mathrm{erf}(-a) = \frac{2}{\pi^{1/2}} \int_0^a \exp(-\zeta^2)d\zeta \qquad (7\text{-}11a)$$

Since the error function is a definite integral it represents a number. Values for the error function are available in many computers and have been tabulated in many handbooks such as the *CRC Handbook of Physics and Chemistry*. A

Table 7-1. Error function values. For negative a, erf(a) is negative.

a	erf(a)	a	erf(a)	a	erf(a)
0.0	0.0	0.48	0.50275	0.96	0.82542
0.04	0.04511	0.52	0.53790	1.00	0.84270
0.08	0.09008	0.56	0.57162	1.10	0.88021
0.12	0.13476	0.60	0.60386	1.20	0.91031
0.16	0.17901	0.64	0.63459	1.30	0.93401
0.20	0.22270	0.68	0.66378	1.40	0.95229
0.24	0.26570	0.72	0.69143	1.50	0.96611
0.28	0.30788	0.76	0.71754	1.60	0.97635
0.32	0.34913	0.80	0.7421	1.70	0.98379
0.36	0.38933	0.84	0.76514	1.80	0.98909
0.40	0.42839	0.88	0.78669	2.00	0.99532
0.44	0.46622	0.92	0.80677	3.24	0.99999

short list of erf is given in Table 7-1. The value of the error function can be approximated to within 0.0005 by the following formula (Vermeulen *et al.*, 1984),

$$\mathrm{erf}(|a|) = [1 - (1 + 0.2784|a| + 0.2314|a|^2 + 0.0781|a|^4)^{-4}] \tag{7-11b}$$

Equation (7-10) is one example of the breakthrough solution used in the superposition results given in Eqs. (7-4) to (7-7). Thus Eq. (7-10) can be used to generate the solution for a variety of situations other than breakthrough from an initially clean column.

It is convenient to write Eq. (7-10) in terms of the Peclet number

$$Pe_z = \frac{zv}{D_m + E_D} \tag{7-12a}$$

where the term $(D_m + E_D)$ is treated as an effective axial diffusivity. To rewrite Eq. (7-10) we define

$$V = \varepsilon_e \, v \, A_c \, t \tag{7-12b}$$

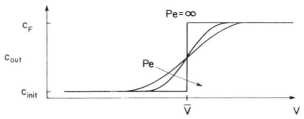

Figure 7-7.   Breakthrough solution for Lapidus and Amundson model, Eq. (7-13).

where V is the volume of solution fed, and

$$\overline{V} = A_c z[\varepsilon_e + (1-\varepsilon_e)\rho_p \ A(T)] \tag{7-12c}$$

$\overline{V}$ is the volume of solution required to saturate a column of length z. In these variables Eq. (7-10) becomes

$$x_A = \frac{c_A}{c_{A,F}} = \frac{1}{2}\left\{1 + \text{erf}\left[\frac{(\text{Pe}_z)^{1/2}(V - \overline{V})}{2(V\overline{V})^{1/2}}\right]\right\} \tag{7-13}$$

This equation also represents the breakthrough curve, X (z,t). Note that the cross-sectional area term, A_c, divides out.

What does the breakthrough curve look like? The results of plotting Eq. (7-13) are shown in Figure 7-7. When the Peclet number becomes infinite (the sum of molecular diffusivity and axial dispersion go to zero), the solution is the same as the solute movement solution for linear isotherms. At smaller Peclet numbers (higher dispersion) there is zone spreading around the wave center predicted by the solute movement theory.

The dispersion solution, Eqs. (7-10) or (7-13), usually gives a very good fit to experimental data for systems with linear isotherms when an effective dispersion coefficient is measured. This gives an effective Peclet number. Once the effective Peclet number has been determined, Eq. (7-10) or (7-13) plus superposition can be used to predict the results for a variety of operating conditions.

Why is this solution able to fit experiments so well when no mass transfer terms are included?

The answer to this question is based on the properties of linear systems. Both dispersion and mass transfer cause zone spreading. The resulting zone spreading for a linear system is identical regardless of which process caused it. Thus a model with no mass transfer resistance can use an effective dispersion coefficient to fit experimental data. The effective dispersion includes molecular diffusion, dispersion and mass transfer effects. Other models including only mass transfer and no dispersion can also fit the experimental data. Note that the ability of a model to fit experimental data does not prove that the model is correct or has included all important terms.

Values of the dispersion coefficient without adsorption and no internal mass transfer can be determined from the correlation developed by Chung and Wen (1968). Their correlation was based on columns packed with non-porous inert beads. Thus there is no mass transfer included.

$$\varepsilon_e \, N_{Pe} = 0.2 + 0.011 \, Re^{0.48} \qquad (7\text{-}14a)$$

where the Peclet number is defined with respect to the particle diameter,

$$N_{Pe} = \frac{d_p \, v}{(D_m + E_D)} \qquad (7\text{-}14b)$$

and the Reynolds number is

$$Re = \frac{\varepsilon_e \, \rho_f \, v \, d_p}{\mu} \qquad (7\text{-}14c)$$

Be sure to note that the Peclet numbers in Eqs. (7-12a) and (7-14b) were defined differently. Equation (7-14a) will predict a value for $(D_m + E_D)$ lower than that observed when mass transfer is present. The difference is a measure of the importance of mass transfer.

The solution for a differential pulse can easily be obtained by substituting

Eq. (7-13) into Eq. (7-7). The error function can be differentiated by using the definition in Eq. (7-11a). The result for a differential pulse is,

$$X_{A \text{ differential pulse}} = \frac{V_F}{4} \left(\frac{Pe_z}{\pi}\right)^{1/2} \frac{(1 + \overline{V}/V)}{(V\overline{V})^{1/2}} \exp\left[\frac{-Pe_z(V - \overline{V})^2}{4V\overline{V}}\right] \qquad (7-15)$$

In chromatography sorption is often quite strong and V is approximately equal to $\overline{V}$ in all parts of the elution zone. If we make the assumption that V is approximately equal to $\overline{V}$ in the preexponential term, Eq. (7-15) first simplifies to

$$X_{A \text{ differential pulse}} = \frac{1}{2} \frac{V_F}{\overline{V}} \left[\frac{Pe_z}{\pi}\right]^{1/2} \exp\left[\frac{-Pe_z(V - \overline{V})^2}{4V\overline{V}}\right] \qquad (7-16a)$$

A further simplification results if $V\overline{V} \approx \overline{V}^2$ in the exponential term. This result is

$$X_{A \text{ differential pulse}} = \frac{1}{2} \frac{V_F}{\overline{V}} \left[\frac{Pe_z}{\pi}\right]^{1/2} \exp\left[\frac{-Pe_z(V - \overline{V})^2}{4\overline{V}^2}\right] \qquad (7-16b)$$

This is a *Gaussian distribution* and is obviously easier to use than either Eq. (7-15) or the error function solutions. The peak maximum occurs when $V = \overline{V}$ (the exponential term is zero). At the peak maximum the concentration is

$$(X_{A \text{ differential pulse}})_{max} = \frac{1}{2} \frac{V_F}{\overline{V}} \left[\frac{Pe_z}{\pi}\right]^{1/2} \qquad (7-16c)$$

Application of these equations is discussed in Example 7-3.

7.5. LINEAR STAGED MODELS FOR CHROMATOGRAPHY

Although chromatographic columns are continuous contact systems and are *not* staged, staged models have been used since the pioneering work of Martin and

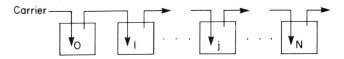

Figure 7-8.   Schematic of staged model.

Synge (1941). (e.g. see King, 1980, Giddings, 1965; or Wankat, 1986). Historically, this occurred because countercurrent distribution (a staged system) was a precursor of the chromatographic theories. The chromatographic column is broken into a series of N stages each with a height H.

$$H = L/N \tag{7-17}$$

The staged model is shown schematically in Figure 7-8. The unsteady state mass balance for stage j for any component is,

$$(c_{j-1} - c_j)dV = V_M \, dc_j + M_s dq \tag{7-18}$$

In this equation V is the cumulative volume of mobile phase flowing in the column, V_M is the volume of mobile phase per stage and M_s is the mass of stationary phase per stage. For a single porosity model we can easily relate V_M and M_s to our usual variables.

$$V_M = \varepsilon_e L \, A_c/N \tag{7-19a}$$

$$M_s = (1-\varepsilon_e)\rho_P \, LA_c/N \tag{7-19b}$$

For linear equilibria, q = Ac, Eq. (7-18) simplifies to

$$\frac{dc_j}{dV} = \frac{c_{j-1} - c_j}{V_M + A_i M_s} \tag{7-20}$$

for each component i.

Equation (7-20) is readily solved for different boundary conditions. For chromatography a pulse of feed of F_i moles of each solute is introduced to stage 0 at volume 0.

$$V_M c_{0,i} + M_s q_{0,i} = F_i, \qquad V = 0 \qquad (7\text{-}21a)$$

and all other stages initially contain no solute.

$$c_{j,i} = 0, \quad j \geq 1 \quad \text{and} \quad V = 0 \qquad (7\text{-}21b)$$

The solution for each solute is then the Poisson distribution which is

$$c_{j,i} = \frac{F_i}{(V_M + A_i M_s)\,(j!)} \left[\frac{V}{V_M + A_i M_s} \right]^j \exp\left[-\frac{V}{V_M + A_i M_s} \right] \qquad (7\text{-}22a)$$

in volume units, or in time units

$$c_{j,i} = \frac{F_i}{\left[V_M + A_i M_s \right](j!)} \left[\frac{u_{si}\, t}{H} \right]^j \exp\left(-u_{s,i}\, t/H \right) \qquad (7\text{-}22b)$$

Continuous distributions are easier to use than the discontinuous Poisson distribution. If the number of stages is large, Eqs. (7-22) can be approximated with Gaussian distributions. At the outlet $j = N$ and the results are,

$$c_i = \frac{F_i}{(V_M + A_i M_s)\,\sqrt{2\pi N}} \exp\left\{ -\frac{[V - V_{peak}]^2}{2\left[V_M + A_i M_s \right]^2 N} \right\} \qquad (7\text{-}23a)$$

where $V_{peak} = (V_M + A_i M_s)N$, or

$$c_i = \frac{F_i}{(V_M + A_i M_s)\,\sqrt{2\pi N}} \exp\left\{ -\frac{(t - t_R)^2}{2\, t_R^2/N} \right\} \qquad (7\text{-}23b)$$

where the retention time $t_R = L/u_{si,} = NH/u_{s,i}$. The predicted shape and properties of the Gaussian distribution are discussed in the next session.

The staged model is convenient, but is not a good model for predicting what will happen when variables are changed. The staged model does not give any indication of how to determine the height of an equilibrium stage, H. For a predictive model a theory which includes mass transfer effects must be included.

7.6. USE OF GAUSSIAN SOLUTION

For long columns and very small pulses the linear chromatography solution for both dispersion and staged models can be written as

$$c = c_{max} \exp(-x^2/2\sigma^2) \tag{7-24}$$

where x is the deviation from the peak maximum and σ is the standard deviation in the same units. This is a Gaussian solution. Giddings (1965) developed a definition of H as

$$H = \frac{d(\sigma^2)}{dz} \tag{7-25a}$$

where z is the distance migrated. For a uniform column of length L this becomes

$$H = \frac{\sigma^2}{L} \tag{7-25b}$$

Then,

$$N = L/H \tag{7-26a}$$

or

$$N = (L^2/\sigma^2) \tag{7-26b}$$

With this extension H and N are defined without referring to the hypothetical staged model. N is a measure of the efficiency of the column.

Any set of consistent units can be used for σ and x. In time units

$$\sigma_t = (LH)^{1/2}/u_s = t_R/N^{1/2} \tag{7-27a}$$

which agrees with Eq. (7-23b). In length units

$$\sigma_l = \sqrt{HL} \tag{7-27b}$$

and in volume units

$$\sigma_v = \overline{V}\left[\frac{2}{Pe_z}\right]^{1/2} = (V_M + A_i M_s)N^{1/2} \tag{7-27c}$$

which corresponds to Eqs. (7-16b) and (7-23a).

The zone spreading measured by σ_t or σ_l is proportional to the square root of the column length. Equation (7-24) is a Gaussian shape as shown in Figure 7-9. The peak maximum exits at retention time t_{Ri} given by the solute movement theory in Eqs. (7-1) or (7-2).

The peak maximum for a differential pulse can be determined from the dispersion model, Eq. (7-16c), and from staged models (see Problem 7-C3). The results are

$$c_{max} = \frac{1}{2}\frac{V_F c_F}{\overline{V}}(\frac{Pe_z}{\pi})^{1/2} = (\frac{F_i}{V_M + A_i M_s})\frac{1}{\sqrt{2\pi N}} \tag{7-28a}$$

A detailed comparison of these results shows that the two models give the same results if,

$$Pe_z = 2N \tag{7-28b}$$

This comparison requires a conversion of the two different nomenclatures (see Problem 7-C8). If N is known the effective dispersion can be calculated or vice versa.

318

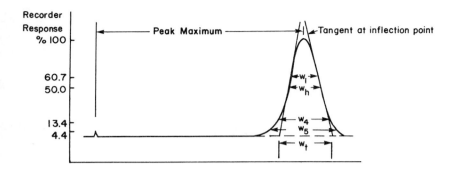

Figure 7-9.   Gaussian response for linear chromatography. Constants for Eq. (7-29):

Width	Constant
w_σ	4
w_h	5.54
$w_{4\sigma}$	16
$w_{5\sigma}$	25
w_t	16

The value of N and hence H (from Eq. (7-17)) can easily be determined from experiments. The value of N is given from the staged model as,

$$N = (\text{constant}) \left[\frac{\text{peak maximum}}{\text{width}} \right]^2 \qquad (7\text{-}29)$$

where the appropriate widths and constants are shown in Figure 7-9. The peak maximum should be measured from the center of the feed pulse. Note that any convenient set of consistent units can be used for the peak maximum and width. One convenient set of measurements is to measure distances on a strip chart recorder. The most convenient calculation is the width at the half height.

In linear systems variances (standard deviations squared) add. In distance units the variance σ_l^2, is proportional to HL. *Thus the H values caused by different zone spreading phenomena (mass transfer, dispersion, extra-column) will add.* Since the purely dispersive effects can be estimated from the Chung and Wen correlation Eq. (7-14) and the mass transfer effects have been correlated (in Eqs. (8-15) to (8-19)), the effect of extra-column zone spreading can be estimated. In a well designed system the extra column effects (mixing in injectors, fittings, distributors, valves, detector, etc.) should be small.

The purpose of chromatography is to separate. In analytical linear chromatography with differential feed pulses the separation of two peaks is often reported as a *resolution*. The resolution is defined as

$$R = \frac{2(t_{R,2} - t_{R,1})}{w_1 + w_2} \tag{7-30}$$

where the terms were shown in Figure 7-3. Note that t_R and w are either in time units or distance on the strip chart, and R is dimensionless. An $R = 1.0$ represents a separation where the two peak maxima are separated by 4σ. For linear isotherms where the peaks are Gaussian this is about a 2% overlap. The retention times can be determined from Eq. (7-1) while the widths can be found as $4\sigma_t$ where σ_t is given by Eq. (7-27a). The resulting "fundamental equation" of linear chromatography is,

$$R = \frac{1}{2} \left[\frac{\alpha_{21} - 1}{1 + \alpha_{21}} \right] \frac{\bar{k}'}{1 + \bar{k}'} N^{1/2} \tag{7-31}$$

where α_{21} is the selectivity defined in Eq. (7-3), and $\bar{k}'$ is the arithmetic average relative retention. The relative retention is

$$k'_i = A_i(T) \frac{\rho_p(1-\varepsilon_e)}{\varepsilon_e} = A_i(T) \frac{M_s}{V_M} \tag{7-32a}$$

Note that $\alpha_{21} = k'_2/k'_1 = A_2/A_1$. For a single porosity model (see Problem 6-C2), $u_{s,i}$ becomes

$$u_{s,i} = \frac{v}{1 + k'_i} \tag{7-32b}$$

Equation (7-31) assumes that N is the same for both components. Substituting Eqs. (7-32a) and (7-32b) into (7-31), we obtain (Giddings, 1965)

$$R = \frac{1}{4} N^{1/2} \frac{\Delta u_s}{\bar{u}_s} \qquad (7\text{-}33)$$

where $\Delta u_s = u_{s1} - u_{s2}$ is the difference in migration velocities and $\bar{u}_s$ is the geometric average of the solute velocities. Equation (7-33) is easy to generalize to other systems such as electrophoresis (see Chapter 11). This equation shows that resolution depends on column efficiency $(N^{1/2}/4)$ times selectivity $(\Delta u_s/\bar{u}_s)$.

The resolution increases as α_{21}, $\bar{k}'$ or N increases. Changing the selectivity, α_{21}, has the most effect. For α_{21} near 1.0, the number of stages (or column length) must be very large to have a reasonable resolution. N starts to increase very rapidly as α_{21} becomes less than about 1.15. For example, increasing α_{21} from 1.1 to 1.2 doubles R at constant N or reduces N by $\sqrt{2}$ at constant R. For large-scale applications α_{21} greater than 1.5 to 2.0 is desirable since N and hence column length will not be excessive. Large α_{21} is desirable since H can be large. The Van Deemter equation discussed later shows that this means a high velocity and hence a high throughput can be used.

Increasing the average relative retention $\bar{k}'$ also increases resolution, but the solute velocities are decreased. Increasing $\bar{k}'$ from ~ 0 to 2 dramatically increases R or decreases N. An optimum $\bar{k}'$ seems to be between 4 and 6. Once $k' > 6$ increases in $\bar{k}'$ have little effect on resolution, but the solvent required increases. Most separations have a k' range from 1 to 10. If the ratio of k' for the last and first peaks is greater than about 30, a satisfactory isocratic elution (no change in solvent) separation is unlikely (Dolan, 1987). Either programming or column switching (see Section 7.10) should be tried. For mixtures of an organic solvent and water, k' decreases by a factor from 2 to 3 for each 10% decrease in the organic fraction (see Figure 7-12, Dolan, 1987). For example, if a component shows a k' of 20 for a 80:20 methanol/water solvent, k' will probably be from 6 to 10 for a 70:30 methanol/water solvent.

Increasing N also increases resolution. If H is decreased by decreasing particle diameter d_p or increasing diffusivity, N will increase. Since decreasing d_p and increasing L both increase pressure drop, there are limits to how much either of these can be changed. When large increases in resolution are needed, the chemistry of the adsorbent should be changed to increase selectivity.

Example 7-3. Linear Chromatographic System

A pulse of anthracene was input into a chromatographic column using isopropanol as the solvent. Column ID = 0.75 cm and the packed length was 80.0 cm. ε_e was estimated as 0.37. N was 266.67. When a pulse was run, the peak maximum exited at 93.79 min. Solvent flow rate was Q = 0.72 ml/min. We wish to build a 50.4 cm column of the same ID and the same packing. Assume H is unchanged. For a 5 minute pulse predict the outlet concentration profile for anthracene. Low concentrations are used and isotherms may be assumed to be linear.

Solution

A. Define. We wish to calculate concentration versus time for this pulse input.

B. Explore. Since N was estimated, the value of H can be calculated. From this H, N and the Peclet number can be calculated for the shorter column. One method of solution is to use the linear dispersion model solution for breakthrough, Eq. (7-13), and from superposition find the solution for a pulse, Eq. (7-6). An alternate solution is to use the Gaussian chromatography solution, Eq. (7-24); however, this will be approximate since the pulse may not be small enough to be considered differential. Although the isotherm value is not given, the necessary parameters can be estimated from the measured retention time.

C. Plan. We will do two solutions. First, Eqs. (7-13) and (7-6) will be used. This involves determining the Peclet number for the 50.4 cm column. After $\overline{V}$ is determined from Eq. (7-12c), values of the breakthrough solution and the pulse solution can be determined.

In the second solution method we will assume that the pulse is small enough that Eq. (7-24) is applicable. After determining the solute velocity from the retention time, the retention time in the 50.4 cm column can be estimated from Eq. (7-2). If x in Eq. (7-24) is the deviation in time from this retention time, σ must be σ_t given by Eq. (7-27b). The profile can now be easily calculated.

D. Do It. The cross sectional area is

$$A_c = \frac{\pi D^2}{4} = \frac{\pi (0.75)^2}{4} = 0.442 \text{ cm}^2$$

Then the superficial velocity $v_{super} = \dfrac{Q}{A_c} = \dfrac{0.72}{0.442} = 1.629$ cm/min

and the interstitial velocity $v = v_{super}/\varepsilon_e = 1.629/0.37 = 4.403$

The H value is: $H = L/N = 80/266.67 = 0.3$ cm

For the 50.4 cm column, $N = L/H = 50.4/0.3 = 168$

and from Eq. (7-28b) the Peclet number is, $Pe = 2N = 336$.

The solute velocity can be determined from Eq. (7-1)

$$u_s = L/t_R = 80/93.79 = 0.853 \text{ cm/min}$$

D2. Calculation for Dispersion Model:

To calculate $\overline{V}$ Eq. (7-12c) is used. The term in brackets is conveniently determined from u_s.

$$u_s = \frac{\varepsilon_e \, v}{\varepsilon_e + (1-\varepsilon_e)\rho_p A(T)}$$

Thus

$$[\varepsilon_e + (1-\varepsilon_e)\rho_p \ A(T)] = \frac{\varepsilon_e v}{u_s} = \frac{1.629}{0.853} = 1.91$$

and

$$\overline{V} = A_c L[\varepsilon_e + (1-\varepsilon_e)\rho_p A(T)] = (0.442)(50.4)(1.91) = 42.55 \text{ cm}^3$$

The breakthrough solution is now easily determined in terms of volumes from Eq. (7-13). The pulse solution from Eq. (7-6) is,

$$\frac{c}{c_F} = X(Pe_z, \ V) - X(Pe_z, \ V - V_F)$$

where the volume of feed is: $V_F = (0.72 \text{ ml/min})(5 \text{ min}) = 3.60$ ml. Substituting Eq. (7-13) into the pulse expression we have,

$$\frac{c_A}{c_{A,F}} = \frac{1}{2}\left\{1 + \text{erf}\left[\frac{(Pe_z)^{1/2}(V-\overline{V})}{2(V\overline{V})^{1/2}}\right]\right\} \tag{7-34}$$

$$-\frac{1}{2}\left\{1 + \text{erf}\left[\frac{(Pe_z)^{1/2}(V-V_F-\overline{V})}{2[(V-V_F)\overline{V}]^{1/2}}\right]\right\}$$

which is

$$\frac{c_A}{c_{A,F}} = \frac{1}{2}\left\{\text{erf}\left[\frac{18.33(V-42.55)}{2(42.55V)^{1/2}}\right] - \text{erf}\left[\frac{18.33(V-46.15)}{2(42.55V-153.18)^{1/2}}\right]\right\}$$

Now we need to calculate. This is easiest to do on a calculator or computer which has the error function built in, or by use of Eq. (7-11b). In

324

the absence of such a tool Table 7-1 or the more complete tables of the normal curve of error (e.g. *Handbook of Chemistry and Physics*) can be used. The calculation can be done in terms of either volume V or time t since these are obviously related.

$$V = Qt = 0.720t \quad \text{or} \quad t = 1.389 \, V$$

The resulting concentrations are shown in the table below and in Figure 7-10.

		Eq. (7-34)	Eq. (7-16b) or Eq. (7-24)
V	t	c/c_F	c/c_F
35.0	48.615	0.0056	0.0093
38.0	52.782	0.0684	0.0773
40.0	55.56	0.190	0.200
42.55	59.1	0.374	0.390
44.0	61.12	0.417	0.435
44.29	61.52		$0.437 = c_{max}$
46.15	64.1	0.354	0.372
50.0	69.45	0.113	0.0964
54.0	75.0		0.00553

D3. Linear Chromatography Solution for Differential Pulse.

For the alternate solution the retention time when the peak maximum exits for a differential pulse would be,

$$t_{R,\text{dif. pulse}} = \frac{L}{u_s} = \frac{50.4}{0.853} = 59.09 \, \text{min}$$

Since the pulse is 5 minutes long the peak will exit 2.5 minutes later (see Eq. (7-2)).

$$t_R = 59.02 + 2.5 = 61.52 \, \text{min}$$

From Eq. (7-27b)

$$\sigma_t = \frac{(LH)^{1/2}}{u_s} = \frac{[(50.4)(0.3)]^{1/2}}{0.853} = 4.56 \text{ min}$$

Now from Eq. (7-24)

$$\frac{c}{c_{MAX}} = \exp(\frac{-x^2}{2\sigma^2}) = \exp\left[\frac{-(t-t_R)^2}{2\sigma_t^2}\right] = \exp\left[\frac{-(t-61.52)^2}{2(4.56)^2}\right]$$

where c_{MAX} is given by Eq. (7-28a).

$$c_{MAX} = \frac{c_F}{2\sqrt{\pi}} \frac{V_F}{V} (Pe)^{1/2} = 0.437 \, c_F$$

Thus Eq. (7-24) becomes,

$$\frac{c}{c_F} = 0.437 \exp\left[\frac{-(t-61.52)^2}{41.59}\right]$$

The results at different times are listed in the table and are shown in Figure 7-10.

E. Check. The results of the two solution methods are not in perfect agreement, but they are reasonably close. Thus although the pulse is not a differential pulse, this assumption is reasonable, and the two models check each other. Equation (7-15) can also be used instead of Eq. (7-24). This result is also reasonably close (see Problem 7-D12). We can also use Eq. (7-29) to estimate N from Figure 7-10. The value of N calculated using the width at half height agrees within 2.5%.

F. Generalization. For differential pulses the linear dispersion model and the linear chromatography model are interchangeable. For finite pulses Eq. (7-6) will be more accurate. However, Eq. (7-28) can often be used *if* the retention time for the peak maximum is adjusted to follow

326

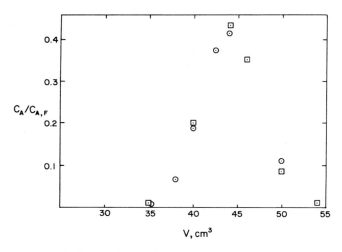

Figure 7-10.   Solutions to Example 7-3 for linear chromatography. ⊙ Dispersion model. ⊡ Differential pulse model.

the center of the feed pulse using Eq. (7-2). Without this adjustment the linear chromatography model would predict a peak maximum at 59.09 minutes which is considerably in error. Obviously, Eq. (7-26) is simpler to use. Note that $c_{max} < c_F$. Eq. (7-28a) will predict $c_{max} > c_F$ for large pulses. In this case the peak will have saturated at $c_{max} = c_F$ and the Gaussian solution cannot be used. As a very rough rule of thumb, if $c_{max} > 0.5\ c_F$ the Gaussian solution should not be used.

7.7. VAN DEEMTER EQUATION

At the low concentrations usually used in analytical chromatography the isotherms are linear. In large-scale applications of chromatography more concentrated solutions are usually separated and non-linear solutions are usually required. However, the linear chromatographic solutions are very useful for the insight they give on the importance of mass transfer and dispersion.

To predict zone spreading, mass transfer and dispersion effects must be included. Lapidus and Amundson (1952) solved a second case where the rate expression is given as,

$$\rho_P(1-\varepsilon_e) \frac{dq}{dt} = k_1 c - k_2 q \tag{7-35}$$

When equilibrium is linear, this equation reduces to Eq. (6-50). The solutions obtained are very difficult to use. A major simplification was made by Van Deemter *et al.* (1956) who assumed linear equilibrium, a very small (differential) pulse of feed, and a long column. Their solution is,

$$c_i = \frac{F_i}{A_c v \varepsilon_e \ (1-k') \ \sqrt{2\pi(\sigma_1^2+\sigma_2^2)}} \exp \left[-\frac{\left[\dfrac{L}{v} (1+k')-t \right]^2}{2(1+k')^2 \ (\sigma_1^2+\sigma_2^2)} \right] \tag{7-36}$$

where F_i is the moles of feed input, A_i is the linear equilibrium constant, k' is given by Eq. (7-32) and

$$\sigma_1^2 = \frac{2L \ (E_D + D_m)}{v^3} \tag{7-37a}$$

$$\sigma_2^2 = 2 \left[\frac{(1-\varepsilon_e)A_i\rho_p}{\varepsilon_e+(1-\varepsilon_e)A_i\rho_p} \right]^2 \frac{L\varepsilon_e}{k_m a_p v} \tag{7-37b}$$

Van Deemter, Zuiderweg and Klinkenberg (1956) then compared this result to the continuous flow staged model written for a chromatographic system, Eq. (7-23b). They found that the height of an equilibrium plate, H, is given as

$$H = A + \frac{B}{v} + Cv \tag{7-38}$$

Equation (7-38) is known as the Van Deemter equation. This equation results from the property of linear systems that variances add. H is proportional to the variance (standard deviation squared) for the chromatographic system.

The A term is caused by eddy dispersion and is the flow contribution to the plate height.

$$A = \lambda \, d_p \tag{7-39}$$

The B term is caused by molecular diffusion

$$B = \gamma \, D_m \tag{7-40}$$

where γ is a labyrinth factor since diffusion paths are not straight. In gas systems the B term can be important, but in liquid systems it is often negligible. The C term includes the mass transfer resistances, and can be expanded as (Giddings, 1965; Snyder and Kirkland, 1979; and see Section 8.3).

$$C = C_m + C_{sm} + C_s \tag{7-41a}$$

C_m is due to extraparticle mass transfer (often called film diffusion).

$$C_m = c_m \, d_p^a / D_m^b \, v^{0.6} \tag{7-41b}$$

The constants a and b are approximately a = 1.4 and b = 2/3 (see Section 8.3). Note that in film diffusion there is a velocity dependence. C_{sm} is due to diffusion in the stagnant mobile phase (often called pore diffusion).

$$C_{sm} = c_{sm} \, d_p^2 / D_{mp} \tag{7-41c}$$

Finally, C_s is due to diffusion in the stationary liquid phase coating the solid or due to diffusion on the solid,

$$C_s = \frac{c_s \, d_c^2}{D_s} \tag{7-41d}$$

where d_c is either the average thickness of the coating or is d_p for adsorbents, and D_s is either the diffusivity in the stationary coating or the diffusivity on the solid.

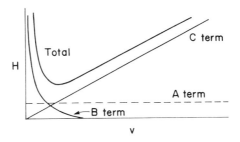

Figure 7-11.   Plot of Van Deemter equation.

The Van Deemter equation is plotted in Figure 7-11 for a gas system where the B term is significant. Note that there is a fluid velocity which minimizes H. Typical values for gas chromatography are A = 0 to 1 mm, B ~ 10 $(mm)^2/s$, and C = 0.001 to 0.01 s which gives $HETP_{min}$ = 0.5 to 2 mm and v_{min} = 1 to 10 ml/s (Moody, 1982). Unfortunately, v_{min} is much too low for commercial applications. Usual operation is at significantly higher velocities where the C term is dominant. Usually, pore diffusion is the controlling mass transfer resistance. Thus combining Eqs. (7-38), (7-41a) and (7-41c), we obtain,

$$H \propto \frac{v \, d_p^2}{D_{mp}} + \text{constant} \qquad \text{(high v)} \qquad (7\text{-}42)$$

The amount of zone spreading, which is measured by H, can be reduced by decreasing particle diameter or increasing the molecular diffusivity. These effects are discussed in detail later.

A variety of other equations for the plate height have been developed (Giddings, 1965; Grushka et al, 1975; Horvath and Lin, 1978). The modified Van Deemter equation

$$H = \frac{B}{v} + C_{sm} \, v + \frac{1}{1/A + 1/(C_m \, v)} \qquad (7\text{-}43)$$

is usually considered more accurate than the Van Deemter equation. Other forms such as the Knox equation (Grushka *et al*, 1975) are considered even more accurate. A very simple form to correlate the effect of velocity is the Snyder equation (Grushka *et al.*, 1975).

$$H = k \, v^n \tag{7-44}$$

where k and n are constants for each packing material.

Detailed analysis of the zone spreading phenomena shows that the theoretical minimum value of H is $H = 2 \, d_p$ (Grushka *et al.*, 1975). H will be in the range from 2.0 d_p to 2.5 d_p under ideal conditions and from 3.0 d_p to 3.5 d_p for real samples (Dolan, 1987). These ranges can be used to rapidly estimate H. For example, for 10 μm particles we would expect H to be in the range from 20 to 35 μm.

In this development the column diameter never appears. Thus, for a *well designed* and *well packed* column there are no theoretical reasons why H should increase as the column diameter increases (in fact, H is often observed to *decrease* as column diameter increases since there are less wall effects). This serves as the basis for scale-up of chromatography to larger sizes. In over-simplified terms, keep length and particle diameter constant and increase column diameter. Note that column diameter is proportional to the square root of throughput (Wankat and Koo, 1988; McDonald and Bidlingmeyer, 1987). The column must be designed so that there is no dead volume where mixing can occur. The feed must be evenly distributed across the column. The column must be packed so that all sections are uniform and channeling is minimized. Failure to follow these principles of good design will cause H to increase. Since N is inversely proportional to H, Eq. (7-31) shows that resolution will decrease if H increases. The zone spreading outside the column caused by fittings, the distributor, valves, the detector etc. is called *extra-column effects*. Since σ^2 values add in linear systems,

$$\sigma_{tot}^2 = \sigma_{col}^2 + \sigma_{ec}^2 \tag{7-45}$$

where σ_{tot}^2 is the actually observed zone spreading. Since $\sigma_{l,col}^2 = HL$ while $\sigma_{l,ec}$ is independent of length, $\sigma_{l,ec}^2$ can be determined by doing two experiments with the same apparatus but with different column lengths. (see Problem

7-D14). In a well-designed apparatus $\sigma_{ec}^2 \ll \sigma_{col}^2$. Note also that the extra-column effects cause zone spreading (σ_{ec}^2), but they do *not* cause separation (N). If good design principles can be followed, theoretical analysis shows that productivity (kg product/hr-kg packing) is significantly higher with short, fat columns packed with small diameter particles and operated with rapid cycles (Wankat and Koo, 1988).

7.8. ROSEN'S SOLUTION

Rosen (1952, 1954) developed an extraordinary solution for linear sorption systems. Assuming dispersion to be negligible and velocity to be constant, he simplified Eq. (6-48) to

$$v \frac{\partial c}{\partial z} + \frac{\partial c}{\partial t} = - \frac{(1 - \varepsilon_e)\rho_p}{\varepsilon_e} \frac{\partial \overline{q}}{\partial t} \tag{7-46}$$

By using the change of variables

$$x = \frac{z(1 - \varepsilon_e)\rho_p}{\varepsilon_e v} \quad , \quad \theta = t - z/v \tag{7-47}$$

he obtained the partial differential equation

$$\frac{\partial c}{\partial x} = - \frac{\partial \overline{q}}{\partial \theta} \tag{7-48}$$

This partial differential equation is coupled to the diffusion equation by the film diffusion equation (6-49). Substituting in the linear isotherm, Eq. (6-4a) and Eqs. (7-47), Rosen obtained the modified film diffusion equation

$$\frac{\partial \overline{q}}{\partial \theta} = \frac{3k_f}{\rho_p(1-\varepsilon_e)R_p} [c - q_s/A] \tag{7-49}$$

where $q_s = q(R_p)$ is the surface concentration of adsorbed material. Rosen assumed sperical particles, $a_p = 3/R_p$. The diffusion equation (6-44a) can be written as

$$\frac{\partial q}{\partial \theta} = \frac{D_{mp}}{r^2} \frac{\partial}{\partial r} \left[r^2 (\frac{\partial q}{\partial r}) \right] \qquad (7\text{-}50)$$

where the same substitutions used to obtain Eq. (7-49) were used.

The average amount adsorbed, $\bar{q}$, can be related to the distribution within the particles, q, by Eq. (6-43b). In Rosen's variables this is

$$\bar{q}(x,\theta) = \frac{3}{R_p^3} \int_0^{R_p} q(r,x,\theta)\, r^2\, dr \qquad (7\text{-}51)$$

Finally, Rosen solved the problem for an initially clean bed with a step input of feed. These initial and boundary conditions are,

$$q(r,x,0) = 0, \quad x \geq 0 \qquad (7\text{-}52a)$$

$$c(0,\theta) = 0 \quad \text{for} \quad \theta = t \leq 0 \text{ and } c(0,\theta) = c_F \quad \text{for} \quad \theta = t \geq 0 \qquad (7\text{-}52b)$$

The solution for other boundary and initial conditions can be obtained by superposition.

Rosen (1952) then solved Eqs. (7-48) to (7-52b). The mathematical details are complex and will be skipped. The exact solution was written in terms of an infinite series which, unfortunately, often has very slow convergence. Rosen (1954) presents numerical solutions.

Rosen (1954) lumped variables in the form

$$\chi = \frac{3D_{mp}\, Az(1-\varepsilon_e)\rho_P}{R_p^2\, v\varepsilon_e} \; , \; v = \frac{D_{mp}\, A(1-\varepsilon_e)\rho_P}{R_p\, k_f} \; , \; \tau = \frac{2\, D_{mp}}{R_p^2} (t - z/v) \qquad (7\text{-}53)$$

He showed that for large χ (long columns) an asymptotic solution is

$$\frac{c}{c_F} = \frac{1}{2}\left\{1 + \text{erf}\left[\frac{\left[\dfrac{3\tau}{2\chi} - 1\right]}{2\left[\dfrac{1 + 5v}{5\chi}\right]^{\frac{1}{2}}}\right]\right\} \tag{7-54}$$

For $\chi > 50$, Eq. (7-54) is within 1% of the exact solution.

To explore the effect of controlling resistances, we can rearrange Eq. (7-54) for long columns to,

$$\frac{c}{c_F} = \frac{1}{2}\left\{1 + \text{erf}\left[\frac{v\varepsilon_e\dfrac{(t - z/v)}{Az(1 - \varepsilon_e)\rho_p} - 1}{2\left[\dfrac{v\varepsilon_e}{z}\left[\dfrac{d_p}{6k_f} + \dfrac{d_p^2}{60\rho_p(1 - \varepsilon_e)D_{mp}A}\right]\right]^{1/2}}\right]\right\} \tag{7-55}$$

If,

$$\frac{d_p}{6\,k_f} \gg \frac{d_p^2}{60\,\rho_p\,(1-\varepsilon_e)\,D_{mp}A} \tag{7-56a}$$

film diffusion controls and the value of D_{mp} is unimportant. This occurs when k_f is small or $D_{mp}A$ is large. Equation (7-55) is simplified for film diffusion control by setting $d_p^2/(60\,\rho_p\,(1-\varepsilon_e)\,D_{mp}A) = 0$. Note that strong adsorption (large A) favors film diffusion control.

If,

$$\frac{d_p^2}{60\,\rho_p\,(1-\varepsilon_e)\,D_{mp}A} \gg \frac{d_p}{6k_f} \tag{7-56b}$$

then pore diffusion controls. This is the more common case. Equation (7-55) is easily simplified by setting $d_p/(6k_f) = 0$.

Equations (7-54) and (7-55) are error function solutions. Thus they predict S-shaped curves which will be similar to the dispersion solutions discussed in Section 7.4. However, there are differences between Eqs. (7-55) and (7-10). The argument of the error function depends linearly on t in Eq. (7-55) while it depend linearly on z in Eq. (7-10). Thus, by careful experimentation it is possible to determine if axial dispersion or mass transfer is the dominant mechanism. Equation (7-55) clearly shows that the total resistance, $[d_p/(6k_f) + d_p^2/(60 \rho_p (1-\varepsilon_e) D_{mp} A)]$, is important. For long columns any combination of pore diffusion and film diffusion which gives the same total resistance will give the same curve. Thus, from a single experiment one cannot delineate the contribution due to pore and film diffusion. The film diffusion coefficient can be estimated from Eqs. (8-15) or (8-16) and D_{mp} can be estimated from Eq. (6-44b).

Rosen's solution can also be applied to pure heat transfer with no adsorption (see Problem 7-E3). A solution similar to Rosen's has been obtained for zeolites with both macropore and micropore diffusion (Cen and Yang, 1986). Carta (1988) solved essentially the same equations as Rosen but for the periodic input of square waves in production chromatography.

7.9. APPLICATION OF THE LINEAR MODELS

The linear models have the unique advantage (or disadvantage depending on how you look at it) that they all predict similar results if they use the same total variance. Thus, once the results have been generated, it is difficult to determine what caused the total variance without independent determination of axial dispersion or mass transfer coefficients. This was illustrated in Example 7-2 where two models gave essentially the same results. Thus the dispersion model, Eq. (7-13), can model systems where mass transfer is important if the Peclet number is adjusted.

Likewise, mass transfer models which do not include dispersion such as Rosen's model and other models (Hougen and Marshall, 1947; Lightfoot et al., 1962; Sherwood et al., 1975; Thomas, 1944, 1948; Hines and Maddox, 1985; and Vermeulen et al., 1984) can model systems where dispersion is important if the mass transfer coefficient is adjusted. The Hougen and Marshall (1947) model assumes that the solute held in the stagnant fluid can be ignored. The result uses J functions which are usually presented in tabular form (Hines and Maddox, 1985; Sherwood, et al., 1975; Vermeulen et al., 1984). The J functions are related to the error function. The Thomas model (Thomas, 1944, 1948; Sherwood et al., 1975; Lightfoot et al., 1962; Vermeulen et al., 1984) based on a kinetic reaction equation can also fit the data well. In the linear limit (the model was derived for Langmuir equilibrium) the Thomas solution for breakthrough is a complementary error function solution which gives results very similar to Eq. (7-13). The Thomas model for Langmuir equilibrium is the basis for many mass transfer solutions for ion exchange. This development is covered in detail elsewhere (e.g. Lightfoot et al., 1962; Sherwood et al., 1975; and Vermeulen et al., 1984).

Since the mass transfer solutions are more complicated to use than the relatively simple dispersion solution, the dispersion solution can be used instead. If a chromatographic experiment is run, N can easily be determined from Eq. (7-29). Then the Peclet number equals 2N. The effect of changing conditions such as particle diameter, velocity or temperature can be determined by calculating H from Eq. (7-17) and then using the Van Deemter equation or other correlations to predict new values for H. Then N and Pe_z can be recalculated and the dispersion solution can be used. Note that the dispersion solution is now applicable to a variety of operating approaches such as breakthrough or elution, not just the pulse solution. Another advantage of the dispersion model is it can easily be written in a two-porosity form (see Problem 6-C5) and thus can correctly model systems where steric exclusion is important.

For more concentrated solutions the isotherms usually become non-linear. For non-linear systems superposition is *not* valid and variances do *not* add. Thus, it is *only* for linear systems that one type of solution can be used to model a system with very different phenomena.

7.10. PROGRAMMING AND COLUMN SWITCHING

Programming or *gradients* are methods used to more rapidly remove slowly moving components. These terms are often used interchangeably and refer to changing a thermodynamic variable which reduces the equilibrium constant. For example, in analytical gas chromatography *temperature programming* is used to remove strongly adsorbed species. This is done by heating the entire column in an oven at a steady rate. Since slow moving species are in the column a lot longer than faster species, the slower species are heated to higher temperatures. According to the Arrehenius relationship, Eq. (6-4b), the linear equilibrium constant A_i will decrease significantly and the species will move faster. Naturally, the column must be cooled before the next feed pulse. Temperature programming is considered in more detail in Problem 7-E2.

In liquid chromatography systems a gradient of some chemical concentration is often used to decrease the equilibrium constant. (Schoenmakers, 1986; Snyder and Kirkland, 1979). This is also called *solvent programming*. In ion exchange, pH and ionic strength changes are often used to remove species from the resin (see Chapter 9). In adsorption and bonded-phase chromatography changes in the solvent polarity are commonly used. For example, if the solvent is water, methanol is often added to help elute strongly adsorbed organic compounds. This is a common method in large-scale chromatography of biologicals. The effect of methanol on the capacity factor k' is illustrated in Figure 7-12 (Majors, 1988). Note the logarithmic dependence of k' on methanol concentration. Gradients can be done in a step-wise or continuous fashion. After all solutes have been removed, the gradient forming chemical must be washed from the column before the next feed pulse.

The reason for programming is easily explained using the system illustrated in Figure 7-13a. The column length or the size of the feed pulse is set by the most difficult separation which is the separation of the two key species A and B. The time to input the next feed pulse and hence the throughput of feed is set by species C and A. Thus, the *easiest* separation controls throughput! The spreading of the solutes can be predicted by Eq. (7-34) or (7-26). Inside the column σ_1, Eq. (7-27b), will be approximately the same if the H values are similar (this is commonly the case). The spread of the peaks exiting the

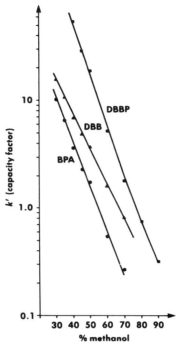

Figure 7-12. Capacity factor k' as a function of methanol concentration in reversed-phase chromatography. Column: ODS reversed-phase; solvent: methanol/water; solutes: DBBP = 4,4'-dibromo-biphenyl, DBB = p- dibromobenzene, BPA = bisphenol A. (Majors, 1988). Reprinted with permission from *LC-GC*, *6*, 16 (1988). Copyright 1988, Aster Publishing Co.

column can be estimated from Eq. (7-27a) which can be written as

$$\sigma_t = \sigma_l/u_s \ .$$
(7-57)

Species C will be spread significantly more than A and B as it exits the column since its velocity is lower.

Solvent programming is illustrated in Figure 7-13b. Now a step addition of solvent S is added after the key components have separated. The velocity of

338

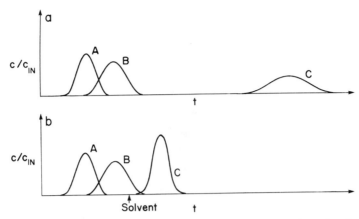

Figure 7-13.   a. Isocratic elution chromatography illustrating the "general elution problem." b. Solvent programming result.

this solvent is easily determined from Eq. (6-23). Since the solvent is chosen so that C is less adsorbed at high S concentrations, species C moves significantly faster. In addition to exiting sooner, the C peak will be spread much less. This is referred to as *compression*. After removing S from the column (which may be difficult if S is strongly adsorbed), the next feed pulse can be input. Comparison of Figures 7-13a and b shows that there can be a considerable increase in throughput. In addition, component C is obtained as a much more concentrated species. It is possible to have $c_{out} > c_F$ (see Problem 7-A9). Both step gradients (Figure 7-13b) and continuous gradients are used. Step gradients are more convenient in large scale systems while continuous gradients are more common in analytical applications (McDonald and Bidling-meyer, 1987).

One particular application of solvent programming which can produce very large increases in solute concentration is *focusing*. To explain this procedure consider the case where a pH gradient is used and assume that the equilibrium constant for solute A decreases as pH increases. The pH wave moves at a velocity u_{pH} in the column. At $(pH)_1$, $u_A(pH_1) = u_{pH}$. Then

$$u_A(pH < pH_1) < u_{pH} < u_A(pH > pH_1) \tag{7-58}$$

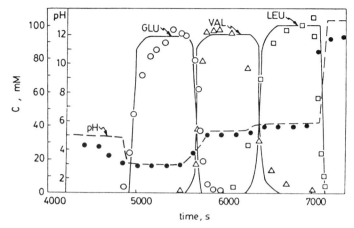

Figure 7-14.   Displacement chromatography of amino acids (GLU = L-glutamic acid; VAL = L-valine; LEU = L-Leucine) using 0.1 M NaOH as displacer on Dowex 50W-X8 cation exchange resin. Solid line is result of model. (Carta *et al*, 1988). Reprinted with permission from *AIChE Symp. Ser., 84* (264), 54 (1988). Copyright 1988, Amer. Inst. Chem. Engrs.

Solute at pH < pH_1 will be overtaken by the pH wave while solute at pH > pH_1 will overtake the pH wave. The result is *focusing* at the pH wave. Focusing was illustrated for thermal waves in Figure 6-11. The result with a pH or solvent gradient will be very similar.

Displacement chromatography is a particular application of gradients which also uses focusing. The column is first equilibrated with a solvent which either does not adsorb or is very weakly adsorbed. The feed pulse is followed by a *displacer* which is more strongly adsorbed than all of the components in the feed. Equations equivalent to Eq. (7-58) will be satisfied for each component. Each component is focused and sharply separated from the other components. This is illustrated in Figure 7-14 (Carta *et al*, 1988). The displacer comes out last. Before the next feed pulse can be input the displacer must be removed from the column. This is often easy to do in ion exchange chromatography (see Chapter 9) but will be difficult in adsorption or partition chromatog-

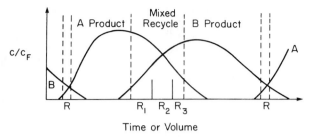

Figure 7-15.   Chromatogram illustrating mixed recycle and recycle of fractions R1, R2, R3. (Wankat, 1986).

raphy when an adsorbate or solute is used as the displacer (see Problem 7-A10). Since each component is focused, the concentrations can be quite high. The solutes thus interact (e.g. as in the multicomponent Langmuir isotherm, Eq. (6-13)). This increases the focusing effect, but in general makes theoretical calculations significantly more difficult. Displacement chromatography is a special case which can be conveniently analyzed (see Section 8.5.1.).

Solvent programming and displacement chromatography require additional chemicals, makes solvent reuse more difficult, and may require excessive washing of the column if the desorbent isotherm is nonlinear. Two alternatives which have been used commercially are *recycle* and *column switching*.

In recycle the solutes are not completely separated in the column. Instead, the overlapping peaks exiting the column are recycled to the feed end. This is illustrated in Figure 7-15 (Wankat, 1986). The advantages of this are the column can be a lot shorter and much more concentrated products are collected. Usually, the entire recycle stream is stored and mixed together. This loses the partial separation which has already been obtained. Better results are obtained if the recycle is done in fractions (R_1, R_2, R_3) which retain the partial separation.

Column switching (Guiochon and Colin, 1986; Wankat, 1986) is illustrated in Figure 7-16 for the three component system illustrated in Figure 7-13a. The feed is input as a pulse into the first column. This column is sized to separate component C. The partially separated A and B peaks are sent to

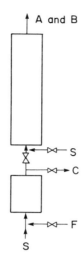

Figure 7-16.   Simple column switching system.

column 2 where they are further separated while component C is withdrawn as product from column 1. Obviously, this allows the next feed pulse to be input sooner and results in significantly less zone broadening of the C peak. The columns can be packed with different sorbents. Use of the linear dispersion or Gaussian models is straightforward for column switching (Agosto *et al*, 1989).

Solvent programming, recycle and column switching are easily extended to separations with more than three components. These methods can be combined (Agosto *et al*, 1989). The first column may be called a *guard column*. The guard column protects the main column from very strongly adsorbed species. Regeneration of the guard column is often done counter-flow to the feed. Many other applications of column switching have been developed (Wankat, 1986).

7.11. LARGE-SCALE CHROMATOGRAPHY

Large-scale applications of chromatography are similar yet quite different than analytical applications. You may have used a gas-liquid chromatograph in chemistry laboratory. A pulse of feed was injected with a syringe in a flowing gas stream, and the outlet concentrations of the separated products were shown on a recorder. After the last product exits, a new pulse of feed was injected. The same ideas are used in large-scale systems, but the objectives have changed. In large-scale chromatography we want to separate and collect the products. Throughput should be as high as possible and the products should be as concentrated as possible. Chromatography is only one of many ways to separate materials and currently it is fairly expensive. McDonald and Bidlingmeyer (1987) suggest using chromatography only as a last resort. Chromatography has become increasingly popular for production of chemicals which cannot be distilled. In biotechnology and pharmaceutical production the compounds cannot be vaporized and liquid chromatography is often the preferred separation method.

Several different types of chromatographic separations have been used for large-scale separations (McDonald and Bidlingmeyer, 1987; Wankat, 1986). Operation in the liquid phase appears to be preferred since many biochemicals cannot be vaporized. In liquid adsorption chromatography the basis for separation is adsorption. The adsorbent can be a polar compound such as silica gel operating in a non-polar solvent such as hexane. In *reverse-phase* operation water or an aqueous phase is the solvent while a non-polar adsorbent is used. The most popular reverse phase packings are C_8 or C_{18} hydrocarbons bonded to silica gel. The majority of large scale applications using migration chromatography are currently reverse-phase. Examples include purification of steroids, hormones, dyes, antibiotics and various other pharmaceuticals (McDonald and Bidlingmeyer, 1987; Wankat, 1986).

In actual practice the peaks spread and solutes overlap considerably. To increase the product purity some of the outlet material may be recycled. These points are illustrated in Figure 7-17 which shows the chromatographic purification of sugars from molasses (Heikkila, 1983). Note that the sucrose is not completely purified and that there are two separate recycle streams. The regeneration of the sorbent is done by feeding fresh solvent (water in Figure 7-17). This removes the solutes from the column, but also dilutes the product. The chromatographic system can fractionate several solutes whereas most adsorption systems produce only one product.

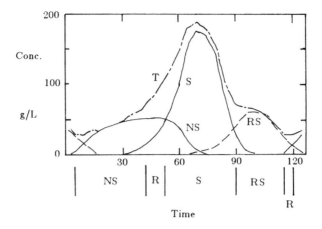

Figure 7-17. Separation results for chromatographic separation of cane molasses. (Heikkila, 1983). T = total, S = sucrose, NS = non-sugars, RS = reducing sugars, R = recycle. Reprinted with special permission from *Chem. Eng.*, *50* (Jan. 24, 1983). Copyright 1983, McGraw-Hill.

One of the most popular methods for large-scale liquid chromatography is to use a reverse phase system with a C-8 or C-18 coating bonded to a porous silica gel in an HPLC system. Packing as small as 10 μm diameter has been used, but larger packings are often used to reduce the pressure drop. An example is shown in Figure 7-18 (Shih, *et al.*, 1983). The elution was done with water until the desired MK peak had exited. After this, the column was regenerated with methanol. Since the MK was quite valuable, no recycle stream was used. Shih *et al.* (1983) noted that the packings vary from batch-to-batch since the process to make these packings is complex. They also noted that some silica leached into the water and had to be removed downstream. Other large-scale applications are reviewed by Wankat (1986). These systems can be purchased as turn-key units from several manufacturers.

Large scale size exclusion chromatography is commonly used industrially for *desalting* proteins. This is the removal of small salt and buffer molecules from the proteins. Hydrophilic gel packings which do not adsorb or

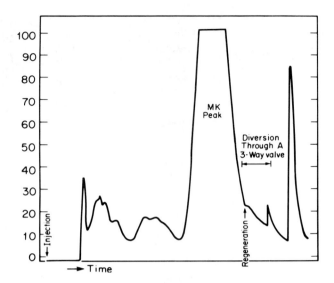

Figure 7-18.   Large-scale chromatographic separation of semisynthetic antibiotic (MK) in 15-cm I.D. column. (From Shih *et al.* (1983). Reprinted with permission from Chem. Eng. Prog., 79(10), 53, 1983. Copyright 1983, American Institute of Chemical Engineers.

denature the protein are often used. Since these gels tend to be compressible, special design procedures are often required (Janson and Hedman, 1982). Rigid particles are used where they are compatible with the chemicals being separated since much higher flow rates and pressure drops can be used. (Hagnauer, 1987).

The usual pressure drop equations are given in Eqs. (8-22) to (8-24). Section 8.5 argues that adsorption systems will have higher productivity if the columns are short and fat, are packed with small diameter particles, and cycling is rapid. These designs can have the same pressure drop, same throughput of feed, and the same separation as more typical designs. Similar arguments can be made for chromatography (Wankat and Koo, 1988). When expensive packings such as bonded phases are used, the reduction in amount of packing can

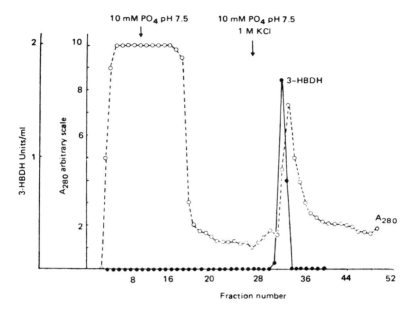

Figure 7-19.   Purification of 3-hydroxybutyrate dehydrogenase by affinity chromatography (Darbyshire, 1981). Reprinted with permission from *Topics in Enzyme and Fermentation Biotechnology*, Section 5, Wiseman, A., Ed., Ellis Horwood, Chichester, 1981. Copyright 1981, Ellis Horwood Ltd.

result in significant cost reductions. Guiochon and Colin (1986) also suggest small diameter packings, but for different reasons.

The on-off, or feed-elute cycle is commonly used for large scale ion exchange (see Chapter 9) and affinity chromatography. These processes can be operated with essentially irreversible sorption during the feed step. Thus the column is loaded with a very large feed pulse. Then nonadsorbed material is washed from column, and the desired product is eluted. Additional separation can be obtained by eluting with step changes in the elutant concentration. An example of a large scale (1.8 liter column) for the affinity chromatography purification of an enzyme is shown in Figure 7-19 (Darbyshire, 1981). Note

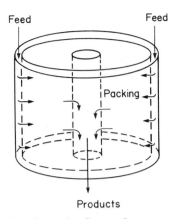

Figure 7-20. Schematic of annular flow column.

that most of the proteins (which absorb at 280 nm) pass through the column without adsorbing. The 1 M KCl was used to desorb the desired enzyme. The product pulse is quite sharp, is significantly purer than the feed, and is much more concentrated than the feed. The use of a 1.8 liter column may not appear to be large-scale, but for many affinity systems it is. The product enzymes may be worth thousands of dollars per kilogram, but the market is small. Darbyshire (1981), Dechow (1989), and Hill and Hirtenstein (1983) contain more information on large scale affinity chromatography.

On-off chromatography does not require long columns or small diameter packings since separation is based on gradient elution not migration. A large area for flow is desireable since larger volumes of fluid can be processed. These considerations have lead researchers to geometries other than cylindrical columns. Annular flow columns shown schematically in Figure 7-20 are available commercially. Flow can be radially inward as in Figure 7-20 or radially outward. These columns have the desired short bed which reduces pressure drop and large cross-sectional area to process large volumes of feed. Feed capacity can be increased by stacking several units on top of each other. Systems similar to this are used commercially for ion exchange and affinity chromatography (Chen and Hou, 1985). The extreme extension of this geometry is to use a membrane hollow-fiber for affinity chromatography

(Brandt *et al*, 1988). Note that other geometries could be used (see Problem 7-B3).

The solute movement theory can be used for a qualitative understanding of the chromatographic separation. This was illustrated in Figures 6-4 and 7-6. Unfortunately, spreading of the zones is always important and must be included in design. For linear systems the models discussed in this chapter are appropriate. For non-linear systems the diffuse wave can be approximately predicted from the solute movement theory. The mass transfer models for non-linear systems discussed in Chapter 8 are used for the shock wave.

A word about economics is in order. Large-scale chromatography is in use for sucrose purification. Sucrose selling price fluctuates, but is usually less than \$0.60/kg. It is obvious that when conditions are favorable large scale chromatography can be used for products with modest selling prices. These favorable conditions are:

1. An inexpensive packing material with a long life, high capacity and high selectivity ($\alpha > 2$) is available.

2. The solvent is either very inexpensive (e.g. water) or is easy to recover.

3. The feed concentration is relatively high.

4. An efficient large-scale chromatographic system is used.

5. Distillation is not feasible or is very expensive.

If some of the first four conditions are not met, large scale chromatography may be feasible only for much more valuable products.

Finally, it should be noted that chromatography is rarely the last separation method used. The desired product exits as a dilute solution in a solvent. Usually this solution needs to be concentrated by membrane separation (see Chapter 12) or evaporation. If the product is desired as a solid, which is usually the case for pharmaceuticals, then an additional crystallization or precipitation step (see Chapters 2 to 4) is needed. Thus chromatography solves one separation problem but adds one or more additional problems.

348

7.12. SUMMARY - OBJECTIVES

In this chapter we have considered chromatographic separations and linear theories to analyze these separations. At the end of this chapter you should be able to:

1. Describe the following chromatographic terms:
   a. Liquid adsorption chromatography
   b. LLC
   c. Bonded-phases
   d. HPLC
   e. Gas-solid chromatography
   f. GLC
   g. Size exclusion chromatography
   h. Affinity chromatography
   i. Programming
   j. Column switching
   k. Reverse-phase

2. Use the solute movement theory to explain both migration and on-off chromatography.

3. Explain and use superposition in linear systems.

4. Use the linear dispersion model.

5. Explain the Van Deemter equation. Use this equation to qualitatively predict the effects of changing different variables and to correlate data.

6. Determine the HETP from experiments. Predict the expected resolution.

7. Use the Gaussian model obtained from staged or continuous contact theory to predict chromatographic separations.

8. Use Rosen's model when the simplified long column solution is appropriate.

9. Explain and solve problems using gradients or column switching.

REFERENCES

Agosto, M., N.H.L. Wang, and P.C. Wankat, "Moving withdrawal liquid chromatography of amino acids", *Ind. Eng. Chem. Res. 28*, 1358 (1989).

Andrews, P., "Estimation of the molecular weights of proteins by Sephadex gel filtration," *Biochem. J., 91*, 222 (1964).

Brandt, S., R.A. Goffe, S.B. Kessler, J.L. O'Connor, and S.E. Zale, "Membrane-based affinity technology for commercial scale purifications," *Bio/Technology, 6*, 779 (1988).

Carta, G., "Exact analytic solution of a mathematical model for chromatographic operations," *Chem. Engr., Sci., 43*, 2877(1988).

Carta, G., M.S. Saunders, J.P. DeCarli, and J.H.B. Vierow, "Dynamics of fixed-bed separations of amino acids by ion-exchange," *AIChE Symp. Ser., 84* (264), 54 (1988).

Cen, P.L. and R.T. Yang, "Analytic solution for adsorber breakthrough curves with bidisperse sorbents (zeolites)," *AIChE J., 32*, 1635 (1986).

Chen, H.-L. and K.C. Hou, "Bioseparation by cartridge chromatography," in G.T. Tsao (Ed.), *Annual Reports on Fermentation Processes*, Vol. 8, Chapt. 3, Academic, Orlando, FL, 1985.

Chung, S.F. and C.Y. Wen, "Longitudinal dispersion of liquid flowing through fixed and fluidized beds", *AIChE Journal, 14*, 857 (1968).

Consden, R., A.H. Gordon, and A.J.P. Martin, "Qualitative analysis of proteins: a partition chromatographic method using paper," *Biochemical J., 38*, 224 (1944).

Craig, L.C. and D. Craig, in A. Weissberger (Ed.), *Technique of Organic Chemistry*, Vol. 3, Interscience, New York, 1956, 149-332.

Darbyshire, J., "Large scale enzyme extraction and recovery", in A. Wiseman (Ed.), *Topics in Enzyme and Fermentation Biotechnology*, Vol. 5, Ellis Horwood Ltd., Chichester, England, 1981, Chapt. 3.

Dechow, F.J., *Separation and Purification Techniques in Biotechnology*, Noyes, Park Ridge, N.J., 1989.

Determann, H., *Gel Chromatography*, 2nd ed., Springer-Verlag, Berlin, 1969.

Dolan, J.W., "Shortcuts for LC measurements," *LC-GC, 5*, 1030 (1987).

Gere, D.R., "Supercritical fluid chromatography," *Science, 222*, 253 (1983).

Giddings, J.C., *Dynamics of Chromatography, Part I, Principles and Theory*, Marcel Dekker, New York, 1965.

Gribnau, T.C.J., J. Visser, and R.J.F. Nivard (Eds.), *Affinity Chromatography and Related Techniques*, Elsevier, Amsterdam, 1982.

Grob, Ř.L. (Ed.), *Modern Practice of Gas Chromatography*, Wiley, New York, 1985.

Grushka, E., L.R. Snyder, and J.H. Knox, "Advances in band spreading theories," *J. Chromatog. Sci., 13*, 25 (1975).

Guiochon, G. and H. Colin, "Theoretical concepts and optimization in preparative scale liquid chromatography," *Chromatography Forum*, 21 (Sept. - Oct. 1986).

Hagnauer, G., "Preparative size exclusion chromatography," in B.A. Bidlingmeyer (Ed.), *Preparative Liquid Chromatography*, Elsevier, Amsterdam, 1987, Chapt.8.

Heikkila, H., "Separating sugars and amino acids with chromatography," *Chem. Eng., 90* (2) 50 (Jan. 24, 1983).

Hill, E.A. and M.D. Hirtenstein, "Affinity chromatography: its application to industrial scale processes," in *Advances Biotechnological Processes,* Vol. 1, A. Mizraki, and A.L. Van Wezel, (Eds.), Alan R. Liss, Inc., New York, 1983, 31-66.

Hines, A.L. and R.N. Maddox, *Mass Transfer. Fundamentals and Applications,* Prentice Hall, Englewood Cliffs, NJ, 1985, Chapt. 14.

Horvath, C. and H.-J. Lin, "Band spreading in liquid chromatography, general plate height equation and a method for the evaluation of the individual plate height contributions," *J. Chromatogr., 149,* 43 (1978).

Hougen, O.A. and W.R. Marshall, "Adsorption from a fluid stream flowing through a stationary granular bed," *Chem. Eng. Prog. 43(4),* 197 (1947).

Ito, Y., R.E. Hurst, R.L. Bowman, and E.K. Achter, "Countercurrent chromatography," *Separ. Purific. Methods, 3,* 133 (1974).

James, A.T. and A.J.P. Martin, "Gas liquid partition chromatography: the separation and micro-estimation of volatile fatty acids. Formic acid to dodecanoic acid," *Biochem. J., 50,* 679, (1952).

Janson, J.C. and P. Hedman, "Large-scale chromatography of proteins," in A. Fiechter (Ed.), *Advances in Biochemical Engineering,* Vol. 125, *Chromatography,* Springer-Verlag, Berlin, 1982, 43.

Johnson, E.L. and R. Stevenson, *Basic Liquid Chromatography,* Varian, Palo Alto, CA, 1978.

King, C.J., *Separation Processes,* 2nd ed., McGraw-Hill, New York, 1980.

Lapidus, L. and N.R. Amundson, "Mathematics of adsorption in beds. VI. The effect of longitudinal diffusion in ion exchange and chromatographic columns," *J. Phys. Chem., 56,* 984 (1952).

352

Lightfoot, E.N., R.J. Sanchez-Palma, and D.O. Edwards, "Chromatography and allied fixed bed separations processes," in H.M. Schoen (Ed.), *New Chemical Engineering Separation Techniques*, Interscience, New York, 1962, p. 9-181.

McDonald, P.D. and B.A. Bidlingmeyer, "Stragegies for successful preparative liquid chromatography," in B.A. Bidlingmeyer, (Ed.), *Preparative Liquid Chromatography*, Elsevier, Amsterdam, 1987, Chapt.1.

McNair, H.M. and E.J. Bonelli, *Basic Gas Chromatography*, 5th ed., Varian, Palo Alto, CA, 1969.

Majors, R.E., "Reader's questions on HPLC columns," *LC-GC*, 6, 16 (1988).

Martin, A.J.P. and R.L.M. Synge, "A new form of chromatogram employing two liquid phases, *Biochem. J.*, 35, 1358 (1941).

Moody, H.W., "The evaluation of the parameters in the Van Deemter equation," *J. Chem. Educ.*, 59, (4), 290 (April 1982).

Perkins, R.V., V.J. Nau, and A. McPartland, "Automatic pH gradient generation for protein and peptide HPLC separations" *LC-GC*, 5, 419 (1987).

Rosen, J.B., "Kinetics of a fixed bed system for solid diffusion into spherical particles," *J. Chem. Phys.*, 20, 387 (1952).

Rosen, J.B., "General numerical solution for solid diffusion in fixed beds," *Ind. Eng. Chem.*, 46, 1590 (1954).

Schoenmakers, P.J., *Optimization of Chromatographic Selectivity*, Elsevier, Amsterdam, 1986.

Sherwood, T.K., R.L. Pigford, and C.R. Wilke, *Mass Transfer*, McGraw-Hill, New York, 1975.

Shih, C.K., C.M. Snavely, T.E. Molnar, J.L. Meyer, W.B. Caldwell, and E.L.

Paul, "Large-scale liquid chromatography system," *Chem. Eng. Prog.*, 79 (10), 53 (1983).

Smith, I. (Ed.), *Chromatographic and Electrophoretic Techniques*, Vol. 1, *Chromatography*, 3rd ed., Interscience, New York, 1969.

Snyder L.R. and J.J. Kirkland, *Introduction to Modern Liquid Chromatography*, 2nd ed., Wiley, New York, 1979.

Stahl, E. (Ed.), *Thin-Layer Chromatography, A Laboratory Handbook*, Academic Press, New York, 1965.

Supina, W.R., "Packed columns/column selection in gas chromatography," in Grob, R.L., (Ed.), *Modern Practice of Gas Chromatography*, 2nd ed., Wiley, New York, 1985, Chapter 3.

Thomas, H.C., Heterogeneous ion exchange in a flowing system," *J. Am. Chem. Soc.*, 1664 (1944).

Thomas, H.C., "Chromatography: A problem in kinetics," *Annals New York Academy of Science, 49*, 161 (1948).

Van Deemter, J.J., F.J. Zuiderweg, and A. Klinkenberg, "Longitudinal diffusion and resistance to mass transfer as causes of nonideality in chromatography," *Chem. Eng. Sci., 5*, 271 (1956).

Vermeulen, T., M.D. LeVan, N.K. Hiester, and G. Klein, "Adsorption and ion exchange," in R.H. Perry and D. Green (Eds.), *Perry's Chemical Engineering Handbook*, 6th ed., McGraw-Hill, New York, 1984, Section 16.

Wankat, P.C., *Large Scale Adsorption and Chromatography*, CRC Press, Boca Raton, FL, 1986.

Wankat, P.C. and Y.M. Koo, "Scaling rules for isocratic elution chromatography," *AIChE Journal, 34*, 1006 (1988).

354

Yau, W.W., J.J. Kirkland, and D.D. Bly, *Modern Size-Exclusion Chromatography*, Wiley, New York, 1979.

Zweig, G. and J. Sherma, (Eds.), *Handbook of Chromatography*, Vol. 2, CRC Press, Cleveland, 1972.

HOMEWORK

A.   *Discussion Problems*

A1.   In your own words explain superposition. How can superposition be used with several solutes?

A2.   Explain the physical measuring of the boundary conditions in Eq. (7-9).

A3.   Explain how the dispersion model with no mass transfer terms can fit column breakthrough data where mass transfer resistances are important.

A4.   When might the B term in the Van Deemter equation be negligible? What type of chromatography is most likely to have a negligible contribution from molecular diffusion. What does Figure 7-11 look like when the B term is negligible?

A5.   In a poorly designed chromatograph the HETP can be significantly greater than predicted by the Van Deemter equation. List several possible causes.

A6.   Explain physically why large molecules exit before small molecules in size exclusion chromatography. Convert Figure 7-2 to a plot of K_d versus log (MW).

A7.   When similar chemicals are separated, the HETP will be approximately the same. This implies that the zone widths inside the columns are approximately the same. However, the widths observed on a strip chart recorder are quite different. Explain why.

A8.   Explain how to use the Lapidus and Amundson model when $v = 0$ and only diffusion occurs.

A9.   Explain how the outlet concentration of species C in solvent programming (Figure 7-13b) can be greater than its feed concentration.

A10.   Displacers used for displacement chromatography with adsorption or partition systems are usually used in high concentrations. Thus, they illustrate strong favorable, non-linear adsorption. Explain why (using solute movement theory) it will be difficult to remove the displacer and reequilibrate the column with solvent.

A11.   Develop your key relations chart for this chapter.

B.   *Generation of Alternatives*

B1.   Develop a problem for linear systems not done in this chapter and show how the solution can be obtained by superposition.

B2.   Brainstorm methods for scaling up capillary gas chromatography to separate tons of feed.

B3.   Develop alternatives to the annular flow column shown in Figure 7-20 which will have short flow paths and high surface areas.

C.   *Derivations*

C1.   Derive Eq. (7-3) using solute movement theory.

C2.   Derive the linear isotherm, effective dispersion model solution Eq. (7-16c) for a differential pulse starting with Eqs. (7-7) and (7-13).

C3.   For the staged model for chromatography, show that c_{max} is given by Eq. (7-28a). Also, show that Eq. (7-22a) satisfies Eqs. (7-20) and (7-21).

356

C4.   Derive Eq. (7-31).

C5.   The Lapidus and Amundson dispersion model with local equilibrium
       was originally solved for a single porosity model. With the assumption
       of local equilibrium $c = c^*$ (or $x = x^*$), the two porosity model can also
       be used. By inspection and analogy determine the two porosity equa-
       tions equivalent to Eq. (7-10) and to Eqs. (7-12c) and (7-13). The result
       you should obtain equivalent to Eq. (7-10) is,

$$x = \frac{c_A}{c_{AF}} = \frac{1}{2}\left\{1 - \mathrm{erf}\left[\frac{z - \dfrac{vt}{1+K_d(\frac{1-\varepsilon_e}{\varepsilon_e})\varepsilon_p+\rho_s(\frac{1-\varepsilon_e}{\varepsilon_e})(1-\varepsilon_p)A}}{\left[\dfrac{4(D_M+E_D)t}{1+K_d(\frac{1-\varepsilon_e}{\varepsilon_e})\varepsilon_p+\rho_s(\frac{1-\varepsilon_e}{\varepsilon_e})(1-\varepsilon_p)A}\right]^{1/2}}\right]\right\}$$

C6.   The Lapidus and Amundson dispersion model with local equilibrium
       can easily be applied to study the zone spreading of thermal waves.
       Develop the appropriate equation for a single porosity model. Do this
       for a step input from $T_{initial}$ to T_F. Use the dimensionless variable
       $\tau_T = (T - T_{initial})/(T_F - T_{initial})$. List the necessary assumptions.

C7.   Although not commonly used, the staged model can be applied to tem-
       perature pulses. Develop this staged energy balance model for adia-
       batic equilibrium stages including the wall heat capacity. Write in
       terms of the dimensionless temperature $\tau_T = (T - T_{initial})/(T_F - T_{initial})$.
       Solve for a pulse of volume V_F of temperature T_F input to stage 0 at V
       = 0.

C8.   Show that Eq. (7-28b) is valid.

C9.   Plot N vs α_{21} for $\bar{k}' = 5$, and R = 1.0. What does this mean in terms of
       column length or allowable velocity?

C10. Write a computer program and use Eq. (7-11b) to calculate erf(a) values for the values of a given in Table 7-1. Compare these numbers with the exact values given in Table 7.1.

C11. Assume that Eqs. (7-53) and (7-54) are correct (trust me). Derive Eq. (7-55).

D. *Single Answer Problems*

D1. The solute velocity for linear systems is easily determined from pulse chromatography experiments. The following data were obtained from a bed 50.4 cm long.

Solute	Retention time, minutes
Naphthalene	43.826
anthracene	59.086
pyrene	81.29

a. Find the solute velocities.

b. If the feed pulse is to be 20 minutes long, how long must the column be to just separate the components? Use the solute movement model.

c. For the column length determined in part b at what time can the next pulse be input to just separate the components?

d. Use the solute movement theory to design a column switching system and repeat parts b and c.

D2. Component A has $A_A = 3.22$ where $A_A = q_A/c_A$. In a chromatograph experiment a small pulse is injected. The peak maximum for component A exits at 12.5 minutes while a non-retained tracer ($q_{tracer} = 0$) exits at 2.8 minutes. Component B in the same experiment exits at 15.6 minutes. Assume isotherms are linear and molecules are small so that $K_d = 1.0$. What is the value of A_B?

D3.   We have done the analysis of an adsorption column and obtained a solution for the breakthrough curve in the form

$$x_A = \frac{c_A}{c_{A,F}} = X(z,t).$$

The analysis used linear isotherms. We now wish to utilize this analysis to determine what happens in *vacancy* chromatography in a column of length L. In *vacancy chromatography* the column is initially saturated at c_0 and then a "negative pulse" of concentration zero is input followed by feed of concentration c_0. Thus feed input is:

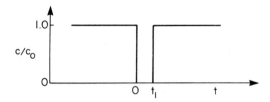

What is the solution for this input in terms of the breakthrough curve solution, $X(z,t)$?

D4.   We have the solution for breakthrough for a linear system.

$$c_A = c_{A,F}\, X(z,t)$$

In terms of X, what is the solution for the following input profile?

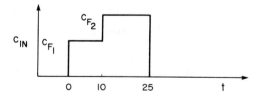

D5.   The purification of hydrogen is a process which can be carried out over Columbia grade L, 18-20 mesh coconut activated carbon. It is desired to remove ethylene from a 1% ethylene feed at 150°F. Predict the time of breakthrough from a 20 cm long tubular column and draw the breakthrough curve which results from the single porosity linear dispersion model developed by Lapidus and Amundson. The system properties are $\varepsilon_e = 0.40$, $\rho_p = 0.52$ g/cm^3, equilibrium q = 117.78 c, $v_{super} = 10$ cm/s, $d_p = 0.10$ cm, $Pe_z = 336$, and $A_c = 1.0$ cm^2.

D6.   For the system of Problem 7-D5, predict the outlet concentration profile if a 10 second pulse of the 1% ethylene feed is input into a 100 cm long column. Other conditions are the same. (Note that Pe_z does change.) You may assume the outlet curve is Gaussian.

D7.   In Example 7-3, the linear dispersion model and the Gaussian chromatography solution are used to calculate the outlet concentration profile of anthracene. It is now desired to see if this same system can separate a solution of anthracene and a molecule of similar size and chemistry. The second component has a linear adsorption coefficient which is 10% greater than that of anthracene. Flow rates, column id, and packing are the same as in Example 7.3.

   a.   Will a reasonable separation occur in an 80 cm long column? (Calculate the resolution R.)

   b.   How long does the column need to be to obtain a proper separation? (That is R = 1.0).

   c.   If the answer to part a is no, what value of A(T) is required for the second component for a reasonable separation (R = 1.0) to occur in an 80 cm long column?

Assume: 1. $(D_m + E_D)$ are the same for both components.
            2. Both components have linear isotherms which are unaffected by each other.

D8.   A liquid chromatograph using 20 μm silica gel is separating acetonaphthalene (A) from dinitronaphthalene (D). k′ values are $k'_A = 5.5$, $k'_D = 5.8$ in a solvent which is 23% methylene chloride, 77% pentane. With an interstitial velocity of 1.0 cm/sec, H is measured as 0.12 cm. We desire a resolution of R = 1.0. What column length is required?

Plot the shape of the outlet acetonaphthalene concentration profile, $c_A/c_{A,max}$ vs. time, for an infinitesimal pulse in a column which gives R = 1.0.

D9. Repeat Problem 6-D2, but for a pulse which is five minutes long.

D10. Repeat Example 7-3 except for a feed pulse which is 12 minutes long.

  a. Use the Lapidus and Amundson dispersion model.

  b. Try to use the Gaussian solution. Why doesn't this work?

D11. A liquid chromatograph using 20μm silica gel is separating acetona-phthalene (A) from dinitronaphthalene (D). $k'_A = 5.5$, $k'_D = 5.8$. At interstitial velocity v = 1.0 cm/s, H = 0.12 cm. At interstitial velocity v = 2.0 cm/s, H = 0.21 cm. For this liquid system the B term in the Van Deemter equation is negligible. Since pore diffusion controls, the C term is

$$C = \frac{c_{sm}\, d_p^2}{D_{sm}}$$

For an infinitesimal pulse we desire a resolution of R = 1.0 at v = 0.5 cm/s in a 100 cm column. What particle diameter should be used? Note: Include both A and C terms. Assume k'_A and k'_D are constant.

D12. In Example 7-3 the Gaussian approximation Eq. (7-16c) or (7-24) was used instead of the somewhat more accurate Eq. (7-15). Recalculate the outlet concentration profile using Eq. (7-15). Compare your results with Example 7-3.

D13. The integral approach illustrated in Example 7-1 gives a point on the shock wave at z = L. Extend this method to obtain other points on the shock wave. Find c and t_{sh} for z = 30 cm. HINT: Set L = 30 cm and adjust the tables in Example 7-1.

D14. In an attempt to determine extra column effects in a chromatograph we do two experiments and determine N for a solute with a linear isotherm.

Experiment 1: $L_1 = 50$ cm, $N_1 = 710$
Experiment 2: $L_2 = 25$ cm, $N_2 = 330$

Except for column lengths, the experiments are identical. Determine H_{col} and $\sigma^2_{1,ec}$.

D15. We are separating methane from helium in an adsorption column packed with 5A zeolite molecular sieve. The particles are 40 to 60 U.S. mesh (250 to 420 μm). The column was 100 cm long and interstitial velocity is 5 cm/s. The feed is 1.1 vol% methane. Use Rosen's model to predict the breakthrough curve if the column is initially clean.

Data: $A = 23.90$ where q and c are in gmole/cm^3,
$D_{mp} = 0.11$ cm^2 /s, $k_f = 2763.0$ cm/s,
$\varepsilon_e = 0.525$ (Cen and Yang, 1986).

Note: Watch your units since q and c are in the same units.

D16. We are testing a column with dilute glucose solutions. The packing is an ion exchange resin in calcium form. Predict the outlet concentration profile from a 1 meter long column. Initially the column contains pure water.

At $t = 0$ start input of $c_F = 3$ g glucose/100 ml.
At $t = 1$ minute start input of $c_F = 5$ g glucose/100 ml.

Data: $\varepsilon_p = 0$, $\varepsilon_e = 0.4$, $H = 0.4$ cm, Equilibrium: $q_G = 0.51\ c_G$
where q_G and c_G are in g/100 ml.
Superficial velocity = 10 cm/min.

E.   *More Complex Single Answer Problems*

E1.   For the fructose-glucose separation discussed in Problem 6-D4, H = 10 cm. (This is very large because of extra column mixing). Assume the feed concentrations of fructose and glucose are equal. Use properties listed in Problem 6-D4.

   a.   If we desire a resolution of R = 1.0 for a differential pulse input, determine the column length required.

   b.   A properly designed analytical system without extensive mixing will have H ~ 0.06 cm. Predict required L for R = 1.0 for a properly designed analytical system with a differential pulse input.

   c.   A 100 cm column is used with a superficial velocity of 15 cm/min. Based on the solute movement theory (Problem 6-D4) there should be perfect separation of the sugars if the feed pulse is 1.48 minutes long and the waiting period between pulses is 1.48 minutes. Suppose we include dispersion effects (H = 0.06 cm) and use t_F = 1.3 minutes and t_{cycle} = 3.0 minutes (a 1.7 minute waiting period). Predict the outlet concentration profiles for three feed pulses. For the products from the second pulse determine the glucose and fructose purities if the cut points are chosen so that $x_{Fructose} = x_{Glucose}$ where $x = c/c_F$. Use the Lapidus and Amundson dispersion model. Why isn't the Gaussian solution valid?

E2.   (Derivation) In analytical gas chromatography it is common to use *temperature programming* to more rapidly elute strongly adsorbed species. In this procedure the feed pulse is input at temperature T_o. The column is operated at this temperature while the fast moving peaks are eluted. At $t = t_o$ the column oven is heated at a constant rate $\partial T/\partial t = b$. This continues until all components have eluted. The oven door is then opened, the system is cooled and the next pulse is input. Equilibrium is usually linear and follows an Arrehenius dependence.

a. Approximate the temperature profile as a series of step changes ΔT at time interval Δt so that $\Delta T / \Delta t = b$ (the heating rate). With this approximation $\partial T / \partial t = 0$ in Eq. (6-58) except at the discrete steps and the solute movement solutions developed in Chapter 6 are applicable. Determine the solute path and estimate the concentration.

b. Use the local equilibrium model to determine the solute path for the temperature gradient $\partial T / \partial t = b$ (Note: in Eq. (6-58) $\partial T / \partial t \neq 0$.)

c. Estimate the concentration along the solute path for Part b.

E3.   (Derivation) With suitable assumptions Rosen's model can be adapted to heat transfer. Derive the appropriate equations which match Eqs. (7-46), (7-49), (7-50), (7-51), and (7-52). Define τ_T as in Problem 7-C6. Determine the lumped variables corresponding to Eq. (7-53). The asymptotic solution remains Eq. (7-54), but with different definitions for the variables. Do this for pure heat transfer with no adsorption. List your other assumptions.

E4.   A 1 meter column is packed with activated alumina. The column initially contains $c = 0.01$ gmole/L of anthracene in cyclohexane. At $t = 0$ a stream of pure cyclohexane at a superficial velocity ($\varepsilon_e v$) of 20 cm/min is input. After 10 minutes a stream containing $c = 0.011$ gmole/L of anthracene in cyclohexane is added at the same velocity. Predict the outlet concentration profile. Data are in Example 7-1.

F.   *Problems Requiring Other Resources*

F1.   The article by Van Deemter *et al.*, (1956) is a classical paper in chromatography. Read this rather long paper and write a two page critical review.

F2.   Another long classical paper is that by Martin and Synge (1941). They used a staged model that was rather different than the one developed here. If the number of stages is large, show that the two staged models are equivalent.

F3.   We are doing size exclusion chromatography of a protein from salts. The protein is quite large and is totally excluded from the packing ($K_d = 0$). A one meter long column packed with particles with an average diameter of 30 μm (30×10^{-6} meters) was used. Operation was at 25°C. Estimated value of $\varepsilon_e = 0.40$. Superficial velocity was 10 cm/min. Assume fluid has the properties of water. Predict the outlet concentration profile if at $t = 0$ a step input from 0 to c_F g/L of protein is introduced. Note: The Chung and Wen correlation given in Eq. (7-14) is accurate for totally excluded species.

Chapter 8

NON-LINEAR THEORIES AND PACKED BED
ADSORPTION SYSTEMS

At higher concentrations adsorption isotherms for most chemicals become non-linear. In this region the linear solutions of Chapter 7 are not valid. The non-linear solutions given in Chapter 6 are useful, but do not include mass transfer and dispersion effects. This chapter will present simple models for one component isothermal, non-linear adsorption. The ramification of these results on design will be explored. When more than one adsorbate is present, the system is usually coupled since the adsorption of one component affects the adsorption of all other components. Nonisothermal systems also show coupled behavior since temperature affects the amount adsorbed. Since the coupled systems are much more complex than uncoupled systems, the models for these systems will not be developed. Instead, only the major results for coupled systems will be discussed.

The basic packed bed system was shown in Figure 6-1. The operation is cyclic with the feed (adsorption) step followed by a regeneration (desorption) step, and a preparation step to prepare the column for the next feed step. During the feed step, adsorption continues until breakthrough occurs. Then the packing is regenerated usually with counter-flow of a hot fluid or by purging at low pressure. Usually the column is *not* completely regenerated but some solute is left in the column. This is done since significantly less desorbent is required. A variety of operating modes are used for adsorption and regeneration and will be explored in this chapter using the theories of Chapters 6 and 7.

8.1 MASS TRANSFER ZONE APPROACH

In actual practice shock waves will spread due to the dispersion and mass transfer terms in Eq. (6-42). However, this spread is opposed by the isotherm

365

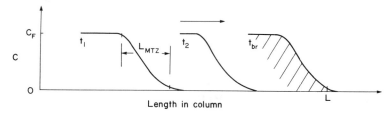

Figure 8-1.   Concentration profiles inside column at different times for constant pattern system.

effect which tends to form shock waves. The net result of these two opposing forces is to form a *constant pattern* wave which does not change shape as it moves in the column. This is shown in Figure 8-1 where the concentration of the fluid inside the bed is shown at different times. Once formed the wave does not change shape as it moves through the column. This behavior will occur whenever the solute movement theory predicts a shock wave.

A common industrial design procedure uses constant pattern analysis based on experimental data. This mass transfer zone approach is based on the original work of Michaels (1952) in ion exchange. What is actually measured are the *breakthrough curves* shown in Figure 8-2 (Weyde and Wicke, 1948). This is the outlet concentration which results from a step input in concentration (Figure 8-2a) or a step decrease in concentration (Figure 8-2b). Note in Figure 8-2a that the breakthrough curves for the longer columns have exactly the same shape. This is constant pattern behavior. Very short columns have a different shape breakthrough curve since the constant pattern is not fully developed. For the elution of a saturated column shown in Figure 8-2b, the waves become more spread for longer columns. This is the *proportional pattern* behavior predicted for nonlinear isotherms in Chapter 6. The *mass transfer zone* or *MTZ* is the region where concentration is changing and thus mass transfer is occurring. For constant pattern behavior the length of the MTZ is constant. The length of the MTZ in time units is easily measured from the breakthrough curve (Figure 8-3). Usually the MTZ is arbitrarily measured from a concentration of 0.05 c_F to 0.95 c_F , since it is hard to tell exactly where the S-shaped pattern starts and ends. We wish to use this data to determine the length of the MTZ

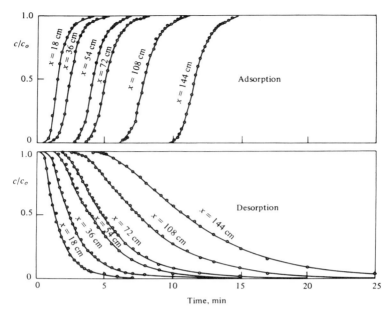

Figure 8-2.   Adsorption and elution of CO_2 on carbon. Reprinted from
               Weyde and Wicke (1940). a. Adsorption breakthrough curves.
               b. Desorption elution curves. v_{super} = 4.26 cm/s.

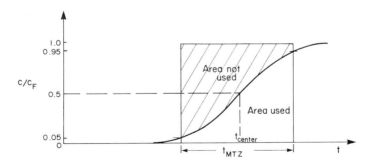

Figure 8-3.   Breakthrough curve for step input.

inside the column. The mass transfer zone must move at the shock wave velocity u_{sh}. Then,

$$L_{MTZ} = u_{sh} t_{MTZ} \qquad (8\text{-}1a)$$

Note that since the shape is not changing, all parts of the wave move at the same velocity. The shock wave velocity can be estimated from Eq. (6-30) or it can be found experimentally. The stoichiometric center of the wave ($c = 0.5c_F$ for a symmetric wave) must also be part of the local equilibrium solution (see Figure 8-3). Then

$$u_{sh} = \frac{L}{t_{center}} \qquad (8\text{-}1b)$$

The advantage of determining u_{sh} from experiments, Eq. (8-1b), is the equilibrium isotherm does not have to be known.

In typical industrial operations adsorption is stopped when breakthrough just starts. This is illustrated by the right side of Figure 8-1. The breakthrough time, t_{br}, can be related to column length, u_{sh} and L_{MTZ}. If breakthrough is defined as $c = 0.05\ c_F$, the center of a symmetric wave has traveled a distance $L - (1/2)\ L_{MTZ}$ (see Figure 8-1). Since the wave center is also the shock solution from the solute movement theory, we can calculate the breakthrough time.

$$t_{br} = (L - 0.5\ L_{MTZ})/u_{sh} \qquad (8\text{-}2)$$

This equation allows us to calculate the breakthrough time as the column length is varied. Since the concentration in the mass transfer zone is varying, the sorbent is not saturated through the entire length of the bed. Only the shaded part of the bed in Figure 8-3 is used. Thus the fractional bed utilization can be determined as,

$$\text{Frac bed util.} = 1 - \frac{L_{MTZ}}{L} \left[\frac{\text{Area not used}}{\text{Total Area in MTZ}} \right] \qquad (8\text{-}3a)$$

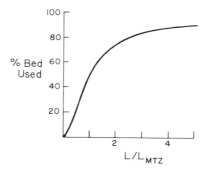

Figure 8-4.   Fraction of bed used as a function of L/L_{MTZ} for constant pattern step. Excerpted by special permission from, Lukchis, G.M., *Chem. Eng. 80*, (13), 111, (1973). Copyright 1973, McGraw-Hill.

The ratio (Area not used)/(Total Area in MTZ) is the fraction of the mass transfer zone which is not useful for adsorbing solute at the saturation concentration. This ratio can be determined from Figures 8-1 or 8-3. The areas are shown in Figure 8-3. If the breakthrough curve is symmetric the ratio is 1/2. Then Eq. (8-3a) simplifies to:

$$\text{Frac bed util.} = 1 - .5(L_{MTZ} / L) \qquad (8\text{-}3b)$$

In both Eqs. (8-3a) and (8-3b) L_{MTZ} must be in length units. The fractional bed use for symmetric beds is shown in Figure 8-4 (Lukchis, 1973).

The amount of solute which can be held by the bed is

$$\text{Capacity} = (\text{Frac bed util.}) \times (\text{Mass of adsorbent}) \times q_{sat} \qquad (8\text{-}4)$$

where q_{sat} is the saturation capacity of the adsorbent for the given feed concentration. The saturation capacity is found from the appropriate equilibrium isotherm calculated at the feed concentration, c_F, or from experiment. The saturation capacity depends on the adsorbent used, the feed concentration, and the temperature. The fractional bed utilization can be increased by increasing L or decreasing the mass transfer zone length. The mass transfer zone length will be shorter for rapid mass transfer rates or small size adsorbent particles. The mass transfer zone tends to be quite large for large molecules such as proteins which have low rates of mass transfer.

A reasonable empirical design approach for favorable type adsorption isotherms (Figures 6-3b or 6-3d) is as follows:

1. For the conditions of the feed step, determine u_{sh} , L_{MTZ}, and q_{sat}. This can be done with a single experiment in a laboratory column.

2. Design the adsorption step using the mass transfer zone approach. Optimum design and theoretical determination of L_{MTZ} is discussed later.

3. Determine the equilibrium isotherm under the conditions of desorption.

4. Design the desorption step (proportional pattern wave) using the solute movement theory.

5. Check the desorption step design with a laboratory experiment.

This combined approach uses the MTZ method where it is valid and it uses the solute movement theory where it is approximately valid.

8.2. CONSTANT PATTERN SOLUTIONS

In this section we will see how the constant pattern shape can be predicted theoretically from a mass transfer analysis. Constant pattern shapes occur when the solute movement theory predicts a shock wave. The isotherm effect which tends to form a shock wave is balanced by the dispersive effects of mass transfer resistances and dispersion terms. The net result is a constant pattern wave which moves at the shock wave velocity, u_{sh}. This pattern will always form when the conditions are right (Cooney and Lightfoot, 1965).

The constant pattern shape greatly simplifies the mathematical analysis. A listing of constant pattern adsorption models is given by Sircar and Kumar (1983). The usual starting equation is the single porosity solute mass balance,

Eq. (6-48), ignoring the dispersion and diffusion term. The system is assumed to be isothermal. Equation (6-48) simplifies to:

$$\frac{\partial c}{\partial t} + \frac{\partial(vc)}{\partial z} + \frac{\rho_P(1-\varepsilon_e)}{\varepsilon_e} \frac{\partial \overline{q}}{\partial t} = 0 \tag{8-5}$$

Since the constant pattern wave has a constant shape, concentration *must* depend only on a single variable. This variable can be a measure of the time or distance from the center of the pattern. The variable τ,

$$\tau = t - z/u_p \tag{8-6}$$

is a measure of time from the center of the pattern which moves at velocity u_p. Since the constant pattern wave depends only on τ, the partial differential equation, Eq. (8-5), can be reduced to an ordinary differential equation. After a few manipulations, the result is,

$$\frac{d}{d\tau} \left[(1 - \frac{v}{u_p})c + \frac{\rho_P(1-\varepsilon_e)\overline{q}}{\varepsilon_e} \right] = 0 \tag{8-7a}$$

Now the solution is obvious,

$$(1 - \frac{v}{u_p})c + \frac{\rho_P(1-\varepsilon_e)\overline{q}}{\varepsilon_e} = \text{constant} \tag{8-7b}$$

If the bed is initially clean then $c = \overline{q} = 0$, and the constant must be zero. Since any uniform initial state can be reached from a clean bed, the constant will always be zero.

We can write Eq. (8-7b) for the conditions after the wave has passed, c_a and $\overline{q}_a$. Dividing Eq. (8-7b) by this form and rearranging, we obtain,

$$\frac{\left[1 - \frac{v}{u_p}\right]c}{\left[1 - \frac{v_a}{u_p}\right]c_a} = \frac{\overline{q}}{q_a} \tag{8-8a}$$

For relatively concentrated gases $v \neq v_a$ since adsorption or desorption changes the gas velocity. For liquids, dilute gases, and exchange adsorption velocity is essentially constant and Eq. (8-8a) simplifies to

$$\frac{c}{c_a} = \frac{\bar{q}}{q_a} \qquad (8\text{-}8b)$$

In the remainder of the development we will assume that velocity is constant. Then $u_p = u_{sh}$. Equation (8-8b) states how c and q must be related because of the mass balance. Since equilibrium has *not* been assumed, c and $\bar{q}$ are *not* in equilibrium. The conditions after the wave, c_a and q_a, will be in equilibrium.

So far, we haven't used the mass transfer expression Eq. (6-50). We will substitute the mass balance result, Eq. (8-8b), and Eq. (8-6) into Eq. (6-50). The result is

$$(1-\varepsilon_e)\rho_P \frac{q_a}{c_a} \frac{dc}{d\tau} = -(k_m \, a_p)\,(c^* - c) \qquad (8\text{-}9)$$

Since there is a constant pattern, c must depend on a single variable and an ordinary differential equation results. To integrate this equation we need a relationship for c^*. The usual method is to assume that this stagnant fluid is in equilibrium with the solid. However, remember $c \neq c^*$. With c^* in equilibrium with q, the isotherm can be used to replace c^* in Eq. (8-9). Then Eq. (8-8b) can be used to replace q with c. This can be done for any isotherm which will give a constant pattern wave.

For example, assume that equilibrium can be fit with a generalized Langmuir expression of the form given in Eq. (6-12a). Then a constant pattern wave will result when a step input of feed is used. Solving for c^* from the Langmuir equation and substituting in Eq. (8-8b), we obtain

$$c^* = \frac{q}{a - bq} = \frac{c(q_a/c_a)}{a - bc(q_a/c_a)} \qquad (8\text{-}10)$$

Substitution of Eq. (8-10) into (8-9) gives an ordinary differential equation.

$$(1-\varepsilon_e)(\frac{q_a}{c_a})\rho_P \frac{dc}{d\tau} = (k_m a_p)[c - \frac{c(q_a/c_a)}{a - bc(q_a/c_a)}] \qquad (8\text{-}11a)$$

The conditions after the wave are the feed values: $c_a = c_F$ and $q_a = q_F$. Thus $q_a/c_a = q_F/c_F = a/(1 + bc_F)$. Substitution of this result into Eq. (8-11a) and simplifying gives

$$\left[\frac{1 + bc_F - bc}{c(b\, c_F - bc)} \right] \frac{dc}{d\tau} = \frac{k_m a_p(1 + b\, c_F)}{\rho_p(1 - \varepsilon_e)a} \tag{8-11b}$$

The integration of Eq. (8-11b) is straightforward. After some algebra the result is,

$$\ln(c_F - c) - \frac{1 + bc_F}{bc_F} \ln\left[\frac{c_F - c}{c} \right] = \frac{k_m a_p(1 + bc_F)}{(1 - \varepsilon_e)\rho_p\, a} \tau + \text{Const.} \tag{8-11c}$$

The column is assumed to be initially uniformly saturated at c_{init}. At time zero a feed of concentration c_F is input. To have a constant pattern wave with a Langmuir isotherm we must have $c_F > c_{init}$. The mass transfer zone can be found by evaluating Eq. (8-11c) from

$$c_{init} + 0.05(c_F - c_{init}) = 0.95c_{init} + 0.05c_F \tag{8-11d}$$

to

$$c_{init} + 0.95(c_F - c_{init}) = 0.05c_{init} + 0.95c_F \tag{8-11e}$$

The result is

$$\Delta\tau = \frac{(1 - \varepsilon_e)\rho_p a}{k_m a_p(1 + bc_F)} \left\{ \ln\left[\frac{0.05}{0.95} \right] \right.$$

$$\left. - \frac{1 + bc_F}{bc_F} \ln\left[\frac{0.05}{0.95} \left[\frac{0.95\, c_{init} + 0.05\, c_F}{0.05\, c_{init} + 0.95\, c_F} \right] \right] \right\} \tag{8-12a}$$

This equation can be interpreted two ways. If we fix the length at the column outlet, $z = L$, then

$$\Delta \tau |_{z=L} = t_{MTZ} \tag{8-12b}$$

If we fix the time at breakthrough, $t = t_{br}$, then

$$\Delta \tau |_{t=t_{br}} = \frac{L_{MTZ}}{u_{sh}} \tag{8-12c}$$

Note that both t_{MTZ} and L_{MTZ} are inversely proportional to $(k_m a_p)$ since $\Delta \tau$ is inversely proportional to $k_m a_p$.

The shape of the constant pattern curve can be obtained by evaluating the constant in Eq. (8-11c) or by evaluating (Eq. 8-11c) from a known point $(c,z)_{known}$ to an arbitrary (c,z). It is often convenient to do this from the center point $c_{1/2} = \frac{1}{2} (c_F + c_{initial})$ at $\tau = \tau_{1/2}$ (Lapidus and Rosen, 1954). This integration assumes the profile is symmetric, but is usually accurate enough. Equation Eq. (8-11c) gives,

$$(\tau - \tau_{1/2}) = \frac{(1 - \varepsilon_e)\rho_p a}{k_m a_p (1 + bc_F)} \left\{ - \ln \left[\frac{2(c_F - c)}{(c_F - c_{init})} \right] \right. \tag{8-13}$$

$$\left. - \frac{1 + bc_F}{bc_F} \ln \left[\frac{(c_F - c)/(c_F - c_{init})}{c/(c_F + c_{init})} \right] \right\}$$

The use of Eqs. (8-12a,b,c) are illustrated in Example 8-1. Typical constant pattern profiles are shown in Figures 8-1, 8-2b and 8-3.

One reason for illustrating this derivation in detail is the same steps can be followed for other equilibrium and mass transfer forms. Any equilibrium form which gives a shock wave with the solute movement theory can be used to replace Eq. (8-10). In addition, a variety of mass transfer expressions can be used instead of Eq. (6-50). Thus the constant pattern solution for almost any type of equilibrium and a variety of mass transfer expressions can easily be developed. This analysis is also applicable to ion exchange (see Problem 9-D5). Unfortunately, this solution is restricted to the constant pattern part of the cycle.

When the equilibrium theory predicts a diffuse wave, a proportional pattern wave results as shown in Figure 8-2b. Since the pattern is not constant, Eq. (8-5) *cannot* be used to simplify Eq. (6-48) to Eq. (8-6). The Thomas solution (Thomas, 1944, 1948; Sherwood *et al.*, 1975; Vermeulen *et al.*, 1984) can be used for the proportional pattern part of the cycle. However, it is complex and restricted to a Langmuir isotherm and a particular type of kinetics. Since the equilibrium solute movement predictions of the diffuse wave are often quite accurate particularly for gas systems, we will use the simple solute movement results for the proportional pattern part of the cycle.

A second limit on the constant pattern solution is the assumption that the column is isothermal. Commercial gas adsorbers are usually adiabatic and have non-negligible values of ΔH_{ads} which often leads to significant temperature increases in the bed during adsorption. During desorption the bed cools down. Since a temperature increase will decrease adsorption equilibrium (see Eq. (6-8)), these effects should be included. Approximate (Leavitt, 1962) and analytical (Sircar and Kumar, 1983) constant pattern methods have been developed for adiabatic systems. Adiabatic systems are discussed in more detail in Section 8.5.2.

In actual practice the MTZ-LUB approach is often used instead of theoretical calculations. This is done since trace components or small temperature changes can have large effects on the breakthrough curve and the MTZ. In addition, since the constant pattern solution ignores dispersion and is based on a lumped parameter mass transfer expression it is not exact. The constant pattern theory is very useful for predicting the effect of changing operating conditions such as velocity, temperature, particle diameter, feed concentration, etc. A semi-empirical procedure where a theoretical result such as Eq. (8-12a) is used to guide experiments and to help correlate data is a better design approach than an entirely empirical design approach.

8.3. MASS TRANSFER CORRELATIONS

In most cases the lumped parameter Eqs. (6-47) or (6-50) are adequate for modeling packed beds. In order to use the theory a good estimate of the mass transfer coefficient $k_m a_p$ is required. k_m is an "effective" mass transfer coefficient. For spherical particles

$$a_p = \frac{6}{d_p} \tag{8-14}$$

where d_p is the particle diameter. For nonspherical particles an equivalent diameter is used.

The mass transfer coefficient is usually correlated in terms of dimensionless groups. A variety of these correlations have been developed (Ruthven, 1984; Sherwood et al., 1975; Yang, 1987). Wakoa and Funazkri (1978) correlated the film coefficient k_f using

$$Sh = 2.0 + 1.1 \, Sc^{1/3} \, Re^{0.6}, \quad 3 < Re < 10^4 \tag{8-15a}$$

where the dimensionless groups are

$$Sh = \frac{k_f d_p}{D_m} \quad \text{Sherwood number} \tag{8-15b}$$

$$Sc = \frac{\mu}{\rho_f D_m} \quad \text{Schmidt number} \tag{8-15c}$$

$$Re = \frac{\rho_f v \varepsilon_e d_p}{\mu} \quad \text{Reynolds number} \tag{8-15d}$$

At low Reynolds numbers the dispersion terms must be corrected for. Wakao and Funazkri (1978) also review a large amount of data to measure k_f. An alternate correlation for the film transfer coefficient is (Sherwood et al., 1975)

$$k_f = 1.17 \frac{v_{super}^{0.585} \, \rho_f^{0.252} \, D_m^{2/3}}{d_p^{0.415} \, \mu^{0.252}}, \quad 10 < R_e < 2500 \tag{8-16}$$

The results obtained from Eqs. (8-15a) and (8-16) will differ somewhat from each other. Since Eq. (8-15) was corrected for axial dispersion, this result should be used if the model includes axial dispersion. If the model ignores axial dispersion a better fit will probably be obtained with Eq. (8-16).

For diffusion inside the pores we really want to solve Eq. (6-44a) with appropriate boundary conditions. This was done in Section 7.8 for Rosen's solution. The appropriate way to sum resistances is shown in Eq. (7-55). Since $a_p = 6/d_p$, the term $d_p/6k_f$ is $1/(k_f a_p)$. Then the other term in the summation in Eq. (7-53) is $1/(k a_p)_{pore}$ (see Eq. 8-19a)). Thus, we would expect an equivalent solution when

$$(ka_p)_{pore} = \frac{60 D_{mp} A(1 - \varepsilon_e)\rho_p}{d_p^2} \qquad (8\text{-}17a)$$

where A is the linear equilibrium constant. For nonlinear systems

$$A = \left[\frac{\partial q}{\partial c} \right]_{avg} \qquad (8\text{-}17b)$$

The equivalence of the solutions to Eqs. (6-44a) and (6-50) disappears for very non-linear systems, at very short times, and for rapid cycling separations. In these situations Eq. (6-44a) should be solved.

For surface diffusion comparison of the solution of Eq. (6-45a) to the solution of the lumped parameter Eq. (6-45b) show a good correspondence when

$$k_s = \frac{60}{d_p^2} D_s \qquad (8\text{-}18a)$$

We often wish to employ a surface diffusion coefficient in equations such as Eq. (6-50) and (6-45c). Then,

$$(ka_p)_{surface} = k_s A(1 - \varepsilon_e)\rho_p = \frac{60 D_s}{d_p^2} A(1 - \varepsilon_e)\rho_p \qquad (8\text{-}18b)$$

This result is also used for nonlinear isotherms by using A defined in Eq. (8-17b). Note the similiarity of the results for pore and surface diffusion.

The effective mass transfer coefficient $k_m a_p$ can be related to the individual coefficients by the usual sum of resistances model if either pore or surface diffusion control transfer inside the particle. For pore plus film diffusion,

$$k_m a_p = \left[\frac{1}{k_f a_p} + \frac{1}{(ka_p)_{pore}} \right]^{-1} \qquad (8\text{-}19a)$$

For use in Eqs. (6-50) or (8-9) this is,

$$k_m a_p = \left[\frac{1}{k_f a_p} + \frac{d_p^2}{60 D_{mp} A(1 - \varepsilon_e)\rho_p} \right]^{-1} \qquad (8\text{-}19b)$$

For liquid systems the surface diffusion term is always neglected, and Eqs. (8-19a) and (8-19b) are appropriate. When surface plus film diffusion occur

$$k_m a_p = \left[\frac{1}{k_f a_p} + \frac{1}{(ka_p)_{surface}} \right]^{-1} \qquad (8\text{-}19c)$$

which is

$$k_m a_p = \left[\frac{1}{k_f a_p} + \frac{d_p^2}{60 D_s A(1 - \varepsilon_e)\rho_p} \right]^{-1} \qquad (8\text{-}19d)$$

If both surface and pore diffusion are important, the sum-of-resistances model cannot be used, and the diffusion equations must be solved simultaneously.

Obviously, to use the correlations in this section we must know both designer specified properties, v and d_p, and physical properties; ε_e, ρ_p, A, ρ_f, D_m, D_{mp}, D_s and μ. The designer specified properties are under the control of the engineer. The properties of the adsorbent; ε_e, ρ_p and A; can be estimated from manufacturer's data, Tables 6-1 to 6-6, and equilibrium data (see Section 6.3). The viscosity can often be estimated from data in Perry and Green (1984) or by methods in Reid *et al.* (1977). Diffusivities can be significantly more difficult to estimate. Methods for estimating the molecular diffusivity are discussed by Perry and Green (1984), Reid et al. (1977) and Sherwood et al. (1975). Extensive tables of parameters for the parameters in theories, and references for experimental values of D_m are given by Marrero and Mason (1972). The effective pore diffusivity D_{mp} can be estimated from Eq. (6-44 a,b), although experimental data is usually required to determine the tortuosity. Surface diffusivities depend on surface coverage and are discussed by (Ruthven, 1984) and (Yang, 1987). Estimation of these values is illustrated in Example 8-1.

Example 8-1. Constant Pattern

Sircar and Kumar (1983) fit data for carbon dioxide, methane, nitrogen and hydrogen adsorption onto BPL activated carbon to a Langmuir isotherm of the form.

$$q = \frac{q_{max} K_A y}{1 + K_A y}$$

where y is the mole fraction adsorbate and q is the moles adsorbate/g adsorbent and adsorbate in the pores is included in q. For methane the parameter values are $q_{max} = 3.65 \times 10^{-3}$; and at 1 atmosphere,

T°C	K_A
25	0.4179
45	0.2550
75	0.1343
95	0.0928

Data: $\varepsilon_e = 0.39$, $\varepsilon_T = 0.763$, $\rho_B = 0.484$ g/cm^3, and $\tau = 8$.

We wish to operate a one meter long adsorption column packed with 1 mm diameter BPL activated carbon particles. The column is initially filled with helium which does not adsorb. Total pressure is 1 atmosphere and temperature is 25°C. A step change in feed gas from an initially pure feed gas to 5 mole % methane is made at t = 0. If the superficial velocity is 55 cm/s, predict the width of the mass transfer zone.

380

Solution

We must first convert the equilibrium data to the form $q = ac/(1 + bc)$. For the gas $c = y \, c_T$ where c_T is gmoles/vol. For an ideal gas $c_T = p/RT$ and $c = y \, p/RT$.

Thus $y = cRT/p = \dfrac{(298.16)(82.057)}{(1)} c = 24466.12 \, c$

$c_T = p/RT = 1/(82.057)(298.16) = 4.087{\times}10^{-5}$ gmoles/cm^3

The equilibrium expression is

$$q = \frac{(q_{max} K \, RT/p)c}{1 + (KRT/p)c}$$

Thus $a = q_{max} \, KRT/p$
    $= (3.65{\times}10^{-3})(0.4179)(82.057)(298.16)/1.0 = 37.32$
and $b = KRT/p = 10,224.4$.
We wish to go from $c_{init} = 0$ to
$c_F = c_T y_F = (4.087{\times}10^{-5})(0.05) = 2.044{\times}10^{-6}$ gmoles/cm^3.

Particle density: $\rho_p = \dfrac{\rho_B}{1 - \varepsilon_e} - \dfrac{\varepsilon_e}{1 - \varepsilon_e} \, \rho_f \approx \rho_B/(1 - \varepsilon_e)$

$\rho_p = 0.484/0.61 = 0.793$ g/cm^3

Since the mass balance was solved without a dispersion term, Eqs. (8-17) to (8-19b) are appropriate.

$$a_p = 6/d_p = 6/0.1 \text{ cm} = 60 \text{ cm}^{-1}$$

Average mole fraction in MTZ in 2.5% CH$_4$

$$\overline{MW} = 0.975(4) + 0.025(16) = 4.30$$

$$\rho_f = \frac{p(\overline{MW})}{RT} = (4.087{\times}10^{-5})(4.3) = 1.757{\times}10^{-4} \text{g/cm}^3$$

For $q = \dfrac{ac}{1 + bc}$, $\dfrac{dq}{dc} = \dfrac{a}{(1 + bc)^2}$

In Eq. (8-19b), $A = \left[\dfrac{dq}{dc}\right]_{avg} = \dfrac{a}{(1 + bc)^2_{avg}}$

$c_{avg} = y_{avg}\, c_T = (0.025)(4.087 \times 10^{-5}) = 1.022 \times 10^{-6}$

$\rho_p\, A = (0.7093)\, \dfrac{(37.32)}{[(1 + (10,224.4)(1.022 \times 10^{-6})]^2} = 28.986$

Reynolds number $Re = \rho_f (v\, \varepsilon_e) d_p / \mu$

From Perry and Green (1984, p 3-248) at 25°C and 1 atm,

$\mu_{He} = 0.000186$ poise, $\mu_{CH_4} = 0.00011$ poise

The mixture viscosity can be estimated (Bird *et al.*, 1961, p.24)

$$\mu_{mix} = \sum_i \dfrac{x_i \mu_i}{\sum_j x_j\, \Phi_{i,j}}$$

where $\Phi_{i,j} = \dfrac{1}{\sqrt{8}}\left[1 + \dfrac{MW_i}{MW_j}\right]^{-1/2}\left[1 + \left[\dfrac{\mu_i}{\mu_j}\right]^{1/2}\left[\dfrac{MW_j}{MW_i}\right]^{1/4}\right]^2$

let He = 1, CH_4 = 2

i	j	MW_i/MW_j	μ_i/μ_j	Φ_{ij}	$\sum x_j \Phi_{ij}$
1	1	1.000	1.00	1.00	
					1.039
	2	0.25	1.69	2.548	
2	1	4.0	0.591	0.3767	
					0.541
	2	1.000	1.00	1.00	

$$\mu_{mix} = \frac{(0.975)(0.000186)}{1.039} + \frac{(0.025)(0.00011)}{0.541} = 0.0001796$$

$$Re = \frac{(0.0001757)(55)(0.1)}{(0.0001796)} = 5.38$$

D_m for CH_4 in He at 25°C is given in Sherwood et al. (1975, p23)

$$D_m = 0.675 \text{ cm}^2/\text{s at 1 atm}$$

From Eq. (6-1c), $\varepsilon_p = \dfrac{\varepsilon_T - \varepsilon_e}{1 - \varepsilon_e} = \dfrac{0.763 - 0.39}{0.61} = 0.61$

Eq. (6-45a) $D_{mp} = \dfrac{\varepsilon_p D_m}{\tau} = \dfrac{(0.61)(0.675)}{8} = 0.0514 \text{ cm}^2/\text{s}$

Use Eq. (8-16) even though Reynolds number is a bit low.

$$k_f = \frac{(1.17)(55)^{0.585}(0.0001757)^{0.252}(0.675)^{2/3}}{(0.1)^{0.415}(0.0001796)^{0.252}} = 24.27 \text{cm/s}$$

$$k_f a_p = (24.27)(60) = 1456.2$$

From Eq. (8-17a), $(ka_p)_{pore} = \dfrac{(60)(0.0514)(28.986)(0.61)}{(0.1)^2} = 5453$

From Eq. (8-19a), $k_m a_p = \left[\dfrac{1}{1456.2} + \dfrac{1}{5453} \right]^{-1} = 1149.3 \text{ s}^{-1}$

Can now determine $\Delta\tau$ from Eq. (8-12a).

$$\Delta\tau = \frac{(0.61)(0.793)(37.32)}{(1149.3)[1 + (10,224.4)(2.044\times10^{-6})]} \left\{ \ln\left[\frac{0.05}{0.95} \right] \right.$$

$$\left. - \frac{[1 + (10,224.4)(2.044\times10^{-6})]}{(10224.4)(2.044\times10^{-6})} \ln\left[\left[\frac{0.05}{0.95} \right]\left[\frac{0.05}{0.95} \right] \right] \right\}$$

$$t_{MTZ} = \Delta\tau = (0.0154)\left\{ (-2.944) - (-287.66) \right\} = 4.381$$

To find $L_{MTZ} = (\Delta\tau) \, u_p$, need $u_p = u_{sh}$.

$$u_p = \frac{(\varepsilon_e v)}{\varepsilon_e + (1 - \varepsilon_e) \rho_p \dfrac{\Delta q}{\Delta c}}$$

where $\dfrac{\Delta q}{\Delta c} = \dfrac{q(c_F) - 0}{c_F - 0}$. Note that q vs c equilibrium data was obtained in a manner consistent with a one porosity mass balance. From the Langmuir isotherm,

$$q(c_F) = \frac{a \, c_F}{(1 + bc_f)} = \frac{(37.32)(2.044 \times 10^{-6})}{1 + (10224.4)(2.044 \times 10^{-6})} = 7.472 \times 10^{-5}$$

then, $\dfrac{\Delta q}{\Delta c} = \dfrac{7.472 \times 10^{-5}}{2.044 \times 10^{-6}} = 36.556$

hence, $u_p = \dfrac{55}{0.39 + (0.61)(0.793)(36.556)} = 3.043$ cm/s

and $L_{MTZ} = (4.381)(3.043) = 13.33$ cm

This is quite short since mass transfer is rapid in gas systems.

We stop the feed step when breakthrough just starts. This occurs when the front of the mass transfer zone reaches the end of the column. From Eq. (8-2) this is

$$t_F = (L - 0.5 \, L_{MTZ})/u_p = (100 - 6.665)/3.043 = 30.67s$$

Note that more than half of this example was involved with correlations to determine physical properties.

8.4. OPTIMIZING FIXED BED SYSTEMS

How long should the column be? What size range of particles should be used? How rapidly should the bed cycle? These questions are all part of the optimization process. A complete optimization requires a complete economic analysis for each particular case. Since this is beyond the scope of this section, we will only partially answer the question by giving general guidelines. The argument will parallel that presented by Wankat (1987) for adsorbers and Wankat and Koo (1988) for chromatography. We will show that beds should be short, small particles should be used, and the beds should cycle rapidly.

As the column becomes longer the MTZ becomes a smaller fraction of the total bed length. Thus the bed utilization increases and more concentrated streams result on desorption. For symmetric mass transfer zones the fractional bed utilization is easily calculated from Eq. (8-3) or Figure 8-4 (Lukchis, 1973). Once the bed length is two or three times longer than the MTZ, further increases in bed utilization are quite modest. Since pressure drop increases as L increases, further increases in column length are usually not justified. When the MTZ is very long, the column-in-series arrangement shown later in Figure 8-15 should be used.

If L is to be set at 2 to 3 times L_{MTZ}, we need to know L_{MTZ}. For a Langmuir isotherm L_{MTZ} can be determined from Eqs. (8-12a and c). The term which has the most effect on L_{MTZ} is the inverse dependence on $k_m a_p$. The mass transfer coefficient can be estimated from Eqs. (8-19) and the area per unit volume, a_p, from Eq. (8-14). When film diffusion controls

$$k_m a_p \rightarrow k_f a_p \tag{8-20a}$$

which can be determined from Eqs. (8-15a) or (8-16). When pore diffusion controls

$$k_m a_p \rightarrow (ka_p)_{pore} = \frac{60 D_{mp} A(1 - \varepsilon_e)\rho_p}{d_p^2} \tag{8-20b}$$

When surface diffusion controls,

$$k_m a_p \rightarrow (ka_p)_{surface} = \frac{60 D_s A(1 - \varepsilon_e)\rho_p}{d_p^2} \tag{8-20c}$$

For liquid systems packed bed adsorbers and chromatographs often have mass transfer inside the particle (pore diffusion) controlling and $k_m a_p$ is inversely proportional to d_p^2. By varying particle diameter, practically any $k_m a_p$ and hence any value of L_{MTZ} can be obtained. The fractional bed use depends on the ratio of L/L_{MTZ}. This ratio can easily be determined. For instance, when a lumped parameter mass transfer expression is adequate and pore diffusion controls, Eqs. (8-12a), (8-12c) and (8-20b) give

$$\frac{L}{L_{MTZ}} \alpha \frac{L}{v \, d_p^2} \tag{8-21}$$

This result is also valid for surface diffusion control.

Pressure drop in the packing is important, particularly when large volumes of gas are processed. For rigid particles the pressure drop can be calculated from

$$\Delta p = \frac{\mu \, v_{super} L}{K \, d_p^2} \tag{8-22}$$

where Δp is in Newtons/m^2. For laminar flow, which is the usual case in packed bed operation, the permeability K can be estimated from (Bird et al., 1960).

$$K = \frac{\varepsilon_e^3}{150(1-\varepsilon_e)^2} \tag{8-23}$$

Equations (8-22) and (8-23) are generally valid for

$$\frac{d_p \, \rho_f \, v_{super}}{\mu} \frac{1}{1-\varepsilon_e} < 10 \tag{8-24}$$

which is usually satisfied in packed bed adsorbers.

Decreasing particle diameter increases Δp as shown by Eq. (8-22). This is the usual argument against decreasing d_p. However, if we keep v_{super} and the ratio (L/d_p^2) constant then Δp is constant. If pore or surface diffusion controls (which is often the case), keeping v_{super} and L/d_p^2 constant will give a constant

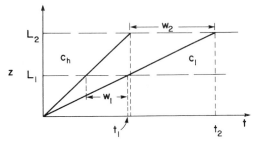

Figure 8-5. Solute movement diagram for diffuse wave. $L_2 = 2L_1$, $w_2 = 2w_1$, and $t_2 = 2t_1$. Thus, $w_2/L_2 = w_1/L_1$, and $t_2/L_2 = t_1/L_1$.

ratio of L/L_{MTZ} (Eq. 8-21). Thus the fractional bed utilization during the constant pattern step will be constant. This assumes that ε_e and the equilibrium isotherm do *not* change as d_p is varied.

During desorption a diffuse wave usually results. Now equilibrium is the controlling factor and particle diameter has little effect. The diffuse wave spread is proportional to the column length. As L decreases, the ratio (diffuse wave width/L) remains constant. This is illustrated in Figure 8-5 which shows a spreading diffuse wave at two different lengths. Thus, if the column is scaled with both v and (L/d_p^2) constant, we will have the same bed utilization, the same separation, and the same pressure drop regardless of the column length.

As the column becomes shorter it will saturate sooner. Thus we must make all parts of the cycle shorter. To scale properly keep the ratio (cycle time) × v/L constant. This is illustrated in Figure 8-5 and Example 8-2. The amount of feed processed per cycle is less, but since there are proportionally more cycles per hour the total amount of feed processed per hour is unchanged. Thus with small particles we use a short bed and obtain the same total separation and the same throughput of feed. The adsorbent productivity (kg product/kg adsorbent, hour) is inversely proportional to L, and will be quite large for columns packed with small particles.

The scaling procedure can be extended to other situations (pore diffusion does not control, turbulent flow, decrease Δp, etc.) by allowing column diameter and hence velocity to vary (Wankat, 1987). This extension is done by taking the ratios of conditions for old and new designs. We assume that the old design is adequate but is not optimized. Thus, from Eq. (8-22),

$$\frac{1}{R_p} = \frac{\Delta p_{old}}{\Delta p_{new}} = \left[\frac{v_{old}}{v_{new}}\right]\left[\frac{L_{old}}{L_{new}}\right]\left[\frac{d_{p,new}}{d_{p,old}}\right]^2 \tag{8-25}$$

where we have assumed that ε_e and fluid properties are constant. If $R_p = 1.0$, the pressure drop will be the same for the two designs.

For a Langmuir isotherm we can find L_{MTZ} from Eqs (8-12a) and (8-12c). Talking the ratios for the old and new designs, we obtain.

$$\frac{1}{R_N} = \frac{(L/L_{MTZ})_{old}}{(L/L_{MTZ})_{new}} = \left[\frac{v_{new}}{v_{old}}\right]\left[\frac{L_{old}}{L_{new}}\right]\left[\frac{k_m a_{p,old}}{k_m a_{p,new}}\right] \tag{8-26a}$$

When $R_N = 1.0$, the fractional bed use (see Figure 8-4) will be constant in the two designs. If pore or surface diffusion controls, Eq. (8-26a) becomes

$$\frac{1}{R_N} = \frac{(L/L_{MTZ})_{old}}{(L/L_{MTZ})_{new}} = \left[\frac{v_{new}}{v_{old}}\right]\left[\frac{L_{old}}{L_{new}}\right]\left[\frac{d_{p,new}}{d_{p,old}}\right]^2 \tag{8-26b}$$

The interstitial velocity v can be related to the volumetric flow rate Q,

$$v = \frac{4Q}{\pi D^2 \varepsilon_e} \tag{8-27}$$

Then the ratio of velocities is

$$\frac{v_{old}}{v_{new}} = \frac{Q_{old}}{Q_{new}}\left[\frac{D_{new}}{D_{old}}\right]^2 \tag{8-28}$$

Inserting Eq. (8-28) into Eqs. (8-25) and (8-26), we obtain

$$\frac{1}{R_p} = \left[\frac{Q_{old}}{Q_{new}}\right]\left[\frac{D_{new}}{D_{old}}\right]^2\left[\frac{L_{old}}{L_{new}}\right]\left[\frac{d_{p,new}}{d_{p,old}}\right]^2 \tag{8-29}$$

For a Langmuir isotherm we can find L_{MTZ} from Eqs (8-12a) and (8-12c). Taking the ratios for the old and new designs, we obtain

$$\frac{1}{R_N} = \left[\frac{Q_{new}}{Q_{old}} \right] \left[\frac{D_{old}}{D_{new}} \right]^2 \left[\frac{L_{old}}{L_{new}} \right] \left[\frac{k_m a_{p,old}}{k_m a_{p,new}} \right] \tag{8-30a}$$

When pore diffusion controls, Eq. (8-30a) simplifies to

$$\frac{1}{R_N} = \left[\frac{Q_{new}}{Q_{old}} \right] \left[\frac{D_{old}}{D_{new}} \right]^2 \left[\frac{L_{old}}{L_{new}} \right] \left[\frac{d_{p,new}}{d_{p,old}} \right]^2 \tag{8-30b}$$

When pore diffusion controls, Eqs. (8-29) and (8-30b) can be considered as two equations with two unknowns and four knowns. The six variables are $1/R_P$, $1/R_N$, (Q_{new}/Q_{old}), (D_{new}/D_{old}), (L_{new}/L_{old}), and $(d_{p,new}/d_{p,old})$. Any four of these can be selected as known. A case study approach to solving Eqs. (8-29) and (8-30a) when pore diffusion does not control is illustrated in Example 8-2. Once the new design has been determined, the adsorbent volume is $\pi D^2 L/4$. Then

$$\frac{(\text{Adsorbent Volume})_{new}}{(\text{Adsorbent Volume})_{old}} = \left[\frac{D_{new}}{D_{old}} \right]^2 \left[\frac{L_{new}}{L_{old}} \right] \tag{8-31}$$

Many commercial adsorption systems use particles in the range of 1 mm. Based on the argument in this section these particles are probably too large, and the columns and cycles are probably too long. There are some practical reasons why smaller particles may be difficult to use. Some of these arguments are:

1. Careful packing procedures are required with small particles. Methods to do this are used commercially.

2. A tighter sieving of small particles is required if axial dispersion is important.

3. The classical rules of thumb for length to diameter have been violated. The columns are now short and fat instead of long and skinny. This will

require a redesign of the end fittings to prevent excessive volumes (see below). Better fluid distribution may be required.

4. Piping and values must be redesigned to reduce volume (see below).

5. The valves must be designed for more rapid cycles. More accurate timing is required.

6. Since the packed column will act as an efficient filter, the feed must be free of suspended solids. However, since cycles are shorter there is less time for suspended solids to build up and clog the bed. Feeds containing suspended solids can be processed in fluidized beds (see Chapter 10).

7. The desired small particle size may not be commercially available, and when they are available may be more expensive than large particles. In addition, the lifetime of small particles may be shorter.

All of these practical arguments are true, but they can usually be taken care of by proper design. There are other conditions where these scaling methods may be useful (Wankat, 1987). Scaling of chromatography systems is quite similiar (Wankat and Koo, 1988), but will not be developed here.

The analysis in Eqs. (8-20) to (8-31) has been concerned only with the packing. As the length of packing L decreases the volume of fluid outside the packing can become important. Referring to Figure 8-6, we see that the extracolumn volume on the feed side is

$$V_{ec,feed} = V_{valve\,1} + V_{pipe} + V_{distributor} + V_{frit} \tag{8-32}$$

The equation for $V_{ec,product}$ will be similar.

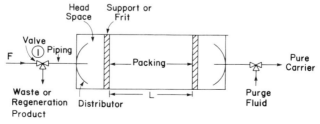

Figure 8-6.   Extracolumn volume in adsorption system.

Consider a very simple two step cycle: Feed and Regenerate. At the end of the feed step, the fluid in volume $V_{ec,feed}$ is unprocessed feed. This material will reduce the recovery of carrier and will contaminate the regeneration product. In addition, the pores of the column contain unprocessed feed. Assuming that the mass transfer zone is symmetric, we obtain

$$V_{pore,feed} = \frac{\pi D^2}{4} [\varepsilon_e + (1-\varepsilon_e) \varepsilon_p] (L - 0.5 L_{MTZ}) \qquad (8\text{-}33)$$

as the volume of unprocessed feed in the pores. The fraction of feed not processed per cycle is

$$\text{frac. feed unprocessed} = \frac{V_{ec,feed} + V_{pores,feed}}{Q t_F} \qquad (8\text{-}34)$$

where $Q t_F$ is the volume of feed during the feed step.

To consider the effect of this unprocessed feed, we can take the ratio of Eq. (8-34) for the new and old designs.

$$\frac{(\text{frac. feed unprocessed})_{new}}{(\text{frac. feed unprocessed})_{old}} = \frac{(V_{ec,feed} + V_{pores,feed})_{new}}{(V_{ec,feed} + V_{pores,feed})_{old}} \frac{Q_{old}}{Q_{new}} \frac{t_{F,old}}{t_{F,new}} \qquad (8\text{-}35)$$

We will consider the simple case where pore diffusion controls and $Q_{old} = Q_{new}$. Then, the previous analysis showed we want $v_{new} = v_{old}$, $D_{new} = D_{old}$, $(L/d_p^2)_{new} = (L/d_p^2)_{old}$, and $t_{F,new}/t_{F,old} = L_{new}/L_{old}$.

First, consider the case where $V_{ec,feed} \ll V_{pore,feed}$ for both designs (this is often true for long columns). Then, Eq. (8-35) becomes

$$\frac{(\text{frac. feed unprocessed})_{new}}{\text{frac. feed unprocessed})_{old}} = \frac{(1 - 0.5 L_{MTZ}/L)_{new}}{(1 - 0.5 L_{MTZ}/L)_{old}} = 1 \qquad (8\text{-}36)$$

This equation equals one since the scaling procedure makes $(L_{MTZ}/L)_{new} = (L_{MTZ}/L)_{old}$. This result shows that the pore volumes scale appropriately. If $V_{ec,feed}$ is not negligible compared to $V_{pores,feed}$; then Eq. (8-35) equals 1 if

$$\frac{(V_{ec,feed})_{new}}{(V_{ec,feed})_{old}} = \frac{L_{new}}{L_{old}} \qquad (8\text{-}37)$$

As the volume of packing is reduced the volume outside the packing must also be reduced.

Actually, Eq. (8-37) is more stringent than practical requirements particularly for dilute systems. For dilute systems Qt_F is often quite large since the shock wave moves very slowly. Equation (8-34) shows that the fraction of feed unprocessed will be small. Practically, changes in this fraction may be unimportant. For concentrated systems changes in the fraction of feed unprocessed is probably important. Then careful design is required to reduce $V_{ec,feed}$.

Example 8-2. Application of Scaling Methods

We have available 0.05 cm diameter BPL activated carbon particles. We wish to repeat the separation in Example 8-1 with the same Δp, the same feed throughput, and the same or better fractional bed use. Find the column diameter, length, feed period, and fluid velocity for the new design.

Solution

Since both film and pore diffusion are important, we will use a case study approach with $(d_{p,new}/d_{p,old}) = 0.5$. We want $R_p = 1$, $R_N \geq 1.0$, and $Q_{new}/Q_{old} = 1$. Equations (8-25) and (8-26a) need to be satisfied. In Example 8-1 $k_m a_p = 1149.3$ s^{-1} was calculated from Eq. (8-19a) where the individual values of k_f and k_{pore} were found from Eqs. (8-16) and (8-17a), and a_p is from Eq. (8-14). Note that the ratio $(k_m a_{p,old}/k_m a_{p,new})$ does not simplify when both pore and film diffusion are important.

Trial-and-Error Case Study Approach:

   a. Guess v_{new}
   b. Calculate $k_f a_p$, $(ka_p)_{pore}$ and $k_m a_p$
   c. Find (L_{old}/L_{new}) from Eq. (8-25) with $R_p = 1$
   d. Calculate R_N from Eq. (8-26a)
   e. If $R_N = 1$, are finished. If not, start over.

Step a. If pore diffusion controlled, $v_{new} = v_{old}$. If film diffusion controls, $v_{new} = 0.75\ v_{old}$ (Wankat and Koo, 1988). Since Example 8-1 showed that pore diffusion was more important than pore diffusion, try

$$v_{super,new} = 0.8\ v_{super,old} = (0.8)(55) = 44\ \text{cm/s}.$$

Step b. Following Example 8-1, $a_p = 6/d_p = 6/0.05 = 120$.

$$k_f = \frac{(1.17)(v_{super})^{0.585}(0.0001757)^{0.252}(0.675)^{2/3}}{(0.05)^{0.415}(0.0001796)^{0.252}} = 3.104(v_{super})^{0.585}$$

Thus, $k_f = 3.104(44)^{0.585} = 28.40\ \text{cm/s}$ and $k_f a_p = 3408.1$. From Eq. (8-17a),

$$(ka_p)_{pore} = \frac{(60)(0.0514)(28.986)(0.61)}{(0.05)^2} = 21{,}811.8$$

Note that $(ka_p)_{pore}$ is not a function of v_{super}. Then from Eq. (8-19a),

$$k_m a_p = \left[\frac{1}{3408.1} + \frac{1}{21{,}811.8}\right]^{-1} = 2947.6$$

Step c. $\dfrac{L_{old}}{L_{new}} = \left[\dfrac{v_{new}}{v_{old}}\right]\left[\dfrac{d_{p,old}}{d_{p,new}}\right]^2 \dfrac{1}{R_p} = (0.8)(4)(1.0) = 3.2$

Thus, $L_{new} = 1.0/3.2 = 0.3125\ \text{m}$

Step d. $\dfrac{1}{R_N} = (0.8)(3.2)\left[\dfrac{1149.3}{2947.6}\right] = 0.998$

or $R_N = 1.002$ which is close enough. The new diameter can be determined from Eq. (8-28)

$$\left[\frac{D_{new}}{D_{old}}\right]^2 = \left[\frac{v_{old}}{v_{new}}\right]\Big/\left[\frac{Q_{old}}{Q_{new}}\right] = \left[\frac{1}{.8}\right]\Big/(1.0) = 1.25$$

$$D_{new} = 1.118\ D_{old}$$

The new value of L_{MTZ} can be found.

$$(L/L_{MTZ})_{new} = R_N(L/L_{MTZ})_{old} = (1.002)\left[\frac{100}{13.33}\right] = 7.52 \text{ cm}$$

Thus $L_{MTZ,new} = L_{new}/7.52 = 31.25/7.52 = 4.16$ cm.
The velocity of the mass transfer pattern is

$$u_{p,new} = u_{p,old}\frac{v_{new}}{v_{old}} = (3.043)(0.8) = 2.434 \text{ cm/s}$$

The feed period can now be determined from Eq. (8-2),

$$t_{F,new} = (L - 0.5\,L_{MTZ})/u_p = (31.25 - 2.08)/2.434 = 11.98 \text{ s}$$

Then,

$$\frac{t_{F,new}}{t_{F,old}} = 0.391 = \left[\frac{L_{new}}{L_{old}}\right]\Big/\left[\frac{v_{new}}{v_{old}}\right] = \frac{(L/v)_{new}}{(L/v)_{old}}$$

The new design is shorter and cycles faster, but has the same separation, same Δp and same throughput. Obviously, the new design uses less packing.

8.5. INTERACTING ADSORPTION SYSTEMS

This series of chapters only skim the surface of theories for adsorption, chromatography and ion exchange systems. The theories were kept simple (remember, this is relative to other theories) by discussing only isothermal, linear adsorption with several solutes or isothermal, non-linear, single solute adsorption. In this section we will briefly look at the results of more complex experiments and theories where there are several interacting solutes or the column is adiabatic. Most of the theories required for these analyses are beyond the scope of this book; however, references for further study will be provided.

394

8.5.1. Interacting Solutes

In general, when there are several solutes they will interact. Thus the equilibrium for one solute depends on the concentration of all solutes. The simplest equilibrium form which expresses this dependence is the multicomponent Langmuir expression,

$$q_j = \frac{q_{MAX}K_jc_j}{1 + \sum\limits_{i=1}^{N}(K_ic_i)}$$ (8-38)

When the concentration of component i increases, the amount of component j adsorbed decreases (i ≠ j). There is *competition* for sites. Equation (8-38) can be adapted to ion exchange also.

The behavior of coupled systems has been extensively studied. The results for adsorption of n-pentane and n-hexane from iso and cyclic hydrocarbons which are not sorbed by the zeolite are shown in Figure 8-7 (Lee, 1972) are typical. The least adsorbed solute, n-pentane, is first adsorbed and is then desorbed as the more strongly adsorbed solute, n-hexane, displaces it. Since it

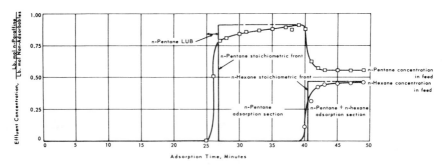

Figure 8-7.   Adsorption of n=pentane and n-hexane on zeolites at 615°F. Feed is 0.4 mole % n-butane, 25.9% n-pentane, 23.9% n-hexane and 49.8% iso and cyclic hydrocarbons. (Lee, 1972). Reprinted with permission from N.N. Li (Ed.), *Recent Developments in Separation Science*, Vol. I, CRC Press, Boca Raton, FL, 75-112, 1972. Copyright 1972, CRC Press.

is being pushed off the adsorbent, the concentration of n-pentane rises to a value above its feed concentration. This behavior often is referred to as *roll-up*. The n-pentane concentration remains at this *plateau* value until the more strongly adsorbed n-hexane starts to breakthrough. Both solutes then go to their feed concentrations.

Three plateaus (initial concentrations of zero, intermediate plateau with high n-pentane concentration, and feed concentrations) are shown in Figure 8-7. In general, for each step change there will be N + 1 plateaus where N is the number of adsorbates. (In ion exchange there will be N plateaus where N is the number of counterions). The two transition zones between the plateaus can be either constant pattern (shock waves) or proportional pattern (diffuse waves). The transitions shown in Figure 8-7 are both constant pattern. When this column is eluted, the two transitions would both be proportional pattern. When there are more components, the patterns can become very complex.

Theoretical calculation for multicomponent systems is difficult. For each solute in adsorption there is an independent mass balance, Eq. (6-42) or (6-48), and a mass transfer relation, Eq. (6-47) or Eq. (6-50). (For ion exchange there are N-1 independent equations since electroneutrality must be satisfied.) All of these equations are coupled by the equilibrium relationship, Eq. (8-38). Thus, all of the equations must be solved simultaneously. This problem has been extensively studied using a complex form of equilibrium theory (Aris and Amundsen, 1973; Helferrich and Klein, 1970; Lightfoot *et al.,* 1962; Rhee, 1971; Ruthven, 1984; Yang, 1987). Although rather complex, this theory is still oversimplified and predicts shock waves instead of the S-shaped constant pattern waves. The theory does correctly predict the plateaus, the transition locations and the types of transitions. To include mass transfer effects numerical models are usually used (Ruthven, 1984; Yang, 1987).

For displacement chromatography (see Section 7.10) there is a simple and useful local equilibrium result (Glueckauf, 1946; Rhee and Amundson, 1982; Wankat, 1986). In displacement chromatography the column is first equilibrated with carrier C. Then a feed pulse of A plus B in C is added. This is followed by a strongly adsorbed displacer D in carrier C. Finally, the column must be reequilibrated by eluting with carrier C.

The strength of adsorption follows D > B > A > C. Thus the displacer pushes out B which pushes out A which pushes out pure C. The result is a series of bands: pure C followed by A in C followed by B in C followed by D in C. This was illustrated in Figure 7-13. Each band is separated by a shock wave. The solute movement diagram is shown in Figure 8-8. The dotted lines represent transient behavior which requires the more detailed theory.

The band widths of A and B must become constant to satisfy a mass balance. This is also observed experimentally. Since the band widths are constant, the shock wave velocities must be equatl.

$$u_{sh,1} = u_{sh,2} = u_{sh,3} \tag{8-39}$$

The concentrations $c_{A,band}$ and $c_{B,band}$ are unknown; however, the concentrations of D are known and the amount adsorbed can be calculated.

$$\frac{\Delta q_D}{\Delta c_D} = \frac{q(c_{D,F}, c_A = 0, c_B = 0) - 0}{c_{D,F} - 0} \tag{8-40}$$

Note that q_D can be calculated despite the coupled isotherm (Eq. 8-38) since D and B never occur simultaneously. We can now calculate $u_{sh,3}$

$$u_{sh,3} = \frac{v}{1 + \dfrac{1-\varepsilon_e}{\varepsilon_e} \varepsilon_p K_{d,D} + \dfrac{1-\varepsilon_e}{\varepsilon_e} (1-\varepsilon_p) \rho_s \dfrac{\Delta q_D}{\Delta c_D}} \tag{8-41}$$

From Eq. (8-39) this is also the value of $u_{sh,2}$. We can write $u_{sh,2}$

$$u_{sh,2} = \frac{v}{1 + \dfrac{1-\varepsilon_e}{\varepsilon_e} \varepsilon_p K_{d,B} + \dfrac{(1-\varepsilon_e)(1-\varepsilon_p)\rho_s}{\varepsilon_e} \dfrac{q(c_{B,band}) - 0}{c_{B,band} - 0}} \tag{8-42}$$

The unknowns are now q_B ($c_{B,band}$) and $c_{B,band}$. These unknowns are related by Eq. (8-42) and the isotherm which is Eq. (8-38) or any other coupled, favorable isotherm. Solving the isotherm and shock velocity equations simultane-

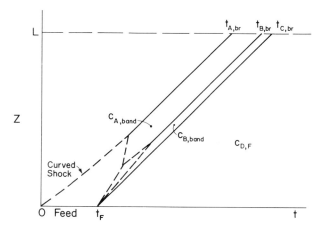

Figure 8-8.   Solute movement diagram for displacement chromatography.

ously, we obtain $c_{B,band}$ and q_B $(c_{B,band})$. This is illustrated for a Langmuir isotherm in Example 8-3. A very similiar calculation can be done for component A to determine $c_{A,band}$ and q_A $(c_{A,band})$.

Since band concentrations are known, we can use a mass balance to find the band widths.

$$c_{A,F} \, t_F = c_{A,band} \, t_{A,band} \qquad (8\text{-}43a)$$

$$c_{B,F} \, t_F = c_{B,band} \, t_{B,band} \qquad (8\text{-}43b)$$

The times the bands breakthrough are easily determined.

$$t_{D,br} = L/u_{sh,3} + t_F \qquad (8\text{-}44a)$$

$$t_{B,br} = t_{D,br} - t_{B,band} \qquad (8\text{-}44b)$$

$$t_{A,br} = t_{D,br} - t_{B,band} - t_{A,band} \qquad (8\text{-}44c)$$

The removal of displacer D with pure C gives a diffuse wave. This wave is easily calculated using the methods of Chapter 6. This step may be a major expense of displacement chromatography because of excessive tailing. In ion exchange chromatography column regeneration may be easy (see Problems 9-D6 and 9-D7).

Note that the only important detail we cannot calculate is the column length necessary to generate the pure bands. This calculation of the dotted lines in Figure 8-8 requires more detailed theories (Rhee and Amundson, 1982).

Displacement behavior will *not* occur if the displacer concentration is too low or D is not strongly enough adsorbed. If A moves faster than $u_{sh,3}$, then the A band will not follow these equations. $u_{sh,A}$ (c_A) will be greater than $u_{sh,3}$ if

$$\frac{\Delta q_A}{\Delta c_A} \Big|_{c_A \ll c_{A,band}} < \frac{\Delta q_D}{\Delta c_D} \Big|_{c_{D,F}} \tag{8-45a}$$

This dilutes the A band. $u_{sh,S}$ ($c_{A,F}$) will be greater than $u_{sh,3}$ if

$$\frac{\Delta q_A}{\Delta c_A} \Big|_{c_{A,F}} < \frac{\Delta q_D}{\Delta c_D} \Big|_{c_{D,F}} \tag{8-45b}$$

and a separate A peak forms. If u_s ($c_A = 0$) > $u_{sh,3}$, the A peak will move completely away from the B band (they will be separated by carrier), and the A peak will have a diffuse tail. This occurs if

$$\frac{\Delta q_A}{\Delta c_A} \Big|_{c_A = 0} < < \frac{\Delta q_D}{\Delta c_D} \Big|_{c_{D,F}} \tag{8-45c}$$

Equations (8-45) assume $K_{d,A} = K_{d,D}$.

Finite mass transfer rates and axial dispersion will broaden the sharp shock waves predicted by the equilibrium theory. The effects of axial dispersion and finite mass transfer rates have been extensively modeled by solving the coupled partial differential equations numerically (Phillips *et al*, 1988).

Example 8 3. Displacement Chromatography

Displacement chromatography has been extensively studied for separation of small biomolecules. We input a 6 minute feed pulse containing 10 mM each of components A and B. The displacer D is input at 40 mM. Predict the band concentrations, the band widths, and the breakthrough times.

Data: $K_{Di} = 1.0$, $\varepsilon_e = 0.4$, $v_{super} = 1$ cm/min, $L = 25$ cm.

Equilibrium: $q_i = \dfrac{a_i \, c_i}{1 + \sum b_j \, c_j}$

where q is mM/ml and c is mM/ml.

$a_A = 3.297$, $b_A = 0.0905$ $(mM)^{-1}$
$a_B = 5.740$, $b_A = 0.1247$ $(mM)^{-1}$
$a_D = 9.203$, $b_D = 0.1501$ $(mM)^{-1}$

(from Phillips *et al*, 1988).

Solution

The shock wave velocity for displacer can be found from Eqs. (8-40) and (8-41). From the equilibrium expression, we obtain

$$\Delta q_D = q_D \ (c_D, \ c_A = c_B = 0) \ = \ 52.56 \ mM/g$$

$$\frac{\Delta q_D}{\Delta c_D} = \frac{52.56}{40} = 1.314$$

For the units of this problem, Eq. (8-41) becomes

$$u_{sh,D} = \frac{v_{super}}{\varepsilon_e + (1-\varepsilon_e) \, \varepsilon_p \, K_{d,D} + (1-\varepsilon_e) \, (1-\varepsilon_p) \, \dfrac{\Delta q_D}{\Delta c_D}} \tag{8-46}$$

$$u_{sh,D} = \frac{1}{0.4 + (0.6) \, (0.4) \, (1.0) + (0.6) \, (0.6) \, (1.314)} = 0.8984 \ cm/min$$

The shock waves for A and B must have the same value. From the Langmuir isotherm

$$\frac{q\,(c_{i,band}\,,\,c_{j\neq i}=0)}{c_{i,band}} = \frac{a_i}{1+b_i\,c_{i,band}} \tag{8-47}$$

Combining this result with Eq. (8-42), we obtain after some algebra.

$$c_{i,band} = \frac{[\varepsilon_e + (1-\varepsilon_e)\,\varepsilon_p\,K_{D,i}] + (1-\varepsilon_e)\,(1-\varepsilon_p)\,a_i - \dfrac{v_{super}}{u_{sh}}}{\dfrac{v_{super}}{u_{sh}}\,b_i - b_i\,[\varepsilon_e + (1-\varepsilon_e)\,\varepsilon_p\,K_{D,i}]} \tag{8-48}$$

Plugging in the numbers, we obtain $c_{B,band} = 27.01$ mM and $c_{A,band} = 16.673$ mM. From Eqs. (8-43),

$$t_{A,band} = t_F\,c_{A,F}/c_{A,band} = (6.0)\,(10.0)/(16.673) = 3.60\ \text{min}$$

and $t_{B,band} = (6.0)\,(10.0)\,/\,(27.01) = 2.22$ min.

From Eq. (8-44a), $t_{D,br} = 25/0.8984 + 6 = 33.83$ min

From Eq. (8-44b), $t_{B,br} = 33.83 - 2.22 = 31.61$ min.

From Eq. (8-44c), $t_{A,br} = 33.83 - 2.22 - 3.60 = 28.01$ min.

Note that the six minute feed band is compressed to 5.82 minutes.

8.5.2. Adiabatic Adsorbers

Until now we have assumed that the column is isothermal or has step changes in temperature. Large columns are often adiabatic not isothermal since a substantial amount of energy may be released when the solute adsorbs. The same amount of energy is later required to desorb the solute. Thus the temperature of the column rises during adsorption and drops during desorption.

To study adiabatic systems the energy balances are required. The energy balance for both phases was given in Eq. (6-51) while the energy transfer equation is Eq. (6-55). The mass and energy balances and the equilibrium relationship are all coupled. The coupling of the energy balance with the mass balance occurs in the heat of adsorption term of Eq. (6-55). Equilibrium is coupled to the energy balance since the equilibrium parameters depend on temperature (Eq. (6-8)). The mass balances are coupled to equilibrium since the mass transfer rate and the amount adsorbed depends on the equilibrium.

Previously, we uncoupled the equations by assuming the column was either isothermal or had negligible heat of adsorption effects. For an isothermal system the energy balances are not required. When the effect of heat of adsorption is negligible, the energy balance can be solved separately. Then the temperature profile can be used to find the equilibrium conditions at any point in the column. This latter method was done for thermal waves in Chapter 6 and in Problems 7-C6, 7-C7, and 7-E3.

The effect of heat of adsorption will be negligible when:

1. $\Delta H_{ads} \sim 0$. This is true for exchange adsorption, displacement adsorption, and ion exchange. In these systems the sorbed species is replaced by another sorbed species. The adsorption and desorption effects balance each other. These processes are usually isothermal.

2. Dilute gas systems. Now $\partial q / \partial t \sim 0$ since there is little adsorbate to adsorb. Although ΔH_{ads} may be substantial, the term $(1-\varepsilon_p)(1-\varepsilon_e)\rho_s\Delta H_{ads}\partial q/\partial t$ in Eq. (6-55) remains small.

3. Most liquid systems. In liquid systems the volumetric heat capacity $(\rho_f C_{pf})$ is large. The energy released by the heat of adsorption is either removed by the flowing liquid or is soaked up by the solid and stagnant fluid with very little increase in temperature. Thus operation is close to isothermal.

4. Pressure swing adsorption systems with very rapid cycles. Temperature does increase during adsorption and decrease during desorption. When the cycle period is on the order of a few seconds or less, the temperature increases and decreases remain very small. These operations are usually treated as isothermal even though strictly speaking they are not.

402

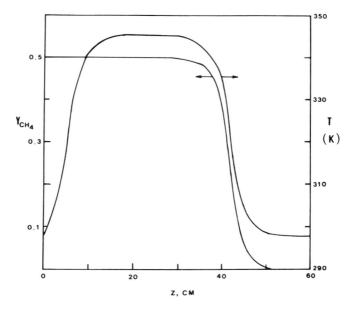

Figure 8-9.   Concentration and temperature profiles for adiabatic adsorption
(Yang, 1987). Bed initially filled with H_2. Feed 50% H_2, 50%
CH_4. Reprinted with permission from R.T. Yang, *Gas Separa-
tion by Adsorption Processes*. Butterworths, Boston, 1987.
Copyright 1987, Butterworths.

Gas systems where items 1, 2 and 4 do not apply will have significant
temperature effects. This is illustrated in Figure 8-9 (Yang, 1987). Note the
large increase in temperature due to the heat of adsorption. Because of the coupling the thermal wave moves slightly ahead of the concentration wave.
Although gas mole fraction y is constant after the concentration wave, q will
vary since T varies. Since all the equations are coupled, the exact solution of
the partial differential equations is difficult. Equilibrium solutions can be
obtained using methods very similar to those used for interacting solutes
(Sweed, 1981; Yang, 1987). Complete solutions including heat and mass
transfer resistances require numerical methods (Ruthven, 1984; Basmadjian,
1983; Yang, 1987). The mass transfer zone will be wider in adiabatic systems

than in isothermal systems. Thus, it is important to include temperature effects either in theoretical calculations or in laboratory experiments.

The behavior of gas systems can be studied qualitatively using the solute movement theory of Chapter 6. When a gas is adsorbed, its density approaches that of a liquid. Thus, if adsorption is strong there will be much more adsorbate on the solid phase than in the fluid. In Eq. (6-23) this means the first two terms in the denominator will be very small compared to the third term. Then,

$$u_s \sim \frac{v}{[(1-\varepsilon_e)/\varepsilon_e](1-\varepsilon_p)\rho_s(\Delta q/\Delta c)} \qquad (8\text{-}49)$$

In most gas systems at modest pressure $(C_{Pf}\rho_f) \ll (\rho_s C_{Ps})$. Thus the amount of energy stored in the solid is much greater than the amount in the gas phase. Then the first two terms in the denominator of Eq. (6-36) will be small compared to the third term. In commercial systems the column diameter is large, W/A_c is small, the wall effect is small, and the fourth term in the denominator of Eq. (6-36) can be neglected. Thus,

$$u_{th} \sim \frac{v}{(1-\varepsilon_e)(1-\varepsilon_p)\rho_s C_{Ps}/\rho_f C_{Pf}\varepsilon_e} \qquad (8\text{-}50)$$

Taking the ratio of Eqs. (8-49) and (8-50) we have,

$$R_T = \frac{\Delta q/\Delta c}{(C_{Ps}/C_{Pf})\dfrac{1}{\rho_f}} \sim \frac{u_{th}}{u_s} \qquad (8\text{-}51)$$

R_T is the *cross-over ratio* (Garg and Ausikaitis, 1983). If $R_T \gg 1$ then the thermal wave moves ahead of the solute wave, while if $R_T \ll 1$ the thermal wave lags behind the solute wave. In both these cases the mass and energy balances are essentially uncoupled. The temperature in the region of the solute wave can be estimated.

The most interesting and complex case occurs when R_T is approximately 1.0. Now the solute and thermal waves travel together and no simplifications are possible. This is the case in Figure 8-9 (Yang, 1987). Although theoretically complex, this operation can be advantageous. Since the loading step is stopped before breakthrough of the solute wave, the thermal wave also remains in the column. The energy released during adsorption is now available for desorption. This principle is commonly used in PSA systems where the cycles are only a few minutes long. Recently, operation with R_T near one has been used in thermally regenerated adsorbers drying ethanol vapor (Ladisch et al., 1984; Garg and Ausikaitis, 1983). The energy required for regeneration can be significantly decreased. Unfortunately, the theory of these systems is beyond the scope of this book.

Adiabatic adsorbers can be designed using the MTZ-LUB approach. Care must be taken that the laboratory columns are equivalent to the large scale system. As the column diameter increases the ratio of wall surface area to column volume decreases. Thus the wall heat transfer term and the wall storage term (the right hand side of Eq. (6-51)) both become less important. In commercial systems with large diameters both these terms are usually negligible. Thus even without insulation the column will effectively be adiabatic. In small diameter laboratory columns the wall effects are relatively much more important. Even with insulation it is difficult to make the wall heat transfer term (term 6 in Eq. (6-51)) negligible. Thus the laboratory and commercial columns are not equivalent. The solution to this problem is to use a large diameter laboratory column (at *least* 3 inches in diameter) and to insulate the column carefully. Then the experimentally measured MTZ will include heat effects. Since the heat effects are approximately the same in the laboratory and commercial columns, this MTZ can be used to design the larger column.

8.5.3. Velocity Effects

Up to now we have usually assumed that the fluid interstitial velocity v is constant. For liquids, the density of the adsorbed material is approximately equal to the liquid density. In addition, changes in pressure or temperature do not markedly change the density. Thus the velocity will remain approximately constant.

For gases there can be large velocity changes. The density of the adsorbed material is approximately the same as a liquid and is much greater than the gas density. Thus, as material adsorbs the gas volume decreases since solute is removed from the gas phase. The velocity must be lower ahead of the solute wave than it is behind the solute wave. This causes self-sharpening or shock type behavior even for linear isotherms. Upon desorption the opposite happens. The gas volume increases, velocity increases, and a spread or diffuse wave results. This velocity effect has been called the *sorption effect,* and it can be calculated quantitatively (Ruthven, 1984; Wankat, 1986).

The sorption effect causes shock and diffuse waves under the same conditions a Langmuir isotherm will. Thus they reinforce each other and are difficult to tell apart. For gas-liquid chromatography (GLC) where the isotherms have the opposite curvature (they are unfavorable), the sorption effect causes a shock wave when the isotherm causes a diffuse wave and vice versa. Thus the sorption and isotherm effects tend to cancel each other in GLC. By tuning the column temperature, GLC peaks can be made to be sharp and symmetrical for concentrated systems where both sorption and isotherm effects are important (Roz *et al.,* 1976). This will be true for any sorbent with an unfavorable isotherm.

In gas systems temperature and pressure changes will also change the density and hence the velocity. If temperature increases, the gas velocity behind the thermal wave increases. Thus hot waves are compressive. For a temperature increase from 20 to 80°C the velocity increase is about 20%. Cooling waves will be dispersive by the same percentage. Changes in pressure will have similar but opposite effects. The pressure effects occur very rapidly and are probably important only with very rapid cycles (1 second or less).

8.6. ADSORPTION - DESORPTION OPERATIONS

Adsorbing the desired solute is often fairly easy. The trick of economical operation is the desorption step. The most commonly used desorption methods are thermal desorption, pressure swing desorption, purge gas desorption and desorption using a desorbent. These methods will be considered separately.

406

8.6.1. Thermal Desorption of Gases

To have continuous treatment of a feed stream at least two columns are required. A fairly typical arrangement is shown in Figure 8-10. The feed gas passes through the operating adsorber where the solute is adsorbed. The treated gas is one product. A small portion of this gas is heated and used to regenerate the column in counter-flow. This can be considered a type of *reflux*. The concentrated gas from desorption is sent to a further separation scheme, exhausted or burned. The operation is timed so that when the first column starts to breakthrough the second column has been regenerated. The columns are then switched and feed goes to the second column while the first column is desorbed. Often the desorbed column is cooled before the feed is switched to it. Many more complex cycles and multi-column arrangements are used (Ruthven, 1984; Wankat, 1986a; Yang, 1987). Note that Figure 8-10 represents a batch operation and *not* steady state. Feed is processed continuously because there is always a clean column to send the feed to.

The solute movement theory for this type of operation was shown in Fig-

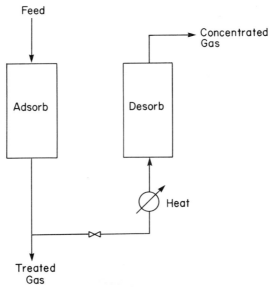

Figure 8-10.   Two column system with thermal desorption.

ure 6-12 for a system with linear isotherms and a negligible heat of adsorption term. This figure is for one of the two columns. The *linear* solute movement theory does not illustrate all of the important features of the cycle shown in Figure 8-11. To do this more complex theories are required. The non-linear isotherm theory with negligible $\Delta H_{ads} \partial \overline{q}/\partial t$ is illustrated in Figure 8-11. Note that the column is not completely regenerated but some solute is left in the column. This is called a *heel* and may be quite large. This diffuse wave is then resharpened by the shock wave during the next cycle. The shock wave in Figure 8-11 is curved. This occurs because the concentrations upstream of the shock wave are continually changing; thus, the last term in the denominator of Eq. (6-23) changes. In practice, the shock wave will result in a constant pattern wave. The MTZ approach can be used to predict the shape of this wave. Partial regeneration means that the entire equilibrium capacity of the column is not available for adsorption. However, partial regeneration is usually much cheaper than complete regneration since an excessive amount of hot gas would be required to completely remove the slow diffuse wave.

Figures 6-12 and 8-11 have assumed that the term $\Delta H_{ads} \partial \overline{q}/\partial t$ in Eqs. (6-53) or (6-55) is negligible. This term will be important in many gas streams and Figures 6-12 and 8-11 will not be valid. A more complex form of the local

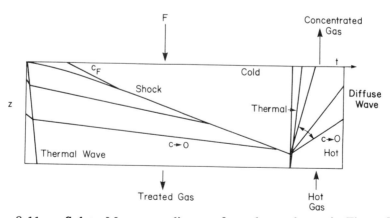

Figure 8-11.   Solute Movement diagram for column shown in Figure 8-10 for non-linear isotherm. The term $\Delta H_{ads} \partial \overline{q}/\partial t$ is assumed to be negligible.

Table 8-1.   Characteristic Temperatures T_o for Various Systems at 1 atm.
Basmadjian (1975a). Reprinted with permission from *Ind. Eng.
Chem. Process Des. Develop., 14*, 328 (1975). Copyright 1975,
American Chemical Society.

System	T_0, °F[a]
CO_2–CH_4–5A molecular sieves	~230
H_2O-air-5A molecular sieves	>600
H_2O-air-silica gel	~250
H_2S–CH_4–5A molecular sieves	~400
Acetone-air-activated carbon	~300

[a] Values are accurate only to ±10% because of uncertainities in the isotherm
slopes and heat capacity values.

equilibrium theory can be used to analyze adiabatic adsorbers when the heat of
adsorption term is important (Pan and Basmadjian, 1971; Basmadjian *et al.*,
1975a,b). The term $\Delta H_{ads} \, \partial \bar{q}/\partial t$ couples the mass and energy balances, and
thus a mathematical uncoupling of the equations is required. The results of
these theories shows that efficient desorption occurs above a characteristic temperature T_o. The characteristic temperature is the temperature at which the
slope of the adsorption isotherm at the origin equals the ratio of heat capacities
C_{Ps}/C_{Pf}. Characteristic temperatures for several systems are given in Table 8-1
(Basmadjian, 1975a). Below the characteristic temperature regeneration is
inefficient and large volumes of purge gas are required. Above the characteristic temperature the regeneration is slightly more efficient, but the reduction in
purge gas volume is very modest. Since heating the purge gas is expensive,
regeneration is usually done slightly above the characteristic temperature. The
use of too low a regeneration temperature also decreases the amount adsorbed
in equilibrium studies (Joshi and Fair, 1988). The regeneration temperature
required for essentially complete equilibrium regeneration is below the characteristic temperature.

The basic system shown in Figure 8-10 can be used for a variety of
separations (Keller, 1982; Kohl and Riesenfeld, 1979; Ruthven, 1984; Wankat

1986), but operation by thermal swing is economical only for feeds with low adsorbate concentrations (usually under 5 mole %). With higher feed concentratios the energy costs for regeneration become excessive (Keller, 1982). Thermal swing cycles do have the advantage of providing high (90 ~ 99%) removal and recovery of adsorbate. Systems similar to Figure 8-10 are used for removal of traces of SO_2, mercury and NO_x from waste gas streams. Zeolite molecular sieves are used for adsorbing SO_2. During desorption the concentration can rise as high as 4% compared to the feed concentration of 2000 to 4000 ppm. A 4% SO_2 stream can be reused to make sulfuric acid. Thus a major advantage of adsorption with thermal desorption is the desorbed solute is at a much higher concentration than in the feed.

Drying of gases with adsorbents is a very common industrial and laboratory practice. You probably did this in chemistry laboratory using a solid such as Drierite which changes color from blue to pink when water is adsorbed. Industrially, activated alumina, silica gel and molecular sieve zeolites are used for adsorption drying. Typical adsorbent properties are listed in Table 8-2 (Basmadjian, 1984). Equilibrium isotherms for drying air using several adsorbents are shown in Figure 8-12. If very low water concentrations are required, molecular sieve zeolites are preferred. Molecular sieve zeolites are more expensive than silica gel and activated alumina, and Table 8-1 shows the zeolites require a higher regeneration temperature. The cheaper adsorbents are often used for less demanding applications, or when the feed gas is very concentrated. A layer of cheap adsorbent such as silica gel followed by molecular sieves is useful to achieve low moisture constant at low cost particularly for concentrated feeds. Basmadjian's (1984) review contains data and information on adsorbent drying.

Regeneration of silica gel and activated alumina is typically done at 100 to 200°C while zeolite molecular sieves require 200 to 300 °C or higher (see Table 8-1 for specific examples). The energy required for the molecular sieve systems is also higher. Counter-flow regeneration, shown in Figures 8-10 and 8-11, uses less energy than co-flow regeneration; however, co-flow regeneration (see Problem 8-A7) is simpler and has lower capital costs. Both are used industrially. A short cooling period (co-flow to the feed step) is often used. Fast cycles increase the adsorbent productivity and smaller equipment is

Table 8-2. Properties of Commercial Desiccants: Manufacturers' Data (Basmadjian, 1984). Reprinted with permission from A.S. Mujumdar (Ed.), *Advances in Drying*, Vol. 3 Copyright 1984, Hemisphere Pub. Co.

Type	Particle size, mm	Density (g/cm^3) Bulk	Density (g/cm^3) Particle	Surface area, m^2/g	Pore Volume, cm^3/g	Pore Diameter, nm	Specific heat J/gK	Maximum heat of J/gK
Activated alumina								
1. Alcoa F-1	<12	0.85	1.42	250	0.40	2.6	-	-
2. Alcoa H-151	3-6	0.85	1.38	360	0.43	4.3	-	-
3. Laporte Actal	6-12,3-6	0.64	1.15	275	0.50	2.8	0.88	2.88
4. Rhone-Poulenc	2-5,5-10	0.77	-	345,315	0.40	-	-	-
5. Kaiser A-201	<12	0.75	1.4	350	0.46	5.2	-	-

Silica gel

6. Davison 03	2	0.72	1.2	750	0.43	2.2	0.92	3.26
7. Davison 59	2-7	0.40	-	340	1.15	14	-	-
8. BASF E	3-5	0.75	-	750	0.43	2.3	1.0	-
9. BASF WF	1-2	0.46	-	370	0.97	10.6	1.0	-
Molecular sieves								
10. Linde 4A	1.6,3.2	0.66	-		-	0.4	1.0	4.19
11. Linde 13X	1.6,3.2	0.61	-		-	1.0	1.0	4.19
12. Davison 513 (4A)	2-5	0.72	1.65		-	0.4	0.96	4.19
13. Davison 542 (13X)	2-5	0.69	-		-	1.0	0.96	4.19
14. Bayer T143 (4A)	1.5-2.5	0.71	1.15		-	0.4	0.92	3.77
15. Bayer W894 (9X)	1-4	0.65	1.05		-	0.9	0.92	3.77

412

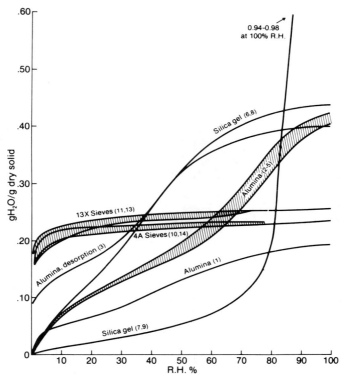

Figure 8-12.   Typical adsorption capacities for removal of water vapor with fresh, activated adsorbents. Numbers refer to Table 8-2. (Basmadjian, 1984). Reprinted with permission from A.S. Mujumdar (Ed.), *Advances in Drying*, Vol. 3. Copyright 1984, Hemisphere Pub. Co.

required. Slow cycles usually have longer adsorbent life and are somewhat simpler to control. The trend has been to shorter cycle periods since major reductions in capital cost can be achieved.

8.6.2. Activated Carbon Solvent Recovery

A modification of the basic system is used for solvent recovery using activated carbon. This has been an extremely common industrial practice since the

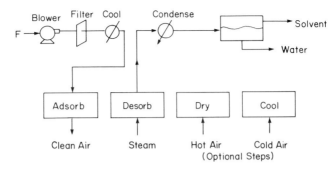

Figure 8-13.   Activated carbon system for solvent recovery using steam desorption.

1920's (e.g. see Mantell, 1950). This is illustrated in Figure 8-13. The air stream containing low amounts of the solvent (from painting, printing, adhesives, coating operations, etc.) is slightly compressed, filtered, cooled to 80 to 90°F and then sent to an activated carbon adsorber. Activated carbon is an excellent adsorbent for a large variety of solvents particularly at the low concentrations encountered in solvent recovery. Concentrations are low since for safety reasons the solvent must usually be kept below 1/4 to 1/2 the lower explosion limit (LEL). Typical values for the LEL of common solvents are (vol %): 3.3; acetone, 2.6; n-butyl alcohol, 1.7; chloroform, non-flammable; ethanol, n-hexane, 1.2; methanol, 6.7; methyl ethyl ketone, 1.9; and toluene, 1.2. The air exhausted is clean. Before breakthrough, the adsorbers are switched and the carbon is regenerated using steam or hot gas. Steam is convenient since condensation of the steam rapidly heats the adsorber, serves as a purge gas, and the steam minimizes fire hazards. The outlet vapor is condensed. If the solvent is immiscible with water the two liquid phases can be separated as shown in Figure 8-13 and the solvent can be reused. The steps to cool and dry the carbon are optional. They are often included since hot activated carbon may catalyze oxidation of the solvent, and water in the bed can interfere with solvent adsorption. Addition of a cooling step usually increases capapcity by about 4%. Usually the MTZ is quite short. Thus shallow (from one to three feet) wide beds can be used. The beds are usually held in horizontal cylindrical vessels. A variety of other adsorber geometries such as cylindrical canisters, pleated cells, flat cells, rotating cylinders and fluidized beds are used (Turk, 1968; Wankat, 1986). Low pressure drop is important since operation of the blower is a major expense. Typical pressure drops are approximately 0.5 inch water per inch of bed. More details are provided by Fulker (1972) and Turk (1968).

Activated carbon is useful for recovering non-reactive solvents with molecular weights in the range of 45 to 200. Lower molecular weight compounds tend to adsorb too weakly, and heavier compounds are difficult to desorb. If traces of heavy compounds are present, a guard bed (a small bed in front of the main bed) is useful to protect the main bed. The guard bed may be periodically replaced instead of trying to regenerate it. If the solvent is miscible or partially miscible with water, distillation is usually used to recover the solvent from water. The distillation system may be more expensive than the adsorbers. Usually, the value of the recovered solvent is expected to pay for the capital and operating costs.

The adsorption step is relatively easy to model. A shock wave results since equilibrium is favorable and very non-linear. The MTZ method can be applied if adjustments for temperature increases are made. Application of the theory to the desorption step requires some modification of the thermal wave velocity to include the latent heat of steam from condensation. The resulting steam wave velocity is (see Problem 8-C5)

$$u_{stm} = \frac{[C_{Pf}(T_a-T_b)+\lambda_w(y_{stm}-y_{w,b})]v}{[1+\frac{\varepsilon_p}{\varepsilon_e}(1-\varepsilon_e)][C_{Pf}(T_a-T_b)+\lambda_w(y_{stm}-y_{w,b})]+\frac{(1-\varepsilon_e)(1-\varepsilon_p)C_{Ps}\rho_s}{\varepsilon_e\rho_f}(T_a-T_b)+\frac{WC_{Pw}}{A_c\rho_f\varepsilon_e}(T_a-T_b)}$$

$$(8-52)$$

$y_{w,b}$ and y_{stm} are the water mole fractions in the vapor before the thermal wave and in the steam, respectively. λ_w is the latent heat of vaporization of water. If steam is not used and there are no condensible vapors, $y_{stm} = y_{w,b} = 0$, and Eq. (8-52) reduces to Eq. (6-36). The condensing steam wave moves considerably slower than the gas velocity v, but considerably faster than a thermal wave calculated from Eq. (6-36).

The diffuse wave which results from desorption is spreadout. Thus it is common to not completely regenerate the bed (as in Figure 8-11). This means that the working capacity is only a fraction of the equilibrium capacity (about 20-33%). For many solvents this gives a working capacity of around 7 to 9 kg of solvent per 100 kg of carbon. This can be used for rough sizing of the adsorber during the feed step. The usual range for steam use is 1 to 5 pounds of steam per pound of adsorbate. Typically, less than 10% of the energy in the steam is used for removal of the adsorbate. About 5% is used for heating the carbon and the steel shell. The rest exits with the hot gas while slow desorption of solvent occurs. A more complete design is usually done using experimental data. Examples of the maximum capacities for different solvents are given in Table 8-3. (Marchello, 1976; Turk 1968). A conservative first estimate of the carbon requirements can be made by assuming the working capacity is 20% of the maximum.

The maximum capacities in Table 8-3 assume that relative humidity of the air is low. The activated carbon does not adsorb water in the same way it adsorbs organic solvents. However, at high relative humidities the water vapor can condense in the capillaries. This condensed water blocks these pores and reduces the capacity of the carbon. As a rough rule of thumb, relative humidities below 50% do not cause problems (Turk, 1968). For higher relative humidities, it may be necessary to partially dry the air by condensation or adsorption, or to operate at a higher temperature where the relative humidity is lower.

Small scale activated carbon solvent recovery adsorbers (less than about 10,000 pounds of carbon) are usually purchased as packaged units. These systems show an economy of scale and become cheaper per pound of carbon as the size increases. In the exponential cost equation for scale-up the exponent is 0.48 (Vatavuk and Neveril, 1983). Larger systems must be custom designed. The exponent becomes 1.20 and there is no economy of scale.

There are many alternatives to steam desorption (Wankat, 1986). All these methods have the advantage of not adding water to the system.

1. Hot gas desorption can be used. This operation will be very similar to the thermal desorption methods discussed previously. The major disadvantage of this approach is that large volumes of hot gas are required to

Table 8-3.   Maximum capacity of activated carbon for various solvents from air at 20°C and 1 atm. (Marchello, 1976; Turk, 1968)

Adsorbate	Maximum Capacity, kg/kg Carbon
Carbon tetrachloride, CCl_4	0.45
Butyric acid, $C_4H_8O_2$	0.35
Amyl acetate, $C_7H_{14}O_2$	0.34
Toluene, C_7H_8	0.29
Putrescene, $C_4H_{12}N_2$	0.25
Skatole,C_9H_9N	0.25
Ethyl mercaptan, C_2H_6S	0.23
Eucalyptole, $C_{10}H_{18}O$	0.23
Ethyl acetate, $C_4H_5O_2$	0.19
Sulfur dioxide, SO_2	0.10
Acetaldehyde, C_2H_4O	0.07
Methyl Chloride, CH_3Cl	0.05
Formaldehyde, HCHO	0.03
Chlorine, Cl_2	0.022
Hydrogen sulfide, H_2S	0.014
Ammonia, NH_3	0.013
Ozone, O_3	decomposes to O_2

transfer the required energy into the adsorber. This method is used commercially when it is important to avoid adding water to the system and in isolated locations where steam is not available. Applications include recovery of easily hydrolyzed esters which react with water and recovery of solvents which form homogeneous azeotropes with water.

2. Vacuum desorption is used commercially for very concentrated gas streams (3 to 50 vol. %) such as the gasoline vapors leaving storage tanks when the tanks are filled. The purpose of pulling a vacuum is to lower the solute partial pressure and thus regenerate the adsorbent. This is shown in Figure 8-14. When the column is evacuated, the non-adsorbed gases are

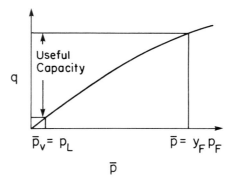

Figure 8-14.   Isotherm illustrating vacuum desorption.

removed first. Thus, $y_{solute} \rightarrow 1.0$ and the partial pressure during evacuation is

$$\bar{p}_{vac} = y_{solute}\, p_{tot,low} \sim p_{tot,low} \qquad (8\text{-}53)$$

whereas $\bar{p}_F = y_F\, p_{tot,F}$. If the feed mole fraction is low, $\bar{p}_F$ will be low. Then the final pressure, $p_{tot,low}$, must be very low in order to have $\bar{p}_{vac} < \bar{p}_F$. The useful capacity (change in amount adsorbed over the cycle) will be quite small. Thus, vacuum desorption in general has been limited to concentrated feeds. For concentrated feeds vacuum desorption can be quite advantageous since the adsorbate can be recovered at quite high purities.

3. An alternative which can be useful for solvents which are difficult to separate from water is to use steam for desorption and then incinerate this waste stream. The incinerator can be used as a boiler to produce the steam required for desorption.

4. The carbon can be regenerated in a kiln. This is commonly used in waste water treatment where high molecular weight organics are adsorbed (e.g. Hutchins, 1979, or Perrin, 1981), but would be unusual in gas treatment.

5. A solvent or supercritical carbon dioxide can be used to extract the adsorbate from the carbon. These methods are currently experimental.

418

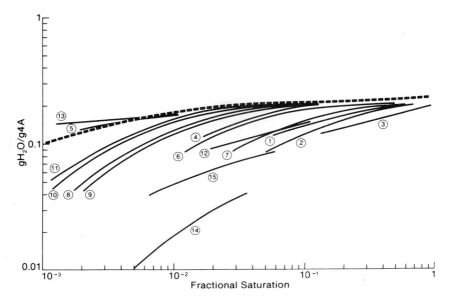

Figure 8-15. Equilibrium isotherms at ambient temperature for water adsorption from organic liquids on 4A molecular sieve. Dotted line is the water vapor isotherm at 25°C. Key: 1. Methylene chloride (1400), 2. Chloroform (970), 3. Carbon tetrachloride (84), 4. Freon 12 (150 at 38°C), 5. Freon 22 (1800 at 38°C), 6. 1,2, dichloroethane (1600), 7. Chlorobenzene (300), 8. Isopropyl alcohol, 9. Acetone, 10. Ethylacetate, 11. Pyridine, 12. Xylene (440), 13. Diethylether (12600), 14. Methyl Alcohol, and 15. Ethanol. Numbers in parenthesis are solubility of water in ppm at 20-25°C. Components not followed with a number are miscible with water (Basmadjian, 1984). Reprinted with permission from A.S. Mujumdar (Ed.), *Advances in Drying*, Vol. 3. Copyright 1984, Hemisphere Pub. Co.

8.6.3. Processing Liquids using Thermal Regeneration

Adsorption is also commonly used for processing liquid streams. Packed beds are used for dilute feeds while simulated moving beds (see Chapter 10) can be used for concentrated systems. Drying of solvents is a major application. Figure 8-15 shows the equilibrum uptake of water on 4A zeolite molecular sieves for a variety of solvents (Basmadjian, 1984). Liquid feed is usually introduced with upwards flow to avoid entrapping gas (Keller, 1982). These systems are regenerated by first draining the column, and then using hot gas with downwards flow to heat the adsorbent. Before the next feed step the bed is normally cooled with gas. Because of vaporization of residual solvent in the bed, energy requirements are relatively high; however, water concentration in the solvents are usually low. Thus the cost per kg of solvent treated is usually modest, and is often cheaper than drying by distillation.

A second application for liquid adsorption is the treatment of drinking water and waste water with activated carbon (For example, see Faust and Aly, 1987). A grade of activated carbon different from that used for gases is commonly used. Parts per million of contaminants can be removed. Since the feed concentrations are low and the equilibrium capacity is high, a very slow moving shock wave results. Thus very long adsorption cycles (several months) can be used. Unfortunately, the mass transfer rates are often very low and the MTZ can be several feet long. Thus long columns or columns-in-series are required. The columns in series idea is illustrated in Figure 8-16. In Figure 8-16a the first column is almost saturated and much of the MTZ is in column 2 which is fresh. Column 3 is unloaded and freshly regenerated carbon is added. In step B the first column has been saturated so the carbon can be removed and fresh carbon can be added. Column 2 is now the lead column while column 3 does the final cleanup. This columns-in-series approach is commonly used whenever the MTZ is long. Stirred tanks are also used (see Chapter 10).

Activated carbon is commonly used for treating drinking water in homes and in bottling plants. In addition to removing traces of impurities, the carbon will remove traces of chlorine. The chlorine does not adsorb but reacts with the carbon,

$$2Cl_2 + 2H_2O + C = CO_2 + 4HCl \tag{8-54}$$

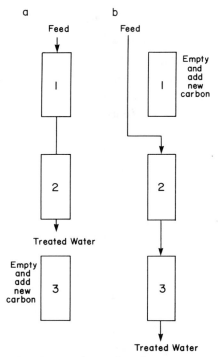

Figure 8-16.   Use of columns in series for waste water treatment with activated carbon.

Note that the product water will be slightly acidic. This is not normally a problem in a bottling plant. In bottling plants fairly pure water is treated and the carbon will last from six months to two years.

In home treatment systems the carbon bed is usually under-the-sink or at the faucet (Anon, 1983). The major problem with home units is homeowners have no way of telling when they are exhausted and may leave the unit onstream too long (see Problem 8-B1).

Another major use of activated carbon is waste water treatment. The compounds removed from waste water are usually in very low concentrations and may have relatively high molecular weights. Examples are chlorinated hydrocarbons, phenol derivatives, and humic acids. It is usually not economical to try and recover these impurities. The usual method of regeneration is to unload the adsorber and send the spent carbon to a kiln (Faust and Aly, 1987; Hutchins, 1979; Perrich, 1981). In the kiln the adsorbed material is burned off the carbon. Naturally, some of the carbon also burns and this carbon must be replenished. Design of systems for wastewater treatment is difficult. There are usually a large number of compounds present, and some of them may be unknown. Also, the feed concentration usually fluctuates considerably. Current design procedure is to use laboratory or pilot plant studies to determine the MTZ under the loading conditions. The MTZ or LUB approach is then used for design. Regeneration conditions are also determined empirically.

8.6.4. Pressure Swing and Vacuum Swing Adsorption

Pressure swing adsorption (PSA) regenerates the column by dropping the pressure and using a portion of the pure product gas as a low pressure purge gas. Vacuum swing adsorption (VSA) regenerates the column at vacuum pressures where the amount adsorbed is quite low. A purge step is often not used in VSA. PSA is illustrated in Figure 8-17a for the simple two-column system known as the Skarstrom cycle (Skarstrom, 1959). When the right column is close to breakthrough, the feed is switched to the left column which has been regenerated. To achieve complete regeneration the volumetric purge-to-feed ratio, γ, must be greater than 1.0. The purge to feed ratio uses volumes calculated at the conditions of each column.

$$\gamma = \frac{V_{Purge}}{V_{Feed}} > 1.0 \text{ , usually } 1.50 > \gamma > 1.05 \tag{8-55}$$

When $\gamma > 1$, a larger volume of gas sweeps through the column during the purge step than during the feed step, and the column is regenerated. The expansion of gas from high pressure, p_H, to the low pressure, p_L, allows the designer to have $\gamma > 1.0$ and still produce product. If the ideal gas law is obeyed the ratio of moles of purge to moles of feed is,

$$\frac{n_{purge}}{n_{feed}} = \frac{p_L}{p_H} \frac{V_{purge}}{V_{feed}} = \gamma \frac{p_L}{p_H} \tag{8-56}$$

Note that the purge can be considered a type of *reflux*.

422

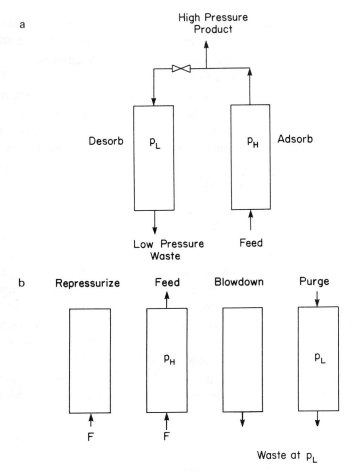

Figure 8-17.   Pressure swing adsorption system. a. Two column system. b. Steps in simple PSA cycle.

Regeneration occurs because of the movement of the solute wave during the purge step. This movement can easily be calculated from Eq. (6-23) or (6-24) for linear systems. The major reason for the movement is the sweeping of a large volume of expanded clean purge gas (high v in Eqs. (6-23) and (6-24)) through the bed. A secondary effect is the reduction of partial pressure when total pressure is reduced (see Figure 8-14).

Each column in Figure 8-17a goes through the four steps shown in Figure 8-17b.

1. Repressurization or compression. Raise pressure from p_L to p_H. Use either feed gas or pure product gas. Use of product gas is advantageous since it provides more reflux.

2. Feed. Adsorb at p_H.

3. Decompression or blowdown. Drop pressure from p_H to p_L. In the simple Skarstrom cycle blowdown is done counter-flow to the feed. A co-flow decompression step can also be used.

4. Purge. Use product gas at p_L to regenerate the column in a counter-flow direction.

The solute movement theory can be used to describe the feed and purge steps which are at constant pressure. The compression and decompression steps require solution of the partial differential equations governing the system. (Chan *et al*, 1981; Ruthven, 1984; Yang, 1987). The theory for linear isotherms shows that the solute wave velocity for the feed and purge steps is given by Eq. (6-24). The waves also move during the repressurization and depressurization steps. The results then look like Figure 8-18. The dotted lines in Figure 8-18 indicate that the exact path is not known when the pressure varies, but the ends of the step are known.

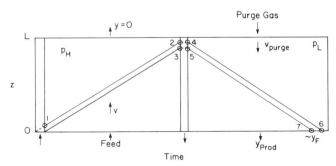

Figure 8-18.   Solute movement theory for PSA. Numbers refer to Example 8-4.

The change in locations of the solute waves during compression and decompression for both PSA and VSA can be determined from,

$$\frac{z_{after}}{z_{before}} = (\frac{P_{after}}{P_{before}})^{-\beta_A} \qquad (8\text{-}57)$$

where the axial distance z must be measured from the closed end of the column and

$$\beta_A = \frac{\varepsilon_e + (1 - \varepsilon_e)\varepsilon_p + (1 - \varepsilon_e)(1 - \varepsilon_p)\rho_s A_{inert}}{\varepsilon_e + (1 - \varepsilon_e)\varepsilon_p + (1 - \varepsilon_e)(1 - \varepsilon_p)\rho_s A_A} \qquad (8\text{-}58a)$$

where the equilibrium is q = Ac. If equilibrium is of the form q = A$\bar{p}$ where $\bar{p}$ is the partial pressure, then

$$\beta_A = \frac{\varepsilon_e + (1-\varepsilon_e)\varepsilon_p + (1-\varepsilon_e)(1-\varepsilon_p)\rho_s\, A_{inert}\, p_{tot}/\bar{\rho}_f}{\varepsilon_e + (1-\varepsilon_e)\varepsilon_p + (1-\varepsilon_e)(1-\varepsilon)\rho_s\, A_A p_{tot}/\bar{\rho}_f} \qquad (8\text{-}58b)$$

where $\bar{\rho}_f$ is the molar density of the gas. If the inert gas does not adsorb, A_{inert} = 0. The term β_A is the ratio of total amount of inert gas which could be stored in the column to the total amount of solute A which could be stored. Compression and decompression steps also change the mole fraction of solute in the gas. This change is,

$$\frac{y_{A,after}}{y_{A,before}} = [\frac{P_{after}}{P_{before}}]^{\beta_A - 1} \qquad (8\text{-}59)$$

The use of these equations and the characteristic diagram is ilustrated in Example 8-4.

In practice the waves are spread by dispersion and slow mass transfer. In usual operating procedures the column is not completely regenerated and only part of the equilibrium capacity can be used. This is illustrated in Figure 8-19. Keeping the mass transfer zone inside the column will make the waste gas more concentrated, and less purge gas is used. The working capacity of the bed

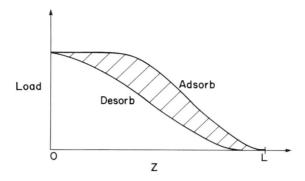

Figure 8-19.   Working capacity in PSA.

is represented by the shaded region in Figure 8-19. The working capacity may be only a few percent of the total capacity of the bed. Very steep, highly favorable isotherms will make the adsorption wave very sharp, but the desorption wave will be very diffuse and spread significantly. The opposite is true for unfavorable isotherms. The optimum isotherm shape will be close to linear. Of course, in most cases the engineer must live with the adsorbents which are readily available.

Pressure swing adsorption systems are used commercially for a variety of gas separations. These include drying air and natural gas, hydrogen purification, separating straight chain hydrocarbons, and purifying nitrogen and oxygen from air. Zeolite molecular sieves, activated alumina, and silica gel are used for drying. Activated carbon or zeolite molecular sieves are used for hydrogen purification while various zeolites are used for the other separations.

A wide variety of PSA and VSA processes are used and are reviewed in detail elsewhere (Ruthven, 1984; Tondeur and Wankat, 1985; Wankat, 1986; Yang, 1987). One and two column systems (Figure 8-17) are commonly used for small-scale applications such as laboratory driers. In larger installations it is very important to have the waste gas as concentrated as possible to avoid loosing product in the waste stream. Multibed systems are used to include pressure equalization steps to recover product gas. A variety of more complex systems using a variety of steps have been developed. In addition to or instead of the 1. repressurization, 2. feed, 3. blowdown, and 4. purge steps, the following steps have been used.

5. *Pressure equalization* involves using the co-current blowdown gas from one column to partially repressurize another column. This step increases the recovery of product, but leads to more complex cycles (Ruthven, 1984; Wankat, 1986; Yang, 1987).

6. *Vacuum regeneration* leads to VSA cycles. VSA would often consist of steps 1, 2, 3 and 6. VSA has the advantages of lower energy use and recovery of a purer adsorbate product. The disadvantages are larger columns with longer operating cycles. Vacuum regeneration is used to obtain both oxygen and nitrogen from air where it has lower operating costs than PSA, but higher capital costs.

7. A high-pressure *rinse* step using a reflux of adsorbate can be useful to remove nonadsorbed gas to produce a purer adsorbate product. This step would normally be done in the same direction as the feed step.

8. Some rapid cycle processes require a *delay* step to allow time for mass transfer.

The designer has a huge number of permutations and combinations of these eight steps to choose from. This allows the designer to use his or her creativity in developing PSA processes.

PSA systems typically operate with gas velocities in the range from 0.01 to 0.5 m/sec. The typical cycle lasts for a few minutes. The adsorber heats up during the feed step and then cools during desorption. For air drying the typical temperature swing is from 2 to 4°C. For more concentrated feeds the temperature swing can be greater than 50°C. Since the cycles are rapid, part or all of the temperature wave stays in the column. Thus part of the energy released during adsorption is stored in the column and is available for desorption. In concentrated systems such as adsorption of nitrogen from air to produce oxygen, the thermal wave will pass out of the column during the feed step, but will

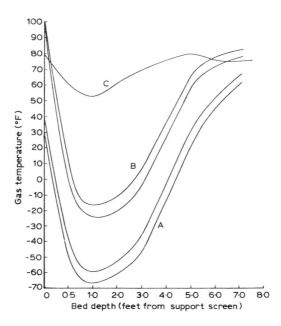

Figure 8-20. Temperature profiles in an industrial-scale zeolite bed for PSA air separation. (A) feed air at 30 and 40°F; (B) feed preheated to 100°F; (C) with heating elements inserted in the beds near the inlet (Collins, 1977).

stay in the column during purge. This occurs because of the reduced gas density during purge. The result is a steady state bed temperature well below ambient. This is illustrated in Figure 8-20 (Collins, 1977).

Example 8-4. PSA solute movement analysis

We wish to remove acetylene from hydrogen gas by pressure swing adsorption. The feed gas is 0.005 mole fraction acetylene. Superficial velocity is 45 cm/sec during the feed step. The column is one meter long. The high pressure is 10 atm while the low pressure is 1 atm. Pick a purge to feed ratio of $\gamma = 1.1$. The cycle is symmetric since a typical 2 column PSA system is used. The cycle is as follows.

Repressurize with feed	0 sec to 2 sec
Feed step at p_H	2 sec to 60 sec
Blowdown	60 sec to 62 sec
Purge at p_L	62 sec to 120 sec

Properties of carbon:	$\rho_s = 2.1$ g/cc,	$K_d = 1.0$
	$\varepsilon_p = 0.336$,	$\varepsilon_e = 0.43$

Equilibrium for acetylene at low partial pressures and 150°F is $q = 35.6$ c where q is gmoles/g adsorbent and c is gmoles/cc fluid. Hydrogen does not adsorb. Use the solute movement theory to predict the outlet mole fraction of acetylene during the purge step (62 sec to 120 sec). What is the minimum column length to have a pure H_2 product?

Solution

A. Define. The four step cycle was shown in Figure 8-17b. We wish to find the outlet concentration profile during the purge step.

B. Explore. The data required for the solute movement theory is presented in the problem statement. We need to trace the movement of solute during the four steps as shown in Figure 8-18. Once the effect of pressurization and depressurization on the acetylene mole fractions has been determined, the outlet concentration profile is easily plotted.

C. Plan. Calculate β_A from Eq. (8-58a). Then the movement of the solute wave during repressurization is found from Eq. (8-57). During the feed step, solute velocity is found from Eq. (6-24) and the net movement of the wave is easily determined. Two solute waves move as shown in Figure 8-18. During blowdown Eq. (8-57) is used for both waves. Solute waves during purge are again calculated using Eq. (6-

24), but velocity must be corrected for the increased purge-to-feed ratio. Finally, Eq. (8-59) is used to calculate the mole fractions.

D. Do It.

$$\beta_A = \frac{\varepsilon_e + (1-\varepsilon_e)\varepsilon_p + (1-\varepsilon_e)(1-\varepsilon_p)\rho_s A_{H_2}}{\varepsilon_e + (1-\varepsilon_e)\varepsilon_p + (1-\varepsilon_e)(1-\varepsilon_p)\rho_s A_A}$$

$$= \frac{0.43 + (0.57)(0.336) + 0}{0.43 + (0.57)(0.336) + (0.57)(0.664)(0.21)(35.6)} = 0.0215$$

The value of β_A is small since A_A is large.

During repressurization Eq. (8-57) is used with z measured from the closed end of the column. Thus $z_{before} = 100$, and

$$z_{after} = 100(10)^{-0.0215} = 95.2$$

which is 4.8 cm from the open end. This is point 1 on Figure 8-18.

Feed step. Interstitial velocity,
$v = v_{super}/\varepsilon_e = 45/0.43 = 104.65$ cm/s. From Eq. (6-24),

$$u_A = \frac{v}{1 + \frac{1-\varepsilon_e}{\varepsilon_e}\varepsilon_p + \frac{1-\varepsilon_e}{\varepsilon_e}(1-\varepsilon_p)\rho_s A_A}$$

$$= \frac{104.65}{1 + \left[\frac{0.57}{0.43}\right](0.336) + \left[\frac{0.57}{0.43}\right](0.664)(2.1)(35.6)} = 1.556 \text{ cm/s}$$

During the 58 seconds of the feed step the acetylene travels

$$(u_A)(58) = 90.24 \text{ cm}$$

Net distance for wave starting at t = 0 is 90.24 + 4.8 = 95.04 cm. This is the minimum column length. Wave starting at t = 2 sec travels to 90.24 cm. These are points 2 and 3 in Figure 8-18.

Blowdown step. Use Eq. (8-57) again measuring z from the closed end of the column. Then to determine point 4 in Figure 8-18,

$$(z_{after})_4 = 4.96 \, (\frac{1}{10})^{-0.215} = 5.21 \text{ cm}$$

which is 94.79 cm from the feed end of column. Calculation of point 5 is similar.

$$(z_{after})_5 = 9.76 \, (\frac{1}{10})^{-0.0215} = 10.32$$

which is 89.68 cm from feed end.

Purge Step. During the purge step the interstitial velocity increases since $\gamma = 1.1$. The new interstitial velocity is,

$$v_{purge} = \gamma v_{feed} = (1.1)(104.65) = 115.1 \text{ cm/sec}$$

The new solute velocity will be

$$u_{A \, purge} = \gamma u_{A \, feed} = (1.1)(1.556) = 1.712 \text{ cm/sec}$$

The breakthrough times (points 6 and 7 on Figure 8-18) are

$$t_6 = \frac{z}{u_A} = \frac{94.789}{1.712} = 55.35 \text{ sec}$$

Total time t_6 is 55.35 + 62 sec = 117.37 sec. For point 7,

$$t_7 = \frac{89.68}{1.712} = 52.38 \text{ sec}$$

Total time t_7 is 52.38 + 62 = 114.38 sec

Concentrations. From 62 to 114.38 sec acetylene has undergone one pressure change from 10 to 1 atmosphere. Since the initial mole fraction was the feed value, Eq. (8-59) gives

$$y_{Prod} = y_{A,after} = y_F(\frac{1}{10})^{-0.9785} = (0.005)(9.517) = 0.0476$$

From 114.38 sec to 117.37 sec the solute wave was first pressurized and then depressurized. These results approximately cancel and $y_{Prod} \sim y_F = 0.005$. This result is not exact because the exact nature of the repressurization and blowdown steps is not known. From 117.37 to 120 sec pure H_2 exits and $y_{Prod} = 0$.

E. Check. Since the exact behavior during repressurization and blowdown are not known, an exact mass balance check is not possible.

F. Generalization. This equilibrium analysis is not complete since the details of the blowdown and repressurization steps are not known. To study these steps in detail would require a detailed study of the gas flow and pressure in the column. The equilibrium analysis also does not include mass transfer and dispersion effects. More complex models are discussed by Ruthven (1984) and Yang (1987). Instead of completely cleaning the bed, we would expect a concentration profile similar to that shown in Figure 8-19. Qualitatively, the results are typical for PSA of dilute gases. The basic equations can be used to study a variety of PSA and VSA cycles.

8.6.5. Regeneration with Purge and Desorbent

In cases where thermal or pressure swing adsorption cycles are inadequate a purge stream (usually not adsorbed) or a desorbent stream (which is a strongly adsorbed component) is used for the regeneration step. This type of operation is common in chromatography (Chapter 7), in ion exchange (Chapter 9), and in simulated moving bed systems (Chapter 10).

432

A common application with gas systems is separating medium molecular weight (C_{10} to C_{20}) straight chain hydrocarbons from branched and cyclic hydrocarbons. The straight chain hydrocarbons can diffuse into 5A zeolite molecular sieves while the branched and cyclic molecules are too large to fit into the cages. Thus the adsorption part of the cycle is simple. Feed is introduced until the straight chain hydrocarbons start to breakthrough. Desorption is more difficult. Once inside the zeolite the linear paraffins are strongly adsorbed even above 350°C. Higher temperatures cannot be used since thermal decomposition becomes excessive. Pressure and vacuum swing operations are useful for the lower molecular weight paraffins ($< C_{10}$), but do not work well for the C_{10} to C_{20} range. The problem with PSA and VSA systems is it is difficult to provide the energy required for desorption during the low pressure purge step.

A variety of commercial purge gas and desorbent processes with different desorption steps have been developed (see Keller, 1982; Ruthven, 1984; Wankat, 1986; Yang, 1987). A general flow sheet is shown in Figure 8-21. In the adsorption step the linear molecules are adsorbed while other molecules are not. In the displace step the non-adsorbed material contained in the external pores is pushed out of the column with desorbent. This step is short. The desorption step is done counter-flow to the feed step. Different commercial processes differ mainly in the desorbent used. For low molecular weight n-paraffins a non-adsorbed gas such as N_2 or H_2 at 600 to 800°F is used. This operation is known as *purge gas stripping*. The mixture of adsorbate and

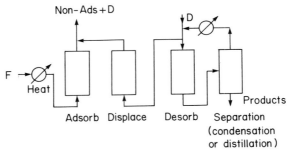

Figure 8-21.   Apparatus for desorption by purge gas stripping or displacement adsorption.

desorbent must then be separated. The separation shown in Figure 8-21 would be done by partial condensation in a device similar to flash distillation. For the harder to desorb C_{10} to C_{20} hydrocarbons a desorbent which is adsorbed is used (this is called *displacement adsorption*). Desorbents have included n-pentane, n-hexane, ammonia and alkylamines. The separation scheme required depends on the desorbent used but is often distillation. Because an additional separation scheme is required, purge gas and desorbent systems are more complicated than PSA or thermal swing. Thus purge gas and desorbent systems are used only when necessary. Distillation will probably be preferred if the relative volatility is greater than 1.2 to 1.3 (Keller, 1982).

In liquid systems a liquid desorbent can be used to extract the adsorbate from the solid. Usually, a solvent which does not adsorb, but has a high affinity for the adsorbate is used. Polymeric resins have been used to recover organics from water (Fox 1979; Fox and Kennedy, 1985; Faust and Aly, 1987) with desorbent regeneration. A variety of flow sheets have been developed for this. One for phenol recovery is shown in Figure 8-22a. Either acetone or methanol is used as a desorbent. The adsorption steps shown in Figure 8-22a consist of adsorption of the waste water feed, then adsorption of water pushed out of column during the start of the desorption, and then *superloading* which is discussed next. The column is desorbed with a solvent such as acetone which essentially pushes the water out in plug flow. Once the acetone and phenol start to breakthrough, the column effluent is sent to a distillation column for separation. The column is reconditioned for the next cycle with a water wash which displaces the weakly adsorbed acetone. The effluent from this step is also sent to the distillation.

The bottoms from the distillation column is an heterogeneous azeotrope which splits into two phases. The phenol phase contains a small amount of water. If necessary, this phenol can be dried with a desiccant. The water phase contains about 10% phenol. What can be done with this very contaminated stream?

The clever answer is to *superload* the adsorption column (Fox, 1979; Fox and Kennedy, 1985). This concept can be understood from the isotherm shown in Figure 8-22b. The resin near the feed inlet is saturated at concentration c_F.

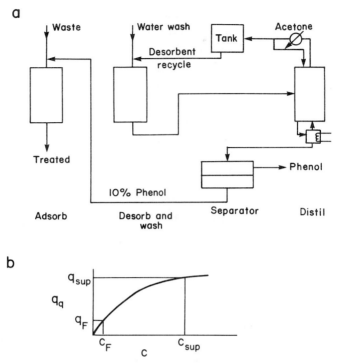

Figure 8-22.   System for phenol recovery using acetone as desorbent. a. Process. b. Isotherm illustrating superloading.

However, since the concentration of the superload stream c_s is much greater than c_F, the resin has considerable capacity remaining to adsorb this stream. This superload capacity is shown in Figure 8-22b. The solute movement theory can be adapted to study the system shown in Figure 8-22a. This is left as Problem 8-C8.

The desorption and purge cycles can produce both a pure non-adsorbed product and a pure strongly adsorbed product. This is a major advantage of these cycles. The major disadvantage of these cycles is they are complex. The processes shown in Figures 8-21 and 8-22a are considerably more complex than the other cycles shown in this chapter. Additional separation devices such as distillation are required.

8.6.6. Systems Without Regeneration

Adsorbents are used in a variety of applications where they are discarded instead of being regenerated. This is economical for some consumer applications, hazardous material adsorption, medical use, and for treating very dilute fluids.

Consumer applications include foods, building materials and water treatment. Very small canisters of a mixture of activated carbon and silica gel are included in some food products such as instant coffees. The carbon will adsorb any objectional organic vapors while the silica gel adsorbs water vapor. Packets of silica gel or zeolites are included with some food products and some consumer goods such as electronics to adsorb moisture. Packets of zeolites are also enclosed in some thermal pane windows to adsorb moisture to prevent fogging. Activated carbon canisters for home water treatment are usually discarded when breakthrough occurs (Anon, 1983).

Adsorbents have been used in the nuclear industry. In these applications the spent adsorbent is often encased in concrete or glass and is then buried. One example of current interest is the adsorption of radon gas by activated carbon. This can be used both for cleanup and for analysis of radon concentrations in buildings. Vermiculite has be used for adsorption of radioactive calcium and strontium from waste water (Wankat, 1986).

Gas masks are another major application of adsorbents where because of the hazardous nature of the adsorbates the adsorbent is not regenerated. Instead, a new canister is used to replace the old canister. Since it is desireable to adsorb a variety of noxious vapors, gas masks are usually designed with series of adsorbents and reactants (e.g. see Mantell, 1950). Gas mask design is obviously an area for experts.

Activated charcoal has a long history of use in medical applications. Two main uses are for treatment of poisoning and digestive tablets. Carbon is also used in animal food to adsorb disease-causing organisms and toxins. Medical applications are discussed in detail by Cooney (1980).

For adsorption of very dilute gases or liquids the use of non-regenerated adsorbents is often attractive even on a large-scale. The non-regenerated sys-

436

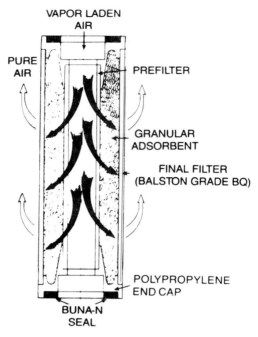

VAPOR LADEN
AIR

PURE
AIR

PREFILTER

GRANULAR
ADSORBENT

FINAL FILTER
(BALSTON GRADE BQ)

POLYPROPYLENE
END CAP

BUNA-N
SEAL

Figure 8-23.   Canister adsorption system used for removal of trace contam-
inants from air. Balston (1986). Reprinted with permission of
Balston, Inc., 703 Massachusetts Ave., Lexington, MA 02173.
Copyright 1986, Balston, Inc.

tem is less expensive since the regeneration facilities and extra plumbing are
not needed. When on-stream life is one or two years, regeneration facilities are
used so seldom that they may not pay for themselves. Non-regenerated adsorption systems are used for removal of trace contaminants from both air and
water, and for removal of traces of solvent with activated carbon. Guard
columns for removal of heavy organics are often designed to have the adsorbent discarded and replaced with fresh adsorbent. As a rule-of-thumb non-
regenerated systems should be considered for concentrations less than 2 ppm.
The adsorbent in a non-regenerated system is often held in a canister or cartridge as shown in Figure 8-23 (Balston, 1986). Additional canisters in parallel

are used for higher flow rates. Canisters are commercially available prepacked with a variety of adsorbents.

8.7. DESIGN CONSIDERATIONS

The packed column system was shown schematically in Figures 6-1 and 8-6. The support and holddown plates need to be sized to prevent movement of the adsorbent. Movement of the adsorbent is likely to cause excessive attrition and adsorbent loss. The support is usually a screen, net or frit. Care should be taken to prevent clogging of the support since this will cause excessive pressure drops.

The distributor should add the feed mixture evenly across the packing. This helps prevent channeling and uneven velocities which will reduce separations. An even withdrawal at the bottom of the column is also desired. The effects of the volume of the piping, distributors etc. was analyzed in Section 8.4.

Both upwards and downwards flow are used. Upward flow may fluidize the particles in the bed causing attrition. Fluidization will not occur if (Ledoux, 1948),

$$\frac{G^2}{\rho_f \, \rho_b \, d_p \, g} < 0.0167 \qquad (8\text{-}60)$$

where G is the mass velocity of the gas in and g is the acceleration due to gravity. Fluidization can also be prevented with a holddown plate. The advantage of upward flow is channeling is probably less of a problem particularly for liquids. Downward flow is useful when a liquid must be drained from the column prior to regeneration.

Pressure drop and particle diameter effects were considered in Section 8.4. Pressure drop is a major consideration particularly in gas systems. Operation of large blowers and compressors is expensive and a maximum pressure drop is often set. Usual design methods have used fairly large particles to keep Δp modest (see Eq. (8-22)). However, small diameter particles have shorter mass transfer zones. When pore diffusion controls, the advantages of both modest pressure drop and short mass transfer zones can be obtained by keeping L/d_p^2 constant. This means short columns packed with small diameter particles with rapid cycling should be used. This is not yet a standard design procedure. Standard design uses particles in the range of 0.1 to 10.0 mm with fairly long columns (a few meters) and long cycles (minutes in PSA to days for thermal cycles).

If Δp, d_p and L are set, then v_{super} can be determined from Eq. (8-22). This allows determination of the appropriate column diameter since v_{super} can also be calculated from the required feed rate, F kg/hr.

$$v_{super} = \frac{F}{A_c \, \rho_f} \qquad (8\text{-}61)$$

This equation allows calculation of A_c and hence diameter.

$$\text{Diameter} = \sqrt{\frac{4}{\pi} \frac{F}{v_{super} \, \rho_f}} = \sqrt{\frac{4}{\pi} \frac{F}{\rho_f} \frac{\mu \, L}{(\Delta p)_{spec} K \, d_p^2}} \qquad (8\text{-}62)$$

Note that feed rate F affects the diameter, but has little effect on column length unless a rule of thumb is used to set the ratio L/Diameter. Usually, two or more columns are used in parallel so that feed can be continuously processed while one column is desorbed.

8.8. SUMMARY - OBJECTIVES

At the end of this chapter you should be able to satisfy the following objectives.

1. Describe the following:

   a. Thermal adsorption systems

   b. PSA

   c. Purge gas stripping

   d. Desorbent Operation

2. Use the linear solute movement theory to explain adsorption separation techniques including:

   a. Trace contaminant removal

   b. PSA

   c. Purge gas stripping

3. Use the nolinear solute movement theory to explain adsorption separation techniques including:

   a. Drying gases

   b. Activated carbon solvent recovery

   c. Activated carbon wastewater treatment

   d. Superloading

4. Use the MTZ-LUB approach to design constant pattern problems.

5. Derive and use constant pattern solutions.

6. Solve displacement chromatography problems using local equilibrium theory with coupled isotherms.

7. Discuss qualitatively:

   a. the optimization of fixed bed systems.

   b. the effect of coupled adsorbates.

   c. the effect of heat of adsorption.

   d. the use of adsorbents in non-regenerated systems.

8. Calculate column diameter and pressure drop, and determine the dimension of systems which will give the same separation, throughput and pressure drop.

REFERENCES

Anon, "Waterfilters," *Consumer Reports, 48* (2), 68 (Feb. 1983).

Aris, R., and N.R. Amundson, *Mathematical Methods in Chemical Engineering,* Vol. 2, *First Order Partial Differential Equations with Applications,* Prentice Hall, Englewood Cliffs, NJ, 1973.

Balston, Inc., Filter Products, Bulletin P-110B, Lexington, MA, 1986.

Basmadjian, D., "The adsorption drying of gases and liquids," in *Advances in Drying,* Vol. 3, Mujumdar, A.S., (Ed.), Hemisphere Pub. Co., Washington, DC, 1984, Chapt. 8.

Basmadjian, D., K.D. Ha, and C.-Y. Pan, "Nonisothermal desorption by gas purge of single solutes in fixed-bed adsorbers. I. Equilibrium theory," *Ind. Eng. Chem., Process Des. Develop., 14,* 328 (1975a).

Basmadjian, D., K.D. Ha, and D.P. Proulx, "Nonisothermal desorption by gas purge of single solutes from fixed bed adsorbers. II. Experimental verification of equilibrium theory," *Ind. Eng. Chem. Process Des Devlop., 14,* 340 (1975b).

Bird, R.B., W.E. Stewart, and E.N. Lightfoot, *Transport Phenomena,* Wiley, NY, 1960, p. 196-200.

Chan, Y.N., F.B. Hill, and Y.W. Wong, "Equilibrium theory of a pressure swing adsorption process," *Chem. Eng. Sci., 36,* 243 (1981).

Collins, J.J., U.S. Patent, 4026, 680 (1977).

Cooney, D.O., *Activated Charcoal: Antidotal and Other Medical Uses,* Marcel Dekker, New York, 1980.

Cooney, D.O. and E.N. Lightfoot, "Existence of asymptotic solutions to fixed-bed separations and exchange equations," *Ind. Eng. Chem. Fundam., 4*, 233 (1965).

Faust, S.D. and O.M. Aly, *Adsorption Processes for Water Treatment*, Butterworths, Boston, 1987.

Fox, C.R., "Removing toxic organics from waste water," *Chem. Eng. Prog. 75*, (8) 70 (1979).

Fox, C.R. and D.C. Kennedy, "Conceptual design of adsorption systems," in *Adsorption Technology*, Slejko, F.L., (Ed.), Marcel Dekker, NY, 1985, 91-165.

Fulker, R.D., "Adsorption" in G. Nonhebel (Ed.), *Processes for Air Pollution Control*, 2nd. ed., CRC Press, Boca Raton, FL, 1972, Chapt. 9.

Garg, D.R. and J.P. Ausikaitis, "Molecular sieve dehydration cycle for high water content streams," *Chem. Eng. Prog.* 79 (4), 60 (1983).

Glueckauf, E., "Contributions to theory of chromatography," *Proc. Roy. Soc. London, A186*, 35 (1946).

Helferrich, F. and G. Klein, *Multicomponent Chromatography*, Marcel Dekker, NY, 1970.

Hutchins, R.A., "Activated-carbon systems for separation of liquids," in P.A. Schweitzer (Ed.), *Handbook of Separation Techniques for Chemical Engineers*, McGraw-Hill, New York, 1979, Section 1.13.

Joshi, S. and J.R. Fair, "Adsorptive drying of toluene," *Ind. Eng. Chem. Rsch*, *27*, 2078 (1988).

Keller, G.E. II, *Adsorption, Gas Absorption and Liquid-Liquid Extraction: Selecting a Process and Conserving Energy*, (Manual 9 in series on Industrial Energy-Conservation, E.P. Gyftopoulos, Editor-in-Chief), MIT Press, Cambridge, MA 1982.

442

Kohl, A. and F. Riesenfeld, *Gas Purification*, 3rd, ed., Gulf Pub. Co., Houston, 1979, Chapter 12.

Ladisch, M.R., M. Voloch, J. Hong, P. Bienkowski, and G.T. Tsao, "Cornmeal adsorber for dehydrating ethanol vapors," *Ind. Eng. Chem. Process Des. Develop., 23,* 437 (1984).

Lapidus, L. and J.B. Rosen, "Experimental investigations of ion exchange mechanisms in fixed beds by means of an asymptotic solution," *Chem. Eng. Prog. Symp. Ser. 50,* (14), 97 (1954).

Leavitt, F.W., "Non-isothermal adsorption in large fixed beds," *Chem. Eng. Prog., 58* (8), 54, (1962).

Ledoux, E., "Avoiding destructive velocity through adsorbent beds," *Chem. Eng.,* 118 (March 1948).

Lee, M.N.Y., "Novel separations with molecular sieves adsorption," in N.N. Li (Ed.), *Recent Developments in Separation Science,* Vol. I, CRC Press, Boca Raton, FL, 1972, 75-112.

Liapis, A.T. and D.W.T. Rippen, "The simulation of binary adsorption in continuous countercurrent operation and a comparison with other operating modes," *AIChE Journal, 25,* 455 (1979).

Lukchis, G.M., "Adsorption systems. Part I: Design by mass transfer-zone concept," *Chem. Eng., 80* (13), 111, (June 11, 1973).

Mantell, C.L., "Adsorption," in J.H. Perry (Ed.), *Chemical Engineer's Handbook,* 3rd ed., McGraw-Hill, NY, 1950, Chapt. 14.

Marchello, J.M., *Control of Air Pollution Sources,* Marcel Dekker, NY, 1976, 232-250.

Marrero, T.R. and E.A. Mason, "Gaseous diffusion coefficients," *J. Phys. Chem. Ref. Data, 1*, 3-118 (1972).

Michaels, A.S., "Simplified method of interpreting kinetic data in fixed bed ion exchange," *Ind. Eng. Chem., 44*, 1922 (1952).

Pan, C.-Y., and D. Basmadjian, "An analysis of adiabatic sorption of single solutes in fixed beds, equilibrium theory," *Chem. Eng. Sci., 26* 45 (1971).

Perrich, J.E. (Ed.), *Activated Carbon Adsorption for Wastewater Treatment*, CRC Press, Boca Raton, FL, 1981.

Perry, R.H., and D.W. Green, (Eds.) *Perry's Chemical Engineers' Handbook*, 6th ed., McGraw-Hill, New York, 1984.

Phillips, M.W., G. Subramanian, and S.M. Cramer, "Theoretical optimization of operating parameters in non-ideal displacement chromatography," *J. Chromatogr., 454*, 1 (1988).

Reid, R.C., J.M. Prausnitz, and T.K. Sherwood, *The Properties of Gases and Liquids*, 3rd ed., McGraw-Hill, New York, 1977.

Rhee, H.-K., "Equilibrium theory of multicomponent chromatography," in *Percolation Processes, Theory and Applications*, A.E. Rodrigues and D. Tondeur (Eds.), Sijthoff and Noordhoff, Alphen aan den Rijn, The Netherlands, 1981, 285-328.

Rhee, H.-K. and N.R. Amundson, "Analysis of multicomponent separation by displacement development," *AIChE Journal, 28*, 423 (1982).

Roz, B., R. Bonmati, G. Hagenbach, P. Valentin, and G. Guiochon, "Practical operation of prep-scale gas chromatogaphic units," *J. Chromatog. Sci., 14*, 367, (1976).

Ruthven, D.M., *Principles of Adsorption & Adsorption Processes*, John Wiley & Sons, New York, 1984.

Sherwood, T.K., R.L. Pigford, and C.R. Wilke, *Mass Transfer*, McGraw-Hill, New York, 1975.

Sircar, S. and R. Kumar, "Adiabatic adsorption of bulk binary gas mixtures: analysis by constant pattern model," *Ind. Eng. Chem. Process Des. Dev., 22,* 271 (1983).

Skarstrom, C.W., "Use of adsorption phenomena in automatic plant-type gas analyzers," *Annals. New York Acad. Sci., 72* (13) 751 (1959).

Sweed, N.H., "Nonisothermal and nonequilibrium fixed bed sorption," in *Percolation Processes, Theory and Applications,* in A.E. Rodrigues and D. Tondeur, (Eds.), Sijthoff and Noordhoff, Alphen aan den Rijn, The Netherlands, 1981, 329-362.

Turk, A., "Source control by gas-solid adsorption and related processes," in A.C. Stern (Ed.), *Air Pollution,* Vol. 3, 2nd ed., Academic Press, New York 1968, 497-519.

Tondeur, D. and P.C. Wankat, "Gas purification by pressure-swing adsorption," *Separ. Purif. Methods, 14,* 157 (1985).

Vatavuk, W.M. and R.B. Neveril, "Part XIV: Costs of carbon adsorbers," *Chem. Eng.,* 131 (Jan. 24, 1983).

Wakao, N., and T. Funazkri, "Effect of fluid dispersion coefficients on particle-to-fluid mass transfer coefficients in packed beds," *Chem. Eng. Sci., 33,* 1375 (1978).

Wankat, P.C., "Cyclic separation techniques," in A.E. Rodrigues, and D. Tondeur (Eds.) *Percolation Processes, Theory and Application,* Sijthoff and Noordhoff, Alphen aan den Rijn, Netherlands, 1981, 443-516.

Wankat, P.C., *Large Scale Adsorption and Chromatography*, CRC Press, Boca Raton, FL, 1986.

Wankat, P.C., "Intensification of sorption processes," *IEC Rsch, 26*, 1579 (1987).

Wankat, P.C. and Y.M. Koo, "Scaling rules for isocratic elution chromatography," *AIChE Journal, 34*, 1006 (1988).

Weyde and Wicke, *Kolloid Z., 90* 156 (1940).

Yang, R.T., *Gas Separation by Adsorption Processes*, Butterworths, Boston, 1987.

HOMEWORK

A. *Discussion Problems*

A1. Explain how feed can be continuously treated in a batch adsorption process by using 2 columns. How would 3 columns be useful?

A2. Explain how each solute movement line in Figure 8-11 is calculated. Sketch the concentration profile (concentration in column versus axial distance) at the end of the feed step and at the end of regeneration.

A3. Sketch the concentration profiles in the columns which are adsorbing in Figure 8-16. Explain why columns in series allows more complete use of the bed.

A4. Explain in your own words how PSA works. Why is temperature often close to constant?

A5. Figures 8-21 and 8-22a show recycle streams. Why might recycle be useful?

A6. Explain in your own words the formation of constant pattern and proportional pattern behavior. Why must the constant pattern wave move at a velocity u_{sh} when v is constant?

A7.　Sketch a co-flow regeneration system for drying a gas. Develop the solute movement diagram for a nonlinear system for co-flow. Compare this with Figures 8-10 and 8-11, and show that counter-flow regeneration requires less energy.

A8.　Explain why a cooling step is often used in drying operations.

A9.　The carbon canisters used on automobiles to prevent evaporative losses of gasoline from the gas tank were developed based on the Skarstrom process. However, pressure is constant. Explain how these canisters work.

A10.　Activated carbon adsorbers for solvent recovery can be regenerated with vacuum instead of steam.

　　a.　Use an equilibrium diagram to explain how this works.

　　b.　Why does this process work best when the feed gas is very concentrated >3%?

　　c.　Systems with vacuum drawn co-flow and counter-flow to the feed have been used commercially. Sketch these two systems discuss the advantages and disadvantages of each.

　　d.　Sometimes a short purge step with hot gas is added to the vacuum purge step. What is the advantage of this? Would co-flow or counter-flow vacuum be advantageous?

These systems are used for treating the gas saturated with gasoline when storage tanks are filled.

A11.　Why is it advantageous to adsorb and then desorb a solvent before incineration instead of just incinerating the feed gas?

A12.　Explain how water can condense in a capillary even though the relative humidity of the air is less than 100%.

A13.　a. Explain the function of superloading.

　　b. The idea of superloading can be generalized. Suppose we have two streams of different composition, but both contain the same solute.

Should the streams be fed separately or mixed together? If fed separately, which stream should be fed first? Explain your answers.

A14. An adsorbent can be included in a muffler to prolong the life of the muffler by preventing corrosion. How does this work? How is the adsorbent regenerated?

A15. Develop your key relations chart for this chapter.

B. *Generation of Alternatives*

B1. Activated carbon is commonly used in water filters for home use. These filters are typically mounted below the sink or on the countertop. Examples of these systems can be seen at a hardware store, a plumbing shop or a Sears store. One major difficulty with these units has been the owner cannot tell when the unit is exhausted (in other words, he can't tell when breakthrough occurs) except by tasting the water. Thus he or she is likely to either discard the cartridge containing the carbon too soon or keep it installed too long. Generate a variety of ways which could be used to cheaply and easily determine when a new cartridge should be installed (see Anon, 1983, for details of these units). Could the homeowner easily regenerate the canister at home?

B2. Your boss has read a copy of this book. He wants to apply the process intensification ideas of reducing particle diameter to an adsorption system for removal of one adsorbate. List all the reasons you can think of why this might be a bad idea. Briefly (1 sentence) explain each reason on your list.

B3. Temperature swings in PSA processes can be 50°C or more for concentrated feeds. This is detrimental. Brainstorm at least five ways to reduce these temperature swings.

C. *Derivations*

C1. Derive Eq. (8-7a) from Eqs. (8-5) and (8-6).

C2. Derive Eq. (8-8b) from Eq. (8-7b).

448

C3. Derive Eq. (8-9) from Eqs. (6-50) and (8-8b).

C4. Develop the constant pattern solution for $\Delta\tau_{MTZ}$ if the Freudlich isotherm, Eq. (6-14), is used with Eqs. (8-9) and (8-8b).

C5. Derive Eq. (8-52). Hint: Treat the steam as a shock and do an energy balance on an element Δz.

C6. Derive Eq. (8-56).

C7. If $u_{th} > u_s$ in drying a gas, show that a cooling step is not required after the regeneration step. Why might a very short cooling step still be desirable before introducing the feed?

C8. Develop the solute movement diagram for superloading. The cycle steps are: 1. feed, 2. superload, 3. counter-flow solvent, and 4. water wash. Equilibrium is shown in Figure 18-22b for steps 1 and 2. Assume solvent is not adsorbed. Assume that adsorption still occurs when solvent is present, but is approximately 1/4 its value from water. Note that the column must be long enough to not breakthrough during both steps 1 and 2.

D. *Single Answer Problems.*

D1. A 0.6 m long laboratory column operates at a superficial velocity of 15 cm/min. A breakthrough curve is measured. The center of the symmetric breakthrough curve is at 57.6 minutes while the width is 8.2 minutes. The laboratory system is designed with minimal extracolumn volume in connecting tubes, valves, detector, etc. The solute is known to follow a Langmuir type isotherm. We wish to operate a system with the same size particles. We want a 90% bed utilization in the unit. Assume pore diffusion controls.

    a. If we operate at the same velocity, how long should the large unit be? What is t_{br}?

    b. If we operate at a superficial velocity of 20 cm/min, how long should the unit be? What is t_{br}?

D2. We are adsorbing anthracene from cyclohexane onto activated alumina.

For a step input from c = 0 to c = 0.012 gmole/L predict L_{MTZ}. Superficial velocity $\varepsilon_e v$ = 25 cm/min. Assume pore diffusion controls. Particles are 0.5 mm in diameter. Use a one porosity model (ε_p = 0).

Data: ε_e = 0.4, $q = \dfrac{22c}{1 + 375c}$, ρ_p = 1.47 kg/L, ρ_f cyclohexane = 0.78 kg/L, K_D = 1.0, D_{mp} = 8.2 x 10^{-7} cm^2/s (this is diffusion inside pores). q is in gmole/kg and c is in gmoles/L. Use Eq. (8-17a).

D3. We have a 100 cm long column packed with 0.1 mm diameter rigid particles. The fluid is water with a viscosity of μ = 1 cp. ε_e = 0.4. Find the superficial velocity for a pressure drop of 100 cm water. Watch your units. This corresponds to SEC with compressible gels.

D4. We have an adequate design using 1.0 mm diameter particles and 75% of the bed is used (L/L_{MTZ} = 2). We wish to increase fractional bed utilization to 85% and reduce pressure drop to 0.9 Δp_{old}. Volumetric flow rate is unchanged. We wish the new length to be 1/2 the old length. What particle diameter is required? What is the required ratio of (D_{new}/D_{old})? Assume pore diffusion controls.

D5. Your boss has decided that the Δp for Example 8-1 will be too high. He wants R_p = 0.75. For the same particle size, same throughput, and the same fractional bed use as Example 8-1, determine D_{new}/D_{old}, L_{new}/L_{bed} and v_{new}/v_{old}.

D6. Repeat Example 8-4 with the following changes in the cycle:
Repressurization is done with pure hydrogen product gas from 0 to 2 secs. (Counterflow to the feed).

Feed Step	2 sec to 63 sec.
Blowdown	63 to 65 sec.
Purge at P_L	65 to 126 sec.

Compare the results with Example 8-4.

D7. A PSA system is being used to remove traces of methane from hydrogen. The feed is 1.1% methane and the remainder is H_2. Feed pressure is 8.9 atm. Column operates at 28.2°C. At this temperature and at low partial pressure equilibrium is linear, $q = 0.6 \bar{p}_{CH_4}$ where q is gmoles CH_4/kg carbon and $\bar{p}_{CH_4}$ is the partial pressure of CH_4 in atmospheres. Hydrogen does not adsorb. We wish to design a simple two bed PSA system to produce 5 nines hydrogen (99.999% pure). Low pressure is 1.1 atm. Use $\gamma = 1.15$. Superficial velocity during the feed step is 50 cm/s. The cycle is symmetric. Repressurization and blowdown both require 5 s. Feed and purge steps are 60 s. Repressurize the column with feed gas.

    a. How long should the column be to prevent breakthrough?

    b. Predict the outlet CH_4 concentration in the waste gas during purge. Carbon Properties: $\rho_s = 2.1$ kg/L, $K_D = 1.0$, $\varepsilon_p = 0.336$, $\varepsilon_e = 0.43$ Assume that the ideal gas law can be used to find $\bar{\rho}_f$. Watch your units in equations for solute velocity.

D8. We are testing the adsorption of unknown pollutants from water onto activated carbon. Superficial velocity in the columns is 12 cm/min.

The following results were obtained.
Col. A. 20 cm long column. $t_{br} = 180$ min, $t_{MTZ} = 200$ min
Col. B. 40 cm long column. $t_{br} = 460$ min, $t_{MTZ} = 200$ min
Both breakthrough curves were symmetric. What is the fractional bed utilization for column B? We want to design a column which will have 90% bed utilization at a superficial velocity of 20 cm/min. Assume that pore diffusion controls. Determine L and t_{br}.

D9. Suppose in Example 8-3 that we want $c_{A,band} = 25$ mM. What value of c_D is required? What are new values of $c_{B,band}$, $t_{A,band}$ and $t_{B,band}$? Other parameters are same values set in statement for Example 8-3.

F. *Problems Requiring Other Resources*

F1. We wish to recover toluene from an air stream using activated carbon. The toluene concentration is 0.30 vol.%. Air flow rate is 50,000 ft^3

STP/min at 90°F. Relative humidity is 10%. We will operate each adsorber for 2 hours for the feed step. Each column will have a 2 ft. bed depth.

Carbon properties: $\rho_B = 515 \text{ kg/m}^3$, $\varepsilon_p = 0.75$, $\varepsilon_e = 0.43$, $C_{ps} = 0.25 \text{ cal/g}°\text{C}$, $K_D = 1.0$

a. Estimate the amount of carbon required for each adsorber. (see Table 8-3).

b. If the superficial velocity of the steam during regeneration is 75 ft/min, estimate the time required for the steam wave to breakthrough. The steam used is saturated steam at one atmosphere.

Chapter 9

ION EXCHANGE

Ion exchange involves the exchange of one ion for another. A common application is water softening where Ca^{+2} and Mg^{+2} ions are removed and replaced by Na^+ ions. Other common applications include water demineralization, sugar refining, hydrometallurgy applications, and a variety of biological separations such as protein fractionation. Ion exchange resins are also used for adsorption, complexations and exclusion separations where ions are not exchanged.

After a short introduction to the basics of ion exchange, we will discuss ion exchange resins and equilibrium. Then ion movement theory and applications will be discussed followed by a brief introduction to mass transfer in ion exchange systems. Finally, design will be briefly considered.

9.1. BASICS OF ION EXCHANGE

For monovalent ion exchange the ion exchange reaction for cations (positive ions) is

$$A^+ + R^-B^+ + X^- = R^-A^+ + B^+ + X^- \qquad (9\text{-}1)$$

In this reaction R^- represent the fixed negatively charged ionic sites on the resin. The oppositely charged ions, A^+ and B^+ are the *counterions* which are exchanging. Ion X^- of the same charge as the fixed group is called the *co-ion*. The co-ions do not appear to enter into the reaction, but in some cases may effect the exchange equilibrium. Equation (9-1) is for *monovalent* ion exchange where all mobile ions have a single charge. An example would be

452

adding KCl to a resin in the Na^+ form. The counterions are K^+ and Na^+ while Cl^- is the co-ion. Anion exchange will be similiar except anions X^- and Y^- will exchange and be counterions while cation A^+ is the co-ion (see Problem 9-A2).

Concentrations in the fluid, c_i, and in the resin, $c_{R,i}$, are usually both measured in equivalents per liter or equivalents/m^3 based on the *total* column volume. Note that some authors use actual resin volume for c_R, and the two definitions will differ by a $(1-\varepsilon_e)$ term.

The total ionic concentration in solution outside the resin is

$$c_T = c_A + c_B \qquad (9-2)$$

while the total concentration of counterions in the resin phase

$$c_{RT} = c_{RA} + c_{RB} \qquad (9-3)$$

Once the resin has been manufactured, the total resin concentration is fixed. This is the concentration of negative charges in Eq. (9-1). Because of the principle of *electroneutrality* (positive and negative charges match), Eq. (9-3) must be satisfied. Thus as counterion B^+ leaves the resin it *must* be replaced or exchanged by another ion, A^+. (Hence the name ion exchange). The total ionic concentration, c_T, can be changed by adding a more concentrated solution to the column. Until this happens Eq. (9-2) must always be satisfied. Increasing the ionic concentration in the feed will cause an *ion wave* in the column. This is a wave where there is a change in the total ionic concentration c_T. After the ion wave, Eq. (9-2) is again satisfied, but with a new value for c_T.

After complete exchange following reaction (9-1), the resin will be entirely in the R^-A^+ form. To regenerate the resin the reaction must be reversed. This can be done by adding a concentrated solution of B^+X^-. Thus a complete ion exchange cycle consists of a *loading* step (A^+ goes on the resin), a *regeneration* step (A^+ removed from the resin), and *wash* step where excess B^+X^- is removed from the column.

For exchange of a *divalent* cation with a monovalent cation the reaction is

$$D^{++} + 2R^-B^+ + 2X^- = R_2^-D^{++} + 2B^+ + 2X^- \qquad (9\text{-}4)$$

Now the divalent ion takes up two fixed sites on the resin. An example is the removal of Ca from water by exchanging it for Na^+. Regeneration can be done with a concentrated NaCl solution.

Equations (9-2) and (9-3) are still valid if c_B and c_{RB} are replaced by c_D and c_{RD}. These equations are valid since the units are in equivalents. In equilibrium equations it will be convenient to define the equivalent fractions of ions in solution

$$x_i = \frac{c_i}{c_T} \qquad (9\text{-}5)$$

and in the resin phase

$$y_i = \frac{c_{Ri}}{c_{RT}} \qquad (9\text{-}6)$$

Note that both equivalent fractions must sum to one.

$$\sum_{i=1}^{C} x_i = 1 , \quad \sum_{i=1}^{C} y_i = 1 \qquad (9\text{-}7)$$

One other interesting phenomena is that the concentration of co-ion, X^-, inside the resin is less than the co-ion concentration outside the resin. This *Donnan exclusion* occurs because the co-ions are repelled by the fixed charges on the resin. The lower c_T, the stronger the Donnan exclusion and the lower the co-ion concentration inside the resin. Donnan exclusion has an important effect on ion exchange cycles. Regeneration is usually done at high concentrations where a significant amount of co-ion is able to diffuse into the resin. When the wash solution where c_T is very low is added, the ionic concentration in solution drops rapidly. The co-ions plus their corresponding counterions are forced out of the resin by the exclusion effect. Thus the effective mass transfer rate during washing is much higher than would be expected.

Non-ionic molecules such as sugars or alcohols have no charge and are not excluded from the resin. Since the co-ion is excluded, the ionic and non-ionic species can be separated by this *ion-exclusion process*. This process is used for sugar purification and does not involve exchange of ions.

9.2. ION-EXCHANGE RESINS

Although different materials are used, the most popular backbone for ion exchange resins is polystyrene. To make the resin insoluble the polystyrene is cross-linked with divinylbenzene (DVB). The greater the percentage of divinylbenzene the less the resin will swell when ions are exchanged, but the resin will be tight and have low mass transfer rates. The range available commercially is from 2 to 12% DVB. A common compromise is to use 8% DVB. The polymer matrix serves to hold the functional side groups which give the resin its fixed charge. By adjusting the chemistry of these functional side groups the behavior of the resin can be changed. This is similar to changing the chemistry of solvents in solvent extraction.

Resin beads are made in two forms: gel and macroporous. The macroporous resins are polymerized in the presence of a third component which is insoluble in the polymer. After removal of the precipitate, large pores remain in the beads. These pores make the inside of the beads more accessible to ions. Macroporous resins can be particularly useful for large ions such as proteins. Unfortunately, the macroporous resins are more expensive, have lower capacity, and are harder to regenerate than gel resins. For both types of beads the external porosity is typically $\varepsilon_e = 0.38$ to .40. Physical properties of gel type resins are given in Table 9-1. Properties of macroporous resins are given by Faust and Aly (1987).

Acidic resins have negative fixed charges and can exchange cations as in Eqs. (9-1) and (9-4). *Basic* resins have positive fixed charges and can exchange anions. Exchangers are also classified as *strong* or *weak*. Strong resins are fully ionized and all the fixed groups are available to exchange counterions. Benzene-sulfonic acid groups on a polystyrene-DVB polymer is the

Table 9-1. Physical Properties of Ion-Exchange Resins. (Miller et al 1984, Vermeulen et al, 1984)

Resin	$\rho_{B,wet}$ (drained) kg/L	% Swelling due to exchange	Max T, °C	pH range	Wet Exchange cap eq/L	Max Flow m/h	Regenerant
Polystyrene -Sulfonic acid							HCl or H_2SO_4 or NaCl
4% DVB	0.75-0.85	10-12	120-	0-14	1.2-1.6	30	
8-10% DVB	0.77-0.87	6-8	150	0-14	1.5-1.9	30	
Polyacrylic acid (gel)	0.70-0.75	20-80	120	4-14	3.3-4.0	20	110% of theory HCl, H_2SO_4
Polystyrene Quaternary Ammonium	0-7	~20	60-80	0-14	1.3-1.5	17	NaOH
Polystyrene -tert-amine (gel)	0.67	8-12	100	0-7	1.8	17	NaOH

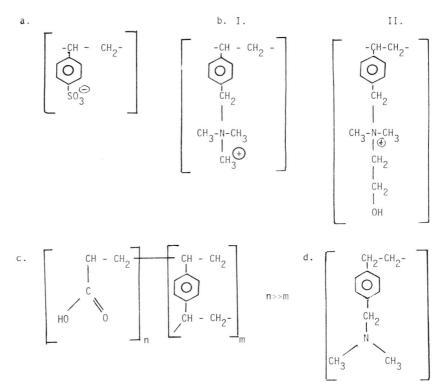

Figure 9-1.   Ion exchange monomers. a. Strong acid. Benzene sulfonic acid. b. Strong base. Quaternary ammonium structures. c. Weak acid. Polyacrylic acid with DVB crosslink. d. Weak base. Tertiary amine on polystyrene.

most common strong acid resin (Figure 9-1a). This is essentially an immobilized sulfuric acid. The commercial resins have dry weight capacities of 5.0 ± 0.1 eq/kg. This corresponds to a typical wet capacity of $c_{RT} = 2.0$ eq/L; although this number will vary as the degree of swelling changes (see Table 9-1). These resins are very stable and can commonly have 20 or more years of service.

The two most common strong base resins are also based on polystyrene-DVB polymers. Now the positively charged fixed groups have a quaternary ammonium structure. Two types are shown in Figure 9-1b. Both of these resins are fully ionized and are essentially equivalent to sodium hydroxide. Typical wet capacities are in the range of $c_{RT} = 1.0$ to 1.4 eq/L. The strong base resins can degrade, and temperatures above 60°C are detrimental particularly at high pH's. See Table 9-1 for other properties.

Weak acid and weak base resins are only partially ionized at most pH's. In effect, this often results in a lower exchange capacity, but makes regeneration easier. Since the weak resins can operate near the stoichiometric requirements of Eqs. (9-1) or (9-4), they require less regenerant than the strong acid and base resins. This can be a major advantage; however, the weak resins are not always applicable.

Weak acid resins are usually copolymers of divinylbenzene and acrylic or methacrylic acid. The polyacrylic acid is shown in Figure 9-1c, and properties are listed in Table 9-1. The weak acid resins have a large number of acid groups which will be partially ionized. These resins can be titrated as shown in Figure 9-2. At low pH's these resins are not useful since the carboxylic acid groups are not ionized and their effective capacities are zero. The weak acid resins have two other disadvantages compared to strong acid resins. These resins swell or contract when ions are exchanged. This swelling can be as high as a 90% increase in volume when H^+ is replaced by the larger Na^+ ion. Swelling can cause excessive pressure drop, resin rupture, and equipment breakage. The resins are chemically stable, but may break from repeated swelling and shrinking cycles. The weak acid resins also are "tight" and ions diffuse slowly. Thus mass transfer resistances inside the resin are high, and the mass transfer zone will tend to be long.

A variety of weak-base resins are commercially available. One type uses the same polystyrene-DVB polymer as strong resins for a backbone, but contains tertiary amine groups (see Figure 9-1d). The amine group can be titrated to give pH curves which are approximately the mirror image of Figure 9-2. The weak base resins are fully ionized at low pH's and not ionized at high pH. The weak base resins can all suffer from oxidation and organic fouling. With a wide variety of resins available, usually one can be found which will be stable under the loading and regeneration conditions.

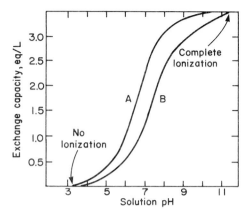

Figure 9-2.   Titration curves for weak acid resins in 0.03M NaCl. A)
Acrylic acid, B) Methacrylic acid. (Anderson, 1979; p. 1-378).
Reprinted with permission from P.A. Schweitzer (Ed)., *Hand-
book of Separation Techniques for Chemical Engineers*, 1979.
Copyright 1979, McGraw-Hill.

A variety of speciality and selective resins are also available for particular applications. (Anderson, 1979; Calmon, 1979; Streat and Cloete, 1987).
Some of these resins have a very high selectivity of one ion because of selective chemical reactions or complexations. Additional details on ion exchange
resins are available in sources such as Anderson (1979); Arden (1968), Calmon
and Gold (1979), Dechow (1989), Dorfner (1972), Helfferich (1962), Kunin
(1960), Naden and Streat (1984), Rodrigues (1986), and Streat and Cloete
(1987).

9.3. BINARY ION EXCHANGE EQUILIBRIUM

For the exchange of monovalent ions shown in Eq. (9-1), the law of mass
action gives an equilibrium constant

$$K = \frac{a_{RA} \, a_B \, a_X}{a_A \, a_{RB} \, a_X} \tag{9-8}$$

460

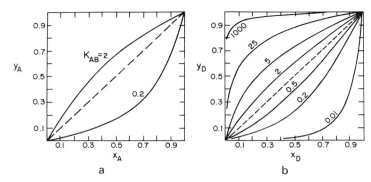

Figure 9-3.   Equilibrium curves for ion exchange. a. Monovalent exchange, Eq. (9-11). b. Divalent-monovalent exchange, Eq. (9-15a). Parameter is $K_{DB} c_{RT}/c_T$

where the a_i are activities. Although this K is a true constant, this equation is not easy to work with since the activities are not known. Activities can be related to concentration by

$$a = \gamma c \qquad (9-9)$$

where γ is the activity coefficient. Substituting Eq. (9-9) into Eq. (9-8), assuming X^- concentrations and activity coefficients are constant and rearranging,

$$K_{AB} = \frac{c_{RA} c_B}{c_A c_{RB}} = \frac{\gamma_A \gamma_{RB}}{\gamma_{RA} \gamma_B} K \qquad (9\text{-}10a)$$

The concentration equilibrium "constant" or *selectivity coefficient*, K_{AB}, will be constant only when the activity coefficients are constant. This is more likely to be true in dilute instead of concentrated solutions.

If we use Eqs. (9-5) and (9-6) the equilibrium can be written in terms of the equivalent fractions of ions, x and y.

$$K_{AB} = \frac{y_A x_B}{y_B x_A} = \frac{y_A (1-x_A)}{(1-y_A) x_A} \qquad (9\text{-}10b)$$

Table 9-2. Approximate Selectivity Constants (Anderson, 1979).

Strong Acid Resins. B = Li^+ 8% DVB				Strong Base Resin. B = Cl^- Medium Moisture			
Ion A	K_{AB}	Ion D	K_{DB}	Ion A	K_{AB}	Ion D	K_{DB}
Li^+	1.0	UO_2^{++}	2.5	OH^- (Type 1)	0.05-0.07	SO_4^{--}	0.15
H^+	1.3	Mg^{++}	3.3	F^-	0.1	CO_3^{--}	0.03
Na^+	2.0	Zn^{++}	3.5	CH_3COO^-	0.2	HPO_4^{--}	0.01
NH_4^+	2.6	Co^{++}	3.7	HCO_3^-	0.4		
K^+	2.9	Cu^{++}	3.8	OH^- (Type II)	0.65		
Rb^+	3.2	Cd^{++}	3.9	BrO_3^-	1.0		
Cs^+	3.3	Ni^{++}	3.9	Cl^-	1.0		
Ag^+	8.5	Mn^{++}	4.1	CN^-	1.3		
		Ca^{++}	5.2	NO_2^-	1.3		
		Sr^{++}	6.5	HSO_4^-	1.6		
		Rb^{++}	9.9	Br^-	3		
		Ba^{++}	11.5	NO_3^-	4		
				I^-	8		

Equation (9-7) for binary exchange was used for the last equality in Eq. (9-10b). Note that K_{AB} is essentially the same definition as a relative volatility or as the separation factor for exchange adsorption (Eq. 6-16). If the activity coefficients are constant, then solving for y_A gives,

$$y_A = \frac{K_{AB}\ x_A}{1 + (K_{AB}-1)x_A} \qquad (9-11)$$

In this form Eq. (9-11) is the same form as the Langmuir isotherm, Eqs. (6-6) and (6-12a). This is an important result. If K_{AB} is constant, theories developed for Langmuir adsorption can be used for binary monovalent ion exchange and vice versa. K_{AB} will be constant for dilute systems where all the $\gamma_i = 1$.

The equilibrium curves for Eq. (9-11) are shown in Figure 9-3a. Approximate values for K_{AB} for both anions and cations are given in Table 9-2.

With weak base resins the resin structure can have a major effect on K_{AB} (Clifford, 1982). Equilibrium data can be checked for fit to Eq. (9-11) as in Eq. (6-12b) and Example 6-1.

For exchange of two monovalent ions

$$K_{CA} = K_{CB}/K_{AB} \tag{9-12}$$

Thus, Table 9-2 can be used to find selectivities for a variety of pairs of ions.

If divalent and monovalent ions are exchanging as in Eq. (9-4) the mass action law gives an equilibrium constant

$$K = \frac{a_{RD} \, a_B^2 \, a_X^2}{a_D \, a_{RB}^2 \, a_X^2} \tag{9-13}$$

If activity coefficients are constant the concentration equilibrium constant, K_{DB}, is

$$K_{DB} = \frac{c_{RD} \, c_B^2}{c_D \, c_{RB}^2} \tag{9-14a}$$

Introducing the equivalent fractions of ions from Eqs. (9-5) and (9-6), we obtain

$$K_{DB} \left(\frac{c_{RT}}{c_T} \right) = \frac{y_D \, x_B^2}{x_D \, y_B^2} \tag{9-14b}$$

Equilibrium now depends on the groups ($K_{DB} \, c_{RT}/c_T$) and will change when the feed concentration is changed. This effect is utilized in water softening and is illustrated in Example 9-2. Substituting in the summation Eqs. (9-7), we have

$$\frac{y_D}{(1-y_D)^2} = (K_{DB} \, c_{RT}/c_T) \frac{x_D}{(1-x_D)^2} \tag{9-15a}$$

or

$$\frac{y_B^2}{1-y_B} = \frac{1}{(K_{DB} \, c_{RT}/c_T)} \frac{x_B^2}{(1-x_B)} \tag{9-15b}$$

Equation (9-15a) is plotted in Figure 9-3b. Note that the curves are symmetric around the y = x axis. These equations are also valid for anion exchange where the charge signs on D, B and R are changed in Eq. (9-4). Note in Figure 9-3b that the shape and relative selectivity can be changed by changing the fluid concentration, c_T. For more accuracy Eqs. (9-15a or b) are easily solved if either x_D or y_D are known (see Example 9-2). A nomograph is also available (Vermeulen et al., 1973).

Approximate values of K_{DB} for strong resins are given in Table 9-2. A large number of mass-action constants are reported by Marcus and Howery (1975), and have been correlated by Vermeulen et al., (1984). For exchange of two divalent ions, E and D,

$$K_{ED} = K_{EB}/K_{DB} \qquad (9\text{-}16a)$$

while for the exchange of a monovalent ion A, and a divalent ion D,

$$K_{DA} = K_{DB}/(K_{AB})^2 \qquad (9\text{-}16b)$$

Thus Table 9-2 can be used to estimate the selectivity for a variety of ion exchange systems.

9.4. ION MOVEMENT THEORY

The solute movement theory developed in Chapter 6 can easily be adapted to binary ion exchange. The most common resins used are gels in which the ions move by diffusion. Because of electroneutrality, there is no volume where ions can sit without being attached to the resin. Thus the development in Eqs. (6-19) to (6-23) is modified to have $\varepsilon_p = 0$ and to use the ion exchange equilibrium in terms of equivalent fractions x and y. The result for any ion is

$$u_{ion} = \frac{v}{1 + \dfrac{1}{\varepsilon_e} \dfrac{c_{RT}}{c_T} \dfrac{\Delta y}{\Delta x} K_E} \qquad (9\text{-}17)$$

where y and x refer to the equivalent fractions of the ion being studied. K_E is an exclusion factor to include the effects of Donnan exclusion and electroneutrality. If the ion is excluded $K_E = 0$ while otherwise $K_E = 1$. For the counterions, A^+, B^+ and D^{++} in Eqs. (9-1) and (9-4), $K_E = 1$. For the co-ions, X^-, K_E is zero at low concentrations. The $(1-\varepsilon_e)$ ρ_s term which appears in the denominator in adsorption calculations (Eq. (6-23)), is not required in ion exchange since c_{RT} is defined in terms of the total volume, and is in equivalents/liter.

Equation (9-17) can represent either shock or diffuse waves. Figure 9-3 shows that when $K_{AB} > 1$ or when $(K_{DB}\,c_{RT}/c_T) > 1$ the equilibrium isotherms have a favorable shape. Then shock waves will result if a solution with low fraction of species A (or D) is displaced by a solution with a high fraction of A (or D). This is exactly the same conditions which give a shock wave for adsorption (see Eq. (6-30) and Example 6-2). For shock waves Eq. (9-17) is

$$u_{sh} = \frac{v}{1 + \dfrac{1}{\varepsilon_e}\,\dfrac{c_{RT}}{c_T}\,K_E\left(\dfrac{y_a - y_b}{x_a - x_b}\right)} \qquad (9\text{-}18)$$

where a refers to after the shock wave and b to before. Both before and after the shock wave liquid and resin are assumed to be in equilibrium.

For a favorable shape isotherm a diffuse wave will result if a solution of high fraction species A (or D) is displaced by a solution of low fraction species A (or D). For the diffuse wave $\Delta y/\Delta x$ is determined from the derivative and Eq. (9-17) becomes,

$$u_s = \frac{v}{1 + \dfrac{1}{\varepsilon_e}\,\dfrac{c_{RT}}{c_T}\,K_E\left(\dfrac{dy}{dx}\right)} \qquad (9\text{-}19)$$

The derivative, dy/dx, can be determined from the appropriate equilibrium equation, such as Eqs. (9-11) or (9-15), or from the slope of the equilibrium curve at the desired x value.

For monovalent ion exchange equilibrium data (y_A vs x_A) does not depend on the total resin capacity, c_{RT}, or the total fluid concentration, c_T. However, both shock and diffuse waves depend on the ratio c_{RT}/c_T. If c_{RT}/c_T is high the resin capacity is large compared to the ionic concentration in the fluid. Waves move slowly since sites on the resin are filled slowly. If c_{RT}/c_T is low, the resin is easily saturated. The waves move quickly in the column. Regeneration usually uses this phenomenon. The ionic concentration of the regenerant may be orders of magnitude higher than the feed concentration. The column will then quickly saturate with the regenerating ion and regeneration is fast.

When the ionic concentration of the liquid is changed, an *ion wave* will pass through the column. A simplified picture of the ion wave is that the resin is already holding all the counterions it can. Counterions can exchange according to Eqs. (9-1) or (9-4), but more equivalents cannot be held up or supplied to the fluid. Thus, for an overall balance the ions are excluded and $K_E = 0$ in Eq. (9-17). The resulting ion wave moves at the interstitial fluid velocity.

$$u_{\text{total ion}} = v \qquad (9\text{-}20)$$

For concentrated solutions this picture is modified since some co-ions can penetrate into the resin. The co-ions take counterions with them. Thus the effective capacity of the resin is greater than c_{RT} and $u_{\text{total ion}} < v$. This effect is usually not large, and will be ignored in our calculations.

For monovalent systems the ion wave does not affect equilibrium, thus $x_{ib} = x_{ia}$ and $y_{ib} = y_{ia}$. The ion wave does change shock and diffuse wave velocities following Eqs. (9-18) and (9-19), respectively. The pattern of shock, diffuse and ion waves for monovalent ion exchange is illustrated in Example 9-1 and in Figure 9-4.

Example 9-1. Ion movement with monovalent ion exchange

We wish to remove K^+ from a liquid using a Duolite C20 (sulfonated polystyrene with 8% DVB - see Figure 9-1a) cation exchange resin at 20°C. The resin is initially in the Na^+ form and will be regenerated with both 0.2 N and 1N NaCl. The initial feed to the column is

0.2N solution with $x_K = 0.70$. The superficial velocity is 5.0 cm/min. A 15 cm laboratory column is used. A pulse of feed is introduced for 15 minutes followed by 5 minutes of 0.2 N NaCl and finally 1.0 N NaCl. Determine the outlet concentration profiles for both K^+ and Na^+.

Solution.

A. Define. The steps of the process are sketched below.

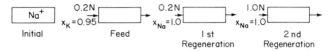

B. Explore. To determine the outlet concentration profile we need to develop the ion movement diagram. This requires calculation of u_{sh}, u_s and $u_{total\ ion}$. Both u_{sh} and u_s require equilibrium data. After the ion wave, both u_{sh} and u_s will change.

C. Plan. The equilibrium data has been measured at 20°C by Bailly and Tondeur (1981). Equilibrium data for a 0.2 N solution was fit very well by a constant equilibrium constant, $K_{KNa} = 1.54$ (Note this is close to the approximate result from Table 9-2. $K_{KNa} = K_{KLi}/K_{NaLi} = 1.45$). We will assume there is no concentration effect on K_{KNa}. Porosity was approximately $\varepsilon_e = 0.4$. The total exchange capacity was 2.38 equivalents/liter.

Since $K_{KNa} > 1.0$ and the bed initially has a zero concentration of K^+, a shock wave will result when the feed is introduced. Equation (9-18) can be used to calculate u_{sh}. For this step $K_E = 1$, $y_{bK} = x_{bK} = 0$, and the fractions after the shock are in equilibrium following Eq. (9-11) with $x_{aK} = x_{Feed} = 0.70$.

The first regeneration is at the same value of c_T so an ion wave is not generated. A diffuse wave following Eq. (9-19) will result. The derivative (dy/dx) comes from Eq. (9-12) and is,

$$\frac{dy_K}{dx_K} = \frac{K_{KNa}}{[1 + (K_{Na}-1)x_K]^2} \qquad (9\text{-}21a)$$

and the resulting diffuse wave velocity is,

$$u_K = \cfrac{v}{1 + \cfrac{1}{\varepsilon_e} \cfrac{c_{RT}}{c_T} K_E \cfrac{K_{KNa}}{[1 + (K_{KNa}-1)x_K]^2}} \qquad (9\text{-}21b)$$

As expected u_K depends on x_K.

The second regeneration step causes an ion wave which follows Eq. (9-20). When this wave intersects the diffuse and shock waves, these waves change since c_T has increased to 1.0 N. The wave slopes are recalculated from Eqs. (9-21b) and (9-18).

D. Do It. Interstitial velocity $v = \dfrac{V_{super}}{\varepsilon_e} = \dfrac{5}{0.4} = 12.5 \ \dfrac{cm}{min}$. Then the shock wave velocity is,

$$u_{sh} = \cfrac{v}{1 + \cfrac{1}{\varepsilon_e} \cfrac{c_{RT}}{c_T} K_E \left(\cfrac{y_a - y_b}{x_a - x_b}\right)}$$

From equilibrium,

$$y_{K,a} = \frac{(x_{K,a})K_{KNa}}{1+(K_{KNa}-1)x_{K,a}} = \frac{(0.7)(1.54)}{1+(1.54-1)0.7} = 0.782$$

Other values are: $\varepsilon_e = 0.4$, $c_{RT} = 2.38$, $c_T = 0.2$, $K_E = 1.0$, $y_{K,b} = x_{K,b} = 0$.

Then $\qquad u_{sh} = \cfrac{12.5}{1 + \cfrac{1}{0.4}\left[\cfrac{2.38}{0.2}\right]\left[\cfrac{0.782-0}{0.7-0}\right]} = 0.365 \ cm/min$

This is plotted on the z vs t diagram in Figure 9-4.

The diffuse wave for the first regeneration step uses Eq. (9-21b) with $\varepsilon_e = 0.4$, $c_{RT} = 2.38$, $c_T = 0.2$, $K_E = 1.0$, and $K_{KNa} = 1.54$.

Thus

$$u_K = \frac{12.5}{1 + \dfrac{45.815}{[1 + 0.54x_K]^2}}$$

Values can be determined for different x_K as shown below.

x_K	u_K ($c_T = 0.2$)	u_K ($c_T = 1.0$) cm/min
0.7	0.497	2.146
0.5	0.424	1.871
0.3	0.358	1.605
0.1	0.296	1.352
0.0	0.267	1.240

This diffuse wave is plotted on Figure 9-4.

The total ion wave is $u_{total\ ion} = v = 12.5$ starting at $t = 20$ minutes. This is plotted on Figure 9-4a. At the intersection points of the total ion wave with the diffuse and shock waves these wave velocities change. Thus we must recalculate u_{sh} with $c_T = 1.0$.

$$u_{sh}(c_T = 1.0) = \frac{12.5}{1 + (\dfrac{1}{0.4})(\dfrac{2.38}{1.0})(\dfrac{0.782-0}{0.7-0})} = 1.635 \text{ cm/min}$$

and the diffuse wave velocity $u_K(c_T = 1.0)$,

$$u_K = \frac{12.5}{1 + \dfrac{8.163}{[1 + 0.54x_K]^2}}$$

The diffuse wave values are given in the table above. These changes in slope are shown in Figure 9-4a.

The solute movement diagram can serve as a guide for the exact calculations. For example, for the shock wave point 1 on Figure 9-4a can be calculated as the point of intersection of shock and ion waves.

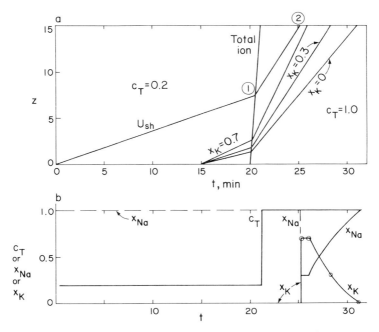

Figure 9-4.   Solute movement and concentration profiles for Example 9-1.
Ion exchange reaction:

$$K^+ + R^-Na^+ + Cl^- \;\rightarrow\; Na^+ + R^- K^+ + Cl^-$$

a. Solute movement diagram. b. Outlet profiles.

That is,

$$u_{sh}(c_T = 0.2)t = u_{total\;ion}(t - 20)$$

or $t = 20.60$ min and $z = u_{total\;ion}(20.6 - 20) = 7.5$ cm. Then point 2 at z
$= L = 15$ is the continuation of the shock wave but at a new value of c_T
and thus a new shock velocity.

$$(15 - 7.5) = u_{sh}(t - 20.60)$$

which gives $t = 25.19$ minutes. Similar calculations can be done for the
diffuse wave at different concentrations.

The outlet concentration and K^+ fractions are plotted in Figure 9-4b. The Na^+ fractions are easily determined from

$$x_{Na} = 1 - x_K$$

E. Check. A basic check is the mass balance on K^+. Does

$$\text{Mass } K_{in} = \text{Mass } K_{out}$$

over the entire cycle? At first, Figure 9-4 may seem to violate this. However, the mass balance

$$(c_{T,in})\,(x_{K,in})\,(t_{in}) = c_{T,out}\,(x_{K,out})\,(t_{out})$$

is satisfied since the outlet total concentration is 5 times the inlet total concentration.

F. Generalization. In general, ion movement and regeneration is faster at higher total fluid concentrations. Thus regeneration is usually done at higher total concentrations. The use of the ion movement diagram as a guide for exact algebraic calculations is generally useful. Of course, the ion movement diagram is then unnecessary, but serves to keep the bookkeeping straight.

Note that both K^+ and Na^+ have shock waves at the same time and have diffuse waves at the same time.

If the column in Example 9-1 were longer, the shock and diffuse waves would intersect. The peak concentration would decrease below $x_F = 0.7$. Also, the shock wave would become curved since x_a and y_a in Eq. (9-18) decrease.

For divalent-monovalent ion exchange following Eq. (9-4), equilibrium depends on c_T. If a divalent ion such as Mg^{++} or Ca^{++} is exchanged for a monovalent ion such as a Na^+, the feed step will usually have $(K_{DB}\,c_{RT}/c_T) > 1.0$. This occurs because c_T is low and K_{DB} is usually > 1.0. Thus, equilibrium is favorable and a shock wave results during the loading step. During the regeneration step a concentrated NaCl solution is used. This greatly increases c_T and now it is possible to have $(K_{DB}\ c_{RT}/c_T) < 1$. Figure 9-3b shows that the isotherm is now unfavorable. Since the divalent ion is being removed with a solution which has a lower fraction x_{Mg} or x_{Ca}, a shock wave again results. This makes regeneration much easier. This behavior is exploited in water softening and will be explored further in Example 9-3.

When the total ion wave passes through the system, a mass balance on a segment of the column shows that $y_{Da} = y_{Db}$. This balance is essentially the same as the balance for thermal waves, Eq. (6-39a), but with $u_{total\ ions} = v$ replacing u_{th} (see Problem 9-C3). Although fractions on the resin are constant, the equivalent fractions in the liquid change since c_T changes. Equations (9-15) can be used to calculate x_D and x_B after the total ion wave passes. These calculations are illustrated in Examples 9-2 and 9-3.

Mass transfer and dispersion have the same qualitative effect on the predicted breakthrough curves for ion exchange as they did for adsorption. Thus the shock waves will be spread out and will form a constant pattern wave as in Figures 8-1 to 8-3. This spreading can be predicted from the mass transfer zone and constant pattern arguments discussed in Chapter 8. For higher values of the particle diffusivity or smaller particles, mass transfer will be more rapid and the breakthrough curve will approach the shock wave shape. For diffuse waves the isotherm shape is usually the controlling effect. Thus the predicted diffuse waves will agree with experimental data except when mass transfer is very slow (for example, with proteins).

The simple theory presented here is not applicable to systems with more than two ions. More complex theories (for example see Helferrich and Klein, 1970; Aris and Amundsen, 1973; or Tondeur and Bailly, 1986) are required since equilibrium depends on the concentration of all ions. These theories are beyond the scope of this book.

Example 9-2. Effect of Total Ion Wave

A 100 cm long bed packed with a strong acid resin is saturated with a feed with $c_T = 0.1$ equivalents/liter. $x_H = 0.4$ and x_{Mg} at 0.6. At $t = 0$

we feed a mixture with $x_H = 0.4$, $x_{Mg} = 0.6$ but $c_T = 0.8$. Superficial velocity is 15 cm/min, $\varepsilon_e = 0.40$, co-ion is Cl^-, $c_{RT} = 2$, and Table 9-2 can be used for selectivities. Determine the effect of this increase in ion concentration.

Solution

An ion wave will pass through the column at velocity

$$u_{ion} = v = v_{super}/\varepsilon_e + 15/0.4 = 37.5 \text{ cm/min}$$

It takes $t_{ion} = L/u_{ion} = 100/37.5 = 2.6667$ min to exit the column. We can do equilibrium calculations to determine the effect of the ion wave. From Eq. (9-16b) and Table 9-2,

$$K_{Mg}H = K_{Mg}Li/(K_{HLi})^2 = 3.1/(1.3)^2 = 1.953$$

Before the wave: $K_{Mg}H \, c_{RT}/c_t = (1.953)\,(2.0)/(0.1) = 39.05$

After: $K_{Mg\,H} \, c_{RT}/c_T = (1.953)\,(2.0)/0.8 = 4.882$

Equation (9-15a) can be used to find y_D before the ion wave. Since $x_D = 0.6$ is known, we can solve for y_D. The result is a quadratic

$$y^2 + b \, y_D + 1 = 0 \tag{9-22a}$$

where

$$b = -\left[2 + \cfrac{1}{\cfrac{K_{DB}}{c_T} \cdot \cfrac{c_{RT} \, x_D}{(1 - x_D)^2}} \right] \tag{9-22b}$$

The solution is

$$y_D = \frac{-b - \sqrt{b^2 - 4}}{2} \tag{9-22c}$$

where we select the minus sign in the quadratic formula since $0 \leq y_D \leq 1$. For this case

$$b = - \left[2 + \frac{1}{(39.05)\,(0.6)/(0.4)^2} \right] = -2.00683$$

and $y_{Mg,b} = 0.9207$

After the ion wave has passed,

$$y_{D,a} = y_{D,b} \tag{9-23}$$

Now $y_{D,a}$ is known and we solve Eq. (9-15a) for $x_{D,a}$. The result is again a quadratic

$$x_D^2 + b' \, x_D + 1 = 0 \tag{9-24a}$$

where

$$b' = - \left[2 + \frac{K_{DB}\, c_{RT}}{c_T} \frac{(1 - y_D)^2}{y_D} \right] \tag{9-24b}$$

and the solution is again given by Eq. (9-22c). Now

$$b' = - \left[2 + (4.882) \frac{(0.0793)^2}{0.9207} \right] = -2.03334$$

Note that the parameter $K_{DB}\, c_{RT}/c_T$ has changed values because of the ion wave. The result from Eq. (9-22c) is $x_{Mg,a} = 0.8333$.

The equivalent fraction of Mg^{++} has increased.

This stream is now pushed out with a feed containing $c_T = 0.8$ and $x_{Mg} = 0.6$. The result will be a diffuse wave. The ion velocity is given by Eq. (9-19) which is

$$u_{D,dif} = \frac{v}{1 + \dfrac{1}{\varepsilon_e} \dfrac{c_{RT}}{c_T} K_E \dfrac{dy_D}{dx_D}} \tag{9-25a}$$

474

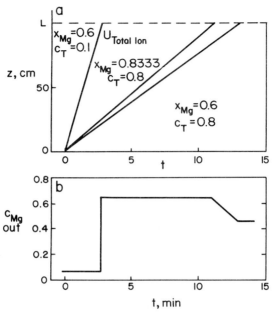

Figure 9-5.   Solution to Example 9-2. a. Ion movement diagram. b. Outlet Mg^+ concentration in equivalents/liter.

We can determine dy_D/dx_D by differentiating Eq. (9-15a). After some algebra, we obtain

$$\frac{dy_D}{dx_D} = \frac{(1-y_D)^3}{1+y_D} \frac{K_{DB} c_{RT}}{c_T} \frac{1+x_D}{(1-x_D)^3} \qquad (9\text{-}25b)$$

When $x_{Mg} = 0.8333$, we know $y_{Mg} = 0.9207$. Then

$$\frac{dy_{Mg}}{dx_{Mg}} (x_{Mg} = 0.8333) = \frac{(1-0.9207)^3}{1+0.9207} (4.882) \frac{1+0.8333}{(1-0.8333)^3} = 0.5017$$

and

$$u_{Mg,dif} = \frac{37.5}{1 + \frac{1}{0.4} \frac{(2)}{(0.8)} (1.0)(0.5017)} = 9.0678$$

Other values are listed in the table.

x_{Mg}	y_{Mg}	$\dfrac{dy_{Mg}}{dx_{Mg}}$	u_{Mg}	$t = L/u_{Mg}$	c_{Mg}
0.8333	0.9207	0.5017	9.0678	11.028 min.	0.6666
0.700	0.85035	0.5567	8.371	11.9455 min.	0.56
0.6000	0.792	0.6128	7.7636	12.881 min.	0.48

The ion-movement diagram and outlet concentration profile are shown in Figure 9-5. Outlet concentration is $c_{Mg} = x_{Mg}\, c_T$.

If c_T after the wave was high enough so that $K_{MgH}\, c_{RT}/c_T < 1$, then a shock wave instead of a diffuse wave would follow the total ion wave. This is illustrated in Example 9-3.

9.5. APPLICATIONS

The most common application of ion exchange is water softening. "Softening" is the removal of "hard" ions such as Ca^{++} or Mg^{++} with "soft" ions such as Na^+. The hard ions have inverse solubility curves; that is, they become less soluble in hot water. When hard water is heated, the calcium and magnesium precipitate out and form a scale. This is not only unsightly it also decreases the heat transfer rate. Hard ions also tend to form a scum with soaps which makes washing clothes, dishes or hands more difficult. When the Ca^{++} and Mg^{++} are exchanged for Na^+, none of these problems occur. However, the removal of Ca^{++} may be detrimental in drinking water since the Ca^{++} seems to decrease the incidence of heart disease (Anon, 1985). Softening is also useful for beet sugar syrups to prevent scaling of pipes and evaporators.

Water softening usually uses a strong acid polystyrene resin with around 8% DVB for cross linking. Packed columns are used and regeneration is done with concentrated salt (NaCl) solutions. The entire process is usually automated. A good idea of this process can be obtained by looking at a home water softener (try the local Sears store or a Sears catalog).

476

Water softeners take advantage of the change in equilibrium for divalent-monovalent exchange when c_T is increased. Both loading and regeneration steps will be operated with shock waves (see Example 9-3). Regeneration is usually done counterflow to the feed direction. Feed flow would usually be downwards while regeneration is done upwards. Regeneration is usually completed in a few hours while the loading step lasts several days. Regeneration is followed by a short wash step to remove excess salt solution from the bed.

Example 9-3. Analysis of Water Softener Cycle.

We wish to soften a water containing 2.0 meq/L Ca^{++} and 9.0 meq/L Na^+ (meq is milliequivalents). Superficial velocity of feed is 10 cm/min. A 2 meter column is used. Regeneration uses 25 wt % NaCl at a superficial velocity of 0.5 cm/min. A strong acid resin with a total wet capacity of $c_{RT} = 2.0$ eq/L and equilibrium parameters given by Table 9-2 should be used. Determine the maximum feed period, the time required for regeneration, and the time required for washing. Also determine the outlet concentration profile during regeneration and wash.

Solution.

A. Define. The process is shown below. Note that counterflow regeneration is chosen.

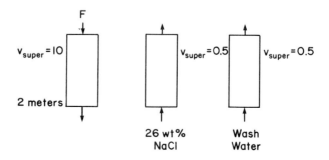

We are to determine the period for each step.

B. Explore. Data is available in Table 9-2; although, we must remember this is only approximate. Several different units are given and must be put into the same units. Since $K_{CaNa}\, c_{RT}/c_T$ probably > 1.0 during the feed, the maximum feed period occurs when the shock wave starts to exit. Thus $t_F = L/u_{sh}$. This does not include the MTZ and thus overpredicts the feed time. The large increase in c_T during regeneration probably makes $(K_{CaNa}\, c_{RT}/c_T) < 1$, and thus a shock wave occurs during regeneration also. The wash step removes excess excluded salt from the bed and; ignoring dispersion, moves at the velocity $u_{total\ ion} = v$.

C. Plan. Preliminary calculations will put all concentrations in units of eq./L.

Feed step. Calculate x_{Ca} in feed. Calculate $K_{CaNa}\, c_{RT}/c_T$ and check if > 1.0. Determine y_{Ca} and u_{sh} from Eq. (9-18) and then $t_F = L/u_{sh}$.

Regeneration. Calculate $(K_{CaNa}\, c_{RT}/c_T)$ and check if < 1.0. Determine effect of ion waves on y_{Ca} and x_{Ca} before u_{sh}. Calculate u_{sh} and $t_F = L/u_{sh}$.

Wash. Calculate $t_{wash} = L/u_{total\ ion}$

Can use following data values. $\varepsilon_e = 0.4$, $K_{CaNa} = (K_{CaLi})/(K_{NaLi})^2 = 1.3$.

D. Do It. For *feed* step $c_T = 2 + 9 = 11$ meq/L $= 11 \times 10^{-3}$ eq/L

$$x_{F,Ca} = 2/11 = 0.1818, \quad x_{F,Na} = 0.8182$$

$$v = v_{super}/\varepsilon_e = 10/0.4 = 25 \text{ cm/min}$$

$$(K_{CaK}\frac{c_{RT}}{c_T}) = (1.3)(\frac{2.0}{11\times10^{-3}}) = 236.4 \text{ which is} \gg 1.0$$

After shock wave $x_{a,Ca} = x_{F,Ca} = 0.1818$

Calculate $y_{Ca^{++}}$ from Eq. (9-15a) or Eq. (9-22)

$$\frac{y_{a,Ca}}{(1-y_{a,Ca})^2} = (K_{CaK}\frac{c_{RT}}{c_T})\frac{x_{a,Ca}}{(1-x_{a,Ca})^2}$$

$$= (236.4)\frac{0.1818}{[1-0.1818]^2} = 64.2$$

Solving for $y_{a,Ca}$ using Eq. (9-22), we obtain $y_{a,Ca} = 0.8827$.

Because of the low concentration of Ca^{++} in the feed and the very high value of $(K_{CaK}\,c_{RT}/c_T)$, the resin contains a much higher fraction of Ca^{++} than the feed.

$$u_{sh} = \frac{v}{1+\dfrac{1}{\varepsilon_e}\dfrac{c_{RT}}{c_T}K_E\dfrac{y_{a,Ca}-y_{b,Ca}}{x_{a,Ca}-x_{b,Ca}}}$$

Before the shock the column is in the sodium form. Thus $y_{b,Ca} = x_{b,Ca} = 0$

$$u_{sh} = \frac{25}{1+\dfrac{(1)\,(2.0)\,(1.0)\,(0.8827)}{(0.4)\,(1.1\times10^{-2)}\,(0.1818)}} = 0.0113 \text{ cm/min}$$

where $K_E = 1.0$ since ions are not excluded. Note the low velocity of the shock wave. This occurs because the resin has a high capacity compared to the liquid concentration, and the resin is selective for Ca^{++}.

$$t_F = \frac{200 \text{ cm}}{0.0113 \text{ cm/min}} = 17,664 \text{ min} = 294.4 \text{ hours}$$

Regeneration: $v = v_{super}/\varepsilon_e = 0.5/.4 = 1.25$ cm/min

To convert 25 wt % to equivalents/L need the density. At 25°C, $\rho_L = 1.194$ g/ml (Perry and Green, 1984, p. 3-83). Pick a basis of 1 liter of solution. Then 1.194 kg solution × 0.25 = 310.4 g NaCl. Since

$MW_{NaCl} = 58.45$, we have $310.4/58.45 = 5.311$ moles which is also 5.311 equivalents. Thus $c_T = 5.311$ equivalents/liter. $x_{Ca,Reg} = 0$ since regenerant is entirely NaCl.

Ratio $K_{CaNa}c_{RT}/c_T = (1.3)(2.0)/(5.311) = 0.49$ which is less than 1.0. Thus, we do get a shock wave when material concentrated in Ca^{++} is removed with regenerant.

The total ion wave moves at velocity $v = 1.25$ cm/min and takes 200 cm/(1.25 cm/min) = 160 min to exit.

When the ion wave passes, $y_{a,Ca} = y_{b,Ca} = 0.8827$, but x_{Ca} changes since c_T has changed. Use Eqs. (9-15a) and (9-24) to calculate $x_{a,Ca}$

$$\frac{x_{a,Ca}}{(1-x_{a,Ca})^2} = \frac{y_{a,Ca}}{(1-y_{a,Ca})^2} \frac{1}{K_{CaNa}\dfrac{c_{RT}}{c_T}} = \frac{0.8827}{(0.1173)^2} \frac{1}{(0.49)} = 130.92$$

We obtain $x_{a,Ca} = 0.9167$ which is a large increase. Before the ion wave, fluid exits with $c_T = 1.1 \times 10^{-2}$ and $x_{b,Ca} = 0.1818$. Immediately after the ion wave fluid exits with $c_T = 5.311$ and $x_{a,Ca} = 0.9167$. This continues until the shock wave when x_{Ca} drops to zero. For the shock wave $y_{b,Ca} = 0.8827$ and $x_{b,Ca} = 0.9167$. After the shock $y_{a,Ca}=x_{a,Ca}=0$.

$$u_{sh} = \cfrac{v}{1 + \cfrac{1}{\varepsilon_e} \cfrac{c_{RT}}{c_T} K_E \left[\cfrac{y_{a,Ca} - y_{b,Ca}}{x_{a,Ca} - x_{b,Ca}}\right]}$$

$$u_{sh} = \cfrac{1.25}{1 + (\cfrac{1}{0.4})(\cfrac{2.0}{5.311})(\cfrac{0-0.8827}{0-0.9167})} = 0.656 \text{ cm/min}$$

This shock wave requires $\dfrac{200 \text{ cm}}{0.656 \text{ cm/min}} = 305.0$ minutes which is 145.0 minutes after the total ion wave exits. Thus solution with $c_T = 5.311$ and $x_{Ca} = 0.9167$ exits for 145.0 minutes.

480

Wash: The wash step has $v = 1.25$. Since the salt contained in the void volume is excluded (the resin is always at capacity), $K_E = 0$ and $u_{wash} = v = 1.25$. (This can also be considered another total ion wave which gives the same result). The wash step requires 160 minutes; however, we can start the wash step so that the wash wave exits shortly after the regeneration shock wave exits. This saves time and regenerant solution.

Summary: Feed step 17,764 min = 294.4 hours
Regeneration 305.0 − 160 minutes = 145.0 minutes = 2.42 hours (see Figure 9-5).
Wash step 160 minutes = 2.667 hours

Total   299.48 hours

$$\% \text{ on stream time} = \frac{294.4}{299.48} \times 100 = 98.3\%$$

The complete solute movement diagram is shown in Figure 9-6.

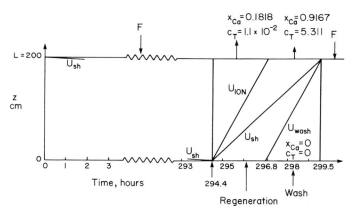

Figure 9-6.   Solute movement diagram for water softener for Example 9-3. Ion exchange reaction:

$$Ca^{++} + 2R^- Na^+ + 2Cl^- \rightarrow 2Na^+ + R_2 Ca^{++} + 2Cl^-$$

E. Check. Since complete regeneration was done, Ca^{++} in should equal Ca^{++} out over a cycle.

During feed: Ca^{++} in $= v_{super} \, A_c \, x_{Ca} \, c_T \, t_F$

$= (10) \, A_C \, (0.1818)(1.1 \times 10^{-2})(17,764) = 355.2 \, A_c$

Ca^{++}out $= v_{super} \, A_c \, [(x_{Ca} \, c_T \, t)_{\text{before total ion wave}}$

$+ \, x_{Ca} \, c_T \, t_{\text{from ion wave to Shock wave}}]$

$= 0.5 \, A_c \, [(0.1818)(1.1 \times 10^{-2})(160) + (0.9167)(5.311)(145.0)] = 353.3 \, A_c$

In = Out within the accuracy of the calculation.

F. Generalization. This example shows a very large increase in both x_{Ca} and c_T when regeneration with a concentrated NaCl solution is used. In addition, the concentrated NaCl solution forms a shock wave which makes regeneration faster and more efficient. Note that the regeneration and wash steps take much less time than the loading step even though the superficial velocity is much lower in the regeneration and wash steps. This large shift in concentration, the speed of regeneration and the formation of shock waves during both feed and regeneration steps are all reasons why water softening has been widely adapted. In addition, the low x_{Ca} and c_T of the feed are very favorable. With higher x_{Ca} and c_T in the feed, the feed shock wave would move faster and the column would load quicker.

Demineralization (or deionization) is also a common industrial ion exchange process. In demineralization the cations are exchanged for H^+ and anions are exchanged for OH^-. The H^+ and OH^- react to form water. Thus, unlike water softening, this process removes ions from the solution. The cation and anion exchange resins are separately regenerated with acid and base. One application of deionization is in the sugar industry where sugar yields can be decreased by first deionizing. A second application is *polishing* (final purification to remove traces of ions) of condensate for high pressure boilers. (e.g. see Streat, 1988)

Demineralization can be done in two beds packed separately with cation and ion exchange resins. However, it is more efficient to use *mixed* beds. A mixed bed contains both anion and cation resins during the feed step. After the feed step is completed, the resins must be separated before regeneration. This can be done by fluidizing the bed with upward water flow. Since different density and size resins are used, the two resins will stratify and can be separated. The ion movement theory plus the MTZ analysis can easily be applied to demineralization systems. Design of the mixed beds requires detailed hydrodynamic data.

Ion exchange is extensively used for recovery of metal ions. This is done both in mining operations and in industrial reprocessing such as plating operations. Examples are recovery of uranium, copper, gold, silver, rare earths, and transuranic elements (for example, see Naden and Streat, 1984 or Streat, 1988). These applications often use moving bed systems which are discussed in Chapter 10.

Ion exchange chromatography is a common separation method in biotechnology (Dechow, 1989; Janson and Helman, 1982; Wankat, 1986). Amino acids, peptides and proteins all have charged groups and can be exchanged on cation or anion exchange resins. Resins with large pores must be used. The operational method for ion exchange chromatography usually uses an *on-off cycle* which was briefly discussed in Chapter 7. In on-off chromatography the equilibrium constant is very large under the feed conditions. Thus, a protein or amino acid which exchanges stays on the resin. There is no migration after an empty site has been found. The off part of the cycle requires changing the conditions so that the protein or amino acid is less attracted to the resin. This can be done by changing either the salt concentration and/or the pH. By using a salt or pH gradient proteins or amino acids can be removed one-by-one. Thus much of the separation may be achieved during the regeneration step. Batch operation in stirred tanks is common since loading can be done in an agitated state which will not clog from particulates (see Chapter 10).

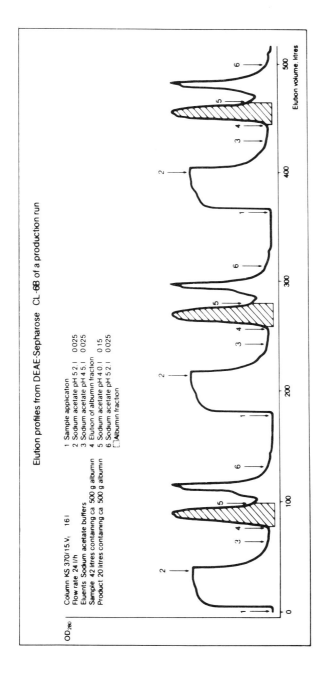

Figure 9-7. Use of ion exchange chromatography for commercial purification of albumin. (Curling *et al.* 1980). By permission of Pharmacia Fine Chemicals AB, Uppsala, Sweden.

An example of the commercial use of ion exchange chromatography for purification of blood plasma proteins is shown in Figure 9-7. Three complete cycles are shown. The first peak (from 1 to 2) is unretained material. After washing the column, the albumin is eluted (4 to 5) by decreasing the pH. The strongly held impurities are removed by further decreasing the pH and increasing the ionic strength. The column is then washed with same buffer solution (#6) as is used for the feed. This prepares the column for the next feed step. The DEAE Sepharose CL-6B is a special cation exchange resin with very large pores (Janson and Hedman, 1982).

The ion movement theory can be applied to on-off chromatography (Wankat, 1986). Shock (constant pattern) waves occur during the loading step. The waves during regeneration depend on the details of the exchange. If the amino acid, peptide or protein has more than one charged group which exchanges, shock waves can also occur during regeneration.

Very large scale applications of ion exchange may not use packed bed systems. In these cases the moving bed systems discussed in Chapter 10 are used.

9.6. APPLICATIONS WITHOUT EXCHANGE: ION EXCLUSION

Ion exchange resins are also used for separations where ion exchange does *not* occur. For example, (the polystyrene-DVB resins will adsorb many organic compounds from water. Macroporous resins are normally used. These adsorption applications were covered in Section 8.6.5.

A second non-exchange application is to separate using *ion exclusion* (Neuman *et al*, 1987; Wheaton and Bauman, 1953). This is illustrated in Figure 9-8 for the separation of sugar (glucose) from sulfuric acid (Neuman *et al*, 1987). Non-charged molecules such as sugars can penetrate into the resin since they are not excluded. Co-ions such as SO_4^{-2} will be excluded from a cation resin by Donnan exclusion effects. If a cation exchange resin in the H^+ from is used, the non-charged sugar molecules have a larger volume available to them than the SO_4^{-2}. Because of electroneutrality, the H^+ must migrate with the

SO_4^{-2}. The result is a chromatographic separation similar to SEC, but the mechanism for separation is different. Note that the sulfuric acid exits first. Ion exclusion is used for separating sugars from salts and acids, separating glycerol from salts, and purification of ethylene glycol by removing salts.

The non-charged (NC) molecules will have a velocity given by

$$u_{NC} = \frac{v}{1 + \dfrac{1}{\varepsilon_e} \, \chi \, K_{d,NC}} \qquad (9\text{-}26a)$$

where χ is the volumetric fraction of the swelled resin taken up by water, and $K_{d,NC}$ is fraction of the volume available to the non-charged molecules. Note that at high concentrations χ and $K_{d,NC}$ will be a function of the ionic concentration. The factor ($\chi \, K_{d,NC}$) can be treated as a distribution coefficient which needs to be determined experimentally. At low concentrations the co-ions are excluded by the Donnan exclusion effect and stay in the external void fraction ε_e.

$$u_{co-ion} = v \qquad (9\text{-}26b)$$

Obviously, the co-ions move faster and can be separated from the non-charged molecules. Because of electroneutrality, a counterion must move with the excluded co-ions.

An example of ion exclusion chromatography is shown in Figure 9-8 where sulfuric acid is separated from glucose (Neuman et al., 1987). The strong cation exchange resin had $\varepsilon_e = 0.40$ and $\chi = 0.766$ in pure water and $\chi = 0.701$ in 0.82 M sulfuric acid. In pure water $u_{NC} = 0.47v$ and separation is relatively easy. As the sample size increases, the local value of c_T increases and Donnan exclusion becomes less effective. Thus, as illustrated in Figure 9-8, the separation deteriorates considerably with larger feed volumes.

Ion exclusion at low concentrations is essentially a linear system with a resin concentration given by,

$$c_R = K_{d,NC} \, \chi \qquad (9\text{-}27a)$$

486

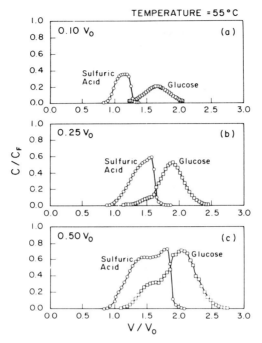

Figure 9-8.   Ion exclusion chromatography separation of sulfuric acid and glucose. V_o = void volume = $\varepsilon_e \, V_{col}$. a. $V_F = 0.10 \, \varepsilon_e \, V_{col}$. b. $V_F = 0.25 \, \varepsilon_e \, V_{col}$. c. $V_F = 0.50 \, \varepsilon_e \, V_{col}$. (Neuman et al., 1987). Reprinted with permission from *Reactive Polymers*, 5, 55 (1987). Copyright 1987, Elsevier.

Thus, at low concentrations the local equilibrium dispersion model, Eqs. (7-12) and (7-13) can fit the outlet concentration profiles. To do this we modify $\overline{V}$ from Eq. (7-12c) to

$$\overline{V} = (A_c z) \left[\varepsilon_e + K_{d,NC} \, \chi \right] \tag{9-27b}$$

The $(1-\varepsilon_e)$ term in Eq. (7-12c) disappears since c_R is based on total bed volume. Equations (7-12a), (7-12b) and (7-13) are unchanged. Superposition principles are valid and the equations for differential pulses (Eqs. (7-15) and

(7-16a,b)) are valid. For small pulses and hence low concentrations this dispersion model fit the glucose data shown in Figure 9-8a (Neuman *et al*, 1987). For larger pulses (higher concentrations in the column) $\chi\, K_{d,NC}$ varies and the model did not fit as well. This model is applied to ion exclusion in Problem 9-D8. With appropriate data Rosen's model (Section 7.8) can also be used to model ion exclusion at low concentrations.

9.7. MASS TRANSFER IN ION EXCHANGE SYSTEMS

Mass transfer in ion exchange systems is considerably more complex than in adsorption. The flux due to electrical transference is (Helferrich, 1962)

$$J_{i\,elec} = -u_i\, z_i\, c_i\, \nabla\phi \qquad (9\text{-}28)$$

where ϕ is the induced electrical potential, c_i is the concentration in moles/liter, z_i the electrical valence and u_i the ionic mobility. For ideal solutions the mobility can be determined as

$$u_i = \frac{D_i\, F}{RT} \qquad (9\text{-}29)$$

where F is Faraday's constant. Equation (9-29) is also valid inside the ion exchange resin.

The net flux is the sum of diffusional flux and the electrical transference flux.

$$J_i = J_{i\,dif} + J_{i\,elec} = -D_i\left(\nabla c_i + z_i c_i \frac{F}{RT}\nabla\phi\right) \qquad (9\text{-}30)$$

This is known as the Nernst-Planck equation. Equation (9-30) is solved along with the condition of electroneutrality,

$$z_A c_A + z_B c_B = \text{constant} \qquad (9\text{-}31)$$

and the condition of no current flow (equal fluxes of equivalents)

$$z_A J_A + z_B J_B = 0 \qquad (9\text{-}32)$$

Even very small deviations from electroneutrality will produce strong electrical fields. If one counterion diffuses faster than the other counterion, the excess flux produces an electrical field. This field slows down the faster counterion and speeds up the slower counterion. The net result is the two fluxes (in equivalents) will be equal, and Eq. (9-32) is satisfied.

Combining Eqs. (9-30) to (9-32) and removing ϕ, the result is

$$J_A = - \left[\frac{D_A D_B (z_A^2 c_A + z_B^2 c_B)}{z_A^2 c_A D_A + z_B^2 c_B D_B} \right] \nabla c_A \qquad (9\text{-}33)$$

This can be considered as

$$J_A = - D_{eff} \nabla c_A \qquad (9\text{-}34)$$

where the effective diffusivity is given by the term in brackets in Eq. (9-33). Note that the effective diffusivity is concentration dependent. If $c_A \ll c_B$ then $D_{eff} = D_A$ while if $c_B \ll c_A$, $D_{eff} = D_B$. Thus the ion of *lowest* concentration controls the transfer.

As the ionic mobilities or diffusivities approach each other there is less effect of the electrical field. If the diffusivities are equal, then $D_{eff} = D_A = D_B$. Typical diffusion constants in gel type resins are on the order of 10^{-7} cm^2/s Some values are given by Vermeulen et al, (1984). For small concentration changes the effective diffusivity will be approximately constant.

In solutions for packed beds we often use a lumped parameter expression such as Eq. (6-50) instead of solving the diffusion equation for the particles. If the effective diffusivity is approximately constant, k_m will be constant and Eq. (6-50) can be applied to ion exchange. In this case the solutions obtained for adsorption in Chapter 8 also apply to ion exchange. The value of k_m needs to be calculated from Eq. (8-19a) with k_f determined from Eqs. (8-15) or (8-16) and k_{pore} from Eq. (8-17a). For ion exchange D_{mp} in Eq. (8-17a) is replaced by D_{eff} from Eqs. (9-33) and (9-34).

If the effective diffusivity is not constant, then k_m will be concentration dependent. Unfortunately, this is often the case. For instance, if an ion exchanger is exchanging ions with different diffusivities, the rates (or k_m values) for loading and elution will be different. Exchange rates are faster when the faster species is initially on the resin (Helferrich, 1962). Theoretical methods for these cases are beyond the scope of this book.

9.8. EQUIPMENT DESIGN CONSIDERATIONS

The design of packed bed ion exchange columns is similar to that of adsorption columns, except the large volume changes which may occur must be designed for (see Table 9-1). The simplest way to allow for expansion and contraction is to leave free space above the packing. When the resin swells, it moves up to occupy the free space. For easy separations such as water softening this approach works well and is inexpensive. The extra mixing which occurs in the free space and because of resin movement is relatively unimportant. The free space can either have a *water* or an *air dome* (Anderson, 1979). Water dome operation is simpler, but involves more mixing. Some free space is also useful for backwashing the column. If the feed step is done with downward flow, the column will fluidize when backwashed. This is useful for removing suspended solids and other crud which will tend to clog the column.

Distribution is very important to prevent channeling, and to minimize dilution. If the feed mixture is denser than the wash liquid, downard flow of the feed with a water dome works well. The denser feed will flow from the distribution pipes and layer directly above the resin. There will be minimal mixing of the feed with the liquid in the water dome. The distributors should be 1 to 2 inches above the resin when the resin is fully expanded. Feeds which are less dense than the wash liquid will mix with the liquid in water dome operation causing significant dilution. Air dome operation is used to minimize dilution. In an air dome the liquid layer is kept 1 to 2 inches above the resin layer. This requires continual adjustment since the resin bed moves up and down. Since it is much simpler to operate, water dome operation is more common.

For more difficult separations a free space may be detrimental. The column expansion of the resin can be accommodated for with floating heads or with balloons (Dorfner, 1972).

Typical beds are from 1 to 3 meters long although special short beds a few cm long using fine mesh resins are available (Eco-Tech, 1983-84; Brown and Fletcher, 1988). The wider the bed the more important fluid distribution is. Once resin swelling has been designed for, scale-up is straightforward. The period of cycles may have to be greater than some minimum time such as 20 minutes to allow the resin time to swell and shrink during the cycle. Since the heat effects balance in an exchange reaction, large systems can be designed directly from laboratory data. If care is taken to have good liquid distribution, the large scale system will often preform better than the lab unit.

For chromatographic separations of biologicals large volume changes are usually not observed. Resins with large pores (~ 1000 $\overset{\circ}{A}$ for proteins) are required. These resins are often compressible and special designs are used (Janson and Hedman, 1982).

9.9. SUMMARY - OBJECTIVES

At the end of this chapter you should be able to meet the following objectives.

1. Define the terms used in ion exchange.

2. Derive the equilibrium expressions from the mass action law. Explain the difference in equilibrium between monovalent exchange and divalent - monovalent exchange.

3. Use ion movement theory for binary ion exchange. Determine the effects of changing total ion concentration.

4. Describe and use ion movement theory for the following processes:

   a. Water softening

   b. Demineralization

   c. On-off ion exchange chromatography

5. Use both ion movement and dispersion models for ion exclusion.

6. Discuss the effect of electrical fields on mass transfer. Apply the solutions of Chapter 8 to ion exchange when the effective diffusivity is constant.

REFERENCES

Anderson, R.E., "Ion-exchange separations" P.A. Schweitzer (Ed.), in *Handbook of Separation Techniques for Chemical Engineers*, McGraw-Hill, NY, 1979, Section 1.12.

Anon., "Hard water may lower heart disease risk," *Chem. Eng. News*, 30, (Sept. 24, 1985).

Arden, T.V., *Water Purification by Ion Exchange*, Plenum, New York, 1968.

Aris, R. and N.R. Amundson, *Mathematical Methods in Chemical Engineering Vol. 2, First Order Partial Differential Equations with Applications*, Prentice Hall, Englewood Cliffs, NJ, 1973.

Bailly, M. and D. Tondeur, "Two-way chromatography. Flow reversal in non-linear preparative liquid chromatography", *Chem. Eng. Sci., 36*, 455 (1981).

Brown, C.J. and C.J. Fletcher, "The Recoflo short bed ion exchange process," in M. Streat (Ed.), *Ion Exchange for Industry*, Ellis Horwood Ltd., Chichester, England, 1988, 392-403.

Calmon, C. and H. Gold, (Eds.), *Ion Exchange for Pollution Control*, CRC Press, Boca Raton, FL, 1979.

Calmon, C., "Specific ion exchangers" in C. Calmon and H. Gold (Eds.), *Ion-Exchange for Pollution Control*, Vol. II, CRC Press, Boca Raton, Florida, 1979, 151.

Clifford, D., "Multicomponent ion-exchange calculations for selected ion separations," *Ind. Eng. Chem. Fundam.*, *21*, 141 (1982).

Curling, J.M., J.H. Gerglof, S. Ericksson, and J.M. Cooney, "Large scale production of human albumin by an all-solution chromatographic process", Joint meeting of the 18th Congress of the International Society of Heamatology and the 16th Congress of the International Society of Blood Transfusion, Montreal, Quebec, Canada, Aug. 16-22, 1980.

Dechow, F.J., *Separation and Purification Techniques in Biotechnology*, Noyes, Park Ridge, N.J., 1989.

Dorfner, K., *Ion Exchangers, Principles and Applications*, Ann Arbor Sci. Pub., Ann Arbor, MI, 1972.

Eco-Tec, Ltd., "Eco-Tec ion exchange systems", 1983 and "Recoflo - A break through in water deionization systems," 1984, 925 Brock Rd. South, Pickering (Toronto), Ontario, Canada, L1W 2X9.

Faust, S.D. and O.M. Aly, *Adsorption Processes for Water Treatment*, Butterworths, Boston, 1987, Chapt. 10.

Helfferich, F., *Ion Exchange*, McGraw-Hill, NY, 1962.

Helfferich, F. and G. Klein, *Multicomponent Chromatography*, Marcel Dekker, NY, 1970.

Janson, J.-C. and P. Hedman, "Large scale chromatography of proteins," in A. Fiechter (Ed.), *Advances in Biochemical Engineering*, Vol. 125, *Chromatography*, Springer-Verlag, Berlin, 1982, 43-99.

Kunin, R., *Elements of Ion Exchange*, Reinhold, NY, 1960.

Marcus, and Howery, *Ion Exchange Equilibrium Constants*, Butterworth, London, 1975.

Miller, S.A., J.D. Darji, and A.W. Michalson, "Liquid-solid systems - ion exchange and adsorption equipment," in R.H. Perry and D. Green (Eds.), *Perry's Chemical Engineer's Handbook*, 6th ed., McGraw-Hill, New York, 1984, 19-40 to 19-48.

Naden, D. and M. Streat, (Eds.), *Ion Exchange Technology*, Ellis Horwood Ltd., Chichester, England, 1984, 563-578.

Neuman, R.P., S.R. Rudge, and M.R. Ladisch, "Sulfuric acid-sugar separation by ion exclusion," *Reactive Polymers, 5*, 55 (1987).

Rodrigues, A. (Ed.), *Ion Exchange: Science and Technology*, Martinus Nijhoff Publishers BV, Dordrecht, The Netherlands, 1986.

Sherwood, T.K., R.L. Pigford, and C.R. Wilke, *Mass Transfer*, McGraw-Hill, NY, 1975, Chapt. 10.

Streat, M. (Ed.)., *Ion Exchange for Industry*, Ellis Horwood, Chichester, England, 1988.

Streat, M. and F.L.D. Cloete, "Ion exchange," in R. Rousseau (Ed.), *Handbook of Separation Process Technology*, Wiley, New York, 1987, Chapt., 13.

Tondeur, D. and M. Bailly, "Design methods for ion exchange processes based on the equilibrium theory," in A. Rodrigues (Ed.)., *Ion Exchange: Science and Technology*, Martinus Nijhoff Publishers BV, Dordrecht, The Netherlands. 1986, 147-198.

Vermeulen, T., G. Klein, and N.K. Hiester, "Adsorption and ion exchange," in R.H.Perry and C.H. Chilton, (Eds.), *Chemical Engineer's Handbook*, 5th ed., McGraw-Hill, NY, 1973, Section 16.

Vermeulen, T., M.D. LeVan, N.K. Hiester, and G. Klein, "Adsorption and ion exchange," in R.H. Perry and D. Green (Eds.), *Perry's Chemical Engineer's Handbook*, 6th ed., McGraw-Hill, NY, 1984, Section 16.

Wankat, P.C., *Large-Scale Adsorption and Chromatography*, CRC Press, Boca Raton, FL, 1986.

Wheaton, R.M. and W.C. Bauman, "Ion exclusion. A unit operation utilizing ion exchange materials," *Ind. Eng. Chem.*, *45*, 228 (1953).

HOMEWORK

A. *Discussion Problems*

A1. As in any field, ion exchange has its own jargon. Define the following terms.

  a) counter-ion
  b) co-ion
  c) electroneutrality
  d) Donnan exclusion
  e) cation
  f) anion
  g) strong and weak exchangers
  h) selectivity coefficient
  i) water softening
  j) demineralization
  k) mixed beds
  l) water dome and air dome operations
  m) ion exclusion
  n) effective diffusivity

A2. Write the reactions analogous to Eqs. (9-1) and (9-4) for anion exchange.

A3. Table 9-2 gives K_{AB} and K_{DB} with selectivities compared to Li^+ and Cl^-. Explain how to determine selectivities with respect to other cations or anions. For example, what is K_{DB} for $Ca^{++} - Na^+$?

A4. In Example 9-1 and Figure 9-4 the shock and diffuse waves will intersect if the column were longer. What happens to the peak concentration when this occurs? If the column is *very* long what is the ultimate peak shape?

A5.   Why must cation and anion exchange resins in a mixed bed be separated before regeneration?

A6.   The equilibrium expressions for monovalent-monovalent, and divalent-monovalent exchange were derived. What does the equilibrium expression for divalent-divalent exchange look like?

A7.   In binary ion exchange if one ion has a diffuse wave the other ion must also have a diffuse wave. The same is true for shock waves. Explain why this is true.

A8.   Explain the differences between size exclusion chromatography and ion exclusion chromatography.

A9.   Develop your key relations chart for this chapter.

C.   *Derivations*

C1.   Equilibrium expressions for monovalent ion exchange and for divalent ion exchange are derived in the text. Derive the equilibrium equation corresponding to Eqs. (9-11) and (9-15a) for trivalent-monovalent ion exchange with the following reaction:

$$T^{+++} + 3R^-B^+ + 3X^- = R_3^-T^{+++} + 3B^+ + 3X^-$$

C2.   Derive Eq. (9-17).

C3.   Derive the result that $y_{D,a} = y_{D,b}$ when a total ion wave passes through a column undergoing divalent-monovalent exchange.

C4.   For divalent-divalent ion exchange show that the equilibrium expression is the same as for monovalent-monovalent ion exchange (that is Eq. (9-11)) if K_{AB} is constant.

C5. For divalent-monovalent exchange show that Eq. (9-16b) is correct.

C6. Derive the equilibrium expression for the general ion exchange reaction,

$$mN^{m+} + nR_m^- B^{m+} + mnX^- = MR_n^- + nB^{m+} + mnX^-$$

where m and n are positive integers.

D. *Single Answer Problems*

D1. A strong base (Type II) ion exchange resin has a resin capacity of C_{RT} = 1.2 eq/L. The total ionic concentration of the solution is 2.0 eq/L. Generate the equilibrium curves for

　　a. CN^- , OH^- exchange

　　b. SO_4^{-2} , NO_3^- exchange

Use the approximate selectivity constants in Table 9-2.

D2. A strong base resin is being used to exchange NO_3^- with Cl^-. The resin capacity is c_{RT} = 1.25 eq/liter. The column is initially in the NO_3^- form. At time t = 0 minutes a feed which has x_{NO_3} = 0.6 enters. This continues for 10 minutes. Then a feed with x_{NO_3} = 0 enters. The total ionic concentration is c_T = 0.85 eq/liter throughout the process. The column is 0.55 meter long. Superficial velocity is 12 cm/min. ε_e = 0.4. Predict the outlet concentration profiles for NO_3^- and for Cl^-. Use Table 9-2 for equilibrium data. Use ion movement theory.

D3. A strong acid ion exchanger is exchanging Ni^{+2} and H^+. Initially c_T = 0.1 eq/L and x_{Ni} = 0.2. Displace this with a fluid with c_T = 5.1 eq/L and x_{Ni} = 0.2. Column is 75 cm long and superficial velocity is 10 cm/min. Predict the outlet concentration profile using ion movement theory.

Data: c_{RT} = 2.1 eq/L, ε_e = 0.4, K_E = 1.0, and selectivity constants are in Table 9.2.

D4. A strong acid resin is being used to exchange Ca^{++} and Mg^{++}. The resin has a capacity of c_{RT} = 2.0 eq/liter. The column is initially in the calcium form. The column is 1 meter long, has a superficial velocity of 10 cm/min, and ε_e = 0.39. The fluid has a total ionic concentration of c_T = 1.0 eq/liter which is constant. At t = 0 a feed which has an equivalent fraction of 0.95 Mg^{++} and 0.05 Ca^{++} is introduced into the column. This continues until t = 30 min when the feed becomes 0.05 fraction Mg^{++} and 0.95 Ca^{++}. Use equilibrium from Table 9-2. Predict the concentration profile for calcium using ion movement theory.

D5. Lapidus and Rosen *(Chem. Eng. Prog. Syp. Ser. 50* (#14), 97 (1954)) studied the breakthrough of Na^+ on Dowex 50X4 resins initially in the H^+ form. For Na^+ concentrations > 120 x 10^{-3} meq/ml constant pattern behavior was observed. Equilibrium data could be fit by the equation n = 60.6c/(1 + 60.6c) where c = meq Na^+ in solution/ml and n = meq Na^+ on resin/ml. The mass transfer expression was

$$\frac{dn}{dt} = k_f \, a_p \, (c - c^*)$$

where $k_f a_p$ was measured as 3.0 ml/(min)(meq) for 50 to 100 mesh particles $(\bar{d}_p$ = 0.446 mm). With a flow rate of 11.0 ml/min in a 15 cm long, 1.4 cm ID column containing 11.65 grams of packing, c/c_F = 1/2 when 335 ml had passed through. Feed concentration c_F = 173 x 10^{-3} meq/ml. ε_e = 0.4.

   a. Calculate L_{MTZ}.

   b. Determine the shape of the constant pattern.

Use the Constant Pattern equations, *but* be careful with your units.

D6. The use of displacement chromatography in ion exchange chromatography can be quite advantageous. The displacing ion can often be removed with little or no diffuse wave by increasing c_T. This high concentration buffer can then be removed with a wash solution. We wish to separate a feed containing Na^+ and NH_4^+ by displacement chromatography. The column is initially preequilibrated with H^+. The displacing ion is Ag^+. Fluid concentration throughout the cycle is $c_T = 0.4$ eq/L. A strong acid resin with $c_{RT} = 2.1$ eq/L is used. The feed is introduced for 10 minutes. The feed is 40 mole % Na^+ and 60 mole % NH_4^+. Co-ion is Cl^-. The column is 75 cm long, has $v_{super} = 20$ cm/min and $\varepsilon_e = 0.39$.

Predict the outlet concentration profiles. Use Table 9-2 to calculate selectivities. See Section 8.5.1. for a description of displacement chromatography.

D7.   A strong-acid resin bed is saturated with an Ag^+ solution $x_{AG} = 1.0$ at $c_T = 0.4$ eq/L. We wish to remove this Ag^+ solution with a concentrated acid solution (H^+) with $c_T = 2.5$ eq/L and $x_H = 1.0$. Predict the outlet concentration profile of Ag^+ in equivalents/liter. Information: Co-ion is Cl^-, $v_{super} = 20$ cm/min, $\varepsilon_e = 0.39$, $c_{RT} = 2.1$ eq/L, Column length = 75 cm. Use Table 9-2 to predict selectivities.

Note: This is the column regeneration step for the displacement chromatography system in Problem 9-D6. However, the two problems can be solved independently.

D8.   Neuman *et al* (1987) studied the ion exclusion chromatography separation of glucose and sulfuric acid on Amberlite IR-118 in the H^+ form. At 55°C they determined the following data for glucose: $v_{super} = 0.61$ cm/min, $L = 61$ cm, $V_{col} = A_c L = 309$ cm^3, $\varepsilon_e = 0.401$, $X = 0.766$, $K_{d,NC} = 0.345$, $(D_m + E_D) = 0.672$ cm^2/min, $V_F = 12.4$ cm^3. (The units in Neuman *et al.* (1987) are somewhat different than the units in this chapter, and the reported values have been adjusted accordingly). Use the Lapidus and Amundson linear dispersion model to predict the glucose outlet concentration. Compare your result with Figure 9-8a.

Chapter 10

MOVING BED AND SIMULATED MOVING BED
SORPTION SEPARATIONS

In most chemical engineering unit operations continuous counter-current flow is used since it is usually the most efficient way to operate. This is the case for equilibrium staged separations. Unfortunately, counter-current movement of solid and fluid is difficult to achieve without extensive mixing of the solid particles. This difficulty has catalyzed considerable research in this area. Counter-current schemes have included flow in open columns, the hypersorption process where solids flow was controlled by the opening and closing of holes in sieve trays, moving belt schemes, countercurrent flow of gas and solids in sieve tray columns with downcomers, pulsed operation in sieve tray columns without downcomers, and magnetically stabilized moving bed systems. The idealized analysis of all these systems will be similar.

In some cases counter-current movement has been abandoned, and *simulated* counter-current flow has been used. The simulated counter-current system uses a series of packed beds and moves the location of all feed and product ports. A close approximation to continuous counter-current movement can be obtained with the simulated systems.

10.1. SINGLE SOLUTE RECOVERY: STAGED SYSTEMS

Three different types of staged systems with countercurrent flow of solids and fluid are currently used commercially for removal of one solute. Since the bed on each stage is fluidized, particulates in the feed will pass through without clogging. Sieve tray columns with downcomers are used commercially for solvent recovery from dilute air streams using activated carbon (Anon, 1977; Wankat, 1986). An example is shown in Figure 10-1. The solid is fluidized on

499

500

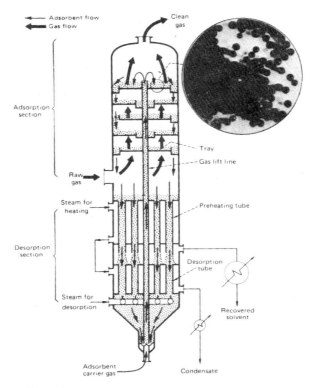

Figure 10-1.   Staged counter-current adsorber with downcomers (Anon, 1977), Reprinted with special permission from *Chem. Engr. 39*, (Aug. 29, 1977). Copyright 1977, McGraw-Hill.

each stage and flows like a liquid on the stage and into the downcomer. These systems were first commercialized in the 1950's, but were plagued by excessive attrition and loss of the carbon. A special very hard, spherical activated carbon is now used and it is claimed that this prevents excessive attrition. Stage efficiencies as high as 90% have been reported in commercial units.

The second type of staged system (called a Cloethe-Streat contactor) used commercially uses *intermittant* operation of sieve tray columns but without downcomers (Cloethe, 1984; Dechow, 1989; Naden and Streat, 1984; Slater, 1981; Streat, 1980; van der Wiel and Wesselingh, 1989; Wankat, 1986;

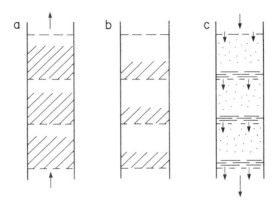

Figure 10-2.   Intermittant counter-current flow of solid and fluid. a. Solid
fluidized while fluid flows. b. Fluid flow stops while solid set-
tles. c. Pulse of fluid carries solid down to next stage.

Wesselingh and van der Meer, 1986). These systems are used for large-scale,
continuous, countercurrent ion exchange for recovering metals and could be
applied in biotechnology. During upflow of the liquid the solids on each stage
are fluidized. To transfer the solids down the fluid flow is stopped, the solids
are allowed to settle, and then a pulse of fluid is used to push the solids down.
This type of operation is illustrated in Figure 10-2. The time dependence of
concentration in a four stage Cloethe-Streat contactor is shown in Figure 10-3
(Dodds et al, 1973). Each stage repeats the same concentration profile each
cycle (this is a cyclic steady state.) The operation is *not* continuous, but closely
approximates continuous countercurrent operation. The number of stages
required or the separation obtained can be estimated from staged models such
as a McCabe-Thiele analysis. A variety of other intermittent, pulsed movement
systems with packed beds during liquid flow are used for continuous ion
exchange (see the next section).

One advantage of the pulsed, intermittent flow contactors is solids and
liquid flows are *decoupled*. Liquid flow rates are chosen to fluidize the solid
resin without eluting it from the bed. For loading columns (columns receiving
the feed) linear fluid velocities in the range from 15 to 23 m/hr are used commercially in uranium processing (Cloethe, 1984). Any desired flow rate of

502

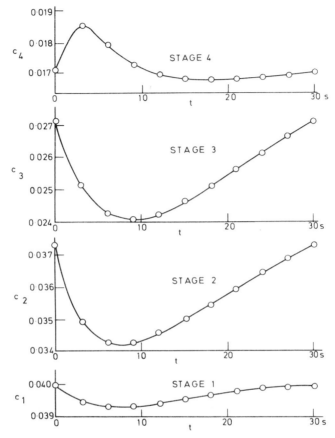

Figure 10-3.   Concentration profiles for a four-stage intermittent fluidized bed ion exchanger. (Dodds *et al*, 1973). Reprinted with permission from *Chem. Eng. Sci.*, *28*, 1233, (1973). Copyright 1973, Pergamon Press.

solids can be obtained by adjusting the time for liquid flow in step A of Figure 10-2. Ratios of liquid flow rate/solid flow rate as high as 300 are commonly used in the uranium mining industry. Such a large ratio would be very difficult to maintain in a continuous countercurrent system. These systems can also treat feeds containing up to 10% suspended solids. Design details and hydraulic considerations are discussed in section 10.5 and in more detail by Wesselingh and van der Meer (1986).

The third type of staged system uses mixers followed by filters, screens, or settlers to separate the resin and liquid. These systems are used for waste water treatment with powdered activated carbon where only one or two stages are required. Agitated staged systems are also used in processing of gold and uranium ores where the feed can contain up to 40% finely suspended solids (Bonsal et al, 1988). In this latter case large resin particles are used so that the resin is easily separated from the suspended solids. Similar systems are used for the batch ion exchange purification of biologicals such as proteins (Dechow, 1989). The stirred tank does not clog with particulates such as cell debris. After the resin is loaded, it is often transferred to a column for gradient elution of the desired solutes. Treybal (1980) discusses agitated tank adsorbers in considerable detail.

All of these staged systems can be designed using the procedures used for other countercurrent staged systems. If the system is isothermal, the design is conveniently done on a McCabe-Thiele diagram which is very similar to the McCabe-Thiele diagrams for absorbers and strippers. (e.g. Brian, 1972; Ruthven and Ching, 1989; Treybal, 1980; Wankat, 1988) A steady-state staged adsorber is shown schematically in Figure 10-4. Since the flow rate of clean adsorbent plus fluid in the pores, S kg/hr, is constant and the flow rate of carrier gas or non-adsorbed solvent, G kg/hr, will often be constant, it is convenient to use mass or mole ratio units. Then solute mass ratio on the adsorbent is q kg solute/kg clean adsorbent plus pore fluid, and in the fluid the mass ratio is Y kg solute/kg solute-free fluid. In these units the adsorbent flow rate and the carrier gas or solvent flow rate are constant.

$$S_j = S , \qquad G_j = G \qquad (10\text{-}1)$$

With these constant overall flow rates, the solute mass balance for the balance envelope shown in Figure 10-4 is

$$Sq_0 + GY_{j+1} = GY_1 + Sq_j \qquad (10\text{-}2)$$

This balance includes solutes in the pores with q. Thus equilibrium must

504

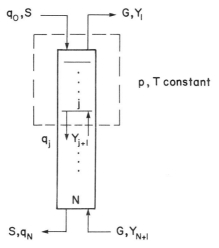

Figure 10-4.   Schematic of staged adsorber.

include the solute in the pores with the amount of solute adsorbed which is essentially a single porosity model. The ratios q and Y can also be in units of moles solute/kg without changing Eqs. (10-1) to (10-3). Equation (10-2) is easily put in the form of an operating line by solving for Y_{j+1}.

$$Y_{j+1} = \frac{S}{G} q_j + (Y_1 - \frac{S}{G} q_0) \qquad (10\text{-}3)$$

This is the equation for a straight line since S/G is constant. The McCabe-Thiele diagram is now easily developed on a Y vs q diagram. This is shown in Figure 10-5a. Note that the equilibrium curve requires both isobaric and isothermal operation. Stage efficiencies can be included in the analysis.

The loaded solid from the adsorber is then sent to a regenerator. Since less solute is adsorbed at higher temperatures and lower pressures, the regeneration is done by operating at higher temperature and/or lower pressure. Thus the mass balances are given by Eqs. (10-1) and (10-2), and the operating line is again Eq. (10-3). Only the concentrations and the equilibrium curve change. The result is shown in Figure 10-5b. The outlet mass ratio Y_1 from the regenerator is usually much higher than the inlet mass ratio into the adsorber. For

505

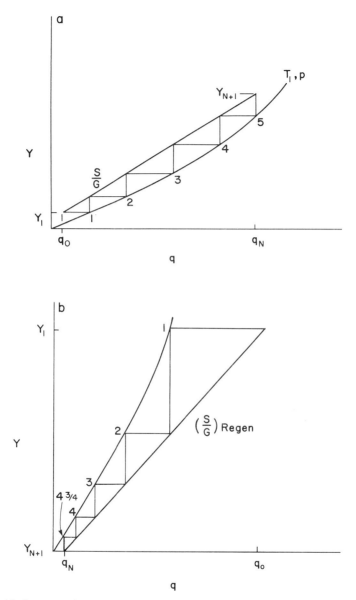

Figure 10-5. McCabe-Thiele diagram for adsorption. a. Loading step. b. Regeneration step.

gases, this high concentration allows recovery of the solute by condensation or absorption. If the solute isn't valuable the concentrated stream can be incinerated. The adsorbent from the regenerator is returned to the adsorber. Note that the combination of an adsorber and a regenerator is similar to the combination of an absorber and a stripper in a gas treating plant.

If the equilibrium curve is straight in either the adsorber or regenerator, then the analysis can be done with the Kremser equation. This analysis is similar to that used for absorbers or extractors and is illustrated in Example 10-1. More details are given by Wankat (1988), or Brian (1972).

Fluid flow rates in regenerators are usually much lower than in adsorbers. With very low gas flow rates the stages will not fluidize properly. Thus regenerators usually use compact moving beds such as those shown in the bottom of Figure 10-1. For liquid systems the intermittent fluidized bed system shown in Figure 10-2 is commonly used for the loading step in ion exchange. The regeneration is usually done in a compact moving bed. The staged model and McCabe-Thiele diagrams can be applied to compact moving beds if an HETP is measured. Then the length of moving bed required is

$$(N) (HETP) = h \tag{10-4}$$

Although this method is commonly used, a theoretically more satisfying approach is to use the mass transfer analysis discussed in Section 10.2.

For ion exchange and exchange adsorption the systems will be isothermal. Stage-by-stage or iterative matrix methods are easily employed for these isothermal systems. If the selectivity K_{ij} is constant, multicomponent systems are easily analyzed using a non-iterative algorithm (Wesselingh and van der Meer, 1986) which is the same algorithm used for distillation with constant relative volatilities (e.g. see Wankat, 1988, Chapter 8). If the operation is not isothermal, then the simple analyses shown in Figures 10-5a and b are not applicable. In this case energy balances must be included. An exact stage-by-stage calculation requires a trial-and-error solution which will be similar to those for non-isothermal absorbers (Treybal), 1980; Smith, 1965). Alternatively, the matrix approach used for absorbers can be applied to staged adsorbers (e.g. Wankat, 1988, Chapt. 15).

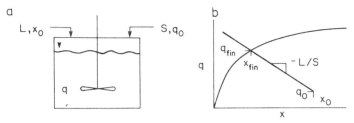

Figure 10-6.   Batch staged sorption. a. Apparatus. L, x_o and S, q_o are initial charges. b. McCabe-Thiele solution.

McCabe-Thiele diagrams can be used to predict the final equilibrium conditions for *batch* stirred tanks. Consider the system shown in Figure 10-6a. L is the charge in kg of liquid to the tank of initial mass fraction x kg solute/kg solution and S is the charge in kg of resin of initial mass ratio q_0 kg solute/kg resin. Then the mass balance is,

$$Lx_0 + S\, q_0 = Lx + Sq \qquad (10\text{-}5)]$$

Solving for q, we obtain

$$q = -\frac{L}{S}\, x + q_0 + \frac{L}{S}\, x_0 \qquad (10\text{-}6)$$

This is a straight operating line as plotted in Figure 10-6b. After a long period of operation, equilibrium will be reached. Then the final values, q_{fin} and x_{fin} are at the intersection of the operating line and the equilibrium curve (see Figure 10-6b). If mass transfer is slow and equilibrium is not reached, a mass transfer rate analysis is required. Equations (10-5) and (10-6) and Figure 10-6b are also applicable to a continuous steady state stirred tank if L and S are flow *rates*.

Example 10-1. Staged analysis

We wish to sorb glucose onto an ion exchange resin in a staged contactor. Feed concentration is 11g/L. We wish an outlet concentration of

1.0 g/L. Inlet resin contains 0.25 g glucose/L. The ratio of volumetric flow rates of resin/solution is 2.5 (L resin/hr)/(L solution/hr). Find the number of equilibrium contacts required.

Solution

We will illustrate the solution using both the McCabe-Thiele method and the Kremser equation. From Problem 6-D4 equilibrium is q = 0.51 c where q and c are in g/L. Assuming that volumetric flow rates of resin, V_R L/hr, and of solution, V_S L/hr, are constant, we obtain the mass balance

$$V_R q_0 + V_S c_{j+1} = V_R q_j + V_S c_1 \tag{10-7}$$

for the column shown in Figure 10-4. This leads to the operating equation,

$$c_{j+1} = \frac{V_R}{V_S} q_j + c_1 - \frac{V_R}{V_S} q_0 \tag{10-8}$$

where $V_R/V_S = 2.5$, $q_0 = 0.25$, $c_1 = 1.0$. Point (q_0, c_1) is on operating line. Equilibrium is $c = 1.961 q$.

Staged Solution

The equilibrium and operating lines are shown in Figure 10-7. Step off stages. Need 7 equilibrium stages.

Kremser Solution

The Kremser equation is easily applied to this problem since operating and equilibrium lines are straight. Many forms of the Kremser equation are available (e.g. see Wankat, 1988). In the units of

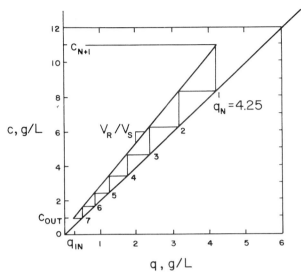

Figure 10-7.   Solution to Example 10-1.

this problem the Kremser equation for the number of equilibrium contacts N is (modification of Eq. (15-30) from Wankat, 1988),

$$N = \ln\left[\left[1 - \frac{m\,V_S}{V_R}\right]\left[\frac{c_{N+1} - c_1^*}{c_1 - c_1^*}\right] + \frac{m\,V_S}{V_R}\right] \Big/ \ln\left[\frac{V_R}{V_S m}\right] \qquad (10\text{-}9)$$

where $m = c/q = 1.961$ and $c_1^* = mq_0 = (1.961)(0.25) = 0.490$. Then

$$N = \frac{\ln\left[(1 - 0.7844)\left[\dfrac{11.0 - 0.49}{1.0 - 0.49}\right] + 0.7844\right]}{\ln\,(1.2749)} \approx 6.81$$

Generalization. Within the accuracy of the graph the two solutions agree. Various forms of the Kremser equation can be used. The Kremser equation is much more convenient when N is specified because outlet concentrations can be calculated directly whereas the

McCabe-Thiele solution will be trial-and-error. Note that the Kremser equation requires constant flow rates and linear equilibrium while the McCabe-Thiele solution can solve problems with non-linear equilibrium. The regeneration step is explored in Problem 10-D5.

10.2. MOVING BED SYSTEMS

Several types of moving bed systems are commonly used commercially. With granular activated carbon for waste water treatment pulsed beds are often used. An example is shown in Figure 10-8a (Storm, 1981). The bed acts as a packed bed during the upward liquid flow step. Then intermittently, the solid is pulsed downward and part of the carbon is removed and sent to a kiln for regeneration. The solute movement theory for operation of a pulsed bed is illustrated in Figure 10-8b. The feed is stopped (time t_p) before breakthrough. The carbon removal pulse has a length l_p. This pulse moves the mass transfer zone back to the starting position, and the feed is started again. This requires that

$$u_{pulse} = l_p/t_p = u_{sh} \qquad (10\text{-}10)$$

where t_p is the feed period between pulses. Note that at time t_p all of the carbon removed is completely saturated. Since the pulsing introduces additional mixing, pulses are usually quite small. Typically, L/l_p is about 20. The resulting operation is then very close to a continuous countercurrent contact. The pulsed beds can usually be operated at considerably higher flow rates (5 to 9 gpm/ft^2) than beds in series (3 to 7 gpm/ft^2) or single beds (1 to 4 gpm/ft^2) (Hutchins, 1981). Thus, although they are somewhat more complex than a packed bed, the pulsed bed systems can be smaller and cheaper.

The Asahi system shown in Figure 10-9 (Arden, 1968; Dechow, 1989; Rodrigues, 1986; Slater, 1980; Streat, 1981; Wankat, 1986) is commonly used for ion exchange systems. During the feed step (Figure 10-9a), the upward flowing water pushes the resin against the top grid and a dense packed bed is formed. Treated water exits at B, and ball valve D is pushed shut which prevents addition of more resin. A small amount of feed water is used to push resin out of cone C into the resin hopper for the next unit. To pulse the resin

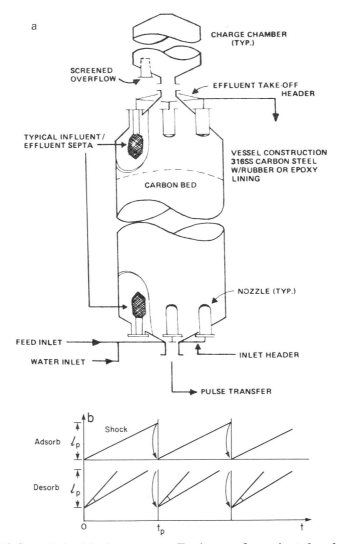

Figure 10-8.   Pulsed bed system. a. Equipment for activated carbon waste-water treatment (Storm, 1981). Reprinted with permission from J.R. Perrich (Ed.)., *Activated Carbon Adsorption for Wastewater Treatment*, 1981. Copyright 1981, CRC Press. b. Solute movement diagram.

512

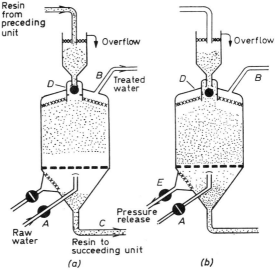

Figure 10-9.   Asahi system for moving bed adsorption and ion exchange.
(Alders, 1968). a. Fluid flow step. b. Addition of new resin.
Reprinted with permission.

downwards, valve A is shut (Figure 10-9b). Resin now drops due to gravity
and valve D opens allowing fresh resin into the vessel. Since a normal ion
exchange cycle consists of feed, regeneration and wash steps; three columns
are required for the Asahi system. Since the three columns have different functions, they are optimized separately. The loading column has a high flow rate
and operates with a slowly moving constant pattern wave. This column can be
wide and short. The regeneration column will have a very low liquid flow rate,
and this column is narrow. Since a diffuse wave occurs during regeneration,
the regeneration column is usually quite long. Washing can be done in a single
mixed tank. The Asahi system has been used extensively for water treatment
and in sugar refining.

An alternate moving bed ion exchange contactor is the Higgins or
Chem-Seps system (Dechow, 1989; Higgins and Chopra 1979; Rodrigues,
1986; Slater, 1981; Streat, 1980; Wankat, 1986) shown in Figure 10-10. All
operations are done simultaneously in the loop. During the liquid flow step the

513

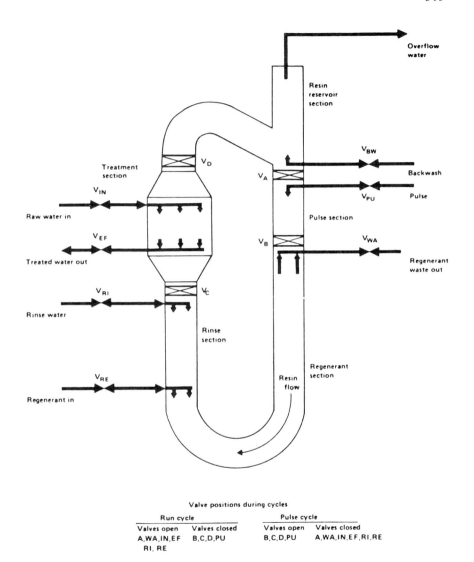

Valve positions during cycles

Run cycle		Pulse cycle	
Valves open	Valves closed	Valves open	Valves closed
A,WA,IN,EF	B,C,D,PU	B,C,D,PU	A,WA,IN,EF,RI,RE
RI, RE			

Figure 10-10. Chem.-Seps semi-continuous ion exchange system. (Higgins and Chopra, 1979). Reprinted with permission from Calmon, C. and Gold., H., (Eds.), *Ion Exchange for Pollution Control*, Vol. 2. Copyright 1979, CRC Press.

resin acts as a packed bed in the treatment, rinse and regenerant sections, but is fluidized in the resin reservoir section where the resin is backwashed to remove suspended solids. The solids movement step uses a counterflow pulse of water to push the resin. The Chem-Seps system has been extensively used for water treatment and hydrometallurgical processes.

A variety of other systems have been developed. Regenerators have quite low liquid flow rates and satisfactory intermittent operation can be obtained in empty pipes (Wankat, 1986). Pulsed upward flow of the solid appears to work well. Fluidized beds can be used when affinity is very high, but there tends to be considerable mixing if the bed is not stabilized (Lochmuller et al, 1988). Truly continuous plug flow of solids can be obtained in magnetically stabilized fluidized beds. (Rosensweig, 1979; Lucchesi et al, 1979; Burns and Graves, 1985, 1987). In these systems either magnetic particles are used as the sorbent or a mixture of magnetic beads and a non-magnetic sorbent are used. The flow of the particles is stabilized with a magnetic field. The advantages of this system are that true plug flow without mixing can be attained and particulates in the feed will not clog the bed as they will in packed or dense moving beds. Unfortunately, the magnetically stabilized systems have proven to be difficult to scale-up and have not yet been commercialized. This technology has been applied both to gas and liquid systems and to adsorption and chromatography systems. It's major use may be in medium-sized equipment for biotechnology. Other designs are reviewed by Slater (1981), Streat (1980) and Wankat (1986).

The countercurrent moving bed systems can be analyzed using a mass transfer analysis. This analysis is more realistic than a staged analysis when the system has continuous contact between solid and fluid. Since the mass transfer approach for moving bed systems is similar to the mass transfer analysis applied to vapor-liquid systems (e.g. see Treybal, 1980; or Wankat, 1988, Chapter 19), only an abbreviated development will be given here. The analysis will assume flow is continuous, and thus will ignore the discrete nature of most of the contactors used commercially. Other presentations of this analysis are given by Treybal (1980) and Wankat (1986). Burns and Graves (1985) use different forward and reverse rate coefficients. Ruthven (1984) includes axial dispersion and gives the solution for linear isotherms.

The column is shown schematically in Figure 10-11a and is assumed to be isothermal. The fluid phase flows at a constant flow rate L kg/hr and flows countercurrent to the solid phase with a flow rate S kg/hr. For a differential element of height dz the mass transfer expression is

$$- \frac{L}{A_c} \frac{dy}{dz} = Ka_p(x - x_E) \qquad (10\text{-}11)$$

where x is the adsorbate mass fraction in the fluid and y_E is the fluid concentration in equilibrium with the solid. The overall mass transfer coefficient K is based on the interfacial area per unit volume, a_p, between solid and fluid. K can be estimated from a sum of resistances model such as Eq. (8-19a), while a_p is given by Eq. (8-14) for spherical particles.

Rearranging Eq. (10-11) we have

$$h = \int_0^h dz = \frac{L}{A_c Ka_p} \int_{x_{out}}^{x_{in}} \frac{dy}{(x - x_E)} \qquad (10\text{-}12a)$$

where we have assumed that $L/A_c Ka_p$ is constant. Equation (10-12a) is often written as

$$h = (HTU)(NTU) \qquad (10\text{-}12b)$$

where

$$HTU = \frac{L}{A_c Ka_p} \qquad NTU = \int_{x_{out}}^{x_{in}} \frac{dy}{(x - x_E)} \qquad (10\text{-}12c)$$

To determine the NTU, $(x - x_E)$ must be determined as a function of x. The equilibrium value is determined from the equilibrium isotherm. The x value can be found from a mass balance using the mass balance envelope

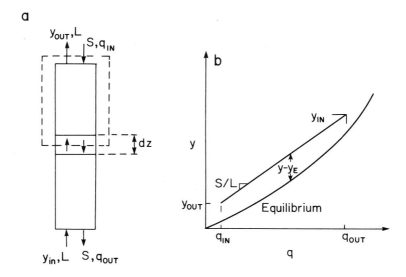

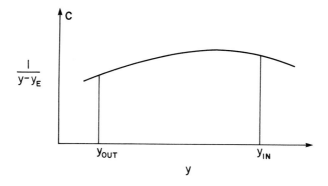

Figure 10-11.   Mass transfer analysis for moving bed systems. a. Schematic of column. b. Determination of $y - y_E$. c. Graphical integration to determine NTU.

shown in Figure 10-11a. The operating equation resulting from this mass balance is,

$$x = \frac{S}{L} q + x_{out} - \frac{S}{L} q_{in} \qquad (10\text{-}13)$$

Both the operating and equilibrium curves can be plotted on a McCabe-Thiele type diagram of x versus q. This is shown in Figure 10-11b for adsorption. The value of $(x - x_E)$ is easily determined as the difference between the operating and equilibrium curves. The NTU integration can be done graphically, numerically, or using Simpson's rule. The graphical integration is shown in Figure 10-11c. Simpson's rule will be

$$NTU = \int\limits_{x_{out}}^{x_{in}} \frac{dx}{x - x_E} =$$

$$\left[\frac{x_{in} - x_{out}}{6} \right] \left[\frac{1}{x - x_E} \Big|_{x_{in}} + \frac{4}{x - x_E} \Big|_{\frac{x_{in}+x_{out}}{2}} + \frac{1}{x - x_E} \Big|_{x_{out}} \right] \qquad (10\text{-}14)$$

Additional accuracy can be obtained if more complicated forms of Simpson's rule are used, or if the integral is divided into parts.

If the equilibrium is linear of the form

$$x = mq + b \qquad (10\text{-}15)$$

then the integration can be done analytically. This result is known as the Colburn equation.

$$NTU = \left[\frac{1}{1 - \frac{mL}{S}} \right] \ln \left\{ (1 - \frac{mL}{S}) \left[\frac{x_{in} - (mq_{in} + b)}{x_{out} - (mq_{in} + b)} \right] + \frac{mL}{S} \right\} \qquad (10\text{-}16)$$

The Colburn equation for adsorbers is similar to the Colburn equation developed for absorbers (e.g. see Wankat, 1988, Chapter 19).

To use Eq. (10-12b) for design the value of the HTU must be known. This requires a value for Ka_p. The value of Ka_p can be determined experimentally or from correlations such as Eqs. (8-15) and (8-17a). In correlations the velocity should be the relative velocity between the solid and fluid.

This analysis includes fluid in the pores with the solid phase. Thus the equilibrium isotherms must also include solute in the pore fluid along with the adsorbed solute. An alternate analysis is to treat the adsorber as a three phase contactor (solid, pore fluid and external fluid) (Wankat, 1986). In most cases the analysis presented here will be adequate. The most serious limitation of this analysis is the isothermal assumption. Non-isothermal systems can be modeled numerically (Liapis and Rippin, 1979).

Example 10-2. Moving Bed Affinity Chromatography

Data for moving bed systems is relatively scarce. Burns and Graves (1987) present the following results for human serum albumin (HSA) sorption by Cibacron Blue F3GA attached to calcium alginate-magnetite beads in a magnetically stabilized fluidized bed.

Feed Concentration = 0.2 mg HSA/ml solution
Input solids = 0.0 mg HSA/g solids
Fluid flow rate = L = 10 ml/min
Solids flowrate = S = 0.5 g/min

$$K = \frac{L}{S} \frac{k_d}{k_a} = 1.6$$

where k_d and k_a are desorption and adsorption rate constants.
Percent HSA adsorbed = 56%
Bed Length, h = 8.0 cm

Find NTU and HTU

Solution

At the low concentration given here adsorption will be linear. Since K = 1.6, k_d/k_a = (1.6) (0.5/10.0) = 0.08 g/ml. This leads to a

Langmuir expression (see Section 6.3), but at low concentrations will be linear. If we write equilibrium as Eq. (10-15) then $b = 0$ and $m = c/q = k_d/k_a = 0.08$ g/ml.

Also: $q_{in} = 0$, mL/S $= \dfrac{(0.08)\,(10.0)}{0.5} = 1.6$, $c_{in} = 0.2$,

$c_{out} = (1-0.56)\,(0.2) = 0.088$ mg/g.

We can solve this either graphically or with the Colburn equation. We will illustrate both. The equations are valid in the units of this problem if S and L are constant. For these dilute solutions they will be.

Graphical Solution: Plot c versus q as shown in Figure 10-12.

> Equilibrium line: $c = mq = 0.08\,q$
>
> Operating line: $c = \dfrac{S}{L}\,q + c_{out} - \dfrac{S}{L}\,q'_{in}$
>
> Slope = S/L = 0.05

Goes through point $(c_{out}, q_{in}) = (0.088, 0)$. Stop at $c_{in} = 0.2$ mg/ml.

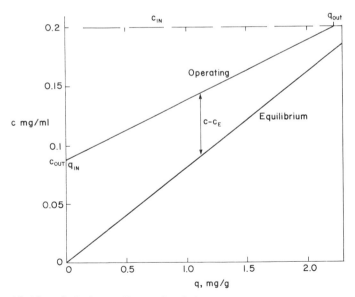

Figure 10-12. Solution to Example 10-2.

In these units Eq. (10-14) becomes

$$NTU = \int_{C_{out}}^{C_{in}} \frac{dc}{c - c_E}$$

$$= \frac{c_{in} - c_{out}}{6} \left[\left[\frac{1}{c - c_E} \right]_{c_{in}} + \left[\frac{4}{c - c_E} \right] \middle| \frac{2}{c_{in} + c_{out}} + \left[\frac{1}{c - c_E} \right]_{c_{out}} \right]$$

where $\dfrac{c_{in} + c_{out}}{2} = \dfrac{0.2 + 0.088}{2} = 0.144$

From the graph we can determine values of $c - c_E$. Then

$$NTU = \frac{0.112}{3} \left[\frac{1}{0.088} + \frac{4}{(0.144 - 0.0896)} + \frac{1}{(0.2 - 0.179)} \right] = 2.47$$

and

$$HTU = h/NTU = 8/2.47 = 3.24 \text{ cm}$$

Colburn Equation Solution: Equation (10-16) in these units is:

$$NTU = \left[\frac{1}{1 - \frac{mL}{S}} \right] \ln \left\{ \left[1 - \frac{mL}{S} \right] \left[\frac{c_{in} - (mq_{in} + b)}{c_{out} - (mq_{in} + b)} \right] + \frac{mL}{S} \right\} \quad (10\text{-}17)$$

$$NTU = \left[\frac{1}{-0.6} \right] \ln \left\{ (-0.6) \left[\frac{0.2}{0.088} \right] + 1.6 \right\} = 2.40$$

Using Eq. (10-12b) we have
HTU = h/(NTU) = 8/2.4 = 3.333 cm
This is a reasonable height which does not indicate excessive backmixing of the resin. Note that the results of the two solutions are essentially equivalent.

10.3. MOVING BED FRACTIONATION

A counter-current system for fractionating two components is shown in Figure 10-13. The solids flow down the column while the fluid flows up. The less strongly adsorbed solute A moves up in zone 1 while strongly adsorbed solute B moves down in this zone. Thus zone 1 purifies solute A. Zone 2 removes solute A from B and thus purifies solute B. In zone 3 solute B is desorbed with desorbent D. Zone 4 serves to remove solute A from the desorbent so that desorbent can be recycled. The desorbent could be water or a solvent.

The solute movement theory can be applied to this system. The solute wave velocities calculated from Eq. (6-23) or (6-24) were with respect to a sta-

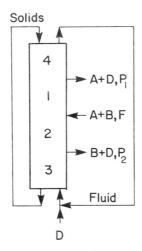

Figure 10-13.   Counter-current separator for fractionation of two solutes.

tionary solid. The appropriate fluid velocity is then the interstitial fluid velocity relative to the solid. Thus

$$v = \frac{v_{super}}{\varepsilon_e} + |v_{solid}|$$ (10-18)

where v_{super} is the superficial fluid velocity and v_{solid} is the superficial solid velocity. Now u_s calculated from Eqs. (6-23) or (6-24) is the solute velocity with respect to the solid. The solute velocity which an observer will see is obtained by subtracting the solids velocity

$$u_{s,cc} = u_s - |v_{solid}|$$ (10-19)

$u_{s,cc}$ is positive when the solute flow is up the column and negative when it flows down.

In a counter-current column the solids velocity is the same in all zones but the superficial fluid velocity varies from zone to zone since feed is added and products are withdrawn. If we set $v_{super,3}$ as velocity in zone 3, then for relatively dilute systems

$$v_{super,2} = v_{super,3} - P_2 / (\rho_f A_c)$$

$$v_{super,1} = v_{super,2} + F/(\rho_f A_c)$$ (10-20)

$$v_{super,4} = v_{super,1} - P_1/(\rho_f A_c)$$

where the product and feed flow rates in kg/min are shown in Figure 10-13. Since v_{super} changes, $u_{s,cc}$ will change from zone to zone. In addition, if the desorbent affects the adsorption of solute then the equilibrium constant A(T) will vary from zone to zone and $u_{s,cc}$ will change. This latter effect is very useful, but is not necessary to make the counter-current column work.

To achieve the separation indicated in Figure 10-13 we want solute A to move upward in zones 1 and 2 and downward in zone 4. Thus

$$u_{A\ cc,1}\ ,\ u_{A\ cc,2} > 0 > u_{A\ cc,4}$$ (10-21)

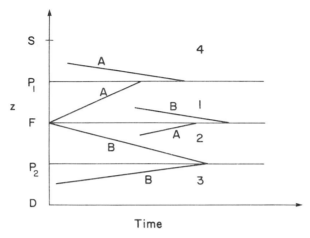

Figure 10-14. Solute movement diagram in continuous countercurrent column for linear isotherms.

Solute B should move downwards in zones 1 and 2 and upwards in zone 3. Thus

$$u_{B\ cc,3} > 0 > u_{B\ cc,1}\ ,\ u_{B\ cc,2} \tag{10-22}$$

Equations (10-21) and (10-22) are an important result since they control the operation of the continuous counter-current column. These equations are valid for both linear and nonlinear isotherms. For nonlinear systems the solute velocities are obviously concentration dependent (see Problem 10-C5). If the system will work, there are ranges of values for P_1, P_2 and D for a given feed flow rate which will satisfy these inequalities. In actual practice it is desirable to choose the flow rates so that all the inequalities are as large as possible.

The appropriate solute waves are shown in Figure 10-14. In the ideal case at steady state there will be no solute A in zones 4, 2 or 3 and no solute B in zones 1, 3 and 4. Because of dispersion and finite mass transfer rates solute A will appear in zones 4 and 2, and B will be in zones 1 and 3. The size of the zones required depends on these dispersion and mass transfer rate effects. In addition, any axial solid or fluid mixing caused by non-perfect flow will require a larger column. Extreme mixing or channeling can destroy the desired separation.

The solute movement theory does not include mass transfer effects. This can be done using the steady-state counter-current theory of mass transfer discussed earlier. A staged analysis can also be used. When there are two adsorbates and a diluent, the analysis will be similar to fractional extraction analysis (e.g. see Brian, 1972; or Wankat, 1988, Chapter 16).

In exchange adsorption (see Figure 6-3e) two adsorbates compete for sites and no diluent is present. A moving bed apparatus can be used to fractionate these solutes. This was done commercially in the 1950's using the Union Oil Co. Hypersorption process (Berg, 1951; Treybal, 1980; Wankat, 1986). This separation had difficulty competing with vacuum distillation and is no longer used. The process was complex both conceptually and mechanically. Since the process is no longer in use, we will not consider it further (see Problem 10-F1 for further study).

Currently, there are no announced moving bed systems being used commercially for fractionation. If separation is easy, other separation techniques such as distillation have been cheaper. If separation is difficult, mixing of the solids must be minimized. Unfortunately, this has been very difficult. New developments such as the magnetically stabilized fluidized beds discussed briefly in Section 10.2 may eventually solve these problems.

10.4. SIMULATED MOVING BED FRACTIONATION

An alternative to moving bed systems is to simulate counter-current movement. This is done with a series of packed bed sections by switching the location of all feed and product withdrawal ports. This is illustrated in Figure 10-15. At time t_1 the product port and all other ports are switched. An observer located at the product port "sees" the solid move down at this time. From time t_1 to t_2 the fluid flows upward. At time t_2 the ports are switched again and the observer "sees" the solid move downward. The net result is the observer "sees" an intermittant counter-current motion of solid and fluid.

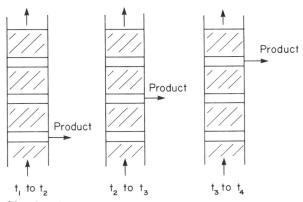

Figure 10-15.   Simulated countercurrent system.

The first simulated counter-current system was the Shanks system which has been applied to leaching, adsorption and ion exchange. The Shanks system uses a series of columns with plumbing arranged so that feed can be input and product withdrawals removed from any column. Thus the counter-current separator shown in Figure 10-13 can be simulated. A modern adaption of the Shanks process simulating the system shown in Figure 10-13 has been extensively commercialized by Universal Oil Products (UOP) (Broughton, 1984-85; Dechow, 1989; Ruthven and Ching, 1989; Wankat, 1986; Storti et al, 1989). UOP used a pilot plant scale system which is a series of columns for scaling up their commercial scale units. The commercial UOP simulated counter-current process, Sorbex, uses a single column with many packed sections and has a rotating valve for distributing feed, desorbent and products. This is shown schematically in Figure 10-16. The UOP process was first commercialized as Molex for separation of linear paraffins from branched-chain and cyclic hydrocarbons using 5A molecular sieves (see Table 6-1). Since then, processes for p-xylene purification (Parex), olefin separation (Olex), and separation of fructose from glucose (Sarex) have been commercialized. Pilot plant scale separations for a variety of other problems have been demonstrated. A large number of patents have been granted on simulated moving bed systems.

The Universal Oil Products system works very well, but is complex and expensive. The rotary valve in particular is expensive since it must be custom

526

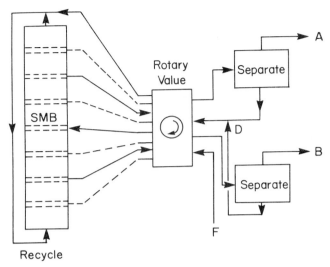

Figure 10-16.   Universal Oil Products Simulated Moving Bed (SMB) System.

designed and machined. Simpler and hence cheaper systems are also commercially available and are commonly used for separation of fructose from glucose. One such arrangement is shown in Figure 10-17 (Wankat, 1986). Here there is one column per zone. Thus, the approach to a truly countercurrent system is only approximate, but the system is simple. The system shown in Figure 10-17 requires 4 solenoid valves per column. In commercial columns a fifth valve may be added to allow backflushing the resin.

The solute movement theory can be used to analyze the simulated counter-current system in two ways. First, if the observer fixes himself at one of the outlet or inlet ports then he sees the solid and entrained fluid transferred downwards in pulses. This observer then sees solids movement in pulses. The average solids velocity this observer sees is given by Eq. (10-10) and the analysis procedure is essentially the same as for a pulsed counter-current system (see Figure 10-7b).

In the second analysis the observer fixes himself on the ground and he sees the solid as stationary. With the fluid flowing up the column, he sees all the inlet and outlet ports move up the column at discrete times. When a port

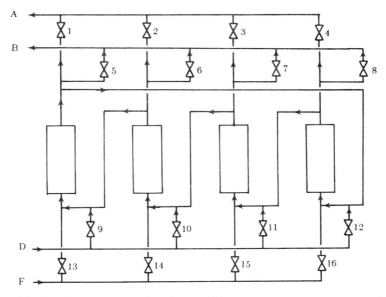

Figure 10-17. Arrangement for SMB with one column per zone and four zones. (Wankat, 1988).

Zone	Inlet Valve Open	Outlet Valve Open
I	13,14,15 or 16	1,2,3 or 4
II	none	none
III	9,10,11 or 12	5,6,7 or 8
IV	none	none

Reprinted with permission from P.C. Wankat, *Large Scale Adsorption and Chromatography*, CRC Press, 1986. Copyright 1986, CRC Press.

reaches the top of the column, it recycles back to the bottom. In between the shifting of port locations, the adsorber is a fixed bed system. Thus the solute wave velocity can be determined from Eqs. (6-23) or (6-24). The fluid velocities in each section will differ. The superficial fluid velocities are given by Eq. (10-20) and the interstitial velocity v equals v_{super}/ε_e. The shifting of ports does not shift the solute waves, but does change the wave velocities since it changes

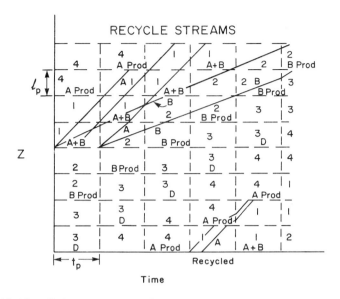

Figure 10-18.   Solute movement is simulated countcurrent system for linear isotherms.

which zone the solute is in. This is illustrated in Figure 10-18. If the desorbent changes the equilibrium constants, this will also change the solute velocities.

Note in Figure 10-18 that the movement of both species is up, but the more strongly adsorbed solute B moves down *with respect to* the port locations. Feed would be introduced continuously at the port marked A + B, but was illustrated for only one time period. The zone numbers corresponding to Figure 10-13 are shown on Figure 10-18. The fluid velocities and hence the solute velocities are different in each zone. When fluid reaches the top of the cascade it is recycled to the bottom. Thus the solute waves are also recycled. If the timing of the switches is appropriate, solute A will appear in zones 1, 2 and the lower section of zone 4, and solute B will appear in zones 1, 2 and the upper section of zone 3. Solute A goes into zone 4 since only a portion of the fluid is withdrawn as product P_1. Solute B goes into zone 3 because of the switching of ports. Dispersion and mixing effects will naturally spread out the solute waves in each zone. Figure 10-18 needs to be studied carefully since the simulated countercurrent motion is somewhat subtle.

To achieve the desired separation we desire to have solute A move up in zones 1 and 2 faster than the port movement and slower than the port movement in zone 4. Solute B should move slower than the port movement in zones 1 and 2 and faster in zone 3. The average velocity of port movement is

$$u_{port,avg} = l_{port}/t_{port} \tag{10-23}$$

where l_{port} is the packing height between ports and t_{port} is the time between switches of ports. The conditions to achieve separation are then

$$u_{A,1} \ , \ u_{A,2} > u_{port,avg} > u_{A,4} \tag{10-24}$$

$$u_{B,3} > u_{port,avg} > u_{B,1} \ , \ u_{B,2} \tag{10-25}$$

These conditions follow the same order as Eqs. (10-21) and (10-22).

How close is a simulated counter-current system to a truly counter-current separator? Although the answer to this depends on the chemical system and the column length, Liapis and Rippin (1979) found that the simulated system had an adsorbent utilization from 79% to 98% that of the truly countercurrent system. With a single zone system they found that from two to four sections were sufficient and that two to four column switches were required to reach a periodic concentration profile. An example of experimental results from a simulated countercurrent system are shown in Figure 10-19 (Neuzil and Jensen, 1978). The average profiles are quite smooth and look very much like the expected shape for a continuous countercurrent system. Because of this similarity, SMB systems are occasionally designed as if they were continuous contact systems, and either the staged or HTU-NTU methods developed previously can be used. A preliminary design can also be done using a staged analysis to determined N in each section and then h from Eq. (10-4). This requires an estimate of HETP. The advantage of this approach is existing multicomponent calculation methods developed for absorption and extraction can be adapted to the SMB. Determination of the number of subsections required

530

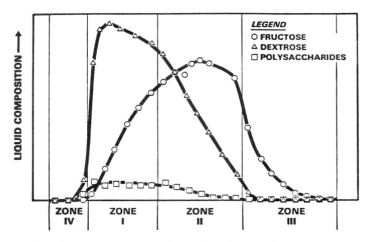

Figure 10-19. Compositions in column for simulated countercurrent system
from Sarex pilot plant. Neuzil and Jensen (1978). Reprinted
with permission.

for each zone requires a detailed time-dependent model (Ruthven and Ching,
1989; Storti et al, 1989).

Comparison of simulated counter-current and truly counter-current systems is of considerable interest. Both systems at steady state can at best do a
complete binary separation. Partial separation of additional components can be
obtained with side withdrawals. The simulated counter-current system could
also be extended to more complex cycles where part of the bed is temporarily
operated as a batch chromatograph. The simulated moving bed system is actually a fixed bed system. Thus flooding (unintentional upwards entrainment of
solid) will not be a problem, but excessive pressure drop may result for small
particles or viscous solutions. The fixed bed will have a lower ε_e and hence a
higher capacity than truly counter-current systems, but this will be offset by the
distribution regions between sections. In moving beds the actual movement of
solids requires means for keeping the bed stable and may result in excessive
attrition, but allows for easy solids replacement or external reactivation. Both
systems have mechanical difficulties to overcome. In the simulated moving
bed these difficulties are the valving, timing and distributors while in an actual

moving bed they involve moving the solids without mixing. Currently, the simulated counter-current systems have been the preferred choice for large-scale adsorption installations to fractionate two solutes.

Example 10-3. Fructose-Glucose Separation in SMB

We wish to use the local equilibrium model to estimate feasible operating conditions for a SMB to separate a dilute fructose and glucose mixture using an ion exchange resin in the calcium form. Do this for a 4 zone system with one section per zone. We arbitrarily choose $t_{port} = 5$ minutes since this is a convenient time. Design for a 5% glucose, 5% fructose feed at a feed velocity

$$v_F = \frac{F}{\rho_f \, A_c} = 1.0 \text{ cm/min.}$$

The superficial velocity in zone 3 should be $v_{super,3} = 20$ cm/min. Use water as the solvent.

Solution

A. Define. The SMB will have the 4 zones shown on Figure 10-13. We need to find product velocities, superficial velocities in each zone, l_{port}, and product concentrations.

B. Explore. This problem is quite open-ended since many different answers will satisfy inequalities (10-24) and (10-25). We will look at the most restrictive of these inequalities and use Eqs. (10-20) to determine values which work. Equilibrium data was given in Problem 6-D4 and u_s was calculated in Problem 6-C3.

C. Plan. Calculate $u_{F,3}$ (solute velocity of glucose in zone 3). Estimate a port velocity which satisfies Eq. (10-25). Then estimate a u_{F1} value to satisfy Eq. (10-25) and calculate $v_{super,1}$ and $v_{super,2}$. Calculate

$u_{G,1}$ and $u_{G,2}$ and check if Eq. (10-24) is satisfied. Determine a $u_{G,4}$ which also satisfies Eq. (10-24). Then determine $v_{super,4}$. The product withdrawal rates can be determined from Eqs. (10-20). This procedure gives a set of feasible operating conditions, and does *not* give optimum operating conditions.

D. Do It. From the solution to Problem 6-C3 and data in Problem 6-D4,

$$u_{F,j} = \frac{v_{super,j}}{\varepsilon_e + (1 - \varepsilon_e) A_F} = \frac{v_{super,j}}{0.4 + (0.6)(0.88)} = 1.078 \, v_{super,j}$$

$$u_{G,j} = \frac{v_{super,j}}{\varepsilon_e + (1 - \varepsilon_e) A_G} = \frac{v_{super,j}}{0.4 + (0.6)(0.51)} = 1.416 \, v_{super,j}$$

In zone 3 $v_{super,3} = 20$ cm/min and $u_{F,3} = 21.56$
From Eq. (10-25) $21.56 > u_{port,avg}$
Arbitrarily, pick $u_{port,avg} = 20$ cm/min
Then, $l_{port} = (u_{port,avg}) \, t_{port} = (20 \text{ cm/min})(5 \text{ min}) = 100$ cm

If we choose $u_{F,1} = 18.5$, Eq. (10-25) will be satisfied.

Then $\qquad v_{super,1} = \dfrac{u_{F,1}}{1.078} = 17.16$ cm/min

$\qquad\qquad v_{super,2} = v_{super,1} - v_F = 16.16$ cm/min

$\qquad\qquad u_{F,2} = (1.078 \, (16.16) = 17.42$ cm/min

For glucose: $u_{G,1} = (1.416) \, v_{super,1} = 24.30$ cm/min

$\qquad\qquad u_{G,2} = (1.416) \, v_{super,2} = 22.88$ cm/min

Eq. (10-24) is satisfied so far, but must also have

$$u_{G,4} < u_{port,avg} = 20$$

Arbitrarily pick $u_{G,4} = 19.0$ cm/min. Then

$$v_{super,4} = \frac{u_{g,4}}{1.416} = \frac{19.0}{1.416} = 13.42 \text{ cm/min}$$

Product withdrawals can be determined from Eq. (10-20).

$$P_1/(\rho_f A_c) = v_{super,1} - v_{super,4} = 3.74 \text{ cm/min}$$

$$P_2/(\rho_f A_c) = v_{super,3} - v_{super,2} = 3.84 \text{ cm/min}$$

Assuming that fructose and glucose are completely separated, the glucose product is diluted to (5%) (1.0)/(3.74) = 1.34%.
Fructose Product is (5%) (1.0)/(3.84) = 1.30%.

E. Check. A check of solute velocities shows that Eqs. (10-24) and (10-25) are satisfied.

F. Generalization. This is clearly not the only solution and not the only solution method. To see the effect of some of the arbitrary choices made in the solution, I tried the following alternate set:

$$u_{port,avg} = 21, \ l_{port} = 105 \text{ cm, and } u_{F,1} = 20.5$$

This gives $v_{super,1} = 19.02$, $v_{super,2} = 18.02$, and $u_{F,2} = 19.42$.

For glucose: $u_{G,1} = 26.93$, $u_{G,2} = 25.5$

Letting $u_{G,4} = 20.5$ then $v_{super,4} = 14.48$

Products: $P_1/(\rho_f A_c) = 4.54$; 1.10% glucose

$$P_2/(\rho_f A_c) = 1.98; \ 2.53\% \text{ fructose}$$

This choice will be harder to operate since solute velocities are significantly closer to the port velocity. If the isotherms have any non-linearity the initial choice is more likely to work. However, there is less overall dilution and significantly less fructose dilution with this set.

10.5 DESIGN CONSIDERATIONS

Each of the contacting methods discussed in this chapter has different design considerations. Fluidized plate columns such as the Cloethe-Streat contactor must operate within certain hydrodynamic limits (Wesselingh and van der Meer, 1985). The lower limits are the fluid velocity must be greater than the minimum fluidization velocity, and the velocity in the holes of the sieve plate must be greater than the settling velocity of the largest resin particles. If we define

$$d^* = d_p/d_{ref} \quad , \quad d_{ref} = \left[\frac{v^2 \, \rho_f}{g \, (\rho_p - \rho_f)} \right]^{1/3} \qquad (10\text{-}26a)$$

$$v^* = v/v_{ref} \quad , \quad v_{ref} = \left[\frac{g(\rho_p - \rho_f)v}{\rho_f} \right]^{1/3} \qquad (10\text{-}26b)$$

where v is the kinematic viscosity and g is the acceleration due to gravity, then the settling velocity is

$$v^*_{settling} = 0.25d^* \quad 3 < d^* < 30 \qquad (10\text{-}27a)$$

and

$$v^*_{settling} = d^{*2}/18 \quad d^* < 1 \; (Re < 1) \qquad (10\text{-}27b)$$

Equation (10-27a) is in the normal range of diameters for ion exchange particles and leads to $v_{settling}$ from 2 to 3 cm/s.

The average hole velocity is

$$v_{hole} = v_{super} \, A_{cs}/A_{hole} \qquad (10\text{-}28)$$

Since usually $A_{hole}/A_{cs} \leq 0.05$, the hole velocity is significantly greater than the superficial velocity. If v_{hole} is less than $v_{settling}$ given by Eqs. (10-26) and (10-27) weeping will occur. Either the number or size of holes can be decreased.

Wesselingh and van der Meer (1985) suggest 0.3 cm holes in laboratory columns and 1.2 cm holes in larger systems.

The minimum fluidization velocity depends on the shape and porosity of the packed bed. The superficial minimum fluidization velocity, v_{mf}, can be determined by equating drag and gravity forces. This velocity can be determined from the solution of

$$(\rho_p - \rho_f)g = \frac{150\,(1-\varepsilon)\mu\,v_{mf}}{d_p^2\,\varepsilon^3} + \frac{1.75\,\rho_f\,v_{mf}^2}{d_p\,\varepsilon^3} \qquad (10\text{-}29a)$$

At low Reynolds numbers the last term is negligible and

$$v_{mf} = \frac{(\rho_p - \rho_f)\,g\,d_p^2\varepsilon^3}{150\,(1-\varepsilon)\,\mu} \qquad (10\text{-}29b)$$

A good rough estimate which is easier to use is (Wesselingh and van der Meer, 1985),

$$v_{mf} = 0.02\,v_{settling} \qquad (10\text{-}29c)$$

The upper limits to successful operation are flooding and insufficient holdup of particles. Flooding occurs when resin particles are carried out of the bed

$$v_{super} \geq v_{settling} \qquad (10\text{-}30)$$

This limit is usually not a problem since holdup becomes too small before Eq. (10-30) is satisfied. As the fluid velocity increases, the fluidized bed expands and holdup decreases. Thus, extremely high stages may be required to hold enough resin for mass transfer. Wesselingh and van der Meer (1985) suggest that holdup is too low if

$$v_{super} > 0.25\,v_{settling} \qquad (10\text{-}31)$$

The pressure drop of the bed is the same as the pressure drop in a packed bed when $v_{super} < v_{mf}$. Thus, Eqs. (8-22) and (8-23) can be used to calculate Δp. Once the bed fluidizes $\Delta p = \Delta p\,(v_{mf})$ is a constant.

The volume fraction particles, e, can be estimated from the Richardson and Zaki relationship (Wesselingh and van der Meer, 1985).

$$\frac{V_{super}}{1-e} - \frac{V_{solid}}{e} = V_{settling} \ (1-e)^{n-1} \qquad (10\text{-}32a)$$

where V_{solid} is the superficial velocity of the solids and n can be determined from

$$\frac{5-n}{n-2.5} = \left[\frac{d^*}{7}\right]^2 \qquad (10\text{-}32b)$$

This last equation leds to n ~ 5 for small particles and n ~ 2.5 for large particles. Wesselingh and van der Meer (1985) give a graphical solution for Eqs. (10-32). At the minimum fluidization velocity e ~ 0.6.

The Cloethe-Streat contactor is somewhat unique in that detailed design procedures have been published in the open literature. Fortunately, Eqs. (10-26) to (10-32) are valid for single fluidized beds such as those occasionally used for on-off chromatography or ion exchange. With the exception of one old paper (Ermenc, 1961), design details for the staged counter current adsorber with downcomers shown in Figure 10-1 have not been published. Hole velocities and fluidization characteristics will be similar to the Cloethe-Streat contactor. What is unique is design of the downcomer. This must be done carefully to avoid fluid bypassing the stages and flowing up the downcomer. In addition, resin attrition can be minimized by designing the system to have smooth edges.

In stirred tank systems the particles are suspended with an impeller. Design details for these systems are discussed by Treybal (1980).

Less information is available about the design of moving bed systems, partially because these systems can be difficult to scale-up. Without a doubt, Exxon has amassed significant information on the design of magnetically stabilized fluidized beds, but most of this information is confidential. Since the project has been dropped, there was apparently difficulty in scaling-up to very large sizes. Burns and Graves (1985) present some sketchy details from their laboratory experiments. Moving beds with intermittant or pulsed solids flow are apparently easier to scale-up and are extensively used (see Figures 10-8a, 10-9 and 10-10). Details for pulsed bed design are sparse, but Hutchins (1981) suggests that

$$L = 20 \, l_p \qquad (10\text{-}33)$$

and a fluid superficial velocity of 5 to 9 gpm/ft^2 be used during the loading step.

Fluidized beds, moving beds and stirred tanks often have different resin requirements than packed beds. Large diameter, dense resins have higher d^* values and hence higher settling velocities. This means that higher fluid velocities and smaller diameter vessels can be used. Unfortunately, larger diameter particles have lower mass transfer rates. Thus, there is a tradeoff between hydrodynamics and mass transfer.

The SMB is really a packed bed, and the packed sections are designed as packed beds. The regions between packed sections and the valve network shown in Figures 10-16 and 10-17 have to be designed to minimize extracolumn volume and mixing. Because it is a fixed bed, the SMB will filter out suspended solids and eventually clog if there are suspended solids in the feed. The moving bed systems all have the advantage that some suspended material can be processed.

10.6 SUMMARY – OBJECTIVES

The purpose of this chapter was to introduce you to moving bed and simulated moving bed adsorption systems. At the end of this chapter you should be able to meet the following objectives.

1. Explain how the following processes work.

   a. Staged moving bed system with downcomers.

   b. Intermittantly operated sieve trays without downcomers.

   c. Asahi and Chem-Seps processes.

   d. Simulated counter-current system.

2. Use the linear solute movement theory to explain adsorption separation techniques including:

    a. Moving bed systems.

    b. Pulsed moving bed systems.

    c. Simulated moving bed systems.

3. Use a stage model for design of staged moving bed systems and for approximate design of both continuous contact moving bed and simulated moving bed systems.

4. Use the mass transfer analysis to design isothermal moving bed systems.

REFERENCES

Anon., "Beaded carbon ups solvent recovery," *Chem. Eng., 39* (Aug. 29, 1977).

Arden, T.V., *Water Purification by Ion Exchange,* Butterworths, London, 1968.

Berg, C., "Hypersorption design. Modern advancements," *Chem. Eng. Prog., 47,* 585 (1951).

Bonsal, R.C., J.-B. Donnet, and F. Stoeckli, *Active Carbon*, Marcel Dekker, New York, 1988.

Brian, P.L.T., *Staged Cascades in Chemical Processing*, Prentice-Hall, Englewood Cliffs, NJ, 1972.

Broughton, D.B., "Production-scale adsorptive separations of liquid mixtures by simulated moving bed technology," *Separ. Sci. Technol., 19,* 723 (1984-85).

Burns, M.A. and D.J. Graves, "Continuous affinity chromatography using a magnetically stabilized fluidized bed," *Biotechnology Progress, 1* (2), 95 (1985).

539

Burns, M.A. and D.J. Graves, "Application of magnetically stabilized fluidized beds to bioseparations," *Reactive Polymers, 6*, 45 (1987).

Cloethe, F.L.D., "Comparative engineering and process features of operating continuous ion exchange plants in South Africa," in Naden, D. and Streat, M. (Eds.), *Ion Exchange Technology*, Ellis Horwood Pub., Chichester, England, 1984, 661-678.

Dechow, F.J., *Separation and Purification in Biotechnology*, Noyes, Park Ridge, NJ, 1989.

Dodds, R., P.I. Hudson, L. Kershenbaum, and M. Streat, "The operation and modelling of a periodic countercurrent, solid-liquid reactor," *Chem. Eng. Sci., 28*, 1233 (1973).

Ermenc, E.D., "Designing a fluidized adsorber," *Chem. Eng., 68*, (11), 87, (1961).

Ford, M.A., "The simulation and process design of NIMCIX contactors for the recovery of uranium," in D. Naden and M. Streat (Eds.), *Ion Exchange Technology*, Ellis Horwood Pub., Chichester, England, 1984, p. 668 to 678.

Higgins, I.R. and R.C. Chopra, "Municipal waste effluent treatment," in C. Calmon and H. Gold (Eds.), *Ion Exchange for Pollution Control*, Vol. II, CRC Press, Boca Raton, FL, 1979, Chapt. 7.

Hutchins, R.A., "Development of design parameters," in J.R. Perrich (Ed.), *Activated Carbon Adsorption for Wastewater Treatment.* CRC Press, Boca Raton, FL, 1981, Chapt. 4A.

Liapis, A.I. and D.W.T. Rippin, "The simulation of binary adsorption in continuous counter-current operation and a comparison with other operating modes," *AIChE Journal, 25*, 455 (1979).

Lochmuller, C.H., C.S. Ronsick, and L.S. Wigman, "Fluidizied bed separators reviewed: A low pressure drop approach to column chromatography," *Preparative Chromatography*, *1*, 93 (1988).

Lucchesi, P.J., W.H. Hatch, F.X. Mayer, and R.E. Rosensweig, "Magnetically stabilized beds. New gas solids contacting technology," Proc. 10th World Petroleum Congress, Vol. 4, SP-4, Heyden & Sons, Philadelphia, 1979, 49.

Naden, D. and M. Streat (Eds.), *Ion Exchange Technology*, Ellis Horwood Pub., Chichester, England, 1984.

Neuzil, R.W. and R.H. Jensen, "Development of the Sarex process for the separation of saccharides," paper 22d, AIChE meeting, Philadelphia, PA (June 6, 1978).

Rodrigues, A. (Ed.), *Ion Exchange: Science and Technology*, Martinus Nijhoff Pub., Dordrecht, The Netherlands, 1986.

Rosensweig, R.E., "Magnetic stabilization of the state of uniform fluidization," *Ind. Eng. Chem. Fundam.*, *18*, 260 (1979).

Ruthven, D.M., *Principles of Adsorption and Adsorption Processes*, Wiley-Interscience, New York, 1984, Chapt. 12.

Ruthven, D.M. and C.B. Ching, "Counter-current and simulated counter-current adsorption separation processes," *Chem. Eng. Sci.* *44*, 1011 (1989).

Slater, M.J., "Recent industrial-scale applications of continuous resin ion exchange systems," *J. Separ. Proc. Technol.*, *2* (3), 2 (1981).

Storm, D.W., "Contacting systems," in J.R. Perrich (Ed.), *Activated Carbon Adsorption for Wastewater Treatment*, CRC Press, Boca Raton, FL, 1981, Chapter 5.

Storti, G., M. Masi, and M. Morbidelli, "On countercurent adsorption separation processes," in A.E. Rodrigues et al (Eds.), *Adsorption: Science and Technology*, Kluwer Academic Publishers, The Netherlands, 1989, 357-381.

Streat, M., "Recent developments in continuous ion exchange," *J. Separ. Proc. Technol., 1* (3), 10 (1980).

Treybal, R.E., *Mass Transfer Operations,* 3rd ed., McGraw-Hill, New York, 1980.

van der Wiel, J.P. and J.A. Wesselingh, "Continuous adsorption in biotechnology," in A.E. Rodrigues et al (Eds.), *Adsorption: Science and Technology*, Kluwer Academic Publishers, The Netherlands, 1989.

Wankat, P.C., *Large Scale Adsorption and Chromatography*, CRC Press, Boca Raton, FL, 1986.

Wankat, P.C., *Equilibrium-Staged Separations,* Elsevier, New York, 1988

Wesselingh, J.A. and A.P. van der Meer, "Counter-current ion exchange," in A. Rodrigues, (Ed.), *Ion Exchange: Science and Technology,* Martinus Nijhoff Publishers BV, Dordrecht, The Netherlands, 1986, 289-318.

HOMEWORK

A.   *Discussion Problems*

A1.   In your own words explain how the intermittant transfer system shown in Figure 10-2 gives counter-current flow. What advantages might this method of operation have compared to using continuous fluidized beds.

A2.   In your own words explain how a simulated counter-current system works. Why does the separation become better as each zone is divided into more column sections?

A3.   Study Figure 10-18. Relate solute movement in Figure 10-18 to zones in Figure 10-13 and to concentration profiles shown in Figure 10-19.

A4.   Relate Eqs. (10-21) and (10-22) to Figures 10-13 and 10-18.

A5.   Show how to include a Murphree efficiency based on the fluid phase in Figures 10-5a and 10-5b.

A6.   Show that the units in Eq. (10-2) are correct for a solute mass balance.

A7.   Explain why the curvature of the isotherms in Figures 10-5a and 10-5b are the opposite of those shown in Figures 6-3b and d even though they could represent the same adsorption system.

A8.   Write a time schedule for switching the valves in Figure 10-17 to simulate a moving bed.

A9.   Sketch a system similar to Figure 10-17, but with 8 columns (2 per zone). Explain the time schedule used for switching the valves. What are the advantages and disadvantages of this system compared to Figure 10-17?

A10. Despite considerable research and development on moving bed and simulated moving bed systems, packed bed adsorbers and chromatographs remain much more common. Discuss why packed beds are more commonly used.

A11. The Cloethe-Streat design for intermittant countercurrent flow of solids and fluid is used commercially for ion exchange processing of uranium solutions. What are the advantages of this design compared to using packed beds? What are the advantages of this designed compared to using a column with sieve trays and downcomers?

A12. Film mass transfer rates in fluidized beds are usually *lower* than those in packed beds. Explain why.

A13. Develop your key relations chart for this chapter.

C. *Derivations*

C1. Derive the solute movement diagram for simulated countercurrent motion if the observer fixes his frame of reference at one of the product ports. (Remember that the product port shifts location every few minutes).

C2. Convert the Kremser equation to the appropriate units for a staged adsorber with a linear isotherm.

C3. (Challenging!) The staged and solute movement theories agree qualitatively. Show that this is true for complete removal of a single solute in a moving bed system for linear isotherms.

    Hint: Start by comparing the slopes of the operating and equilibrium lines in Figure 10-5a to achieve $Y_1 \sim 0$.

C4. Derive the equation to relate Y to c.

C5. Expand Eqs. (10-21) and (10-22) or Eqs. (10-24) and (10-25) to include the concentration dependence of the solute velocities. Using a typical favorable equilibrium isotherm, explain why satisfaction of this set of equations is more difficult for nonlinear systems than for linear systems.

D. *Single Answer Problems*

D1. A staged adsorber (as shown in the top section of Figure 10-1) is used to adsorb propane from hydrogen on a silica gel at 40°C. The adsorber operates at a total pressure of 2 atmospheres. Inlet silica gel is pure ($q = 0$). Inlet gas is 0.10 mole fraction propane. Outlet gas should contain 0.005 mole fraction propane. Use a $S/G = 1.5 \times (S/G)_{min}$, and determine the number of equilibrium stages required. S = kg/hr clean silica gel, G = kg/hr of H_2.

    Equilibrium data was given in Problem 6-D1 for a single porosity model.

D2. A Cloethe-Streat intermittant contact fluidized bed system is to be used for recovery of U_3O_8 on a strong acid resin initially in the H^+ form.

The feed is 0.10 g/liter of U_3O_8 in aqueous solution. An outlet concentration of 0.002 g/l is desired. The recycled resin from the elution column contains 1.0 g/liter of U_3O_8. Equilibrium data (Ford, 1984) are given below,

c,g/l	0.0030	0.0111	0.0330	0.0560	0.1010
c_R, g/l	8.2	14.7	25.0	30.6	38.0

If (liquid flow rate, liter/hr)/(solid flow rate, liter/hr) = 300, find

  a. The outlet concentration of the resin.

  b. The number of equilibrium stages required (Assume the flows are continuous).

D3. We wish to use a DEAE Sephadex A-50 ion exchanger to sorb bovine serum albumin in a batch stirred tank system. The tank is charged with 10 kg of dry resin which is initially clean. The total liquid charge is 60,000 kg and is 1.2×10^{-3} weight fraction protein which is 1.2 mg protein/g solution in an aqueous solution. Find the final concentration in the tank and on the resin after equilibrium is attained. Equilibrium data is given in Example 6-1. What fraction of the protein is recovered on the resin?

D4. A staged contractor is being used to soften water. The feed contains 2.0 meq/L Ca^{+2} and 9.0 meq/L Na^+. A strong acid resin with $c_{RT} = 1.7$ eq/L is used. A Murphree stage efficiency based on liquid concentrations of 80% is expected. The system has four real stages. Entering resin is entirely in the Na^+ form. We desire an outlet product which is 0.01 meq/L Ca^{+2}. What ratio (liquid flow rate/solids flow rate) is required?
Equilibrium data is available in Table 9-2.

D5. The resin from Example 10-1 is regenerated in a staged contactor with 4 equilibrium stages. The inlet resin concentration is $q_0 = 4.52$ g/L while outlet is $q_N = 0.25$ g/L. Entering solution is pure hot water. At the higher temperature of operation equilibrium is $q = 0.05$ c. What value of V_R/V_S is required?

D6.   Example 10-2 presented one set of data from Burns and Graves (1987). For another experiment under different condtions they found:

Feed concentration = 1.0 mg HSA/ml solution

Input solutes = 0 mg HSA/g solids

Fluid flowrate = 10.0 ml/min

Solids flowrate = 0.5 g/min

$$K = \frac{L}{S} \frac{k_d}{k_a} = 3.1$$

% HSA adsorbed = 25%

Bed length, h = 5.0 cm

Find NTU and HTU. Speculate on why HTU increased.

D7.   We wish to regenerate calcium alginate beads which contain human serum albumin (HSA) in a moving bed column. Regeneration is done by changing pH and ionic strength so that equilibrium is linear and becomes $m = c/q = 1.2$. The inlet regenerant is pure, $c_{in} = 0$ mg HSA/ml and inlet solids have $q_{in} = 2.24$ mg HSA/g adsorbent. Solids flow rate $S = 0.5$ g/min and $L = 1.0$ ml/min. We desire $q_{out} = 0.05$ mg HSA/g adsorbent. HTU = 10.0 cm. Find the height of the column and c_{out} in mg HSA/ml.

Note: This problem represents the regeneration of the beads from Example 10-2.

D8.   A 4 zone SMB is being used to separate pyrene and anthracene. The system will have one column per zone. Each of the 4 columns is 150 cm long. The value of $t_p = 937.5$ s. $\varepsilon_e = 0.37$. Measurements in a packed bed give solute velocities: $u_p = 0.0664$ v and $u_A = 0.1066$ v. Isotherms are linear. The following superficial velocities are used:

$$v_{super,3} = 1.0 \text{ cm/s}, \ v_{super,2} = 0.666 \text{ cm/s},$$

$$v_{super,1} = 0.814, \ v_{super,4} = 0.444$$

a.   Does this satisfy Eqs. (10-24) and (10-25)?

b.   Determine the time required and the distance travelled for pyrene and anthracene to exit the SMB.

c.   Determine the product velocities where $v_{Prod} = P/\rho_f A_c$.

546

D9. We wish to fluidize a polystyrene-sulfonic acid ion exchange resin. The spherical beads have a diameter of 0.7 mm. The resin density is 0.82 g/cm^3 when they are wet but have been drained. $\chi = 0.75$. Fluid is water at 25°C where $\rho_f \sim 1.0$ g/cm^3 and $\mu = 0.94$ cp. The acceleration due to gravity at sea level is $g = 980$ cm/s^2.

Calculate:　　a. Reference velocity and diameter

　　　　　　　b. d*

　　　　　　　c. $v_{settling}$

　　　　　　　d. If $v_{super} = 2.0$ cm/s and $v_{solids} = 0$, determine e.

F. *Problems Requiring Other Resources*

F1. The hypersorption process is an interesting historical example of a process which was used commercially, but is now obsolete. Study the hypersorption process (Berg, 1951; Treybal, 1980; Wankat, 1986) and write a report on this process. In your report answer the following questions:

Why is the process no longer used?

What were the major problems with hypersorption?

Could modern adsorbents or techniques be used to make hypersorption competitive?

If you were employed by a major petroleum or petrochemical company, would you recommend a major research program to develop a modern hypersorber?

Why or why not?

NOMENCLATURE CHAPTER 11

a	angle in two-dimensional system (Figure 11-7b)
c	solute concentration
$c_{i,o}$	bulk molar concentration
C_p	specific heat
D_{eff}	effective axial dispersion coefficient, cm^2/s
e	electron charge, 1.602×10^{-19} coulombs
E	electric field strenght, volts/m
f_c	friction coefficient
F	force, Newtons
F	Faraday's constant
g	acceleration due to gravity, m^2/s
Gr	Grashof number, Eq. (11-12)
h	characteristic length, e.g. R_p or 1/2 distance beteen plates, m
I	current, amps
k	Boltzmann constant, 1.386×10^{-23} J/K
k_T	thermal conductivity
L	distance traveled, Eq. (11-32)
L	length, m
n_i	maximum number of peaks in development direction i
n_{2D}	maximum number of peaks in two-dimensional development
N	number of plates
N_A	Avagadro's number, 6.02×10^{23}

p	$-d\mu/dz$, Eq. (11-44)
P	power, watts
Q	net charge, coulomb
r	radial direction, m
R	resolution
R	resistance, ohms
Ra	Rayleigh number, Eq. (11-12)
R_p	radius, m
t	time,s
t_{exper}	time of experiment, s
T	absolute temperature, K
u	migration velocity, cm/s
u_{osm}	electroosmosis velocity
u_s	solute velocity from Eq. (6-22)
v_{buffer}	buffer velocity, cm/s
V	voltage, volts
W	width, m
y	direction between electrodes
$y_{i,net}$	net lateral movement, Eq. (11-33)
$y_{recycle}$	distance recycle stream shifted
Y_i	location of peak center
z_i	valence
Z_i	migration distance or location of peak center

Greek

β	coefficient volumetric expression, Eq. (11-11)
ΔR_p	shear boundary is at $R_p + \Delta R_p$
ΔT	characteristic temperature difference, K
ε	dielectric constant of medium
ε_o	permittivity free space, $8.85 \times 10^{-12}\ C^2/Jm$
ζ	zeta potential, value ψ at $R_p + \Delta R_p$
ζ_{wall}	zeta potential of wall
η	viscosity
κ	Debye-Huckel constant, Eq. (11-6), m^{-1}
λ_i	ionic equivalent conductivity, Eq. (11-9d)
μ	electrophoretic mobility, m^2/Vs
μ_{osm}	electrophoretic mobility of layer next to wall
ρ	fluid density, kg/m^3
$\bar{\rho}$	average fluid density
σ_c	electric conductivity, $(ohm \cdot cm)^{-1}$
$\sigma_{l,i}$	standard deviation in length units for component i
ψ	electrical potential
ψ_o	electric potential at surface of particle

Chapter 11

ELECTROPHORETIC SEPARATION METHODS

Electrophoresis is a method which uses the different migration rates of charged molecules or particles in an electric field for separation. The method was first developed by Arne Tiselius (1937) who received the Nobel prize in 1948 because of the tremendous impact of electrophoresis on biochemical separations. A large number of variants of electrophoresis have been developed and will be introduced in this chapter. These methods are used extensively for laboratory scale biochemical separations such as protein and polynucleotide separations. Despite numerous efforts, scale-up has had minimal success mainly because of thermal convection caused by Joule heating of the system.

First, the basic concepts and theory of electrophoresis will be presented followed by a discussion of phenomenon which complicate the simple picture. Then, some of the wide variety of electrophoresis processes will be briefly explained and possibilities for scale-up will be explored. Isotachophoresis which is essentially a displacement chromatography version of electrophoresis will be explained theoretically and scale-up will be discussed. Isoelectric focusing which has developed as a separate technique will be explained. Finally, electrochromatography will be briefly described. Chapter 7 is a prerequisite for this chapter since chromatographic approaches to zone spreading will be used. Since electrophoretic methods are not currently used on a large-scale, this chapter should be considered a progress report.

11.1. THEORY OF ELECTROPHORESIS

The theory of electrophoresis is well understood, but can rapidly become quite complex. We will first start with a physical picture of the basic reasons why

550

Table 11-1. SI Units for Electrical Terms

Charge, Q:	Coulomb (C) = Amp · second
	Coulomb = Joule/volt = Nm/V
Dielectric constant, ε:	dimensionless
Electric field, E:	Volt/meter
Energy:	Joule (J) = Newton meter
Force, F:	Newton (N) = kg m/s^2
Power, P:	Watt (W) = Joule/second
Pressure, p:	Pascal (Pa) = N/m^2
Viscosity, η:	Pascal·second = Ns/m^2
Permittivity free space:	$\varepsilon_o = 8.85 \times 10^{-12}$ C^2/Jm
Coulomb's law:	$F = \dfrac{1}{4\pi\varepsilon_0}\dfrac{Q\,Q'}{\varepsilon r^2}$

electrophoresis works. Then a simplified mathematical treatment of the forces involved in electrophoresis will be presented, and finally the complicating factors which reduce the separation will be identified.

We will use SI units for electrical terms. Great care must be taken when comparing with equations in other units since the equations may differ. Some of the SI conversions are listed in Table 11-1. The proportionality factor $1/(4\pi\varepsilon_0)$ for Coulomb's law is required for SI units, but does not occur in other units.

11.1.1. Basic Concepts of Electrophoresis

Electrophoresis is essentially based on different rates of migration in an electric field. Charged molecules or particles have a force exerted on them by the electric field. If the net charge on the particle is Q, then the force is QE where E is the electric field strength. Because of this force, the particle will accelerate towards one of the electrodes. Particles with a net positive charge move towards the cathode (the negative pole) while particles with a net negative charge move towards the anode (the positive pole). The acceleration caused by this electrophoretic attraction is opposed by friction, electrophoretic retardation and a relaxation effect. At steady state the sum of the forces is zero and the particle moves at a constant migration velocity u. This is usually written as

$$u = \mu E \qquad (11\text{-}1)$$

where the migration velocity u is in m/s or cm/s, the field strength E is in volts/m or volts/cm, and the electrophoretic mobility μ is in m^2/volt·s or cm^2/volt·s. The electrophoretic mobility can be either positive or negative depending upon the sign of the net charge on the molecule. The essential purpose of the theory is to predict μ.

Electrophoresis is useful for separating a variety of biochemicals because these molecules have net charges. For example, the general formula for an amino acid is

$$NH_2 - \underset{\underset{R}{|}}{C} - COOH$$

where R is a functional group. At low pH values the α-amino group will be in the protonated form, NH_3^+, while at high pH values the carboxylic acid group will be in the form COO^-. Since both groups can be ionized simultaneously, the amino acid can have a positive, negative or neutral charge. In addition, the R group may be charged (see Lehninger, 1970, for details). Amino acids are the basic building block of proteins; thus, a protein will usually contain a large number of positive and negative charges. The net charge on the protein will determine which electrode the protein migrates towards. There is one pH value where the net charge on the protein is zero and $\mu = 0$. This is the isoelectric point or pI of the protein. A short list of pI values for amino acids and proteins is given in Table 11-2. Isoelectric focusing uses a pH gradient in the column and focuses each protein at its isoelectric point.

A second major group of biochemicals which are often separated by electrophoresis are the polynucleotides such as RNA and DNA. These molecules are phosphoric acid esters of 5-carbon sugars with a base attached.

There are only five principal bases in polynucleotides all of which are purines or pyrimidines (see Lehninger, 1970 for details). Since the phosphate groups are usually very negatively charged, the polynucleotides usually migrate to the anode. The polynucleotides often have an almost constant charge-to-size ratio, and thus sieving gels are used to utilize frictional forces (see Section 11.2.2.).

Table 11-2. Molecular Weights and Isoelectric Points
(Blackshear, 1984; Lehninger, 1970; Reeder, 1987; Righetti, 1983)

Compound	Mol. Wt.	pI(25°C)
Aspartic Acid		2.77
L-glutamic acid		3.22
β-aspartyl-histidine		4.94
Triglycine		5.59
Histidine		7.47
Lysine		9.74
Arginine		10.76
Ovalbumin	43,000-45,000	4.70
Bovine albumin	68,000	4.95 ± 0.02 (4°C)
β-Lactoglobulin	18,400	5.14 (A)/5.39 (B)
		5.45 ± .02 (B at 4°C)
Mysosin	2,000,000–2,120,000	6.2 – 6.6
Myglobin (horse)	16,950–17,800	7.33 ± 0.01
		7.58 ± 0.02 (4°C)
Ribonuclease	13,700	8.88 ± 0.03
Cytochrome c	11,700-12,500	9.28 ± 0.02
Human fetal brain cells		4.38
Escherichia coli		5.6
Normal liver cells		6.5

11.1.2. Forces in Electrophoresis

A relatively simple theory of electrophoresis can be developed by considering a force balance. The development given here will follow that of Hiemenz (1986) while more detailed analyses are given by Overbeek and Bijsterbosch (1979) and O'Brien and White (1978).

The force which causes electrophoretic migration is the electrophoretic attraction force.

$$\text{Electrophoretic Attraction} = QE \tag{11-2}$$

where Q is the net charge on the molecule or the particle. The primary force which deaccelerates the particle is the friction force

$$\text{Friction Force} = -f_c \, u \tag{11-3a}$$

where f_c is the friction coefficient. For spherical particles at very low Reynolds numbers in free liquids f_c can be determined from Stokes law

$$f_c = 6 \pi \eta R_p \tag{11-3b}$$

where η is the viscosity of the medium and R_p is the radius of the particle or molecule. In stabilizing media such as gels or paper f_c needs to be determined experimentally.

For isolated ions we can set the sum of these two forces to zero. Solving for velocity, we have

$$u = \frac{Q E}{f_c} \tag{11-4a}$$

which for spherical ions is

$$u = \frac{Q E}{6 \pi \eta R_p} \tag{11-4b}$$

Since the charge on an ion is $Q = z\,e$ where e is the electron charge, 1.602×10^{-19} coulombs, and z is the valence, Eq. (11-4b) become

$$u = \frac{z\,e\,E}{6\,\pi\,\eta\,R_p} \qquad (11\text{-}4c)$$

Comparing Eqs. (11-4c) and (11-1), we obtain the mobility of an isolated ion

$$\mu = \frac{z\,e}{6\,\pi\,\eta\,R_p} \qquad (11\text{-}4d)$$

Note that viscosity should be in Pa·s (Ns/m^2) = 0.001 centipoise so that units work.

For charged colloidal particles the picture is significantly more complicated, and there are additional forces. (See Hiemenz, 1986, for a detailed explanation). In order to carry an appreciable current there must be small electrolytes in solution. The electric field exerts a force on these ions; however, since the ions are quite small and are hydrated the force is transferred to the water. This causes an electroosmotic flow of water with respect to the particles which retards the particle movement. To determine this *electrophoretic retardation force* we must look at the environment of large charged molecules or particles. This environment is shown schematically in Figure 11-11 for a negatively charged spherical particle (the picture will be similiar for a positively charged particle). To have electroneutrality the negatively charged particle must have an appropriate number of positively charged ions associated with it. These positively charged counterions distribute around the particle. The conbination of negative and positive charges is called the *double layer*. The electrical potential has a value ψ_o at the particle surface. However, there is a layer of liquid one or two molecules thick which is bound to the particle and moves with the particle. The fluid starts to move at the *shear boundary* ($R_p + \Delta R_p$ in Figure 11-1). The potential has a value ζ (the *zeta potential*) at the shear boundary. The zeta potential is the value observed in experiments and ζ controls the electrophoretic mobility of particles. Usually ζ is measured by measuring the electrophoretic mobility of the particles.

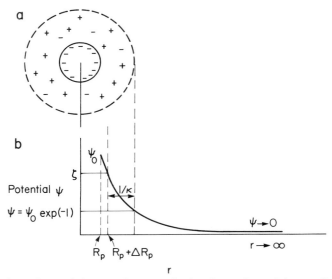

Figure 11-1.   Potential around a negatively charged particle. a. Schematic.
b. Potentials at different values of κ.

The zeta potential is unknown but is proportional to the electric potential
at the surface of the sphere ψ_o. The electrical potential drops from a value of
ψ_o at the surface of the particle to zero at an infinite distance according to the
Poisson-Boltzmann distribution

$$\psi = \psi_o \exp\left[-\kappa\left(r-R_p\right)\right] \tag{11-5a}$$

which is shown in Figure 11-1b. The potential at the surface of the sphere, ψ_o,
is

$$\psi_o = \frac{Q}{4\,\pi\,\varepsilon_o\,\varepsilon\,R_p} \tag{11-5b}$$

where Q is the total charge on the particle and SI units are being used. The
term κ

$$\kappa = \left[\frac{1000\,e^2\,N_A\sum\left(c_{i,o}\,z_i^2\right)}{\varepsilon_o\,\varepsilon\,k\,T}\right]^{\!\frac{1}{2}} \tag{11-6}$$

is the Debye-Huckel constant. The summation term is twice the ionic strength. In this equation e is the elementary charge which is 1.602×10^{-19} coulombs, N_A is Avogadro's number 6.02×10^{23}, $c_{i,o}$ is the bulk molar concentration of the ion, z is the charge number of the ions including the sign, ε is the dielectric constant of the medium, k is the Boltzmann constant, 1.38066×10^{-23} J/K, T is the absolute temperature, and $\varepsilon_o = 8.85 \times 10^{-12}$ Coulomb^2/Joule m. The units of κ are m^{-1}. This can be seen by writing out the SI units in Eq. (11-6).

$$\kappa = \left[\frac{(1000 \frac{L}{m^3}) (C)^2 (\frac{1}{mole}) (\frac{mole}{L})}{(C^2/Jm) \left[\frac{J}{K} \right] K} \right]^{\frac{1}{2}} = m^{-1}$$

The thickness of the double layer is imprecisely set at $1/\kappa$ (see Figure 11-1b). Then κR_p is the ratio of the particle diameter to the thickness of the double layer. Typical values of $1/\kappa$ in aqueous solution are (Overbeek and Bijsterbosch, 1979): $c = 10^{-5}M$, $1/\kappa = 1.0 \times 10^{-7}m$; $c = 10^{-3}M$, $1/\kappa = 1.0 \times 10^{-8}m$, and $c = 10^{-1}M$, $1/\kappa = 1.0 \times 10^{-9}m$.

The electrophoretic retardation force can be determined several different ways. The general solution first developed by Henry is

$$\text{Electrophoretic Retardation Force} = \left[4\pi \varepsilon_0 \varepsilon \zeta R_p f(\kappa R_p) - Q \right] E \qquad (11\text{-}7a)$$

Values for $f(\kappa R_p)$ at various values of ζ are given by Hiemenz (1986). For small particles with $\kappa R_p < 0.1$ this simplifies to Huckel's solution.

$$\text{Electrophoretic Retardation Force} = \left[4\pi \varepsilon_0 \varepsilon \zeta R_p - Q \right] E \qquad (11\text{-}7b)$$

For large particles with $\kappa R_p > 100$ Henry's solution simplifies to Smoluchowski's solution

$$\text{Electrophoretic Retardation Force} = \left[(1.5) 4\pi \varepsilon_0 \varepsilon \zeta R_p - Q \right] E \qquad (11\text{-}7c)$$

There is a fourth force which occurs because the double layer is distorted since the charged particle and the ion atmosphere move in opposite directions. The distorted atmosphere exerts a force on the particle which is known as the *relaxation effect*. If we are willing to assume that the relaxation effect is negligible, we can easily determine μ. This assumption is usually made in simplified treatments, but more exact numerical solutions include the relaxation effect (Overbeek and Bijsterbosch, 1979). We sum Eqs. (11-2) and (11-7), and solve for μ. The general result is

$$\mu = \frac{u}{E} = \frac{4\pi\,\varepsilon_0\,\varepsilon\,\zeta\,R_p}{f_c}\,f(\kappa\,R_p) \tag{11-8a}$$

while if $\kappa R_p < 0.1$ we obtain

$$\mu = \frac{4\pi\,\varepsilon_0\,\varepsilon\,\zeta\,R_p}{f_c} \tag{11-8b}$$

and if $\kappa R_p > 100$ we obtain

$$\mu = \frac{6\pi\,\varepsilon_0\,\varepsilon\,\zeta\,R_p}{f_c} \tag{11-8c}$$

For free solution systems at low Reynolds numbers Eq. (11-3) can be inserted for f_c in Eqs. (11-8). The general result is

$$\mu = \frac{u}{E} = \frac{2\,\varepsilon_0\,\varepsilon\,\zeta\,f(\kappa\,R_p)}{3\,\eta} \tag{11-9a}$$

while if $\kappa\,R_p < 0.1$ we have

$$\mu = \frac{2\,\varepsilon_0\,\varepsilon\,\zeta}{3\,\eta} \tag{11-9b}$$

and if $\kappa\,R_p > 100$ we obtain

$$\mu = \frac{\varepsilon_0\,\varepsilon\,\zeta}{\eta} \tag{11-9c}$$

Note that some references present these equations in cgs units. The cgs result can be obtained by dividing Eqs. (11-9) by $4\,\pi\,\varepsilon_0$.

559

Table 11-3. Mobilities in Aqueous Solution
(Everaerts et al, 1976; Karol and Karol, 1978)

Ion	μ, cm^2/Vs
H^+	36.2×10^{-4}
C_s^+	8.13×10^{-4}
Rb^+	8.03×10^{-4}
K^+	7.67×10^{-4}
NH_4^+	7.6×10^{-4}
$CH_3NH_3^+$	6.0×10^{-4}
$(CH_3)_2NH_2^+$	5.4×10^{-4}
$(CH_3)_3NH^+$	4.8×10^{-4}
$(CH_3)_4 N^+$	4.7×10^{-4}
Li^+	4.02×10^{-4}
$(C_2H_5)_4 N^+$	3.6×10^{-4}
$(C_4H_9)_4 N^+$	2.0×10^{-4}
NO_3^-	-7.4×10^{-4}
Cl^-	-7.9×10^{-4}
Br^-	-8.1×10^{-4}
OH^-	-20.5×10^{-4}

Typical values for μ in free solution are 5×10^{-4} cm^2/sV (5×10^{-8} m^2/sV) for small ions and 1×10^{-5} cm^2/sV (1×10^{-9} m^2/sV) for proteins. Table 11-3 lists values for small ions (Everaerts et al, 1976; Karol and Karol, 1978). Note that μ decreases as the size of the ion increases. Hydrogen and hydroxyl ions are unique in their high mobilities. For small ions mobilities are usually not reported in the literature. Instead, *ionic equivalent conductivities*, λ_i, are usually reported and are related to mobility by (Newman, 1973)

$$\lambda_i = |z_i| F^2 \mu_i \tag{11-9d}$$

where F is Faraday's constant, z_i is the charge number of species i, and λ_i is the ionic equivalent conductance, mho $\cdot$ cm^2/equiv.

From these equations we can deduce quite a bit about the electrophoretic behavior of a molecule or particle. From Eqs. (11-9) and (11-1) it is clear that particles are retarded by high viscosities, and particles with higher ζ potentials move faster. The dependence of the ζ potential on operating variables can be deduced from Eqs. (11-5a) to (11-6). Remember that ζ is the value of ψ at the shear boundary $(r=R_p+\Delta R_p)$. The value of ψ_o and hence ζ increases as the charge Q increases or the particle radius R_p decreases. For practical purposes ζ and hence μ and u are proportional to the charge to size ratio Q/R_p. Since the net charge Q on a molecule is very dependent on the pH, ζ, μ, and u are very dependent on pH. Both the thickness of the double layer, $1/\kappa$, and ζ decrease rapidly as the concentration or the valence of the electrolytes increase. Increasing temperature increases $1/\kappa$ and hence ζ and decreases the viscosity η, and thus both μ and u are increased. Of course, temperature is limited by the stability of the molecule and convection effects.

Example 11-1. Double Layer Thickness and Zeta Potential

a. Estimate the double layer thickness in a 0.005 M solution of NaCl at 25°C.

b. A 10^{-6}m diameter particle has a measured mobility of 1 $\times 10^{-9}$ m^2/sV in a 0.005 M aqueous solution of NaCl at 25°C. What is the value of ζ?

Solution

Part a. At 25°C, $\varepsilon = 78.30$ for water (Dean, 1985, 10-99).

$$\sum (c_i \, z_i^2) = c_{Na} \, (z_{Na})^2 + c_{Cl} \, (z_{Cl})^2 = 2 \, z^2 \, c = 2(1.0)^2 \, (0.005) = 0.01$$

Then, from Eq. (11-6)

$$\kappa = \left[\frac{(1000) \, (1.602 \times 10^{-19})^2 \, (6.02 \times 10^{23}) \, (0.01)}{(8.85 \times 10^{-12}) \, (78.30) \, (1.38066 \times 10^{-23}) \, (298.16)} \right]^{\frac{1}{2}}$$

which gives

$$\kappa = 2.327 \times 10^8 \text{ m}^{-1} \quad \text{and} \quad \frac{1}{\kappa} = 4.297 \times 10^{-9} \text{ m}$$

Part b. $\kappa R_p = (2.327 \times 10^8 \text{ m}^{-1}) \ (1 \times 10^{-6} \text{m}) = 232.7$
Use Eq. (11-9c). Rearranging, we have

$$\zeta = \frac{\mu \eta}{\varepsilon_0 \varepsilon}$$

For water at 25°C, $\eta = 0.890 \times 10^{-3} \ \frac{\text{N s}}{\text{m}^2}$ (Dean, 1985, p. 10-99).

$$\zeta = \frac{\left[0.89 \times 10^{-3} \ \dfrac{\text{N s}}{\text{m}^2}\right] (1 \times 10^{-9} \text{ m}^2/\text{sV})}{(8.85 \times 10^{-12} \text{ C}^2/\text{Jm}) \ (78.30)} = 0.001284 \ \frac{\text{N Jm}}{\text{V C}^2}$$

which is

$$\zeta = 0.001284 \ \frac{\text{J}^2}{\text{C}^2 \text{ V}} = 1.284 \times 10^{-3} \text{ V}$$

where we have used the conversions in Table 11-1.

It should be noted that it is important to check the units. Also, the stoichiometry and equilibrium of the dissociation must be considered when calculating $\sum (c_i \, z_i^2)$ for more complex ions.

11.1.3. Complicating Factors in Electrophoresis

Unfortunately, the operation of elecrophoretic separations is not as simple as the preceeding section may imply. The first complicating factor is Joule or resistance heating. The power generated in a resistance is

$$P = IV = I^2 R \tag{11-10}$$

where I is the current in amps, V is the voltage in volts, and R is the resistance in ohms. Then the power consumption P is in joules/sec = watts. This power is dissipated by heating the electrophoresis cell. This I^2R heating is undesireable since the local differences in temperature causes local differences in density and hence convection cells. In addition, large increases in temperature may destroy fragile biochemicals.

Convection caused by Joule heating can destroy the separation developed by different migration rates. The temperature gradient can be related to density changes by assuming that density is linear in temperature

$$\rho = \bar{\rho} - \bar{\rho} \beta \, (T - \bar{T}) \tag{11-11}$$

where β is the coefficient of volumetric expansion. The occurrence of thermal convection depends upon the value of the Rayleigh number (for example, see Ostrach, 1977).

$$Ra = \frac{\beta \, \bar{\rho}^2 \, C_p \, g \, h^3 \, \Delta T}{k_T \, \eta} = \frac{\bar{\rho} \, g \, C_p \, h^3 \, \Delta \rho}{k_T \, \eta} \tag{11-12}$$

The amount of convection depends upon the value of the Grashof number.

$$Gr = \frac{\bar{\rho}^2 \, \beta \, g \, h^3 \, \Delta T}{\eta^2} = \frac{\bar{\rho} \, g \, h^3 \, \Delta \rho}{\eta^2} \tag{11-13}$$

The second equation in both Eqs. (11-12) and (11-13) is obtained by substituting in Eq. (11-11). In these dimensionless groups $\bar{\rho}$ is the average fluid density, g is the acceleration due to gravity, h is a characteristic length such as the half distance between parallel plates or the pore radius, k_T is the thermal conductivity, C_p is the specific heat of the fluid, σ_c is the electrical conductivity in $1/(ohm-cm)$, and ΔT is a characteristic temperature difference. The Grashof number is the ratio of buoyancy to viscous forces while the Rayleigh number is the Prandtl number $(C_p \eta / k_T)$ times the Grashof number. For very small Rayleigh numbers there will be no convection, while for larger Rayleigh numbers convection occurs. The critical Rayleigh number depends on the geometry (Ostrach, 1977). The convection becomes stronger as the Grashof number increases.

Many ingenious methods have been developed to control or prevent convection. Efficient cooling helps reduce ΔT and prevents thermal degradation. Biochemicals are often electrophoresized near 4°C since they are stable at this temperature and water has a density maximum at 4°C which means that $\beta = 0$. Usually, the difference between plates is kept small (small h), or the electrophoresis is done in small tubes or in the pores of a gel, membrane, paper or capillary. Another method of keeping Ra and Gr small is to increase the viscosity η. Rotation of the apparatus or the fluid has been used as a way of stabilizing the fluid so that convection cells do not occur. The critical Rayleigh number is larger in horizontal equipment than in vertical equipment; thus, horizontal chambers can have the plates further apart and still not have convection (Ostrach, 1977). Finally, electrophoresis has been done in space where g is very small. Equipment to keep both Gr and Ra small is explored in Section 11.2. where a variety of different electrophoresis methods are explored.

The introduction of a gel or membrane to stop convection can add an additional complicating factor. This is *sieving* of the molecules or particles. The migration of molecules in a gel is hindered since the pores of the gel are not straight. If the pores are not a lot larger than the molecule there will be additional frictional forces between the molecule and the gel which will retard the migration of the molecule. The larger the molecule the more this sieving effect hinders the migration. If the molecule is too large it cannot enter the gel at all and u = 0. These sieving effects can be very helpful since they allow one to separate molecules with the same charge to size ratio. The application of sieving effects is discussed in Section 11.2.2.

Electroosmosis is another complicating factor in electrophoresis. Fixed charges on the chamber walls or on the gel are subject to a force because of the electric field. Since the charges are fixed, the fluid moves. This fluid movement is electroosmosis (Vanderhoff and Micale, 1979). The electroosmosis velocity can easily be calculated. For instance, for electrophoresis between two parallel walls which are charged, μ can be determined from Eq. (11-9c). Substituting this into Eq. (11-1), we obtain

$$u_{osm} = \mu_{osm} \, E = \frac{\varepsilon_o \, \varepsilon \, \zeta_{wall} \, E}{\eta} \qquad (11\text{-}14)$$

Equation (11-9c) is used because the wall can be considered as a particle with infinite radius and hence κR_p is very large. The effect of electroosmosis is to reduce the separation. The amount of reduction depends upon the geometry and will be discussed in Section 11.2. Electroosmosis can be reduced or eliminated by using walls or gels which have no residual charge. This can be done by coating the walls with a material such as methylcellulose which has a very low zeta potential.

11.2. METHODS FOR ELECTROPHORESIS

Electrophoresis has been blessed with a huge number of variants designed to avoid some of the problems discussed in the previous sections. Two major variants, Isotachophoresis and Isoelectric focusing, have to a large extent become considered as separate techniques. These methods are discussed in Sections 11.3 and 11.4. In this section a number of variants of the basic electrophoresis method will be discussed. Many of these methods are probably of interest only as analytical methods, and thus will be discussed rather briefly. Those methods which may have applications in large scale separations will be discussed in more detail.

11.2.1. Moving Boundary Electrophoresis

Moving boundary electrophoresis is the original method developed by Tiselius (1937) for separating proteins. It is now used mainly for measuring electrophoretic mobilities since more recent methods are easier to use and provide better separations. The apparatus is shown schematically in Figure 11-2. The cell is U-shaped with rectangular cross-section. Protein solution in buffer is initially added to one arm and the bottom of the cell while the other arm is filled with pure buffer solution. The voltage is applied and electrophoresis proceeds. Each protein migrates according to Eq. (11-1) where μ is determined by Eq. (11-9a, b, or c). Since the protein solution is denser than the buffer, the density gradient is stable and convection is prevented.

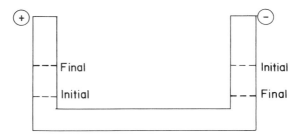

Figure 11-2.   Moving boundary electrophoresis.

Analysis is based on determining the migration of bands of different density. This is usually done by using an optical system which measures the deflection of light as it passes through liquid with a gradient of the index of refraction. The commonly used methods are schlieren and interference optics. These methods are specialized and expensive (for a brief introduction see Bier, 1974).

Only the fastest moving component in each direction can be recovered as a pure component. This limitation is one of the major reasons that moving boundary electrophoresis has been replaced by other electrophoretic methods. The chromatographic analog of moving boundary electrophoresis is frontal analysis which is also rarely used.

11.2.2. Gel, Membrane and Paper Electrophoresis

One common method of preventing convection is to do the electrophoresis in a stabilizing porous media such as a gel, a membrane, or on paper. These methods are usually operated as *zone electrophoresis* which is analogous to elution chromatography. Since zone electrophoresis is quite similiar regardless of the porous media used, we will explain the method for the most common approach which is gel electrophoresis. A laboratory gel electrophoresis cell is shown in Figure 11-3a. A thin layer of gel is polymerized onto a support plate. The gel is connected to the electrode compartments by filter paper bridges. The support plate, which is usually Mylar or glass, is placed on a coolant plate so

566

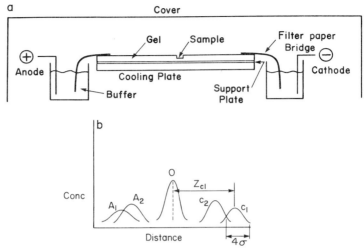

Figure 11-3. Zonal gel electrophoresis. a. Apparatus. b. Observed concentrations. A_1 and A_2 are anions, 0 = zero charge, C_1 and C_2 are cations.

that Joule heating can be removed. The gel layer is kept quite thin (usually less than 5mm) to have better heat dissipation and for increased mechanical strength. The entire apparatus is covered to control evaporation and for safety reasons (high voltages may be used). A variety of modifications to the basic apparatus are used, but they do not change the function of the device. These modifications include the use of vertical slabs or tubes, and two-dimensional methods (see Sections 11.2.5. and 11.2.6.).

In zonal gel electrophoresis a small sample is placed in a sample well in the center of the gel slab. When the current is turned on, the solute molecules start to migrate towards the anode or the cathode. Since the width of the feed sample is quite small, each solute migrates as a zone with a velocity u_i given by Eq. (11-1). The zones eventually become separated from each other. The operation is stopped before the fastest migrating species reaches the bridges to the electrode compartments. In analytical applications the products are often detected directly on the gel by UV absorbance, fluoresence, or other methods (see Andrews, 1986; or Melvin, 1987; or Righetti, 1983). For preparative applications the solutes need to be recovered from the gel. Recovery can be done by scrapping some of the gel into a beaker, by blotting onto paper, or by eluting electrophoretically or with flow. The final concentrations observed will have a Gaussian shape as shown in Figure 11-3b. (see Section 11.2.3).

The stabilizing media should have certain properties. It should be inert and not react with the species being separated. There should be no residual charges on the media since charges may ion exchange with the species being separated and will cause electroosmotic flow. The pores of the media must be at least as large as the molecules being separated or the molecules will not enter the media. If the pores are only slightly larger than the largest molecules being separated, then the larger molecules will be retarded by frictional forces and these molecules will no longer follow Stoke's law. However, this sieving effect is useful since sieving separates on the basis of size while electrophoresis without sieving separates on the basis of the charge to size ratio. To use sieving, gels with known and different pore sizes are polymerized.

The most common electrophoresis in use today is *polyacrylamide gel electrophoresis (PAGE)*. Polyacrylamide is an excellent anti-convective gel. It is easy to polymerize in place, and it can be polymerized with a variety of pore sizes. In addition, there is very little residual charge on the polymer. To make a PAGE plate, acrylamide (see Figure 11-4a) is polymerized directly as a slab on the support plate. The acrylamide is cross-linked with NN'methylene bisacrylamide (bis). An initiator such as ammonium or potassium persulphate and a catalyst such as N,N,N',N', tetramethylenediamine (TEMED) are required. The polymerization is a vinyl type polymerization which produces a random coil polymer. The pore size can be controlled by varying the total monomer concentration T (% acrylamide + % 'bis') or the degree of cross-linking C (% 'bis' / % T x 100). Reducing %T increases the pore size, but the maximum attainable size is about 80 nm. Gels more dilute than this become mechanically unstable. Pores also become larger if %C is increased to 30%C which corresponds to gels in the range of 200 to 250 nm. This is done at a constant %T which is often about 15w/v% acrylamide. The pores become larger at high crosslinker concentrations because a "bead-like" structure is formed instead of the usual three-dimensional lattice. Recipes for the gels and buffer solutions are

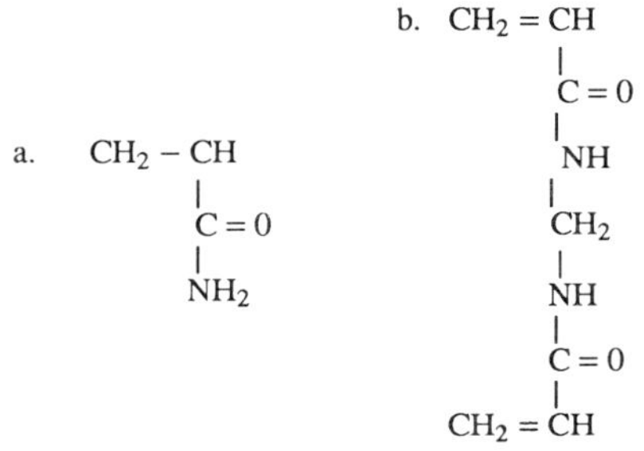

b. $CH_2 = CH$
$|$
$C = 0$
$|$
NH
$|$
CH_2
$|$
NH
$|$
$C = 0$
$|$
$CH_2 = CH$

a. $CH_2 - CH$
$|$
$C = 0$
$|$
NH_2

c. $CH_3 - (CH_2)_{10} - CH_2\ OSO_3^-\ NA^+$

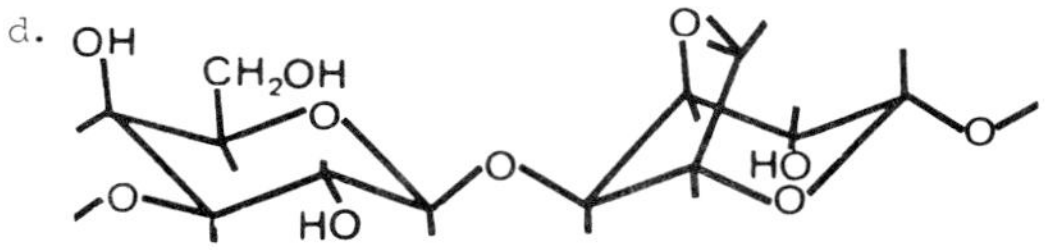

Figure 11-4. Chemicals used in gel electrophoresis. a. acrylamide monomer. b. NN' methylene bis acrylamide (bis.). c. Sodium dodecyl sulphate (SDS). d. Agarobiose (1,3 linked β-D galactopyranose and 1,4 linked 3,5 anhydro-α-L- galactopyranose).

given by Andrews (1986) and Blackshear (1984). The gel slab can be polymerized with a gradient in pore size so that molecules will slow down and eventually stop when they reach a limiting pore size. This is called *pore limit electrophoresis* (Gianazza and Righetti, 1979).

A modification of PAGE which is commonly used is to use a *stacking gel* which is also called *disc gel electrophoresis* (Ornstein, 1964; Davis 1964). In this case a very dilute stacking gel (2.5 w/v% acrylamide) is placed on top of the separating gel (15 % acrylamide) in a vertical tube. Thus the gel is discontinuous (disc). The sample is placed between a leading chloride buffer which migrates rapidly and a trailing glycinate buffer which migrates slowly. In the stacking gel this combination leads to the electrophoresis equivalent of displacement chromatography. (In other words isotachophoresis occurs in the stacking gel. The theory behind this method is explored in Section 11.3.) The sample is then concentrated in the stacking gel. The separating gel operates at a higher pH which causes the glycine to dissociate and hence move faster. In the separating gel the glycine move immediately behind the chloride and the sample molecules separate as in zone electrophoresis. Andrews (1986) and Blackshear (1984) give recipes for the gels and buffer solutions.

Another common method used for PAGE is to treat proteins with sodium dodecyl sulphate (SDS) (see Figure 11-4c). This method was first developed by Maizel (1966) and modern methods are spelled out by Andrews (1986) and Blackshear (1984). When a solution of proteins at pH 7 is treated with 1 w/v% SDS and 0.1M mercaptoethanol to destroy disulfide bonds, the polypeptide chain is unfolded and the protein is converted to a rod-like molecule. What is remarkable is that with very few exceptions 1.4 grams of SDS will be bound to each gram of protein. The result is that each protein is converted into a complex with the same charge-to-mass ratio, and all complexes have essentially the same electrophoretic mobilities in free solution. The SDS-protein complexes are different sizes and can be separated on the basis of protein size by using the sieving property of polyacrylamide gels. SDS-PAGE is commonly used as an analytical method and to estimate relative masses. The method is also used to look for subunits since breaking the disulphide bonds breaks apart subunits.

Other gels are also used for electrophoresis. Agarose gels are used because they can have larger pores than polyacrylamide gels and thus can separate larger molecules. Agarose is a polymer of D-galactose and 3,6 anhydrogalactose. The repeating unit in agarose, agarobiose, is shown in Figure 11-4d. The alternating sugar groups are substituted with sulphate, methoxyl, pyruvate, and carboxyl groups, and this substitution has a major effect on the gel properties. Chains are held together by hydrogen bonds. For vertical slabs an agarose concentration as low as 0.8 w/v% can be used. Molecules as large as 50×10^6 molecular weight can migrate into the gel. For horizontal slabs concentrations as low as 0.2 w/v% are mechanically stable and will admit molecules as large as 150×10^6 molecular weight into the gel. Agarose gels are commonly used for electrophoresis of DNA. The agarose gels do contain sulphate and carboxylic acid groups which are charged and can cause electroosmosis. This can be minimized with an alkali pretreatment. In addition, the properties of agarose gel are very temperature dependent and precise temperature control is important to obtain reproducible results. Agarose gels are used in pulsed electrophoresis which is discussed in Section 11.2.5. Polyacrylamide-agarose composite gels are sometimes used for electrophoresis of RNA, DNA, and large proteins. The composites have intermediate properties.

The first gel used for gel electrophoresis was starch (Smithies, 1955). Starch is cheap and easy to use, but is not commonly used today. It is difficult to control pore size with starch and there are negative side chains which can interact with the protein and cause electroosmotic flow. Recipes for starch gel electrophoresis are given by Andrews (1986).

Filter paper was the first anti-convective medium used for zone electrophoresis. The filter paper replaces the gel in Figure 11-3a. This method is convenient and simple, but has disadvantages. The paper has fixed negative charges which interact with proteins and cause electroosmotic flow. An advance over paper is the use of cellulose acetate membranes since the hydroxyl groups have been esterified. Cellulose acetate membranes are advantageous for analysis since the membrane can be made transparent with a mineral oil of the appropriate refractive index.

11.2.3. Zone Spreading in Zonal Electrophoresis

Zonal electrophoresis is similiar to elution chromatography. The linear zone spreading analysis of Section 7.6. has been extended to electrophoresis (Giddings, 1966; Jorgenson and Lukacs, 1981). A modification of their analyses will be presented here. For linear systems with a pulse of feed we expect a Gaussian solution such as Eq. (7-24). This is

$$c_i = c_{max,i} \exp \left[- \frac{(z - Z_i)^2}{2 \sigma_{l,i}^2} \right] \tag{11-15}$$

where $\sigma_{l,i}$ is the standard deviation of the electrophoresis system and Z_i is the location of the peak maximum. The width of the zone is then $4\sigma_{l,i}$. This is shown in Figure 11-3b. The net velocity observed by a molecule is the sum of electrophoretic migration and electroosmotic flow.

$$u_{net} = \mu E + \mu_{osm} \, E \qquad (11\text{-}16a)$$

For homogeneous solutions $E = V/L$ where L is also the maximum length of migration. Then Eq. (11-16a) becomes

$$u_{net} = \mu \, V/L + \mu_{osm} \, V/L \qquad (11\text{-}16b)$$

The migration or retention time for a species migrating an average distance Z_i is

$$t_{R,i} = Z_i/u_i = \frac{Z_i \, L}{(\mu_i + \mu_{osm}) \, V} = t_{exper} \qquad (11\text{-}17a)$$

where the migration distance is given by

$$Z_i = u_i \, t_{exper} = \left[\mu_i \, \frac{V}{L} + \mu_{osm} \, \frac{V}{L} \right] t_{exper} \qquad (11\text{-}17b)$$

Because batch electrophoresis is not normally run as an elution system, the retention time of all peaks is equal to the experimental time, t_{exper}, and is the same. If the peaks are eluted out the end of the column, then $Z_i = L$ and $t_{R,i} = L/u_i$.

The Einstein relationship for spreading due to diffusion can be extended to all the linear dispersion processes in the electrophoresis system.

$$\sigma_{l,i}^2 = 2 \, D_{eff,i} \, t_{R,i} = 2 \, D_{eff,i} \, t_{exper} \qquad (11\text{-}18)$$

where D_{eff} is the effective axial dispersion coefficient in the electrophoresis system. Combining Eqs. (11-17a) and (11-18), we obtain

$$\sigma_{l,i}^2 = \frac{2 \, D_{eff,i} \, Z_i \, L}{(\mu_i + \mu_{osm}) \, V} \qquad (11\text{-}19)$$

Equation (11-19) can be combined with Eq. (7-26b) with a migration distance Z_i to obtain,

$$N_i = Z_i^2/\sigma_i^2 = \frac{(\mu_i + \mu_{osm})VZ_i}{2D_{eff,i}\,L} = \frac{\left[\mu_i \dfrac{V}{L} + \mu_{osm} \dfrac{V}{L}\right]^2 t_{exper}}{2D_{eff,i}} \qquad (11\text{-}20)$$

Note that as long as the value of V/L is high a large N is achieved. The time of the experiment, t_{exper}, is usually set so that the fastest migrating species travels a distance L. This is often a dye added as a marker.

$$t_{exper} = \frac{L}{u_{max}} = \frac{L^2}{\left[\mu_{max} + \mu_{osm}\right]V} \qquad (11\text{-}21a)$$

Then Eq. (11-20) becomes

$$N_i = \frac{V}{2D_{eff,i}} \frac{(\mu_i + \mu_{osm})^2}{(\mu_{max} + \mu_{osm})} \qquad (11\text{-}21b)$$

This result is somewhat suprising since it says that the efficiency of the electrophoretic system (N_i) does not depend on the migration length Z_i. Note that if we let the marker dye determine L or t_{exper}, then the marker we choose helps determine N. Equation (11-21b) implies that the marker should have a mobility close to that of the sample. The easiest way to increase N in electrophoresis is to increase the applied voltage V.

Since N depends on the experimental time, a somewhat better comparison is the rate of generation of plates in plates/sec,

$$\text{Generation of plates} = \frac{N_i}{t_{exper}} = \frac{2D_{eff,i}}{\left[\mu_i \dfrac{V}{L} + \mu_{osm} \dfrac{V}{L}\right]^2} \qquad (11\text{-}22)$$

where Eq. (11-20) was used. The higher the generation of plates the more efficient the device is.

573

The resolution R between different zones can also be determined. Resolution is again defined by Eq. (7-30). Equation (7-33) gives a convenient way to determine R. Substituting Eqs. (11-20) and (11-16) into Eq. (7-30), we obtain

$$R = \frac{1}{4} \, \overline{N}^{1/2} \, \frac{\Delta u_s}{\overline{u}_s} = \frac{1}{4} \, \frac{V}{L} \left[\frac{t_{exper}}{2 \overline{D}_{eff}} \right]^{1/2} (\mu_1 - \mu_2) \qquad (11\text{-}23)$$

which simplifies when t_{exper} is given by Eq. (11-21a) to

$$R = \frac{1}{4} \left[\frac{V}{2 \overline{D}_{eff} \, (\mu_{max} + \mu_{osm})} \right]^{1/2} (\mu_1 - \mu_2) \qquad (11\text{-}24)$$

In these equation μ_i is the electrophoretic mobility of species i; and $\overline{\mu}$, $\overline{N}$, and $\overline{D}_{eff,i}$ are the arithmetic average values. Note that resolution can be increased by increasing V.

This analysis of zone spreading is also applicable to free-flow and capillary electrophoresis (see Section 11.2.4.).

Example 11-2. Batch Electrophoresis

A batch electrophoresis experiment is done in PAGE where $\mu_{osm} = 0$. The measured mobilities and diffusivities of the two proteins of interest are:

$$\mu_A = 1.050 \times 10^{-5}, \quad \mu_B = 1.033 \times 10^{-5} \text{ cm}^2/\text{Vs},$$

$$D_A = D_B = 1.5 \times 10^{-7} \text{ cm}^2/\text{s}$$

The experiment is run at E = 125 volts/cm for 2.5 hours. Assume the width of the feed well is very small. Determine the location of the peaks (distance from feed well), the peak widths, and the resolution of the two proteins.

Solution

This problem is a straight forward application of the theory developed in this section. The migration distance is:

$$Z_i = u_i \, t_{exper} = \mu_i \, E \, t_{exper}$$

which is

$$Z_A = (1.05 \times 10^{-5}) \, (125) \, (2.5 \text{ hr}) \left[\frac{3600 \text{ s}}{\text{hr}} \right] = 11.81 \text{ cm}$$

and

$$Z_B = (1.033 \times 10^{-5}) \, (125) \, (2.5) \, (3600) = 11.62 \text{ cm}$$

From Eq. (11-18),

$$\sigma_{l,i}^2 = 2 \, D_{eff} \, t_{R,i} = (2) \, (1.5 \times 10^{-7}) \, (2.5) \, (3600) = 0.0027 \text{ cm}^2$$

which gives $\sigma_{l,i} = 0.0520$ cm which is the same for both proteins.

$$\text{Width} = 4 \, \sigma_l = 4(0.052) = 0.208 \text{ cm}$$

Then From Eq. (11-23),

$$R = \frac{1}{4} \, \frac{V}{L} \left[\frac{t_{exper}}{2 \, D_{eff}} \right]^{\frac{1}{2}} (\mu_1 - \mu_2) = \frac{1}{4} \, E \left[\frac{t_{exper}}{2 \, D_{eff}} \right]^{\frac{1}{2}} (\mu_1 - \mu_2)$$

which is

$$R = \frac{125}{4} \left[\frac{2.5 \times 3600}{2 \, (1.5 \times 10^{-7})} \right]^{\frac{1}{2}} (1.050 \times 10^{-5} - 1.033 \times 10^{-5}) = 0.9202$$

The resolution can be increased by increasing E and by increasing t_{exper} (assuming the plate is long enough so that $L > Z_A$).

11.2.4. Affinity Electrophoresis and Immunoelectrophoresis

Affinity electrophoresis and immunoelectrophoresis are two related methods which are commonly used for biochemical analysis. In affinity electrophoresis the gel contains immobilized ligands which can interact with the migrating species (Horejsi, 1984; Andrews, (1986). The ligand is often chosen to have a specific biochemical affinity for the species of interest, and thus is similiar to affinity chromatography (see Section 7.1.). Agarose gel is normally used because the chemistry of binding a large variety of compounds to agarose is well known. Usually, the affinity interaction retards the movement of the desired species. Thus, affinity electrophoresis would be a useful complement to a normal electrophoresis run since the affinity electrophoresis experiment could separate compounds which would form a single zone in normal electrophoresis.

A variety of immunoelectrophoresis methods are used for clinical analyses. In classical immunoelectrophoresis a slab containing 1 to 2% agarose is formed and the proteins (antigens) are separated as in typical gel electrophoresis. Then, suitable antibodies are placed in a trough parallel to the path of migration of the species. The antibodies then diffuse through the gel to the antigen zones. When antibodies and antigens react they form precipitate if there is sufficient but not excess of the two reactants. This is the equivalence region shown in Figure 11-5a. Arcs of precipitates are observed. These arcs and the various steps in the process are illustrated in Figure 11-5b. If a single antibody is used it will react preferentially with a single antigen and the resulting pattern will be simple. If a broad spectrum of antibodies are used it will react with most or all of the proteins and a very complex pattern of precipitate arcs will form. Introductions to classical immunoelectrophoresis are given by Andrews (1986), Bier (1974) and Melvin (1987).

Rocket electrophoresis is a modification of classical electrophoresis developed by Laurell (1966). In rocket electrophoresis the agarose sheet contains the antibody of interest before the electrophoresis is started. As the electrophoresis proceeds precipitate forms whenever the amounts of antigen and antibody are in the equivalence region. The result are the patterns shown in Figure 11-5c which have been called "rockets". The height of a rocket depends

576

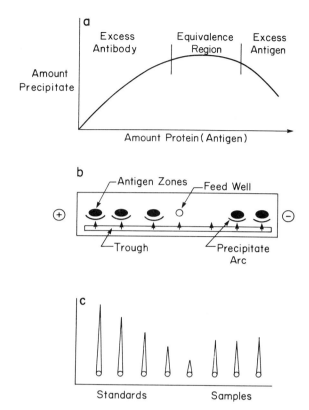

Figure 11-5.   Immunoelectrophoresis. a. Precipitation between antigen and
antibodies. Amount of antibody is fixed. b. Classical immunoelectrophoresis. c. Rocket electrophoresis.

upon the antigen concentration in the feed. Thus, the method can be made
quantitative by running a series of standards of known antigen concentration at
the same time as the unknown samples are run.

11.2.5.   Free Solution and Capillary Electrophoresis

Free solution electrophoresis is done without a supporting medium. Obviously, moving boundary electrophoresis is an example of free solution electro-

phoresis. Free solution electrophoresis can also be done with zonal development and in small capillaries. The application of free solution electrophoresis of most interest to chemical engineers is continuous two-dimensional electrophoresis which is discussed in Section 11.2.7.

The use of a free solution is essential for electrophoresis of very large molecules such as some proteins, RNA, and DNA. (Molecules of molecular weight less than 150×10^6 are usually done in agarose gels.) In addition, the electrophoresis of particles must be done in free solution. This is of particular importance for the separation of whole cells. In free solution electrophoresis there is no gel or paper to stabilize flow. To prevent convection thin chambers are normally used. This makes the h^3 term in the Rayleigh number, Eq. (11-12), small, and makes efficient cooling easier so that ΔT is also small. Since the critical Rayleigh number is higher for horizontal plates than for vertical plates (Ostrach, 1977), the plates are usually laid horizontally.

The zone spreading analysis developed in Section 11.2.3. is applicable to zonal free solution electrophoresis. Special coatings can be applied to the walls of the chamber to keep μ_{osm} and hence u_{osm} small. Then, Eqs. (11-23) and (11-24) show that higher resolutions will be obtained with high applied voltages. The effective axial diffusivity is kept small by use of thin chambers.

Microscope electrophoresis is a free solution method which does electrophoresis of colloidal particles between two microscope slides (Bier, 1974). The migration of particles is directly observed with a microscope. This method was in use before moving boundary electrophoresis was developed and is still used for determining μ of particles.

Capillary electrophoresis is currently a hot area of research for analytical chemists (Gordon et al, 1988; Jorgenson, 1987). Commercial capillary electrophoresis systems became available in late 1988. In capillary electrophoresis (also called capillary zone electrophoresis and high-performance capillary electrophoresis) capillaries which are 25 to 75 μm in inside diameter are used. With capillaries of this small size cooling is quite efficient and the Rayleigh number is quite small. In addition, the walls act to inhibit convective motion. Capillaries above 80 μm show a significant decrease in performance. With capillaries smaller than 80 μm operation can be done without convection even at voltages as high as 30,000 volts. To dissipate the Joule heating caused by 30,000 volts capillaries up to one meter long are used. Obviously, at this high voltage stringent safety precautions are necessary. According to Eqs. (11-20) and (11-23), both N and R will be high at these high voltages. Experiments routinely show 300,000 to 400,000 plates if very small samples with concentrations as low as 10^{-5} M are used, and up to one million plates have been observed. The analysis uses a sample from 1 to 10 nL, and the analysis time can be as short as ten minutes. Short analysis time is very important when many samples need to be analyzed. The method has been extremely successful with small molecules, but significantly less successful with proteins since proteins adsorb to the walls of the capillary. This can be controlled by modifying the walls of the capillary by appropriate surface treatment. Appropriate surface coatings are also useful to control electroosmosis. Electroosmosis is often desireable since it acts as a "pump" which causes fluid flow with an almost flat velocity profile (Gordon *et al*, 1988). Protein adsorption can also be controlled by operating under basic conditions where both the wall and the proteins are negatively charged. High concentrations of salts in the buffer will also reduce interactions with the wall. Currently, protein analysis must be considered as qualitative not quantitative. These methods are all part of current research programs (Gordon *et al*, 1988; Jorgenson, 1987).

Large scale application of free solution electrophoresis is currently done in two-dimensional systems (see Section 11.2.7.). Large-scale application of

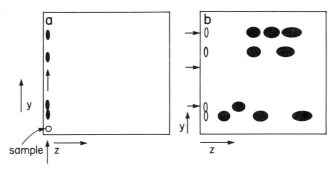

Figure 11-6.   Sequential two-dimensional separation. a. First development. b. Second development.

capillary electrophoresis would be of considerable interest, but has major obstacles to overcome before it becomes a reality. Because of the small sample size and low concentration required for high N in small capillaries, a very large number of capillaries would have to be bundled in parallel. Each of these capillaries has to be essentially identical or the separation observed in each will be different. The capillary walls must be quite thin or the volumetric efficieny will be rather low (porosity will be very low). One possible way around these problems would be to form the capillaries in a microporous material such as the polymer blocks being used for chromatography. In addition, methods of eluting the separated components would need to be developed.

11.2.6. Sequential Two-Dimensional Methods

Even with a very large N, molecules with the same electrophoretic mobilities will not separate. In addition, biological mixtures often have thousands of components which is more than can be separated and observed in a single electrophoretic experiment. To overcome these problems a variety of sequential two-dimensional methods have been developed for analysis. The basic idea behind sequential two-dimensional development is illustrated in Figure 11-6. The sample is developed in the first direction using an electrophoretic or chromatographic technique. Then the plate is developed in the second direction using a different technique which utilizes a somewhat different mechanism for separation. For example, if the first development uses ordinary electrophoresis the second development could use SDS-PAGE. Then the first development is essentially separating on the basis of the charge to size ratio while the second development is separating on the basis of size only. Molecules with the same size-to-charge ratio will not separate during the first development, but will separate during the second development if the molecular sizes are different. It is important that different experimental conditions be used for the two runs; otherwise, nothing is gained from doing development in two directions.

Two-dimensional methods can also separate many more compounds than one-dimensional systems as long as the two developments are independent.

Giddings (1984) showed that the maximum number of compounds n_{2D} that can be detected by a two-dimensional method is

$$n_{2D} = n_1 \, n_2 \qquad \qquad (11\text{-}25)$$

where n_1 and n_2 are the maximum number of peaks which can be detected by the two separate developments. If the two developments are not independent n_{2D} will be significantly less than predicted by Eq. (11-25).

Sequential two-dimensional separations can be traced back to Haugaard and Kroner (1948) who did paper chromatography followed by paper electrophoresis. Since paper chromatography separates by a combination of adsorption and ion exchange while paper electrophoresis separates on the basis of ion exchange and electrophoresis, the two developments are close to independent. A modification of this method which uses paper electrophoresis followed by paper chromatography has become commonly known as fingerprinting and is used for producing peptide maps (Ingram, 1956; Melvin, 1987). A large variety of similiar sequential two-dimensional methods have been reviewed by Smith (1968, 1979). These include paper electrophoresis followed by transferring the spots to a starch gel and then doing starch gel electrophoresis, starch gel electrophoresis followed by paper or thin layer chromatography, cellulose acetate electrophoresis followed by electrophoresis on DEAE paper, and other methods.

O'Farrell (1975) acheived a major breakthrough in sequential two-dimensional separations by doing iso-electric focusing first followed by SDS-PAGE. Since isoelectrical focusing separates based on the isoelectric point (see Table 11-1 and Section 11.4.) and SDS-PAGE on molecular size, the two developments are independent. This was the first sequential two-dimensional method with completely independent developments. In addition, both methods are high resolution methods with high values of n_1 and n_2 in Eq. (11-25). The predicted value of n_{2D} is as high as 5000. A large number of related techniques have since been developed (Andrews, 1986; Gianazza and Righetti, 1979; Lester et al, 1981; Dunn and Burghes, 1983). These include isoelectric focusing followed by a variety of electrophoretic methods such as: PAGE, gel pore-gradient electrophoresis, immunoelectrophoresis, and isotachophoresis.

A one or two-dimensional method which is rather different than the methods discussed up to now is *pulsed gel electrophoresis* which is being developed as a method for separating very large DNA molecules (Schwartz, 1987). The basic idea in pulsed gel electrophoresis is to change the direction of the field so that the DNA molecules must change direction. In the two-dimensional pulsed gel system there are two pairs of electrodes which are arranged perpendicular to each other. Every time the field is switched (or pulsed) the long DNA molecule changes direction. Different size molecules can adjust to the pulsing with different relaxation times. Smaller molecules can follow the change in direction quicker and thus should move faster. Thus, the method can be tuned to separate different size molecules. This method has caused considerable excitement since it is capable of separating yeast chromosomes. The method was first announced in 1983 and a commercial instrument is available for analytical separations.

There are many other possible combinations of two-dimensional development methods. Giddings (1984) estimated that there are from 10^4 to 10^6 distinguishable two dimensional methods. Obviously, not all of these combinations will be advantageous. Problem 11-B1 encourages you to generate some ideas of your own.

Zone spreading in sequential two-dimensional systems can be described by an extension of the methods used for one-dimensional systems (Giddings, 1984). The variance for a one dimensional system is given by Eq. (11-18). For a two dimensional system there will be variances in both directions.

$$\sigma_{y1}^2 = 2 D_{y1}\, t_1 \ , \ \ \sigma_{z1}^2 = 2 D_{z1}\, t_1 \tag{11-26}$$

where subscript 1 refers to the first development. After both developments, the total variances will be

$$\sigma_y^2 = \sigma_{y1}^2 + \sigma_{y2}^2 = 2 D_{y1}\, t_1 + 2 D_{y2}\, t_2 \tag{11-27a}$$

$$\sigma_z^2 = \sigma_{z1}^2 + \sigma_{z2}^2 = 2 D_{z1}\, t_1 + 2 D_{z2}\, t_2 \tag{11-27b}$$

The solution for the total concentration is the sum of the Gaussians in the y and z directions.

$$c_i(y,z) = c_{i,max} \exp \left[-\frac{(y - Y_i)^2}{2\,\sigma_y^2} - \frac{(z - Z_i)^2}{2\,\sigma_z^2} \right] \qquad (11\text{-}28)$$

where n is the total moles of solute and Y_i and Z_i are the location of the peak (or spot) center. Note that $Y_i = u_{i,1}\,t_1$ and $Z_i = u_{i,2}\,t_2$. Equation (11-28) represents an elliptical spot on the y-z plane. The widths of the spot are $w_y = 4\,\sigma_y$ and $w_z = 4\,\sigma_z$. The four effective dispersion coefficients can be different. Since developments 1 and 2 may represent completely different processes on different media, it is reasonable that σ_1 and σ_2 will be different. These effective dispersion coefficients can be measured from experiments.

11.2.7. Continuous Two-Dimensional Electrophoresis

Continuous two-dimensional electrophoresis is the current focus of efforts to scale up electrophoresis so that it can be used for commercial separations. The basis of continuous two-dimensional electrophoresis is illustrated in Figure 11-7a. The feed is introduced at the top of the plate and flows downward while subject to an electric field which is perpendicular to the flow direction. In the simplest version of the process all species have the same vertical velocity. The horizontal veolcities are given by Eq. (11-1) and depend upon the electro-phoretic mobilities. The net velocity of each component is the vector addition of the vertical and horizontal velocities (see Figure 11-7b).

$$\tan a = \frac{u}{v_{buffer}} \qquad (11\text{-}29)$$

The result is a continuous, steady state, multicomponent separation. The one-dimensional zone spreading analysis developed in Section 11.2.3. can be applied with slight modifications to the continuous two-dimensional apparatus. The separation is occurring only in the y direction in Figure 11-7a. The x direction is a non-selective displacement. Thus, the maximum number of com-

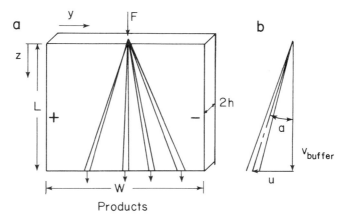

Figure 11-7.   Continuous two-dimensional electrophoresis. a. Apparatus. b. Vector addition of velocities.

ponents which can be separated is n_1. When Eqs. (11-14) to (11-24) are applied to the continuous two-dimensional apparatus the retention time is the same for all components.

$$t_R = L/v_{buffer} \qquad (11\text{-}30)$$

Now, u is the velocity in the y direction, $E = V/W$, σ^2 is measured in the y direction, and z_i is the distance of migration in the y direction which is $z_i = u_i \, t_R$. Although the transformation of the one-dimensional equations to the continuous two-dimensional form is left as Problem 11-C1, the final result for resolution is given below

$$R = \frac{1}{4} \left[\frac{L}{2 \, \overline{D}_{eff} \, v_{buffer}} \right]^{\frac{1}{2}} (\mu_1 - \mu_2) \frac{V}{W} \qquad (11\text{-}31)$$

Comparison with Eq. (11-23) shows that there is considerable similarity between one-dimensional and continuous two-dimensional electrophoresis.

The basic process shown in Figure 11-7a has been used for paper electrophoresis (Durrum, 1951; Strain and Sullivan, 1951). If there is no adsorption or ion exchange, the results are two-dimensional electrophoresis and the theory presented earlier can be used to predict the location of peaks and the amount of zone spreading. If ion exchange or adsorption occur, the separation is a combination of these effects plus electrophoresis. The paper in Figure 11-7a can obviously be replaced with a variety of gels (Smith, 1968). If sieving occurs in the gel, then separation will be a combination of size and charge effects. One can also use size exclusion chromatography particles (this is different than having a gel since the space between particles is available to all molecules) to produce a combination of size exclusion chromatography and electrophoresis (Epstein, 1977). The devices with paper and gels have relatively low flow rates, and apparently have not been scaled-up to much larger sizes.

The major scale-up efforts have been made for continuous, two-dimensional electrophoresis in free solution. Early versions of this method were demonstrated by Svensson and Brattsten (1949) in Sweden and Grassman and Hannig (1950) in West Germany. The flow rates can be significantly greater than in gel or paper, and particles can be separated. The basic apparatus is the same as Figure 11-7a. This process has attracted considerable attention and has been extensively reviewed (Hannig, 1978; McCann et al, 1973; Just and Werner, 1979; Kolin, 1979; and Wankat, 1984-85). Scale-up is difficult because of the need to control convection and the relatively low resolving power of the system at modest voltages. Early efforts at scale-up were aimed at the basic apparatus shown in Figure 11-7a. Since no stabilizing medium is used, a thin chamber (0.6 to 1.5 mm) with cooling on both sides is used. The apparatus has usually been used vertically, but horizontal operation is probably preferable since the critical Rayleigh number is much higher. Use of chambers with a width less than 5mm will stabilize the flow, but limits the separation which can be acheived. Special 'fan' collectors need to be used for these very narrow designs (Kolin, 1979). Currently obtainable volumetric throughputs using the basic apparatus are about 4 mL/hr. A commercial apparatus called the Elphor VaP 21 is available from Bender and Hobein of Munich (Mosher et al, 1987). This device is quite versatile and can also be used for isotachophoresis and isoelectric focusing (see Sections 11.3. and 11.4.).

Devices similiar to Figure 11-7a have been flown in the space shuttle as a way to prevent thermal convection since gravity is very small (Morrison et al,

1984). Both the Rayleigh and Grashoff numbers, Eqs. (11-12) and (11-13), will be small since g is small. This approach works, but is rather expensive.

Once it became clear that the basic geometry had almost insurmountable difficulties, a variety of clever methods were devised to overcome these difficulties. Perhaps the first attempts to stabilize the flow was the addition of a density gradient (Philpot, 1940; Mel, 1964). Chemicals such as sucrose or cesium chloride are added to the carrier fluid in layers of increasing density. Migration is then normal to the density gradient in either a vertical or an horizontal device. If the added density gradient is steep enough, thermal convection can be prevented. A related approach is to add a thickening agent such as methylcellulose to increase the viscosity, η (Dobry and Finn, 1958). This reduces the Rayleigh number in Eq. (11-12) and may prevent convection. If convection occurs it will be reduced since the Grashof number in Eq. (11-13) becomes smaller. However, increasing viscosity also decreases μ_i (see Eq. (11-9c)), and probably decreases resolution (Eq. (11-31)). Unfortunately, both these methods require addition of chemicals to the separating mixture and these chemicals must eventually be removed.

The fluid can also be stabilized by superimposing a rotational flow perpendicular to the migration direction. The most direct way of doing this was developed by Philpot (1973). Philpot's device is shown schematically in Figure 11-8 (Philpot, 1973; Beckwith and Ivory, 1988; Mosher et al, 1987). Carrier fluid flows vertically between two concentric cylinders which are separated by a gap of about 3 to 5mm. The inner cylinder is the cathode and is fixed. The outer cylinder serves as the anode and rotates at speeds up to 150 rpm. This rotation produces a steady angular flow in the annulus which is superimposed on the vertical parabolic flow. Feed is introduced into the carrier along the entire circumference of the inner cylinder. Migration of the molecules is radially outward, and product is collected at different radial positions but around the entire circumference of the annulus. Despite the 5mm distance between cylinders, 29 separate fractions are collected in the commercial Biostream device. Since the feed is introduced along the entire circumference of the inner cylinder, the feed rate which can be processed is much higher than with the parallel plate device shown in Figure 11-7a. This device can process protein solutions at throughputs greater than two liters per hour which

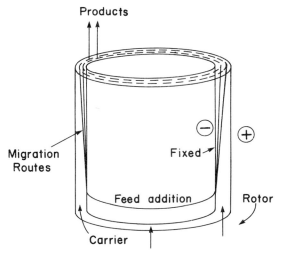

Figure 11-8.   Philpot-Harwell rotating electrophoresis device.

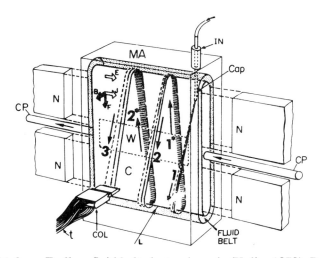

Figure 11-9.   Endless fluid belt electrophoresis (Kolin, 1979). Reprinted with permission from P.G. Righetti, C.J. van Oss, and J.W. Vanderhoff (Eds.), *Electrokinetic Separation Methods*, Elsevier/North Holland Biomedical Press, Amsterdam, 1979. Copyright 1979, Elsevier/North Holland Biomedical Press.

corresponds to a maximum of 150g of protein per hour. On the other hand, the resolution and the number of components which can be separated is higher in the parallel plate device. About a 20°C temperature increase is observed in the flowing liquid, but thermal convection is totally prevented. To prevent thermal degradation of proteins the feed is first chilled to about 2°C. The short 15 to 60 second residence time also helps to prevent protein degradation. Beckwith and Ivory (1988) presented a detailed analysis of the solute trajectories. The Philpot-Harwell device is commercially available from Harwell as the Biostream separator. Unfortunately, further scale-up of the device is likely to be difficult.

Kolin (1979) devised an alternate method of superimposing a rotational flow on the flowing axial fluid. Kolin put a magnet inside the loop of fluid to produce a rotational flow which represses thermal convection. Several different devices were developed; one of the more sophisticated, a racetrack design, is shown in Figure 11-9 (Kolin, 1979). The combination of rotational flow and particle migration causes a helical flow path for all particles. The addition of a carrier flow in the same direction as the electrical field serves to change the pitch of all particles. The particles can be made to form several loops; then

$$\text{Distance Traveled, } L = n \times \text{circumference} \qquad (11\text{-}32)$$

where n is the number of turns traveled. This is equivalent to recycling the fluid. According to Eq. (11-31), larger L increases resolution. Thus, this device has excellent resolution but limited throughput. Further scale-up will probably be difficult.

A rather different approach is to use continuous free flow two-dimensional electrophoresis with a series of recycles to produce what is effectively a continuous, steady-state, countercurrent electrophoresis (Gobie et al, 1985). A schematic of this device is shown in Figure 11-10. Feed is introduced in the center and purge at the two ends. These are the only locations where fresh solution is added; thus, products withdrawn from the bottom will not be excessively diluted. Liquid leaving the bottom of the apparatus is recycled to the top where it provides the buffer flow. The recycle streams are

588

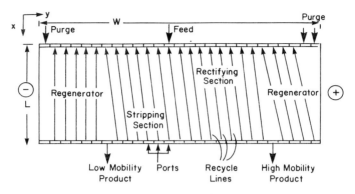

Figure 11-10. Recycle two-dimensional electrophoresis operating as a continuous countercurrent electrophoresis system. Modified from a Figure in Gobie *et al.* (1985).

shifted one or more ports back. This shift is important since it essentially produces the countercurrent motion. The solute retention time for one pass is given by Eq. (11-30) and the solute migration velocity in the y direction is given by Eq. (11-16a) where $E = V/W$. The net lateral movement of a solute i is

$$y_{i,net} = u_{i,net}\ L/v_{buffer} - y_{recycle} \tag{11-33}$$

where $y_{recycle}$ is the distance the recycle stream is shifted. If $y_{i,net} > 0$, then the net solute migration is to the right. These solutes will eventually exit as high mobility product. All solutes with $y_{i,net} < 0$ (includes positive charge and no charge) will have net migration to the left. These solutes eventually end up as low mobility effluent. The regenerators shown in Figure 7-9 have the same purposes as zones 3 and 4 in counter-current adsorbers (Figure 10-11). The right regenerator where $y_{i,net} < 0$ for all components is analogous to zone 4 while the left regenerator where $y_{i,net} > 0$ for all components is analogous to zone 3. These regenerators allow the use of reflux at both ends and elute without excessive dilution. The slope of the left regenerator must be adjusted if there are positively charged solutes in the feed. The device shown in Figure 11-10 acts as a steady-state, countercurrent separator and separates the feed into two products. Thus, it is a binary separator. Because of the large amount of recycle, separation should be quite sharp even for solutes with close to the same mobility. This approach is still experimental, and is it not clear if this apparatus can be scaled-up.

11.3. ISOTACHOPHORESIS (DISPLACEMENT ELECTROPHORESIS)

Isotachophoresis can be considered as a displacement form of electrophoresis, and it has an analogous relationship to zonal electrophoresis as displacement chromatography does to elution chromatography. The theory of isotacho- phoresis was developed in 1897 by Kohlrausch, but serious developmental work did not begin until the 1940's when A. J. P. Martin and F. M. Everaerts collaborated on the process (see Everaerts et al, 1976; and Everaerts and Verheggen, 1987). The method did not become popular until the late 1960's. Currently, it is a fairly common analytical technique and has considerable potential as a large-scale method. When stacking gels are used in electro- phoresis (see Section 11.2.2.), the stacking gel is operating as an isotacho- phoresis system.

In isotachophoresis the sample is placed between a leading (L) and a trailing (T) electrolyte. The pH of the mixture is adjusted so that all solutes (such as amino acids or proteins) have the same charge. To be specific we will assume they are all cations. The leading electrolyte is chosen to have a higher mobility than all the solutes and the trailing electrolyte is chosen to have a lower mobility than all the solutes. Thus, L is analogous to the solvent and T to the displacer in displacement chromatography. Recipes for leading and trailing electrolytes are given by Everaerts et al (1976) and Holloway and Battersby (1984). After the current is turned on, a series of zones are formed with sharp boundaries between the zones. The zones are in the order L, fastest solute, next fastest solute,..., slowest solute and then T, (See Figure 11-11a). Each zone is concentrated and contains essentially pure solute in solution plus the coun- terion. Operation is with constant current. Since the mixture is concentrated and is not homogeneous, the field strength E is *not* constant but varies from zone to zone. The field strength is lowest in zone L and highest in zone T, (see

590

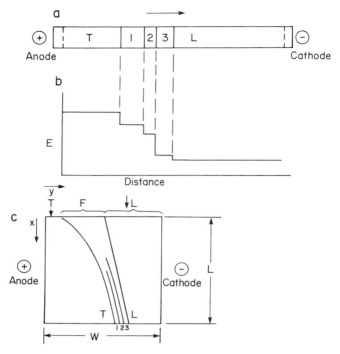

Figure 11-11. Isotachophoresis of cations. a. Schematic of bands. b. Electric field strength. c. Continuous two-dimensional system.

Figure 11-11b). Since Joule heating is proportional to E, the temperature becomes highest in the terminating electrolyte zone. Thus, vertical equipment should be arranged with L on the bottom, T on top, and downwards migration. Isotaccphoresis can be done in paper, gels, capillaries, and free solution (Andrews, 1986; Everaerts et al, 1976; Everaerts and Verheggen, 1987; Holloway and Battersby, 1984; Mosher et al, 1987). Paper, gel and capillaries are operated in batch mode while free solution is usually operated continuously. Modified electrophoresis equipment is usually used.

The theory of isotachophoresis is presented in considerable detail by Everaerts et al (1976). In this section we will present a simplified theory for dilute systems with completely ionized salts which closely follows the development of Karol and Karol (1978). In isotachophoresis pure bands with constant concentrations are observed experimentally. To satisfy a mass balance each band must have constant velocities

$$u_L = u_1 = u_2 = u_3 = \cdots = u_T \tag{11-34}$$

which is analogous to Eq. (8-39) developed for displacement chromatography. Substituting in Eq. (11-1), we obtain

$$\mu_L\, E_L = \mu_1\, E_1 = \mu_2\, E_2 = \cdots = \mu_T\, E_T \tag{11-35}$$

Equation (11-35) is known as the isotachophoretic condition. This equation differentiates isotachophoresis from the other electrophoretic methods. Since the mobilities are in order $\mu_L > \mu_1 > \mu_2 > ... > \mu_T$, the field strengths in each band must be in the reverse order, $E_T > E_n > ... > E_1 > E_L$, (see Figure 11-10b). Any solute molecule diffusing into a slower band experiences a field strength which is higher, and thus the solute is accelerated back into the correct band. Thus there is a focusing effect which keeps the bands sharp despite diffusional effects.

The total current I is the sum of the current carried by cations and anions.

$$I = c_i\, u_i\, z_i\, e\, N\, A_c + c_-\, |u_-|\, z_-\, e\, N\, A_c \tag{11-36}$$

where z is the valence, $e = 1.6 \times 10^{-19}$ Coulomb, and ze is the charge on each ion. N is Avogadro's number 6.022×10^{23}, A_c is the cross-sectional area of the apparatus, and c is the concentration in g moles/cm^3. Note that eN = F, Faraday's constant. Electroneutrality requires that

$$c_i\, z_i = c_-\, z_- \tag{11-37}$$

Substituting this condition into Eq. (11-36), we obtain

$$I = c_i\, z_i\, e\, (u_i + |u_-|)\, N\, A_c \tag{11-38}$$

which becomes

$$I = c_i\, z_i\, E_i\, N\, A_c\, e\, (\mu_i + |\mu_-|) \tag{11-39}$$

when we substitute in Eq. (11-1). Since the current I is constant, Eq. (11-39) is valid for i = L,1,2,...,T. Setting Eq.(11-39) equal for components L and i, and substituting in Eq. (11-35) to remove the field strengths, we obtain

$$c_{i,band} = c_L \; \frac{(\mu_L + |\mu_-|) \, \mu_i \, z_i}{(\mu_i + |\mu_-|) \, \mu_L \, z_L} \tag{11-40}$$

This result, which is valid for isotachophoresis of dilute systems with completely ionized salts, allows the calculation of the concentration in each band. Obviously, if c_L is fairly high then c_i in the band will also be high. Note that c_i does not depend on the feed concentration of component i. Thus, if the feed is dilute rather high concentration ratios can be achieved. In fact, the solubility of proteins places a limit on the value of c_L which can be used (Holloway and Battersby, 1984). The band widths can be determined from a mass balance which is

$$c_{F,i} \text{ (feed width)} = c_{i,band} \text{ (bandwidth)} \tag{11-41}$$

This is analogous to Eq. (8-43) developed for displacement chromatography.

This solution is oversimplified since it ignores the transient period before the bands are fully formed. Thus it is again analogous to the theory used for displacement chromatography where the transient period was also ignored. Everaerts et al (1976) give a more detailed analysis.

Because of electroneutrality there can be no gaps between bands. If one or more bands are quite narrow it can be difficult to recover the solute as a pure component. *Spacers* can be advantageous in this case. A spacer is an ion with a mobility in-between the mobilities of the two solutes of interest. The spacer will then separate these solutes. Since the spacer concentration is controlled by the experimenter, Eq. (11-41) shows that the spacer band can be any desired width. Unfortunately, finding appropriate spacers may require a lot of trial and error. A variation of the spacer method is the *field step method* (Mosher et al, 1987). In this method the feed is introduced into a buffer of low conductivity which is sandwiched between two buffers of high conductivity. The field strength is high in the low conductivity buffer and thus the solutes migrate quickly in this buffer. In the high conductivity buffers the field strength and the solutes slow down; thus, solute accumulate at the two interfaces. This approach is thus a binary separation.

Isotachophoresis has considerable potential as a preparative method. The capacity is much greater than in conventional electrophoresis or isoelectric focusing (Karol and Karol, 1978). Because of the focusing and concentrating effects, rather large feed pulses can be used in batch operation. In continuous operation the feed port can be quite wide. A commercial free-flow electrophoresis apparatus, the Elphor VaP 21, is readily adaptable to continuous, free-flow isotachophoresis (see Section 11.2.7.). In continuous isotachophoresis as shown in Figure 11-11c the feed is introduced between the leading and terminating electrolyte ports (Mosher et al, 1987). Electrophoretic migration is in the y direction while everything flows at the same velocity in the x direction. Capacity of the commercial instrument is up to 5g protein per hour. In the field step method the Elphor VaP has processed proteins at the rate of 30g per hour.

Example 11-3. Continuous Two-Dimensional Isotachophoresis

Continuous two-dimensional isotachophoresis is run in an apparatus similar to Figure 11-11c. The leading electrolyte is 0.04 N H^+. The trailing electrolyte is 0.01 N Li^+. The coion is Cl^-. The feed contains 0.01N RbCl and 0.01 N KCl. The apparatus has L = W = 12 cm. The trailing electrolyte is input from y = 0 to y = 2.5 cm (measured from the anode), the feed is then input for 7.0 cm, and then the leading electrolyte (see Figure 11-11c). Find the Rb^+ and K^+ concentrations in the bands and the band widths once steady state has been obtained. Data is available in Table 11-3.

Solution

Equation (11-40) can be applied. From Table 11-3,
$\mu_L = 36.2 \times 10^{-4}$, $\mu_{Rb} = 8.03 \times 10^{-4}$, $\mu_K = 7.67 \times 10^{-4}$, $\mu_{Li} = 4.02 \times 10^{-4}$

and $|\mu_{Cl}| = 7.9 \times 10^{-4}$ cm^2/Vs. Then from Eq. (11-40),

$$c_{Rb,band} = (0.04) \frac{(36.2 + 7.9)\ (8.03)}{(8.03 + 7.9)\ (36.2)} \frac{(1)}{(1)} = 0.0248 \text{ N}$$

$$c_{K,band} = (0.04) \frac{(36.2 + 7.9)\ (7.67)\ (1)}{(7.67 + 7.9)\ (36.2)\ (1)} = 0.0240 \text{ N}$$

From Eq. (11-41),

bandwidth RbCl = (0.01) (2.5 cm) / (0.0248) = 1.0081 cm

bandwidth KCl = (0.01) (2.5) / (0.0240) = 1.0415 cm

The order of the ions will be H$^+$, Rb$^+$, K$^+$, and then Li$^+$. Determination of other details about the operation such as the distance required to reach steady state and the exit locations of the bands require more complicated theories (Evereaerts *et al*, 1976).

11.4. ISOELECTRIC FOCUSING

Isoelectric focusing is electrophoresis in a pH gradient. Remember that the size and sign of the charge on proteins depends on the pH, and at the isoelectric pH (called the pI) the protein has no net charge. This is shown in Figure 11-12a. Note that at pH values lower than the pI the proteins have a positive charge, and they will migrate towards the cathode. At pH values higher than the pI the proteins have a negative charge and will migrate towards the anode. For isoelectric focusing the pH gradient is set up with low pH values at the anode and high pH values at the cathode (see Figure 11-12b). Thus, in a stationary pH gradient proteins will migrate until they reach pH = pI and then they stop since there is no force on the protein. At this point the mobility $\mu = 0$ since $\zeta = 0$. Since proteins from both higher and lower pHs migrate to the pI position, the protein is focused at the pI. The final separation achieved is an

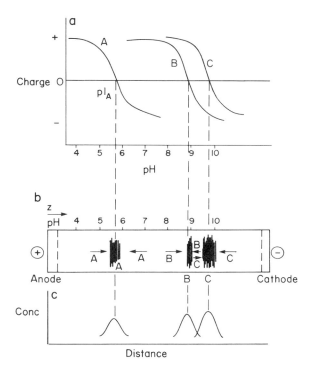

Figure 11-12. Isoelectric Focusing. a. Effect of pH on charge of proteins. b. Focused bands. c. Concentrations.

equilibrium separation with each protein focused at its pI. This is shown schematically in Figures 11-12b and 11-12c. Molecules which differ by as little as 0.02 pH units can be separated. The resulting bands can be very concentrated compared to the feed concentrations. Isoelectric focusing is a very powerful separation method which has been extensively used for separation of biological compounds.

We will first briefly consider the history of isoelectric focusing since that will clarify the difficulties which had to be overcome to make the technique successful. Then, a simple zone spreading theory will be presented. Finally, a variety of preparative methods for isoelectric focusing will be reviewed.

11.4.1. History and Basic Ideas

Righetti (1983) has presented a detailed and very readable account of the history of isoelectric focusing. In 1954-1955 A. Kolin developed a method for focusing ions in a continuous pH gradient stabilized with a sucrose density gradient. His pH gradients were produced by placing the sample between acidic and basic buffers, applying the electric field and allowing diffusion to produce the pH gradients. Unfortunately, the pH gradients were transient and long-term focusing runs were not possible.

In the late 50's and early 60's Harry Svensson (now Rilbe) did fundamental theoretical work which predicted the requirements of a stable isoelectric focusing system (Svensson, 1961, 1962a, 1962b; Rilbe, 1973). To generate a stable pH gradient a carrier ampholyte was required. A carrier ampholyte is:

1. Amphoteric. That is, the sign of the charge on the molecule is pH dependent. Amphoteric compounds will reach an equilibrium position in a pH gradient.

2. A carrier. This means that the species can carry current which requires that it be a good conductor, and that it can 'carry' pH which requires that it be a good buffer. The value of $|pI - pK_1|$ should be small.

3. In addition, the carrier ampholyte should be quite soluble, have no effect on the sample, and be easily separable from the sample.

Whilst developing the theory Svensson searched through chemical catalogs for appropriate compounds. He was partially successful, but no appropriate compounds were found in the very important range between pH 5 and 7. The first seven compounds listed in Table 11-2 are from Svensson's list (Svensson, 1962a). Svensson then found that peptides formed from cleaving proteins could be used to form a partially successful carrier ampholyte.

Svensson encouraged Olof Vesterberg to join in the search for a suitable carrier ampholyte. In 1964 Vesterberg was successful. He coupled acrylic acid to a series of amines to produce a series of compounds with pI and pK values in the range from 3.5 to 10 (Vesterberg, 1969). Subsequent work extended the pH range from 2 to 11. These carrier ampholytes are commercially available as Ampholine from LKB. Later, Serva and Pharmacia developed different carrier ampholytes.

Once carrier ampholytes were available applications immediately followed. Since much of the equipment was developed from existing electrophoresis designs, equipment development was rapid. Preparative systems include gel, density gradient, free flow and recycling systems. These are discussed in Section 11.4.3.

In 1982 Righetti's group (Bjellqvist et al, 1982) announced the development of immobilized pH gradients. Acrylamide derivatives of the structure

$$CH_2 = CH-CO-NH-R$$

where R is either a carboxylic or tertiary amino group will form a series of buffers with different pK values (Dunn, 1987). When these buffers are mixed with acrylamide and Bis (see Section 11.2.3.), they can be polymerized to form a gel with a pH gradient. Since the compounds forming the pH gradient are part of the solid matrix, the pH gradient is completely stable. These gels are available as Immobiline gels from LKB. The use of immobilized pH gradients has generated considerable excitement, but is currently only of use with PAGE. Thus, carrier ampholytes must be used with other gels and in free solution. The use of carrier ampholytes and immobilized gels simultaneously has proven to be advantageous since the carrier ampholytes increase the rather low conductivity of the immobilized pH gradients (Righetti et al, 1987).

11.4.2. Theory of Isoelectric Focusing

Once focusing is complete, isoelectric focusing is a steady state process where the electrical focusing effect is just balanced by diffusion. The mass balance at steady state for any component which focus is (Righetti, 1983; Svensson, 1961)

$$\frac{d\,(c\,\mu\,E)}{dz} = \frac{d}{dz} D \frac{dc}{dz} \qquad (11\text{-}42)$$

This equation is not valid for compounds which do not focus (neutral or not amphoteric compounds). It is convenient to set z=0 at the center of the focused band with positive z towards the cathode (see Figure 11-12b). Doing the first integration we obtain

$$c\,\mu\,E = D\,\frac{dc}{dz} \qquad (11\text{-}43)$$

where the constant of integration must be zero since the protein concentration is zero outside the focused zone. The left hand side is Cu which is flow of protein into the zone due to the electrophoretic force. The right hand side is the diffusion away from the zone.

Before doing the next integration, we need to know how μ varies with distance z. Define

$$p = -\frac{d\mu}{dz} = \frac{-d\mu}{d(pH)}\,\frac{d(pH)}{dz} \qquad (11\text{-}44)$$

Because of the choice of axis, d(pH)/dz is positive. The value of d(pH)/dz can be determined experimentally by locating marker compounds such as those listed in Table 11-2. $d\mu/d(pH)$ is always negative since ζ in Eqs.(11-9) decreases from positive to negative as pH increases. Thus, p in Eq. (11-44) is an inherently positive quantity. p is considered to be a constant since the focused bands are quite narrow. Then $d\mu/d(pH)$ will be approximately constant and d(pH)/dz can be linearized. At the center of the band (z=0) $\mu = 0$. Integrating Eq. (11-44), we obtain

$$\mu = -pz \qquad (11\text{-}45)$$

After substituting this result into Eq. (11-43), we obtain

$$\frac{dc}{c} = -\left[\frac{p\,E}{D}\right] z\,dz \qquad (11\text{-}46)$$

If p, E and D are all constant in the focused zone, Eq. (11-46) can be integrated.

$$c = c_{max} \exp \left\{ \frac{-p E z^2}{2D} \right\} \qquad (11\text{-}47)$$

When z=0, c = c_{max} which is the maximum concentration in the focused zone. Equation (11-47) is a Gaussian distribution and is shown in Figure 11-12c.

Comparing this result with Eq. (7-24), we see that the standard deviation for isoelectric focusing is

$$\sigma = \sqrt{D/p\,E} \qquad (11\text{-}48a)$$

Substituting in Eq. (11-44), we also have

$$\sigma = \sqrt{\frac{D}{E \left[-\dfrac{d\mu}{d(pH)} \dfrac{d(pH)}{dz} \right]}} \qquad (11\text{-}48b)$$

The standard deviation will be small for molecules which have low diffusivities and high values of $d\mu/d(pH)$. These conditions are both valid for proteins which means that isoelectric focusing will give sharp bands for proteins. However, D is the effective diffusivity in the isoelectric focusing system. Thus, it is important to stabilize the system to prevent convection. This is done with a gel, density gradient, thin chambers, or other methods.

The conditions required for adequate resolution can be derived from this Gaussian solution (Righetti, 1983; Rilbe, 1973). If the peak to peak distance between two adjacent zones is equal to three times the average value of $\bar{\sigma}$, then the peaks will overlap but will be definitely resolved. This leads to the difference in pH of the two peaks being

$$\Delta pH = \Delta z \, \frac{d(pH)}{dz} = 3\bar{\sigma} \, \frac{d(pH)}{dz} \qquad (11\text{-}49)$$

Substituting in Eq. (11-48b), we obtain the following condition for adequate resolution.

$$\Delta \, pI = 3 \, \sqrt{\frac{\overline{D} \, [d(pH)/dz]}{E \, [-d \, \mu/d(pH)]}} \qquad (11\text{-}50)$$

This result shows that the required difference in pI values of the two proteins is less for molecules with low diffusivity and high values of $-d\mu/d(pH)$, and less for systems with shallow pH gradients and high field strengths. The estimated minimum value of ΔpI is about 0.02 pH units with carrier ampholytes. One advantage of immobilized pH gradients is that quite shallow pH gradients can be generated to maximize the resolution of proteins with close to the same pI. The minimum value of ΔpI may be as low as 0.002 pH units (Dunn, 1987).

Example 11-4. Isoelectric Focusing

An IEF experiment is done with a combined immobilized pH gradient on PAGE and carrier ampholytes. Operation is at steady state at 25°C and E = 80 V/cm. We observe horse myglobin at 5.12 cm from the anode and histidine at 7.84 cm from the anode. We wish to separate two quite similar proteins whose pI is about 7.4. When we do IEF of one of these proteins the peak width is 0.21 cm. What is the minimum value of ΔpI for which we can still separate the two proteins?

Solution

The pH gradient can be determined from the two marker compounds horse myglobin and histidine. From Table 11-2
$pI_{myglobin} = 7.33$ and $pI_{hist} = 7.47$.

Then $\dfrac{d(pH)}{dz} = \dfrac{7.47 - 7.33}{7.84 - 5.12} = 0.0515$ pH units/cm.

Since the proteins we want to separate are similar, $D / \left[\dfrac{-d\mu}{d(pH)} \right]$ will be approximately equal for them. We can combine width = 4σ with Eq. (11-48b),

$$\text{width} = 4 \sqrt{\left[\dfrac{D}{-\left[\dfrac{d\mu}{d\,pH} \right]} \right] \left[\dfrac{1}{E \dfrac{d(pH)}{dz}} \right]} \qquad (11\text{-}51)$$

Then,

$$\dfrac{D}{\left[-\dfrac{d\mu}{d(pH)} \right]} = \left[\dfrac{\text{width}}{4} \right]^2 E \dfrac{d(pH)}{dz} \qquad (11\text{-}52)$$

From the measured width and pH gradient,

$$\dfrac{D}{\left[-\dfrac{d\mu}{d(pH)} \right]} = \left[\dfrac{0.21\ \text{cm}}{4} \right]^2 80 \dfrac{V}{cm} (0.0515) \dfrac{pH\ units}{cm} = 0.01136$$

Now Eq. (11-50) gives,

$$\Delta pI = 3 \sqrt{\dfrac{\bar{D}}{(-d\mu/d(pH))} \dfrac{d(pH)/dz}{E}}$$

or

$$\Delta pI = 3 \sqrt{(0.01136)\,(0.0515/80)} = 0.0081\ \text{pH units}$$

Note that this is within the guidlines for the minimum ΔpI value when immobilized pH gradients are used.

11.4.3. Methods of Preparative Isoelectric Focusing

A variety of methods for preparative IEF have been developed. Most of these methods are based on modifications of electrophoresis systems. In fact, many commercial electrophoresis systems are designed so that electrophoresis, isotachophoresis and isoelectric focusing can all be done in the same apparatus.

Gel isoelectric focusing is commonly used for small-scale preparative applications (Andrews, 1986; Dunn, 1987; Fawcett, 1973; Radola, 1984; Righetti, 1983; Righetti et al, 1987). In IEF sieving is undesireable since sieving will slow down the attainment of the steady-state. Thus, a gel with large pores is desired. Either PAGE polymerized to form a continuous layer or beads of Sephadex or Biogel are used. The continuously polymerized PAGE systems allow the use of immobilized pH gradients, but the recovery of products is more difficult (Dunn, 1987; Radola, 1984). The PAGE systems dominate analytical applications, but are less commonly used for preparative applications. Although columns can be used, slabs are preferable since cooling is more efficient. A variety of units are commercially available (Radola, 1984). Gel thicknesses of up to about 5mm are used since beyond this thickness thermal gradients start to skew the zones. Granulated gels such as Sephadex G-200 or Biogel are commonly used for preparative IEF. Recovery of the proteins is easier, and these gels can be used in two-dimensional devices such as those discussed next (see Figure 11-13).

Two-dimensional free-flow electrophoresis equipment is easily adaptable to isoelectric focusing (Fawcett, 1973; Just and Werner, 1979; Righetti et al, 1980; Righetti, 1983). A comparison between free-flow electrophoresis and free-flow isoelectric focusing is shown in Figure 11-13 (Fawcett, 1973). Ampholyte is added to all the entering streams in Figure 11-13b and focuses as it flows down the column. Prefocusing the ampholyte will speed up the focusing of the sample. Note that free flow isoelectric focusing can be advantageous since a wider band can be fed and the products are concentrated into narrow bands while in electrophoresis the bands are spread. Obviously, more than two solutes can be separated. The free-flow apparatus is also very good for separating cells or particles (Just and Werner, 1979). Several variants of the basic apparatus have been developed and are discussed in detail by Righetti (1983).

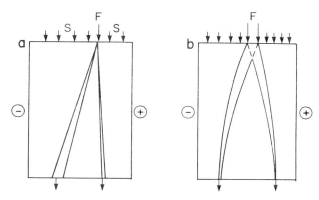

Figure 11-13. Diagrammatic representation of continuous flow systems. a. electrophoresis, b. Isoelectric focusing. Liquid flows at right angles to the electric field. From Fawcett (1973).

Density gradients can be used to stabilize IEF from convection (Fawcett, 1973; Righetti, 1983). Density gradients can be done in batch systems, and commercial instruments based on Svensson's design are available. However, the main interest for chemical engineers is in continuously flowing two-dimensional systems. One way of doing this is illustrated in Figure 11-14 (Fawcett, 1973). A sucrose density gradient is used to increase the density at

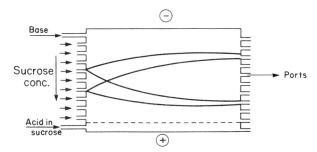

Figure 11-14. Continuous-flow density gradient isoelectric focusing apparatus. Cathode along the top, anode in side limb. Density gradient flows from left to right. Modified from Fawcett (1973).

the bottom of the system. If the system is cooled from the bottom only, the temperature gradient will help stabilize the system.

One problem with the devices shown in Figures 11-12b and 11-14 is the residence time may be too short to complete focusing. If the flow rate is decreased, throughput obviously drops. If the voltage is increased, cooling can be a problem. One solution to this problem is to use the continuous flow, recycling IEF apparatus shown in Figure 11-15 (Righetti et al, 1980; Righetti, 1983; Bier *et al*, 1986; Mosher et al, 1987). This device uses a compact focusing cell with a cathode to anode distance of 3 cm. The cooling is done in a separate heat exchanger which cools the recirculating streams. This arrangement effectively uncouples the focusing and cooling functions which are done simultaneously in Figures 11-13 and 11-14. The flow channels in the focusing cell can

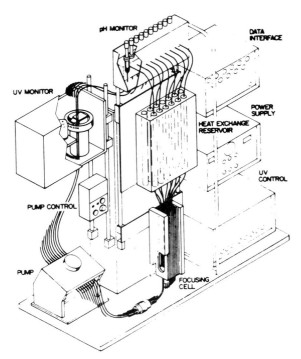

Figure 11-15.   Continuous flow, recycling isoelectric focusing.

be separated by PVC filters or Nylon screens. Operation is batch since a sample is added and recirculated until separation has been acheived; then, the products are withdrawn. Recently, it has been found that separation is improved if a thin film of fluid is focused with no membranes, filters or screens (Mosher et, 1987). This modification allows for a continuous pH gradient instead of the step gradients obtained with ten separate channels. The continuous flow, recycling IEF system is available commercially.

11.5. ELECTROCHROMATOGRAPHY

If one is doing electrophoresis with a stabilizing medium, it is very appealing to try chromatography simultaneously. This simultaneous electrophoresis and chromatography is called electrochromatography, and was tried by both Durrum (1951) and Strain and Sullivan (1951). These experiments used paper as a support medium in a two-dimensional apparatus. Because of the charged groups on the paper, some ion exchange chromatography is almost unavoidable. The combination of chromatography and electrophoresis can be used to separate compounds which would be difficult to separate by electrophoresis alone. Nerenberg and Pogojeïf (1969) applied an axial electrical field to a Sephadex size exclusion column. With this one-dimensional system they found a significant increase in resolving power compared to SEC alone. Epstein (1977) did combined SEC and electrophoresis in a continuous two dimensional system. He found that the Sephadex gel helped to stabilize the system and prevent convection. (Sephadex beads are commonly used in IEF to prevent convection, see Section 11.4.3.) None of these methods appear to have been adopted on a large scale.

O'Farrell (1985) developed the *counteracting chromatographic electrophoresis* method. This method has caused considerable interest particularly among chemical engineers since the method appears to have promise for large scale separations. An extensive review and analysis has been published by Locke and Carbonell (1989).

The apparatus for counteracting chromatographic electrophoresis is

606

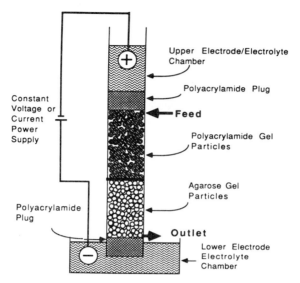

Figure 11-16. Apparatus for counteracting chromatographic electrophoresis (Locke and Carbonell, 1989). Reprinted with permission from *Separation and Purification Methods, 18*, 1 (1989). Copyright 1989, Marcel Dekker.

shown in Figure 11-16 (Locke and Carbonell; 1989). The pH is adjusted so that the desired proteins have a negative charge; then, all the desired proteins migrate upwards to the anode. At the same time a downwards flow of feed and buffer solution is superimposed on the system. The net velocity of a protein molecule is then

$$u_{net} = \mu\,E + \mu_{osm}\,E - u_s \qquad (11\text{-}53)$$

where u_s is given by Eq. (6-22) with the adsorption parameter $A = 0$. Usually, the electroosmotic flow will be negligible, $\mu_{osm} = 0$. The top layer of particles, polyacrylamide in Figure 11-16, is chosen so that all of the desired proteins are excluded from the pores, $K_d = 0$. The flow rate and electrical field are adjusted so that the net movement of desired protein is downwards in this layer. The second layer of particles, agarose in Figure 11-16, is chosen so that the desired protein can enter all the pores, $K_d = 1$. With the proper choice of velocity and electrical field the net velocity of the desired protein given by Eq. (11-53) will be positive in the agarose. The result will be focusing of the desired protein at the interface of the two gels. As the protein concentration increases significantly in the focused zone, the electrical conductivity will increase. Thus, the electrical field E will locally decrease and μE in Eq. (11-53) will decrease. At high enough protein concentrations the net velocity will become zero or negative. The result is the development of an equilibrium zone containing quite concentrated protein in the agarose gel layer. As more protein is added the size of this equilibrium zone will increase.

The engineer can adjust operating conditions so that proteins which are not desired will not focus at the gel boundary. If these proteins have a positive charge, there is no upward force and they will be swept downwards to the cathode. Negatively charged proteins will not focus if they have a net upwards velocity in the polyacrylamide layer which can happen if $K_d > 0$. These proteins also will not focus if they have a net downwards velocity in the agarose layer which can occur if $K_d < 1$. The result is the equilibrium zone will be both significantly concentrated in the desired protein, and will be somewhat purified. This method will probably not separate very similiar proteins.

An obvious extension which O'Farrell (1985) tried is to have a series of layers of gels with different sixe exclusion limits. These layers can easily be generated by mixing two gels with different pore sizes. Different proteins will then focus at different borders. O'Farrell showed that the protein could be moved from one equilibrium zone to another by changing the voltage.

The method appears to have promise as a preparative technique since O'Farrell (1985) reported that the capacity was 1000 times that of electrophoresis. Collection of the proteins could be done through side taps placed at the borders of different gel layers. Feed can be added for quite a long time if the equilibrium zones have a concentration significantly greater than the feed concentration. This will usually be the case since protein feeds are often quite dilute. One possible problem is precipitation of the protein if the concentration becomes too high. Continuous operation could be achieved by continuously withdrawing a small side stream from each equilibrium zone.

11.6. SUMMARY - OBJECTIVES

This chapter is an introduction to electrophoretic separation methods and a progress report on large-scale applications. At the end of this chapter you should be able to:

1. Understand and explain the basic concepts of electrophoresis, isotachophoresis, isoelectric focusing, and electrochromatography.
2. Predict the zone spreading for electrophoresis, isotachophoresis, and isoelectric focusing.
3. Be familiar with analytical applications of the electrophoretic methods.
4. Explain the advantages and disadvantages of various preparative methods.

REFERENCES

Andrews, A.T., *Electrophoresis*, 2nd ed., Oxford University Press, Oxford, 1986.

Beckwith, J.B. and C.F. Ivory, "The influence of diffusion on elution profiles in the Philpot-Harwell electrophoretic separator", *Chem. Eng. Commun. 54*, 301 (1987).

Bier, M., "Electrophoresis", in B. Karger, L.R. Snyder and C. Horvath, (Eds.), *An Introduction to Separation Science*, Wiley, New York, 1974, Chapter 17.

Bier, M., N.B. Egen, G.E. Twitty, R.A. Mosher, and W. Thormann, "Preparative electrophoresis comes of age," in C.J. King and J.D. Navratil (Eds.), *Chemical Separations*, Vol. I, *Principles*, Litarvan Literature, Denver, 1986, p. 133-151.

Bjellqvist, B., K. Ek, P.G. Righetti, E. Granazza, A. Gorg, R. Westermeier, and W. Postel, *J. of Biochem. Biophys. Methods, 6*, 317 (1982).

Blackshear, P.J., "Systems for polyacrylamide gel electrophoresis", in W.B. Jakoby (Ed.), *Methods in Enzymology*, Vol. 104, *Enzyme and Related Techniques*, Part C, Academic Press, Orlando, FL, 1984, p. 237-255.

Davis, B.J., "Disc electrophoresis II. Method and application to human serum proteins," *Annals N.Y. Acad. Sci., 121*, 404 (1964).

Dean, J.A. (Ed.), *Lange's Handbook of Chemistry*, 13th ed., Marcel Dekker, New York, 1986.

Dobry, R. and R.K. Finn, "Engineering problems in large-scale electrophoresis", *Chem. Engr. Prog., 54*,(4) 59 (1958).

Dunn, M.J., "Electrophoresis in polyacrylamide gels", in J.W. Jorgenson and M. Phillips (Eds.), *New Directions in Electrophoretic Methods*, ACS Symp. Series No. 335, ACS, Washington, DC, 1987, Chapt. 2.

Dunn, M.J. and A.H. Burghes, *Electrophoresis, 4*, 97-116 (1983).

Durrum, E.L., "Continuous electrophoresis and ionophoresis on filter paper" *Journal ACS, 73*, 4875 (1951).

Epstein, I., "An apparatus for continuous separation of macromolecules by combined electrophoresis and gel filtration", *Chromatographia, 10* (2), 65 (1977).

Everaerts, F.M., J.L. Beckers, and Th.P.E.M. Verheggen, *Isotachophoresis. Theory, Instrumentation and Applications*, Journal of Chromatography Library, Vol. 6, Elsevier, Amsterdam, 1976.

Everaerts, F.M. and Th.P.E.M. Verheggen, "Capillary isotachophoresis", in J.W. Jorgenson and M. Phillips (Eds.), *New Directions in Electrophoretic Methods*, ACS Symp. Ser. No. 335, ACS, Washington, DC, 1987, Chapt. 14.

Fawcett, J.S., "Isoelectric focusing", in E. Reid (Ed.), *Methodological Developments in Biochemistry*, 2. *Preparative Techniques*, Longmans, London, 1973, Chapter 7.

Gianazza, E. and P.G. Righetti, "Electrophoresis in gels of graded porosity and two-dimensional techniques", in P.G. Righetti, C.J. van Oss, and J.W. Vanderhoff (Eds.), *Electrokinetic Separation Methods*, Elsevier/North Holland Biomedical Press, Amsterdam 1979, p. 293-311.

Giddings, J.C., "Generation of variance, theoretical plates, resolution, and peak capacity in electrophoresis and sedimentation", *Separ. Sci., 4*, 181 (1969).

Giddings, J.C., "Two-dimensional separations: concept and promise", *Anal. Chem., 56*, 1258A (1984).

Gobie, W.A., J.B. Beckwith and C.F. Ivory, "High resolution continuous flow electrophoresis", *Biotechnol. Prog., 1*, (1), 60 (1985).

Gordon, M.J., X. Huang, S.L. Pentoney, Jr., and R.N. Zare, "Capillary electrophoresis," *Science, 242*, 224 (1988).

Grassman, W. and K. Hannig, "Ein Enfaches Verfahren zur Kontinuirlichen Trennung von Stoffgemischen Auf Filterpapier Durch Electrophorese" *Naturwissenschaften, 37*, 397 (1950).

Hannig, K. "Continuous free-flow electrophoresis as an analytical and preparative method in biology", *J. Chromatogr., 159*, 183 (1978).

Haugaard, G. and T.D. Kroner, "Partition chromatography of amino acids with applied voltage", *Journal ACS, 70*, 2135 (1948).

Hiemenz, P.C., *Principles of Colloid and Surface Chemistry*, 2nd ed., Marcel Dekker, New York, 1986.

Holloway, C.J. and R.V. Battersby, "Preparative isotachophoresis", in W.B. Jakoby (Ed.), *Methods in Enzymology*, Vol. 104, *Purification and Related Techniques*, Part C, Academic Press, Orlando, 1984, Chapt. 15.

Horejsi, V., "Affinity electrophoresis", in W.B. Jakoby (Ed.), *Methods in Enzymology*, Vol. 104, *Enzyme Purfication and Related Techniques*, Part C, Academic Press, Prlando, FL, 1984, p. 275-281.

Ingram, V.M., "A specific chemical difference between the globins of normal human and sickle-cell anemia haemoglobin", *Nature, 178*, 792 (1956).

Jorgenson, J.W., "Capillary zone electrophoresis", in J.W. Jorgenson and M. Phillips (Eds.), *New Directions in Electrophoretic Methods*, ACS Symp. Ser. No. 335, ACS, Washington, DC, 1987, Chapt. 13.

Jorgenson, J.W. and K.D. Lukacs, "Zone electrophoresis in open-tubular glass capillaries", *Anal. Chem. 53*, 1298 (1981).

Just, W.W. and G. Werner, "Cell separation by continuous flow electrophoresis and isolectric focusing", in P.G. Righetti, C.J. van Oss, and J.W. Vanderhoff (Eds.), *Electrokinetic Separation Methods*, Elsevier/North Holland Biomedical Press, Amsterdam (1979), 143-167.

Karol, P.J. and M.H. Karol, "Isotachophoresis", *J. Chem. Educ., 55*, 626 (1979).

Kolin, A., "Endless belt continuous flow deviation electrophoresis", in P.G. Righetti, C.J. van Oss, and J.W. Vanderhoff (Eds.), *Electrokinetic Separation Methods*, Elsevier/North Holland Biomedical Press, Amsterdam (1979), 169-220.

Laurell, C.-B., "Quantitative estimation of proteins by electrophoresis in agarose gels continuing antibodies", *Anal. Biochem., 15*, 45 (1966).

Lehninger, A.L., *Biochemistry*, Worth, New York, 1970.

Lester, E.P., P.F. Lemkin, and L.E. Lipkin, "New dimensions in proteins analysis", *Anal. Chem., 53*, 390A (1981).

Locke, B.R. and R.G. Carbonell, "A theoretical and experimental study of counteracting chromatographic electrophoresis," *Separ. Purific. Methods, 18*, 1 (1989).

McCann, G.D., J.W. Vanderhoff, A. Strickler and T.I. Sacks, "Separation of latex particles according to size by continuous flow electrophoresis", *Separation Purific. Methods, 2*, 153 (1973).

Maizel, J.V., Jr., "Acrylamide-gel electrophorograms by mechanical fractionation: radioactive adenovirus protein", *Science 151*, 989 (1966).

Mel, H.C., "Stable-flow boundary migration and fractionation of cell mixtures. I. Apparatus and hydrodynamic feedback principles", *J. Theoret. Biol., 6*, 307 (1964).

Melvin, M., *Electrophoresis*, in Analytical Chemistry by Open Learning Series, Wiley, Chichester, England, 1987.

Mosher, R.A., W. Thormann, N.B. Egen, P. Couasnon, and D.W. Sammons, "Recent advances in preparative electrophoresis", in J.W. Jorgenson and M. Phillips (Eds.), *New Directions in Electrophoretic Methods*, ACS Symp. Ser. No. 335, ACS, Washington, DC, 1987, Chapt. 16.

Morrison, D.R., G.H. Barlow, and C. Cleveland et al., *Adv. Space Res., 4*, 67 (1984).

Nerenberg, S.T. and G. Pogojeff, "Preparative electrochromatography and electrophoresis using adopted Sephadex and other columns," *Am. J. Clin. Path., 51*, 728 (1969).

Newman, J.T., *Electrochemical Systems*, Prentice-Hall, Englewood Cliffs, N.J., 1973, Chapt. 11.

613

O'Brien, R.W. and L.R. White, "Electrophoretic mobility of a spherical colloidal particle," *J. Chem. Soc. Faraday Transactions, II, 74*, 1607 (1978).

O'Farrell, P.H. "High resolution two-dimensional electrophoresis of proteins", *J. Biol. Chem., 250*, 4007 (1975).

O'Farrell, P.H. "Separation techniques based on the opposition of two counteracting forces to produce a dynamic equilibrium," *Science, 227*, 1586 (March 29, 1985).

Ornstein, L., "Disc electrophoresis I. Background and theory," *Annals N.Y. Acad. Sci., 121*, 321 (1964).

Ostrach, S., "Convection in continuous-flow electrophoresis", *J. Chromatogr., 140*, 187 (1977).

Overbeek, J.Th.G. and B.H. Bijsterbosch, "The electrical double layer and the theory of electrophoresis", in P.G. Righetti, C.J. van Oss and J.W. Vanderhoff (Eds.), *Electrokinetic Separation Methods*, Elsevier/North-Holland Biomedical Press, Amsterdam, 1979, p. 1-32.

Philpot, J.St.L., "Apparatus for continuous-flow preparative electrophoresis", in E. Reid (Ed.), *Methodological Developments in Biochemistry, 2. Preparative Techniques*, Longmans, London, 1973, Chapter 8.

Philpot, J.St.L., "The use of thin layers in electrophoretic separations", *Trans. Faraday Soc., 39*, 38 (1940).

Radola, B.J., "High-resolution preparative isolectric focusing", in W.B. Jakoby (Ed.), *Methods in Enzymology*, Vol. 104, *Enzyme Purification and Related Techniques*, Part C, Academic Press, 1984, Chapter 13.

Reeder, D.J., "Development of electrophoresis and electrofocusing standards", in J.W.Jorgenson and M. Phillips (Eds.), *New Directions in Electrophoretic Methods*, ACS Symp. Ser. No. 335, ACS, Washington, DC, 1987, Chapt. 7.

Righetti, P.G., *Isolectric Focusing: Theory, Methodology and Applications*, Elsevier Biomedical, Amsterdam, 1983.

Righetti, P.G., E. Gianazza, and K. Ek, "New developments in isoelectric focusing", *J. Chromatogr., 184*, 415, (1980).

Righetti, P.G., C. Gelfi, and E. Gianazza, "Immobilized pH gradients: recent developments", in J.W. Jorgenson and M. Phillips (Eds.), *New Directions in Electrophoretic Methods*, ACS Symp. Ser. No. 335, ACS, Washington, DC, 1987, Chapt. 3.

Rilbe, H., "Historical and theoretical aspects of isoelectric focusing," *Ann. N.Y. Acad. Sci. 209*, 11, (1973).

Schwartz, D.C., "Pulsed electrophoresis", in J.W. Jorgenson and M. Phillips (Eds.), *New Directions in Electrophoretic Methods*, ACS Symp. Ser. No. 335, ACS, Washington, DC, 1987, Chapt. 12.

Smith, I. (Ed.), *Chromatographic and Electrophoretic Techniques*, Vol. II. *Zone Electrophoresis*, 2nd Ed., William Heineman Ltd., 1968.

Smith, I., "Zone electrophoresis on paper, thin layers and pevikon block", in P.G. Righetti, C.J. van Oss, and J.W. Vanderhoff (Eds.), *Electrokinetic Separation Methods*, Elsevier/North Holland Biomedical Press, Amsterdam (1979), p. 33-53.

Smithies, O., "Zone electrophoresis in starch gels: group variations in the serum proteins of normal human adults", *Biochem. J. 61*, 629 (1955).

Strain, H.H. and Sullivan, J.C., "Analysis by electromigration plus chromatography", *Anal. Chem. 23*, 816 (1951).

Svensson, H., "Isoelectric fractionation, analysis, and characterization of ampholytes in natural pH gradients. I. The differential equation of solute concentrations at a steady state and its solution in simple cases", *Acta Chem. Scand. 15*, 325 (1961).

Svensson, H., "Isoelectric fractionation, analysis, and characterization of ampholytes in natural pH gradients. II. Buffering capacity and conductance of isoionic ampholytes", *Acta Chem. Scand. 16*, 456 (1962a).

Svensson, H., "Isoelectric fractionation, analysis, and characterization of ampholytes in natural pH gradients. III. Description of apparatus for electrolysis in columns stabilized by density gradients and direct determination of isoelectric points", *Arch. Biochem. Biophys. Suppl. 1*, 132 (1962b).

Svensson, H. and I. Brattsten, "An apparatus for continous flow electrophoresis", *Arkiv. Kemi. 1*, (47), 401 (1949).

Tiselius, A., "A new apparatus for electrophoretic analysis of colloidal mixtures", *Trans. Faraday Soc., 33*, 524 (1937).

Vanderhoff, J.W. and F.J. Micale, "Influence of electroosmosis", in P.G. Righetti, C.J. van Oss, and J.W. Vanderhoff, (Eds.), *Electrokinetic Separation Methods*, Elsevier/North-Holland Biomedical Press, Amsterdam, 1979, p. 81-93.

Vesterberg, O., "Synthesis and isoelectric fractionation of carrier ampholytes", *Acta Chem. Scand., 23*, 2653 (1969).

Wankat, P.C., "Two-dimensional separation processes", *Separ. Sci. Technol., 19*, 801 (1984-85).

HOMEWORK

A. *Discussion Problems*

A1. Define the following terms.

    a. Moving boundary electrophoresis

    b. Zone electrophoresis

    c. Isoelectric focusing

    d. Isotachophoresis

    e. Paper electrophoresis

    f. SDS-PAGE electrophoresis

    g. Immunoelectrophoresis

    h. Rocket electrophoresis

    i. Fingerprinting

    j. Capillary electrophoresis

    k. Free flow electrophoresis

    l. Recycle electrophoresis

    m. pI

    n. Electrical double layer

    o. Zeta potential

    p. Electroosmosis

    q. Carrier ampholyte

A2. Explain why the "rockets" shown in Figure 11-5c form.

A3. Why is isolectric focusing a more robust separation method than electrophoresis?

A4. Explain why the two developments should be independent in sequential two-dimensional systems?

A5. Why is two-dimensional electrophoresis currently the system of choice for scale-up?

A6. Continuous operation of counteracting chromatographic electrophoresis would not completely purify the desired proteins. Explain why there would be more impurity than in batch operation.

A7. Develop your key relations page for this chapter.

B. *Generation of Alternatives*

B1. Brainstorm at least 20 different sequential two-dimensional development methods. A matrix may be useful for doing this.

C. *Derivations*

C1. Transform the one-dimensional zone spreading Eqs. (11-15) to (11-24) to the continuous two-dimensional system shown in Figure 11-7a.

C2. Equation (11-15) can be derived by solving the appropriate partial differential equations. The Lapidus and Amundson dispersion model (see Section 7.4) can be used to develop the solution. Do this derivation.

NOTES: 1. Use Eq. (7-10).

2. $A(T) = 0$ and $v = u_{i,net}$ (Eq. (11-16b)).

3. Use superposition Eq. (7-7) and the definition of erf in Eq. (7-11a).

C3. Units are a problem and need to be practiced.

a. Show that ψ_o in Eq. (11-5b) is in volts.

b. Show that the units in Eq. (11-4b) are correct.

c. Show that the units in Eq. (11-9b) are correct.

D. *Single Answer Problems*

D1. A 1×10^{-9} m diameter particle has a measured mobility of 1×10^{-8} m^2/sV in a 0.0001 M aqueous solution of $Na_2 SO_4$ at 25°C. What is the value of ζ?

D2. A protein is run in a PAGE electrophoresis apparatus for 3 hours at 2000 volts. The plate is 20 cm long. The center of the protein spot is measured at 8.54 cm from the feed well and the spot width is 0.103 cm. Estimate μ and D for the protein at the conditions of this experiment.

D3. Tiselius (1937) reported the following data on two proteins: $A = R.$ Phycocyan and $B = R.$ Phycoerythrin.

$$pI_A = 4.85 \qquad\qquad pI_B = 4.25$$

$$\left[\frac{d\mu}{dpH} \right]_A = -\,10.2 \times 10^{-5} \text{ (at pI)} \qquad \left[\frac{d\mu}{dpH} \right]_B = -\,14.2 \times 10^{-5} \text{ (at pI)}$$

μ is in cm^2/s volt.

The proteins are to be separated in a continuous flow, two-dimensional free solution apparatus (see Fig. 11-7). The apparatus dimensions are $L = 10$ cm, $W = 5$ cm and $h = 0.3$ cm. The feed entry is 0.1 cm wide. Voltage is 900 volts. Average fluid velocity $v_{buffer} = 0.2$ cm/s. The apparatus is horizontal and has efficient cooling from the bottom. Assume there is no thermal convection and no electroosmosis.

a.) At pH 4.25 estimate μ_A and μ_B. Determine the angles a_A and a_B. Estimate the width of the zones at the exit and the locations of the peak maximums if $D = 4 \times 10^{-7}$ cm^2/s for both proteins. If the observed width is 0.9 cm, calculate D_{eff}.

b.) Repeat part A at pH 4.55. Assume the values of $d\mu/d(pH)$ are constant.

D4. A sequential 2D experiment is done for a protein which has $D_{y,1} \sim 10^{-8}$ and $D_{y,2} \sim 2 \times 10^{-7}$ cm^2/s. Assume $D_{y,1} = D_{z,1}$ and $D_{z,2} = 5 \times 10^{-6}$. The first development is for 4 hours and the second is for 10 hours.

a. What are the widths w_y and w_z of the spot?

b. If the spot center is at $Y = 5.0$ cm, $Z = 10.6$ cm, plot the constant concentration line where $c = 0.5\, c_{max}$ on a y,z plane.

D5. We wish to separate various ammonium ions by isotachophoresis. NH_4^+ is used as the leading ion and $(C_4H_9)_4\, N^+$ as the trailing ion. Initial concentration of NH_4^+ and $(C_4H_9)_4\, N^+$ are both 0.03 N. The feed contains 0.01N $CH_3NH_3^+$, 0.0025N $(CH_3)_3\, NH^+$ and 0.006N $(C_2H_5)_4\, N^+$. The feed band is 2 cm long. The experiment is operated as a batch experiment in free solution Cl⁻ is the anion. Once the bands have been formed, determine the concentrations of $CH_3NH_3^+$, $(CH_3)_3 NH^+$, $(C_2H_5)_4 N^+$ and $(C_4H_9)_4 N^+$. Also, find the widths of the $CH_3 NH_3^+$, $(CH_3)_3 NH^+$ and $(C_2H_5)_4 N^+$ bands. Data is in Table 11-3.

D6. An isotachophoresis experiment is done to determine μ_{Na}. The leading electrolyte is NH_4^+ of concentration 0.01 N. Trailing electrolyte is $(C_2 H_5)_4 N^+$ initially at 0.005 N. The co-ion is Cl⁻. The feed band is 3 cm wide and contains 0.005 N NaCl. After the experiment is at steady state, the Na⁺ band is 1.8703 cm wide. What is μ_{Na^+} (in cm²/Vs)? Data is in Table 11-3.

D7. The two proteins in problem 11-D3 are to be separated in a batch IEF system. The system length is 10 cm. pH varies linearly from pH 3.0 to pH 5.0 over this length. Note that this is a very easy IEF separation. Assume $D_{eff} = 0.0004$ cm²/s which is high for an IEF system.

a.) Determine the field strength E required to achieve an acceptable separation (Eqs. 11-49 and 11-50).

b.) At the field strength calculated in part A determine σ_A, σ_B and the widths of the two zones. (width = 4σ).

c.) If E = 80 volts/cm, determine σ_A and σ_B and the widths.

D8. An isoelectric focusing experiment was done on a cooled plate. The following data were obtained at steady state at E = 100 V/cm:

Observed Compound	Distance from anode, cm
Ovalbumin	6.2
β-aspartyl-histidine	7.0
Evans blue (pI = 5.35)	8.5
Congo red (pI = 5.80)	10.1

See Table 11-2 for additional data on these compounds.

a. We wish to separate two similar proteins whose pI is about 5.2, $D = 2 \times 10^{-7}$ cm^2/s,

$$\frac{d\mu}{d(pH)} = -1.5 \times 10^{-5} \; \frac{cm^2}{s \; V \; (pH \; unit)}$$

What difference in pI values is required to obtain two resolved peaks?

b. If another protein is observed at 9.1 cm, what is its pI?

D9. A continuous flow, two-dimensional, free solution, IEF system is used for separating proteins. The carrier ampholyte is prefocused. Assume that steady state is obtained. Dimensions: L = 20 cm, W = 10 cm, 2h = 0.5 cm. There are 50 outlets and each covers 0.2 cm of the width. From a given outlet the product is well mixed. Operation is at 25°C. The pH gradient varies from 3 at the anode to 10 at the cathode. Assume the gradient is approximately linear. Assume cooling is adequate and there is no convection. Ports are numbered starting with 1 at the anode.

a. Which port(s) does protein A of Problem 11-D3 exit from if V = 375 volts?

b. Which port(s) does protein B of Problem 11-D3 exit from if V = 375 volts?

Part III
MEMBRANES

NOMENCLATURE CHAPTERS 12 AND 13

a, a'	terms in quadratic equation
a	constant for diffusivity, Eq. (12-75)
a	constant for osmotic pressure, Eqs. (12-18b,c)
A	area of membrane, m^2 or cm^2
A_{cs}	cross-sectional area for flow, m^2 or cm^2
A_m	area of a membrane in ED stack, m^2
b	constant, Eq. (12-64)
b, b'	terms in quadratic equation
c, c'	terms in quadratic equation
c	concentration. Either weight or molar or equivalents (ED) g/L, g/cc, gmoles/L, g equivalents/L
c_b	bulk concentration
c_g	gel concentration
c_{in}	inlet concentration
c_m	concentration in membrane
c_{out}	outlet concentration
c_p	permeate concentration
c_{2m}	solute concentration in membrane
c'_{2m}	solute concentration in membranes on high pressure side
c''_{2m}	solute concentration in membrane on low pressure side
c_{2p}	solute concentration in permeate
c_w	wall concentration

623

c_{2w}	solute concentration at wall
$C_{P,L}$	heat capacity liquid, cal/g°C
$C_{p,v}$	heat capacity vapor, cal/g°C
d,D	diameter, cm or m
d_{eq}	Equivalent diameter, Eq. (13-12).
d_p	particle diameter in gel layer, m
D	Diffusivity, cm²/s
D_{1m}	solvent diffusivity in membrane, cm²/s
D_{2m}	solute diffusivity in membrane, cm²/s
D_o	parameter for diffusivity, Eq. (12-75)
E	energy, joules
f	Fanning friction factor, Eq. (13-10b,c)
f_{12}, f_{23}	friction factors, Eqs. (13-86) and (13-87)
F	flow rate, gmoles/time or g/time
F_{in}	inlet flow rate, kg moles/s or m³/s
F_{out}	outlet flow rate, kg moles/s or m³/s
F_p	permeate flow rate, cm³/s, m³/s or kg moles/s
$F_{Recycle}$	recycle flow rate
F	Faraday. 96,500 amp·sec/equiv
h	half height between parallel plates, cm
H	hydrodynamic permeability, Eq. (13-96)
ΔH_f	latent heat of freezing, Eq. (12-19)
i	current density, amp/m²

I	current, amps
j_D	Colburn j-factor, Eq. (13-10a,b)
J_{asy}	asymptotic volumetric flux, Eq. (13-19)
J_{init}	initial flux
J_{solv}, J_1	volumetric solvent flux, $cm^3/cm^2 s$ or L/m^2 day
J'_{solv}, J'_1	mass solvent flux, $g/cm^2 s$
J_{solute}, J_2	solute flux, $g/cm^2 s$
$J_{2,dif}$	solute flux due to diffusion
k	mass transfer coefficient, cm/s
k^I_{solute}	feed mass transfer coefficient
k^{II}_{solute}	dialysate mass transfer coefficients
k^T	total mass transfer coefficient in dialysis
K_A	solubility parameter, Eq. (12-15)
K_g	gel permeability, Eq. (12-38)
K_{solute}	solute permeability
K_{solv}	solvent permeability
K_1	$= c_{1m}/c_{1p}$, solvent distribution coefficient
K_2	solute distribution coefficient, Eq. (13-78)
L	length, cm or m
L_{ii}, L_{ij}	phenomenological coefficients, Section 13.6
m	exponent for flux decay, Eq. (13-19)
m	mobility, Section 13.6
M	$= c_w/c_b$, concentration polarization modulus

MW	molecular weight
n	total moles solute, Section 12.5.
n	number of tubes or cells
n	constant in Eq. (12-18c)
N	number of molecules or particles
N_A	Rate of transfer, cm^3/s
p	pressure, atm, bar, psi, mmHg, kPa
p_h, p_H	high pressure
p_L	low pressure
p_P	permeate pressure
Δp_m	effective pressure driving force across membrane, Eq. (13-94)
$\bar{p}$	partial pressure
$\bar{p}_1$	partial pressure on liquid side for pervaporation
$\bar{p}_2$	partial pressure on vapor side for pervaporation
P	permeability of gas, cm^3 (STP) $cm/cm^2 s$ (cm Hg)
$q_1, q_2,$	molar flow rates on high pressure and permeate sides
q_p	permeate molar flow rate
Q	charge, coloumbs
Q	volumetric flow rate, cm^3/s or L/hr
Q_d	dialysate volumetric flow rate
Q_F	feed volumetric flow rate
r	radial direction
R	radius, cm
R	resistance per cell, ohms

R	retention
R	gas constant
R°	inherent retention $= 1 - c_p/c_w$
R_{app}	apparent retention $= 1 - c_p/c_b$
R_{energy}	gas constant in energy units, (Example 13-1)
R_p	pore radius, cm
R_{press}	gas constant in pressure units, (Example 13-1)
Re	Reynolds number $= d\, u_b\, \rho/\mu$
S^*	Henry's law constant, Eq. (12-76)
Sc	Schmidt number $= \mu\, \rho/D$
t	time, s or days
t_g	gel layer thickness, cm
t_m	membrane thickness, cm
T	absolute temperature, K
T_f, T_f^*	freezing temperature of solution and pure solvent, K
T_{in}	inlet temperature
T_{out}	outlet temperature
T_{ref}	reference temperature
u	velocity in x direction, cm/s
u	center of mass velocity of pore fluid
u_b	bulk velocity, cm/s
u_{in}	inlet average velocity, cm/s
v	velocity in y or r direction, cm/s
v_i	partial molar volume, Eq. (13-63)

v_w	velocity through wall, cm/s
v_1	partial molar volume of solvent, gmoles/cm^3
$v_{solvent}$	partial molar volume of solvent, gmoles/cm^3
V	voltage, volts
V	volume, cm^3 or L
VP	vapor pressure
w	width, cm
x	axial distance, cm
x	distance into membrane, cm
x	liquid mole fraction
X_i	force on component i, Section 13.6
y	direction perpendicular to parallel plates
y	gas or vapor mole fraction
y'	y/h
y_h	gas mole fraction on high pressure side
y_{in}	inlet mole fraction
y_{out}	outlet mole fraction
y_p	permeate mole fraction
y_1	mole fraction on high pressure side
y_2	mole fraction on permeate side
$y_{2,0}$	eqs. (13-44a,c)
Y_i	external force on component i, Section 13-6
z	feed mole fraction

Greek Letters

α	selectivity, K_{solv}/K_{solute} in RO
α_{AB}	selectivity, P_A/P_B, in gas permeation
α'_{AB}	selectivity, Eq. (12-81), in pervaporation
γ_w	fluid shear rate, Eqs. (13-15) and (13-17)
δ	boundary layer thickness, cm
ε	porosity
η_m	manifold efficiency, ED
η_s	semipermeability membrane efficiency, ED
η_w	water transfer efficiency, ED
θ	cut $= F_p/F_{in}$
θ_{Tot}	total cut in recycle system, F_p/F_{new}
λ	latent heat of vaporization, cal/g or cal/gmole
λ	tortuosity
μ	viscosity, poise or pascal-sec.
μ_i	chemical potential of species i
ν	kinematic viscosity $= \mu/\rho$
ξ	efficiency of current utilization, Eq. (12-67)
ξ	$v_w^3\,h\,x/3u_{in}\,D^2$, Section 13.5
π	osmotic pressure, atm
π	Pi, 3.141592654....
ρ	density, g/cm^3
$\hat{\rho}$	molar density, gmoles/cm^3 or kgmoles/m^3
ω	angular velocity, radians/s

Chapter 12

INTRODUCTION TO MEMBRANE SEPARATIONS

A variety of membrane separation processes such as reverse osmosis, ultrafiltration, gas permeation, and electrodialysis are becoming increasingly popular in industry. This popularity is due to the simplicity of the processes, the gentle nature of the separation (high temperatures and phase changes are not required), the usual low energy requirements, and the often low capital and operating costs. In this chapter all of the membrane separation processes will be introduced. Simple equations for understanding and designing the processes will be presented. The emphasis will be on understanding the physical nature of the processes. Chapter 13 builds on the basics presented in this chapter and presents more detailed analyses of the processes occurring in membrane separators.

12.1. BASIC CONCEPTS

A membrane is a physical barrier between two fluids. In over 99% of the cases of current industrial interest the membrane is made from a polymer. This polymer is cast or spun or extruded to form a continuous film without holes in the desired geometry. The simplest geometry used for membrane separators is the stirred cell shown in Figure 12-1. The fluid enters into the upper chamber. Part of the feed stream is transferred through the membrane to the lower chamber. With a perfect membrane only species A will transfer through the membrane while species B will remain in the upper chamber. Either species may be the desired product. The stirrer is used to improve mass transfer rates and prevent the buildup of species B at the membrane surface.

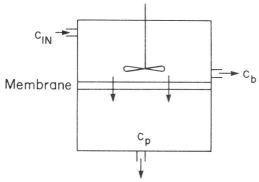

Figure 12-1.   Stirred cell membrane system

The flux through the membrane can be written as

$$\text{Flux} = \frac{\text{Transfer rate}}{\text{Transfer area}} = \frac{\text{Permeability}}{\text{Thickness}} (\text{Driving Force}) \qquad (12\text{-}1)$$

Flux is defined either as J = (Volume)/(area)(time) or as J' = (mass)/(area)(time). Obviously, these two fluxes are related by $J' = J\rho_p$ where ρ_p is the permeate density. The flux depends linearly on both the permeability (a constant which indicates how "tight" the membrane is) and the driving force. The driving force depends upon the type of separation. For instance, in gas permeation the driving force is the pressure difference across the membrane. The membrane can separate two gases because the permeabilities are very different. Note that, in general, both gases do transfer through the membrane, but one of them transfers at a much higher rate. Thus, most membrane separators are not equilibrium processes but are *rate processes*. The flux also depends inversely upon the thickness of the membrane. The thinner the membrane the higher the flux.

High fluxes are usually very desirable since the transfer area required will be lessened. Thus we want a high driving force. In the cases of gas permeation, reverse osmosis (used for purifying water) and ultrafiltration (used for concentrating large molecules) this means a high pressure drop across the membrane. The membrane must be mechanically strong to withstand these high pressures. Mechanical strength requires a thick membrane. However,

a   Feed Phase

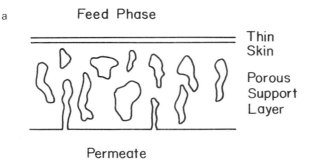

Thin
Skin

Porous
Support
Layer

Permeate

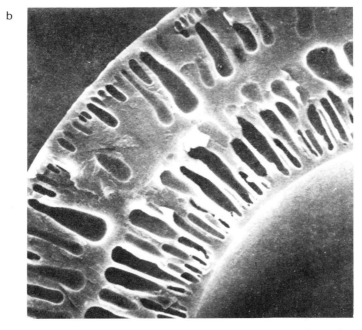

Figure 12-2.   Asymmetric membrane. a. Schematic. b. Scanning electron microscope photograph. (Warashina *et al*, 1985). Part b reprinted with permission from *Chem. Tech*, 558 (1985). Copyright 1985, American Chemical Society.

Eq.(12-1) shows that thick membranes will have low fluxes and hence large areas will be required to achieve the desired transfer rate. A fundamental problem which stopped the commercial use of membranes for many years was how to make a membrane which was thin enough to have high fluxes while at the same time it was mechanically strong.

The solution to this problem was found in the late 1950's and early 1960's by Sidney Loeb and S. Sourirajan (Loeb and Sourirajan, 1960, 1963). Their solution was to make a membrane which was *asymmetric* or *anisotropic*. This type of membrane is illustrated in Figure 12-2. The membrane was cast to have a very dense thin layer or skin on one side. This layer was typically 0.1 to 1.0 microns thick. The thin skin does the actual separation of the species. Thus in Eq.(12-1) the *thickness* term is very small. The thin skin is supported by a much thicker porous layer. This layer provides the required mechanical strength, but it is so porous that no separation occurs in this layer. These membranes can be operated at pressure drops in excess of 1000 psig. The Loeb-Sourirajan membrane was made from cellulose acetate for desalination of water by reverse osmosis. Methods for casting these membranes are reviewed by Kesting (1985) and Soltanieh and Gill (1981). The use of asymmetric membranes has been extended to a variety of other polymers and to other membrane separation methods. The history of membrane separations is discussed by Lonsdale (1982). Not all membrane separators use asymmetric membranes. The exceptions will be discussed in the individual sections.

A variety of different polymers have been used commercially for membrane systems. The polymers used can be classified into three categories: *rubbery polymers, glassy polymers,* and *ion exchange membranes*. Rubbery polymers such as silicone rubber operate above the glass transition temperature, T_g, of the polymer. As a generalization, rubbery polymers have high fluxes of organics and low flux of water. Glassy polymers such as polycarbonate operate below T_g. These polymers can be either amorphous or partially crystalline. Glassy polymers are selective for water. Ion exchange membranes are essentially ion exchange resins (see Chapter 9) made in membrane form. Ion exchange membranes are very selective for water.

The most common structures are shown in Figure 12-3 (Kesting, 1985;

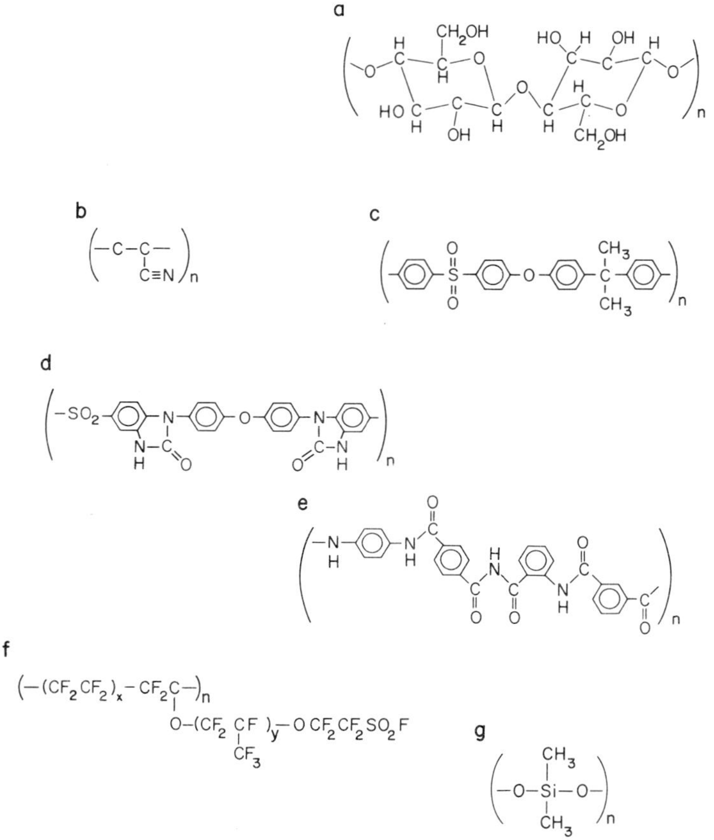

Figure 12-3.   Polymers used for membrane separators. a. Cellulose (D,UF).
b. Polyacrylonitrile (D,UF). c. Polysulfone (GP,RO,UF,ED). d.
Polybenzimidazolone (RO). e. Polyamide (from terephthalic
acid m-amino benzamide and m-phenylene diamine) (RO,UF).
f. Nafion (Donnan dialysis). g. Silicone (GP). Key: GP = Gas
Permeation, D = Dialysis, RO = Reverse Osmosis, UF =
Ultrafiltration, ED = Electrodialysis

Pusch and Walch, 1982; Soltanieh and Gill, 1981; Ward *et al.*, 1985). Additional examples of polymers used for membranes are discussed by Kesting (1985), Lloyd and Meluch (1985), Finken (1985), Pusch and Walch (1982), and Ward *et al.*, (1985). For example, Figure 12-3 shows only one of the possible polyamides (Kesting, 1985; Pusch and Walch, 1982). The cellulose (Figure 12-3a) and cellulose acetate membranes were the first commercially successful membranes. Although still commonly used, considerable research has gone into developing membranes with better chemical and thermal resistances. Polysulfone (Figure 12-3c) and Nafion (Figure 12-3f) have outstanding resistances to chemicals. Polystyrene cross-linked with divinylbenzene (Figures 9-1 a and b) also has excellent chemical resistance and is used as a backing for composite membranes and as the basis for electrodialysis membranes.

With a high flux rate species B which does not transfer through the membrane may build up to a high concentration at the surface of the1 membrane. This is called *concentration polarization* and is illustrated in Figure 12-4. Since the transfer rate of species B through the membrane is low, the permeate concentration is low, $c_p \ll c_b$. Species A (which might be the solvent) has a high flux through the membrane. Thus, there must be a convective flow towards the membrane. This convective flow carries B to the membrane surface. Since the flux of B is low, the concentration of B will build up at the membrane wall. Thus, a concentration gradient is produced. This buildup of B

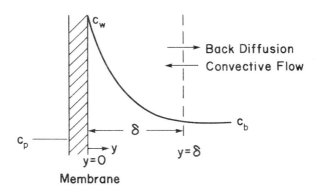

Figure 12-4.   Build-up of retained species at membrane wall (concentration polarization).

is counteracted by diffusion into the bulk fluid. If diffusion rates are high as is true in most gas systems, then the concentration buildup will be modest and concentration polarization will not be a problem.

In liquid systems diffusivities are small and $c_w > c_b$. Concentration polarization is detrimental for several reasons. The high c_w value means that any liquid that leaks through the membrane will be at a high concentration of B and thus will increase c_p. The high wall concentration also increases the osmotic pressure (see Section 12.4.) which reduces the driving force for transfer of solvent. High concentrations of solute can also cause gelling or fouling at the membrane surface which will drastically decrease flux (see Section 12.5.). To avoid concentration polarization we can use stirring, turbulence, high shear rates, or very thin channels.

12.2. MEMBRANE MODULES

The general design requirements for any membrane system can now be listed.
1. Thin active layer of membrane.
2. High permeability for species A and low permeability for species B.
3. Stable membrane with long service life.
4. Mechanically strong.
5. Large surface area of membrane in small volume.
6. Concentration polarization eliminated or at least controlled.
7. Easy to clean if necessary.
8. Inexpensive to build.
9. Low operating cost.

This list of desirable design conditions is general. Items specific to each of the membrane devices will be discussed later. A historical perspective on membrane modules with many early advertisements is given by Kremen (1986). Currently, spiral wound and hollow fiber systems have most of the market.

The simplest geometry for a membrane separator is the stirred cell shown in Figure 12-1. Stirred cells are commonly used in laboratories, but the membrane surface area is small. Thus for large scale commercial applications other

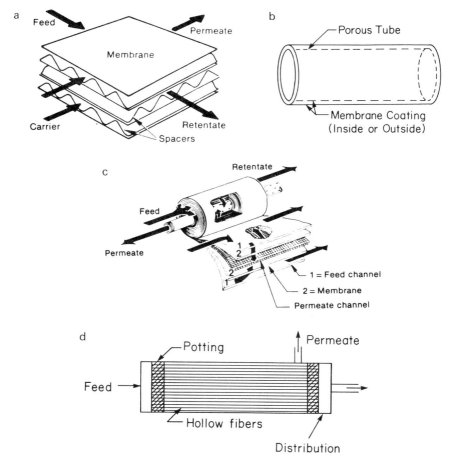

Figure 12-5.   Geometries of commercial membrane systems. a. Plate-and-
frame. b. Tubular. c. Spiral wound. d. Hollow fiber.

geometries are required. The most commonly used commercial systems are
shown in Figure 12-5. The plate-and-frame system is similar to a plate-and-
frame filter press with a series of flat membrane sheets. The area per volume
ratio is significantly higher than stirred cells but lower than spiral wound or
hollow fiber systems. The sheets can be quite close together to reduce concentration polarization. The major advantage of plate-and-frame systems is they

can be taken apart for cleaning if necessary. Their major application has been in the food industry where fouling is a major problem. The plate-and-frame geometry is also used for electrodialysis.

Cylindrical geometries are also used. In the tubular system shown in Figure 12-5b the membrane is coated on the inside or outside of the porous support tube. Typical inside diameters are in the range from 1 cm to 1 inch. A bundle of tubes can be packaged together as in a shell-and-tube heat exchanger, but the area/volume ratio is low. The main advantage of tubular systems is they can be mechanically cleaned by forcing a sponge ball through the tubes. Thus tubular systems compete with plate-and-frame systems for dirty or fouling applications. Design details of these systems are given by Stana (1977).

The spiral wound system shown in Figure 12-5c is a way of increasing the area/volume ratio of flat plat devices. Two feed channels, two membranes, and a permeate channel are layered and wrapped around a central porous tube several times. Spiral wound systems made from cellulose acetate are commonly used for reverse osmosis. This design is a good method for achieving large area/volume (about 300 ft^2 per ft^3) with membrane materials which cannot easily be extruded into hollow fibers. Concentration polarization is controlled by using thin channels and wrapping the membrane around plastic netting which induces turbulence. Unfortunately, these systems cannot be used for treating very dirty or fouling systems since they are not easy to clean. Design details are given by Kremen (1977). Spiral wound is one of the two most popular configurations.

The hollow fiber system shown in Figures 12-5d and 12-6 is also one of the two most popular designs. The fibers are extruded from polymers such as Nylon or polysulfone. A typical reverse osmosis hollow fiber would have a inner diameter of 42 microns, an outer diameter of 85 microns, and a 0.1 to 1.0 micron skin on the outer surface (Applegate, 1984). For gas permeation the fibers are made somewhat larger to reduce the pressure drop inside the tubes. For ultrafiltration the fibers are much larger (500 to 1100 micron i.d.) and the skin is on the inside of the fiber. These numbers indicate that a considerable amount of engineering design can be done with the fibers. The fibers can have fairly thick walls and with flow radially inward large pressure gradients can be

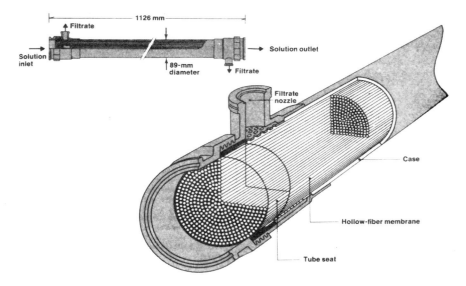

Figure 12-6. Details of hollow-fiber module. (Warashina *et al*, 1985). Reprinted with permission from *Chem. Tech.*, 558 (1985). Copyright 1985, American Chemical Society.

handled. The major advantage of the hollow fiber systems is that a huge number of fibers (4.5×10^6) can be packed inside a 25.4 cm (10 inch) diameter cartridge. Thus the area/volume ratio is very high (about 5000 ft^2 per ft^3) and costs are kept down. A major disadvantage of hollow fibers is particulate solids can permanently clog the tiny fibers. Thus dirty fluids must be thoroughly cleaned before being sent to the hollow fiber separator. Details of hollow fiber systems are given by Orofino (1977) and Caracciolo *et al.*, (1977).

All of the basic systems are usually built in a few basic modular sizes. A "module" is a complete unit such as a hollow fiber separator capable of processing a given amount of fluid with a given separation. The details of a hollow fiber module used for ultrafiltration are shown in Figure 12-6 (Warashina *et al.*, 1985). A single module is often not sufficient for the required flow rate and/or separation. Thus modules are cascaded in a variety of ways to produce the desired separation. One advantage of modular construction is the modules

640

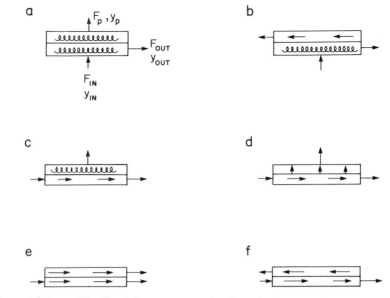

Figure 12-7.   Idealized flow patterns for flow inside module. a. Completely
mixed. b. Mixed on feed (high pressure side). c. Mixed on permeate (low pressure) side. d. Cross-flow. e. Co-current. f.
countercurrent.

can be constructed in a plant instead of being field constructed. This is usually
significantly cheaper. One disadvantage of modular construction is that there is
probably very little economy of scale.

The flow patterns inside the module have a large effect on the outlet concentrations and flow rates of the high and low pressure products. Several idealized flow patterns are shown in Figure 12-7. The completely mixed case, Figure 12-7a, is the easiest to analyze but the least advantageous for separation.
The system which is mixed on the feed side, Figure 12-7b, is close to the flow
pattern which occurs for most hollow fiber systems for gas permeation and
reverse osmosis. Figure 12-7c shows the idealized flow pattern of a hollow
fiber system for ultrafiltration where the feed is inside the fibers. The solution
is well-mixed on the permeate side. Plate-and-frame and spiral wound systems
can have a modification of the cross-flow system, Figure 12-7d, or they could

be modifications of the co-current flow system, Figure 12-7e or the counter-current flow system, Figure 12-7f. The countercurrent flow pattern will be most advantageous and has been used to design experimental fractionation systems.

Once the flow pattern is known external mass balances can be combined with Eq. (12-1) to solve for the outlet concentrations and flow rates. For a completely mixed system Eq. (12-1) is the same everywhere. Mass balances for perfectly mixed systems will be illustrated throughout this chapter. These are the easiest balances to solve, and since perfectly mixed gives the least separation the design will be conservative. For the other flow patterns the driving force varies throughout the module and an integration is required. These external mass balances are developed in Chapter 13.

Cascade schemes are shown in Figure 12-8. When the capacity of a single module is insufficient, the obvious solution is to connect two or more modules in parallel (Figure 12-8a). If a single module is unable to remove the desired amount of permeable species A, the series arrangement shown in Figure 12-8b can be used. The parallel-series arrangement is useful when both high flow rates and high recoveries of A are desired. Note in Figure 12-8c that the number of modules in parallel can be decreased as more fluid is removed. A commonly used alternative is the recycle system in Figure 12-8d. This system keeps flow rates high to decrease concentration polarization and it allows for a high recovery of the permeable species. Recycle systems are commonly used in batch operation to process liquids. Recycle systems can also be put in parallel to increase the capacity. When the selectivity of the membrane is too low to produce a pure enough permeate, the permeate in series arrangement shown in Figure 12-8e can be used. The engineer would prefer to obtain a better membrane instead of staging the permeate since permeate staging requires an extra pump or compressor. Thus operating costs will be high. Note that a recycle stream will often be used for the stream that does not pass through the membrane. If both streams need to be put in series the counter-current cascade shown in Figure 12-8f can be used. This countercurrent cascade is similar to other countercurrent cascades discussed in this book except that additional energy must be input before each stage. This occurs because the rate process is unable to reuse the energy from stage-to-stage. Because of this,

642

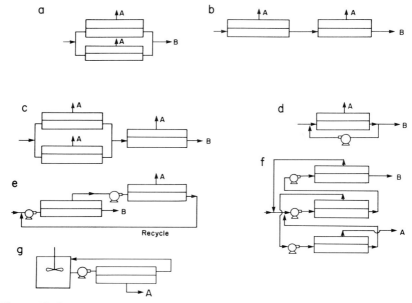

Figure 12-8.   Cascades for membrane separators. a. Parallel. b. Series. c. Parallel-series. d. Recycle. e. Permeate in series. f. Countercurrent fractionation. g. Batch. Species A is more permeable and species B is less permeable.

operating costs will be high and the use of this countercurrent cascade in a membrane process will be unusual. In the batch operation shown in Figure 12-8g recovery in a single pass is insufficient, and operation is continued until enough of the more permeable species has been recovered. Batch systems are common in applications such as food processing where frequent cleaning is required. Modifications of these cascades used for gas permeation are shown in Figure 12-11.

In the remainder of this chapter the different membrane separation systems will be considered individually. The presentation starts with gas permeation since in many ways it is the simplest of the membrane processes. Then the liquid systems reverse osmosis, ultrafiltration and dialysis are considered. Electrodialysis uses electrical forces to separate liquids containing ions, and thus this process introduces new concepts. Following this, pervaporation which involves vaporizing a liquid at the membrane surface will be considered. Finally, the experimental liquid-membrane systems will be briefly discussed.

12.3. GAS PERMEATION

In gas permeation two or more gas species are separated based on different permeabilities in a membrane. Although any of the devices shown in Figure 12-4 could be used, hollow fiber and spiral wound systems are used commercially. The hollow fiber systems have the advantage of very large surface to volume ratios. The hollow fibers can have an i.d. up to 200 microns in diameter. The larger the i.d. the lower the pressure drop inside the tubes (a surprisingly important design consideration), but the lower the area/volume ratio. The wall thickness can be from 25 to 250 microns depending upon the pressures which must be withstood (Henis and Tripodi, 1983). The skin is from 0.1 to 1.0 microns thick and is formed on the outside of the hollow fiber. Thus flow is radially inward since this allows the fiber to withstand much higher pressures. Shell-and-tube separators similar to Figure 12-6 are used. The hollow fiber systems are currently being used commercially for recovery of hydrogen and carbon dioxide, and nitrogen generation from air.

The spiral wound configuration is also used commercially for carbon dioxide recovery using cellulose acetate membranes. This configuration has the advantages of a lower pressure drop in the direction of flow, and the technology to build the system is less complex. However, the area/volume ratio is much lower than in hollow fiber systems. A variety of both hollow fiber and spiral wound applications are discussed by Spillman (1989).

The basic flux equation written in words in Eq. (12-1) becomes

$$J_A = \frac{F_{P,A}}{A} = \frac{P_A \, \Delta\bar{p}_A}{t_m} \tag{12-2}$$

where J_A is the volumetric flux, $F_{P,A}$ is the steady state volumetric transfer rate of species A through the membrane, A is the membrane area, P_A is the permeability of the membrane for species A, the driving force $\Delta\bar{p}$ is the change in the partial pressure of the species across the membrane, and t_m is the thickness of the membrane skin. Obviously, consistent units must be used. The usual units for permeability are $cm^3[STP]cm/cm^2$ s (cm Hg). Since the partial pressure is the mole fraction times the total pressure , $\bar{p}_A = y_A p_{tot}$, Eq. (12-2) can also be written as

$$J_A = \frac{F_{P,A}}{A} = \frac{P_A(p_h y_{h,A} - p_p y_{p,A})}{t_m} \qquad (12\text{-}3)$$

In this equation p_p is the total permeate pressure, p_h is pressure on high pressure side, $y_{h,A}$ is mole fraction A on high pressure side and $y_{p,A}$ is the mole fraction A in the permeate. This equation often has to be applied point-by-point since y and p can vary. With a large pressure difference across the membrane, it is possible to have $y_{p,A} > y_{out,A}$ and still have transfer of this species through the membrane. In order to obtain separation of different gases the permeability of the membrane must be significantly different for the two gases. The selectivity of the membrane

$$\alpha_{AB} = \frac{P_A}{P_B} \qquad (12\text{-}4)$$

should be greater than 20 or preferably 40.

For the completely mixed system in Figure 12-7a the external mass balance at steady state is

$$F_{in} y_{in} = F_{out} y_{out} + F_P y_P \qquad (12\text{-}5)$$

where F is the molar flow rate and y is the mole fraction. This mass balance is often written as

$$y_{in} = (1 - \theta) y_{out} + \theta \, y_P \qquad (12\text{-}6)$$

where the *cut* θ is the permeate flow rate divided by the feed flow rate.

$$\theta = F_P/F_{in} \qquad (12\text{-}7)$$

The cut is usually one of the design parameters. With θ specified, we can solve Eq. (12-6) for y_{out}

$$y_{out} = \frac{y_{in} - \theta\, y_P}{1 - \theta} \qquad (12\text{-}8)$$

For gas permeators concentration polarization is usually not a problem since diffusivities are high and can probably be neglected. Thus the flux equations apply to bulk concentrations since the wall concentration equals the bulk concentration at each point. The external mass balance, Eq.(12-5), and the flux, Eq. (12-3), can be solved simultaneously for the completely mixed separator shown in Figure 12-6a (Hwang and Kammermeyer, 1975). For a binary gas Eq. (12-3) can be written for both species A and B. In molar units the result for component A is,

$$F_p y_p = \frac{P_A A \hat{\rho}_A}{t_m}\left[p_H y_{out} - p_L y_p \right] \qquad (12\text{-}9a)$$

while for component B,

$$F_p (1 - y_p) = \frac{P_B A \hat{\rho}_B}{t_m}\left[p_H(1 - y_{out}) - p_L(1 - y_p) \right] \qquad (12\text{-}9b)$$

where $\hat{\rho}_A$ and $\hat{\rho}_B$ are the molar densities at the permeate conditions, and A is the area for mass transfer. Dividing Eq. (12-9a) by (12-9b), we obtain

$$\frac{y_p}{1 - y_p} = \alpha_{AB}\, \frac{\hat{\rho}_A}{\hat{\rho}_B}\, \frac{y_{out} - \left[\dfrac{p_L}{p_H}\right] y_p}{(1 - y_{out}) - \dfrac{p_L}{p_H}(1 - y_p)} \qquad (12\text{-}10)$$

Substituting in Eq. (12-8) we have

$$\frac{y_p}{1 - y_p} = \alpha_{AB}\, \frac{\hat{\rho}_A}{\hat{\rho}_B}\left[\frac{\dfrac{y_{in} - \theta\, y_P}{1 - \theta} - \dfrac{p_L}{p_H} y_P}{1 - \dfrac{y_{in} - \theta\, y_P}{1 - \theta} - \dfrac{p_L}{p_H}(1 - y_p)} \right] \qquad (12\text{-}11)$$

Once fractions are cleared, Eq. (12-11) becomes

$$a \, y_p^2 + b \, y_p + c = 0 \tag{12-12}$$

where

$$a = \left[\frac{\theta}{1-\theta} + \frac{p_L}{p_H} \right] \left[\alpha_{AB} \frac{\hat{\rho}_A}{\hat{\rho}_B} - 1 \right] \tag{12-13a}$$

$$b = (1 - \alpha_{AB}) \frac{\hat{\rho}_A}{\hat{\rho}_B} \left[\frac{p_L}{p_H} + \frac{\theta}{1-\theta} + \frac{y_{in}}{1-\theta} \right] - \frac{1}{1-\theta} \tag{12-13b}$$

$$c = \alpha_{AB} \frac{\hat{\rho}_A}{\hat{\rho}_B} \left[\frac{y_{in}}{1-\theta} \right] \tag{12-13c}$$

and then

$$y_p = \frac{-b \pm \sqrt{b^2 - 4ac}}{2a} \tag{12-14}$$

The root which gives y_p between zero and one is used. For ideal gases $\hat{\rho}_A/\hat{\rho}_B = 1$ and the equations simplify. Alternate manipulations of these equations are shown in Example 12-1.

The permeate concentration increases as the membrane selectivity increases, the pressure ratio p_H/p_L increases, or the cut θ decreases. These effects are illustrated in Section 13.4. We will see that the completely mixed module provides the worst separation and countercurrent is best.

Example 12-1. Gas Permeation.

We wish to remove CO_2 contaminating CH_4. At 35°C and $p_H = 20$ atm the permeability of cellulose acetate membrane is (Chern *et al*, 1985) P_{CO_2} $= 15 \times 10^{-10}$ and $P_{CH_4} = 0.48 \times 10^{-10}$ [cc (STP) cm]/[cm^{2}s cm Hg]. The unit 10^{-10} [cc (STP) cm]/[cm² s cm Hg] is defined as 1 Barrer. The gas is perfectly mixed on both sides of the membrane. The high pressure feed gas is 90 mole % CH_4 and 10 mole % CO_2. The permeate pressure is 1.1 atm, and the cut $\theta = 0.5$. Determine the membrane selectivity, y_{p,CO_2}, the CO_2 flux and the CH_4 flux if $t_m = 1$ μm.

Solution

Selectivity, $\alpha_{CO_2-CH_4} = \dfrac{P_{CO_2}}{P_{CH_4}} = \dfrac{15}{0.48} = 31.25$. The permeate mole fraction $y_p = y_{p,CO_2}$ can be determined from Eqs. (12-12) to (12.14). From Eq. (12-13),

$$a = \left[\frac{0.5}{1-0.5} + \frac{1.1}{20} \right] (31.25 - 1) = 31.91$$

$$b = (-30.25) \left[\frac{1.1}{20} + 1 + \frac{0.1}{0.5} \right] - 2 = -39.96$$

$$c = (31.25) \left[\frac{0.1}{0.5} \right] = 6.25$$

Where we have assumed $\hat{\rho}_A/\hat{\rho}_B = 1.0$. Then from Eq. (12-14)

$$y_P = \frac{39.96 \pm \sqrt{1596.8 - (4)\,(31.91)\,(6.25)}}{63.82}$$

Since $0 \le y_P \le 1$, use the minus sign. $y_P = 0.183$. Now using mass balance Eq. (12-8)

$$y_{out} = \frac{0.1 - 0.5\,(0.183)}{0.5} = 0.0168$$

The CO_2 flux can be found from Eq. (12-3).

$$J_{CO_2} = \frac{15 \times 10^{10} \left[\dfrac{cc\ (STP)\ cm}{cm^2\ s\ cm\ Hg} \right]}{(1\ \mu m)\ (10^{-4}\ cm/1\ \mu m)} \left[\frac{76\ cm\ Hg}{1\ atm} \right]$$

$$\times \left[(20)\ (0.0168) - (1.1)\ (0.183) \right] atm = 1.535 \times 10^{-4}\ \frac{cc\ STP}{cm^2\ s}$$

where $y_{h,CO_2} = y_{out}$ since the module is well mixed.

$$J_{CH_4} = \left[\frac{0.48 \times 10^{-10}}{10^{-4}} \right] (76)\ [20\ (0.9832) - (1.1)\ (0.817)] = 6.85 \times 10^{-4}$$

Notes: 1.) Most of the CO_2 is removed, yet permeate gas is still mainly CH_4. This is important since driving force for CO_2 transfer remains positive.

2.) Since the module is perfectly mixed, $y_{h,A} = y_{out}$ in Eq. (12-3).

3.) $J_{CH_4} > J_{CO_2}$ despite much higher CO_2 permeability. This occurs because of the much higher driving force for CH_4

4.) Appropriate conversion factors are required.

5.) Concentration polarization (see next section) is assumed to be negligible.

6.) Note that transfer of CO_2 is "uphill" in the sense that CO_2 mole fraction is higher on the permeate side. The pressure drop allows this direction of mass transfer since $\bar{p}_{in,CO_2} > \bar{p}_{p,CO_2}$.

7.) Since other flow configurations such as counter-current will give higher y_p and lower y_{out}, this design is conservative.

A large literature has developed on the subject of membrane permeabilities (Chem *et al.*, 1985; Finken, 1985; Hwang and Kammermeyer, 1975; Kesting, 1985; Koros and Chern, 1987; Rogers, 1985; Stannett *et al.*, 1979; Stern, 1976; Stern and Frisch, 1981). A simplified picture following Baker and Blume (1986) will be presented here. The permeability is the product of the solubility of the gas in the membrane and the diffusivity of the gas in the membrane.

$$P_A = K_A D_A \qquad (12\text{-}15)$$

The solubility parameter K can be considered an Henry's law constant which links the concentration of a species in the membrane to the partial pressure in the adjacent gas. For simple gases the solubility increases as the gas diameter increases because the gas becomes easier to condense. This is illustrated in Figure 12-9a where the Lennard-Jones collision diameter is used as a measure of the size of the gas. As the diameter of the permeate molecule increases, the diffusivity normally decreases becauses large molecules interact more with the polymer chains. This effect is illustrated in Figure 12-9b. Figures 12-9a and b are for natural rubber membranes. The values of K and D depend upon the polymer, but the general behavior will be similar to that shown in these figures. The permeability is the product of K and D. This product is shown in Figure 12-9c for several different polymers. The diffusivities of most gases in rubbery polymers are approximately the same; thus, selectivity comes from solubility differences. In glassy polymers both diffusivity and solubility differences are important in determining selectivity. Listings of permeabilities for several gases in a variety of polymers are given by Koros and Chern (1987), Pusch and Walch (1982), Stannett *et al.* (1979), and Stern (1986).

Figure 12-9c helps to explain why purification of hydrogen from carbon monoxide, nitrogen or methane; and separation of carbon dioxide are currently the major industrial successes. Hydrogen and carbon dioxide have significantly greater permeabilities than the gases they are separated from since H_2 has a high diffusivity and CO_2 has a high solubility. Development of membranes for other separations is more difficult since more specific interactions between the permeant and the polymer are probably required to achieve high selectivities. One way to do this is to use "carriers" which will complex with the desired gas to help transport it across the membrane (Baker and Blume, 1986).

650

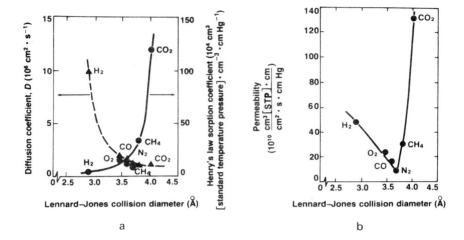

a

b

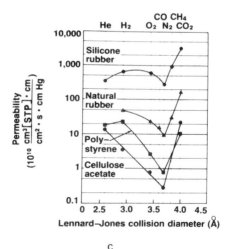

c

Figure 12-9.   Permeation of gases in polymer membranes (Baker and Blume, 1986). a. Diffusivity and solubility in natural rubber. b. Permeability in natural rubber. c. Permeabilities in four polymers. Reprinted with permission from *Chem. Tech.*, 232 (1986). Copyright 1986, American Chemical Society.

Obtaining a membrane with high permeability is not sufficient to have an economical commercial separator. In addition, we must be able to form the membrane into a geometry which will be able to withstand fairly high pressures, will have high area/volume ratios, and will have a thin active skin with no holes. Spiral wound cellulose membranes and hollow fiber polysulfone membranes satisfy the first two requirements. The third requirement is much more difficult. The thinner the skin the more likely there will be imperfections or pores which are much larger than the gas molecules being separated. The gas flows through these pores by convective flow driven by the pressure gradient across the membrane. Unfortunately, this gas does not undergo separation mechanism and the concentration of this gas will be the same as that on the high pressure side of the membrane. Although significant strides have been made in producing more perfect membrane skins, this approach has not yet made thin skinned membranes which are perfect enough for hydrogen purification. A surface porosity as low as 10^{-6} will lower the separation factor of H_2 compared to CO for polysulfone membranes from 40 to approximately 5 (Henis and Tripodi, 1983). This value is not high enough to obtain pure hydrogen.

Two methods are used in commercial separators to circumvent this problem. For CO_2 purification cellulose acetate membranes are used with a fairly thick skin. This reduces the permeability, but with CO_2 this is less critical since CO_2 has a very high permeability (see Figure 12-9c). The second solution used for H_2 purification is to coat an asymmetric polysulfone membrane which inherently has a high separation factor with a layer of silicone rubber (Henis and Tripodi, 1983, Finken, 1985; Schell, 1985) and Stern (1986). The silicone rubber layer serves to seal the defects. These resistance model (RM) membranes are illustrated schematically in Figure 12-10. The silicone rubber has a very high permeability (but low selectivity). The permeabilities [cm^3 (STP) cm/cm^2 s cm Hg] of silicone rubber are 5.2×10^{-8} and 2.5×10^{-8} for H_2 and CO, respectively. The polysulfone has permeabilities of 1.2×10^{-9} and 3.0×10^{-11} for H_2 and CO, respectively (Finken, 1985). The RM membrane will have its permeability reduced slightly, but has a selectivity > 30 which is high enough for commercial H_2 purification. Note in Figure 12-10 that it is difficult to determine exact values for t_m for either layer. Experimentally, it is

652

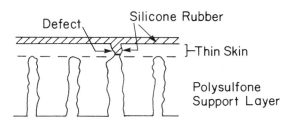

Figure 12-10. Resistance model (RM) gas permeation membrane.

easiest to measure the ratio P/t_m and to not separate the terms. Other commercial applications are discussed by Schell (1985) and Stern (1986).

A first cut at design of a gas permeator can be made once the permeabilities, pressure drop, thickness of the active layer, and area per volume of the spiral wound or hollow fiber system are known. To determine the amounts and compositions of both high and low pressure products the flow patterns inside the separator and the product cut must be specified. These details are discussed in Chapter 13.

The single stage systems shown in Figures 12-5 to 12-7 are often not optimal and modifications of the cascades shown in Figure 12-8 are often used. Three cascades used commercially for gas permeation are shown in Figure 12-11 (Spillman, 1989). The two-stage process with recycle shown in Figure 12-11a is used to improve recovery of the slower permeating species at the cost of additional compression and membrane area. If the concentration of the permeating species is very high, the "premembrane" shown in Figure 12-11b can be useful for bulk removal. According to Eq. (12-3) a low permeate pressure will decrease membrane area or increase product recovered; however, if recompression is required a low permeate pressure increases recompression costs. One compromise is the two stage process shown in Figure 12-11c where the permeate pressures are different. Since gas compression is done in stages, the two permeate pressures are chosen to match the compression scheme.

Currently, gas permeators are speciality items which would be ordered from the manufacturer. The permeators are often ordered as a turn-key device. That is, the purchaser specifies required operating conditions including the inlet

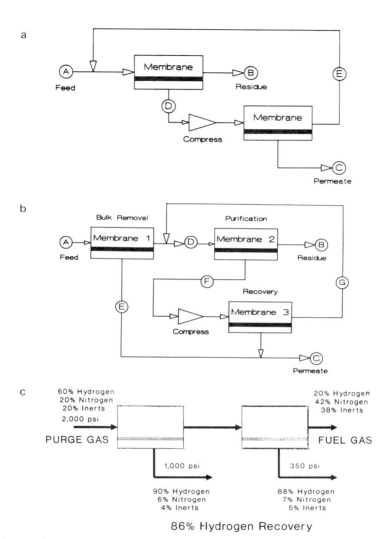

Figure 12-11.   Cascades for gas permeation (Spillman, 1989). a. Two stage with recycle to improve recovery of the slower permeating species. b. Three stage showing addition of a "premembrane" for bulk removal. c. Two stage with different permeate pressures. Reprinted with permission from *Chem. Eng. Prog.*, *85*(1), 41 (1989). Copyright 1989, Amer. Inst. of Chem. Eng.

gas composition and flow rates, temperature and pressure, and the required outlet gas composition for both high and low pressure gases. The manufacturer then designs and builds a system which he guareentees will meet the required specifications. Unfortunately, this arrangement is not as full-proof to the purchaser as it sounds. If the actual operating conditions are different than specified, the guareentee may be voided. In addition, the supplier will tend to over-design to be sure he meets the specifications. Finally, turn-key units tend to be more expensive than systems where the buyer does the design. It is best if the buyer knows as much as possible about the separator even when he is buying a turn-key system. This allows the buyer to write a more advantageous contract and to do a better job bargaining. Additional factors which can be important in design are discussed in Chapter 13.

The economics of gas permeation separation compared to competing processes is discussed in detail by Spillman (1989). He concludes:

1. Membranes are efficient concentrators, but are not efficient in producing 100% purity.

2. Only optimized systems including multi-stage processes such as those shown in Figure 12-11 should be used in economic comparisons.

3. Recompression costs are very important and must be included in the analysis.

4. Since the technology is changing very rapidly, economic analyses can become rapidly outdated.

5. Hybrid systems (membranes plus another separation) are often advantageous. This occurs since membranes work best at low concentrations of the permeating species while systems such as absorption work best at high concentration. Examples of hybrid systems for air separation are given by Beaver et al (1988) and Gienger and Ray (1988).

12.4. REVERSE OSMOSIS (RO)

Reverse osmosis (RO) is a process which reverses the normal direction of osmosis by increasing the pressure of the concentrated stream. Obviously, this definition is useless unless we know what osmosis is. Thus we need to digress slightly into the thermodynamics of membranes.

Osmosis is the flow of *solvent* through a semipermeable membrane from the less concentrated to the more concentrated region. A "semipermeable membrane" is a membrane which allows solvent to pass but completely prevents the flow of certain solutes or ions in solution. The osmotic flow is a natural occurrence as the system tends to come to equilibrium and equalize chemical potentials. The osmotic flow can be decreased by applying a pressure to the concentrated solution. The higher the applied pressure the less the osmotic flow. When the flow stops, the applied pressure is the *osmotic pressure* which is given the symbol π. At higher pressures flow will be reversed and we will transfer solvent from the concentrated to the dilute solution. This is *reverse osmosis*.

As long as the membrane is perfectly semipermeable, the osmotic pressure is a thermodynamic property of the solution and is independent of the membrane properties. The osmotic pressure can be measured directly, although it is often much more convenient to estimate it from other thermodynamic quantities. Osmotic equilibrium requires that the chemical potentials of the solvent on both sides of the membrane are equal.

$$\mu_{1,\text{solvent}} = \mu_{2,\text{solvent}} \tag{12-16}$$

Note that the equilibrium condition is on solvent *only*. Since solute does not pass through the membrane, solute is not in equilibrium. Thermodynamic arguments can now be used to derive equations which allow calculation of the osmotic pressure (for example, see Reid, 1966). Assuming that the liquid is incompressible and that activities can be estimated from vapor pressure measurements, the result is

$$\pi v_{\text{solvent}} = RT \ln \left[\frac{VP_{\text{pure solvent}}}{VP_{\text{solution}}} \right] \tag{12-17}$$

where v_{solvent} is the partial molar volume of the solvent. Equation (12-17) is usually quite accurate, but is not always convenient to use since it requires

656

Table 12-1.   Osmotic pressure of aqueous sucrose
solutions at 30°C (Reid, 1966).

	π in atmospheres		
c, gmoles/liter	Van't Hoff Eq. (12-18a)	Eq. (12-17)	Experimental Data
0.991	20.3	26.8	27.2
1.646	30.3	47.3	47.5
2.366	39.0	72.6	72.5
3.263	47.8	107.6	105.9
4.108	54.2	143.3	144.0
5.332	61.5	199.0	204.3

vapor pressure data of solutions. A simpler result is obtained by assuming that the solution is dilute and that Raoult's law is valid. This result is the van't Hoff equation,

$$\pi = cRT \tag{12-18a}$$

where c is the molar concentration of solute in solution (moles/volume). Although very convenient, the van't Hoff equation is often incorrect. This is illustrated in Table 12-1 which presents the calculated and experimental values for the osmotic pressure of aqueous sucrose solutions (Reid, 1966). For this system Eq. (12-17) is quite accurate while the van't Hoff equation seriously underestimates the osmotic pressure. If the solution dissociates or associates in solution Eq. (12-17) remains valid, but Eq. (12-18a) should not be used. Although the van't Hoff equation may be invalid it is often useful to assume a linear dependence on concentration

$$\pi = a\,c \tag{12-18b}$$

where a is an empirically determined constant, and c may be in any desired units. For macromolecules the osmotic pressure increases much faster than linearly, and can often be represented as (Wijmans *et al.*, 1984),

$$\pi = ac^n \qquad (12\text{-}18c)$$

where a is a constant and n>1. Often n is approximately 2.

The osmotic pressure of solutions is not widely tabulated and vapor pressure data may not be available. Fortunately, the osmotic pressure can be related to freezing point depression which is easy to measure and is widly tabulated (e.g. in *Handbook of Chemistry and Physics*). The osmotic pressure is related to freezing point depression by (Reid, 1966),

$$\pi = \frac{\left[T_f^* - T_f \right] \Delta H_f \, T}{v_{solvent} \, T_f \, T_f^*} \left[\frac{R_{press}}{R_{energy}} \right] \qquad (12\text{-}19)$$

where T_f^* is the freezing point temperature of pure solvent, T_f is the freezing point temperature of solution of the desired mole fraction and ΔH_f is the latent heat of freezing of the solvent. The ratio R_{press}/R_{energy} is the ratio of gas constants in pressure and energy units. This conversion is required to obtain π in pressure units (see Problem 12-F2). Note that both Eqs. (12-18a) and (12-19) predict π depends linearly on T. Use of Eq. (12-19) is illustrated in Example 13-1.

The flow in reverse osmosis is driven by pressure differences. Although concentration polarization is usually important in reverse osmosis (see Figure 12-4), for the moment we will assume that the solutions are perfectly mixed so that there is no concentration buildup. Then $c_w = c_b$ (This development follows that of Blatt *et al*, 1970). Equation (12-1) becomes

$$J_{solv} = \frac{K_{solv}}{t_m}(\Delta p - \Delta \pi) \qquad (12\text{-}20a)$$

where K_{solv} is the permeability of the membrane to the solvent (usually water), Δp is the pressure drop across the membrane, and $\Delta \pi$ is the osmotic pressure difference across the membrane. Note that the pressure driving force is reduced by the osmotic pressure difference. As the solution becomes more

658

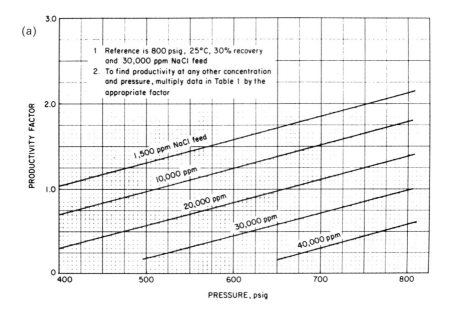

(a)

PRODUCTIVITY FACTOR

1 Reference is 800 psig, 25°C, 30% recovery and 30,000 ppm NaCl feed
2. To find productivity at any other concentration and pressure, multiply data in Table 1 by the appropriate factor

1,500 ppm NaCl feed

10,000 ppm

20,000 ppm

30,000 ppm

40,000 ppm

PRESSURE, psig

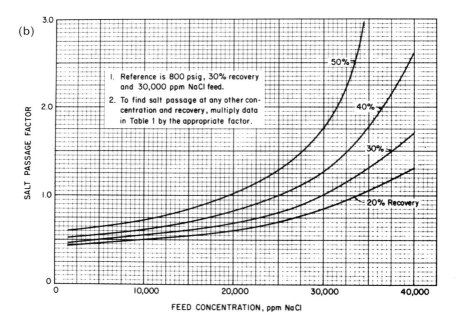

(b)

SALT PASSAGE FACTOR

1. Reference is 800 psig, 30% recovery and 30,000 ppm NaCl feed.
2. To find salt passage at any other concentration and recovery, multiply data in Table 1 by the appropriate factor.

50%

40%

30%

20% Recovery

FEED CONCENTRATION, ppm NaCl

concentrated, π increases and higher pressures are required to achieve acceptable fluxes.

Real membranes are partially permeable. Thus there will be some solute flux through the membrane. Neglecting concentration polarization, the flux of solute is

$$J_{solute} = \frac{K_{solute}}{t_m}(c_b - c_p) \qquad (12\text{-}21)$$

where K_{solute} is the permeability of the membrane to the solute, and c_p is the permeate concentration. Conservation of mass requires that

$$J_{solute} = c_p\, J_{solution} \approx c_p\, J_{solv} \qquad (12\text{-}22)$$

which relates the two flux equations. Experimentally the rejection coefficient

$$R^\circ = \frac{c_b - c_p}{c_b} = 1 - \frac{c_p}{c_b} \qquad (12\text{-}23)$$

is often reported. Combining Eqs. (12-20a) to (12-23), we obtain the rejection coefficient R° with no concentration polarization

$$R^\circ = \frac{\alpha(\Delta p - \Delta\pi)}{1 + \alpha(\Delta p - \Delta\pi)} \qquad (12\text{-}24a)$$

Figure 12-12.   Reverse osmosis results (Caracciolo *et al*, 1977). a. Effect of pressure and feed concentration on production from a DuPont B10 hollow fiber RO system for desalinating water. Productivity at reference conditions (referred to as Table 1) is 1500 gpd. b. Effect of feed concentration and recovery on salt passage for a DuPont B10 hollow fiber RO system for removing NaCl from water. Salt passage at reference (referred to as Table 1) is 1.5 wt%. Reprinted with permission from S. Sourirajan (Ed.), *Reverse Osmosis and Synthetic Membranes* (1977). Copyright 1977, National Research Council of Canada, Ottawa.

where α is the selectivity,

$$\alpha = K_{solv}/K_{solute}$$ (12-24b)

For a perfectly impermeable membrane the selectivity is infinite and R=1. For membranes with finite selectivity some increase in the observed rejection coefficient can be obtained by increasing Δp. This also increases the solvent flux. This pressure effect is illustrated in Figure 12-12a (Caracciolo et al, 1977) for a hollow fiber membrane.

Concentration polarization is usually important in reverse osmosis. Equation (12-20) remains valid except we must now calculate $\Delta\pi$ using the concentrations across the membrane. Referring to Figure 12-4, $\Delta\pi = \pi(c_w) - \pi(c_p)$. Since $c_w > c_b$, $\Delta\pi$ increases and solvent flux decreases as concentration polarization increases. Equation (12-21) changes since the bulk fluid concentration c_b is replaced by the wall concentration c_w. This is usually written as

$$J_{solute} = \frac{K_{solute}}{t_m}(Mc_b - c_p)$$ (12-25)

where M is the *polarization modulus* defined as

$$M = c_w/c_b$$ (12-26)

As M increases the solute flux increases since any solution which leaks through the membrane is more concentrated.

The solvent flux, Eq. (12-20a), can be written in terms of M if we assume that π is proportional to concentration (Eq. (12-18b)). This makes the osmotic pressure difference

$$\Delta\pi = M\pi(c_b) - \pi(c_p)$$

and Eq. (12-20a) becomes

$$J_{solv} = \frac{K_{solv}}{t_m}\left[\Delta p - (M\pi(c_b) - \pi(c_p))\right]$$ (12-27)

Note that this predicts that solvent flux decreases as M increases. Combining Eqs. (12-22), (12-23), (12-25) and (12-27), we obtain an expression for the rejection coefficient when there is concentration polarization.

$$R = 1 - \frac{M}{1 + \alpha[\Delta p - (M\pi(c_b) - \pi(c_p))]} \qquad (12\text{-}28)$$

As expected R decreases as M increases except when the selectivity α is infinite. Equation (12-28) reduces to Eq. (12-24a) when M=1. Additional manipulations of these equations are illustrated in Example 12-2.

Example 12-2. Reverse Osmosis of Na_2CO_3

An experimental RO membrane is being used to produce a waste stream which is Na_2CO_3 solution. The pure water flux at 30°C is measured as $J_{solv} = 1500$ L/m^2 day when $\Delta p = 25$ atm. With the Na_2CO_3 solution, operation is at 30°C with $p_h = 50$ atm and $p_L = 1$ atm. Both permeate and feed sides of the membrane are assumed to be perfectly mixed.

   a. For an ideal membrane (R = 1) find J_{solv} when M = 1 and when M = 1.2.

   b. For a real membrane we measure $c_p = 0.005$ when M = 1. Find J_{solv} when M = 1 and when M = 1.2.

Solution

A. Define. The problem is clearly defined in the problem statement.
B. and C. Explore and Plan. Although the definition is clear, the path to solution is not. We obviously need to determine osmotic pressure. Equation (12-17) is accurate. Vapor pressure data (Perry and Green, 1984), p. 3-73) at 30°C is:

wt% $Na_2 CO_3$	0	5%	10%	15%	20%	25%	30%
VP, mm Hg	31.82	31.2	30.4	29.6	28.8	27.8	26.4

From the pure water flux we can find K_{solv}/t_m from Eq. (12-20a). Then for part a J_{solv} is obtained from Eq. (12-20a) when M = 1.0 and from Eq. (12-27) when M = 1.2. For the real membrane with M = 1, c_p can be found from Eq. (12-23). Then J_{solv} is determined from Eq. (12-20a). We can also use the measured value of R to find $\alpha = K_{solv}/K_{solute}$ from Eq. (12-24a). This gives us K_{solute}/t_m. This value is needed when M = 1.2. Combining Eqs. (12-22), (12-25) and (12-27) we can solve for c_p. Once c_p is known Eq. (12-27) is used to find J_{solv}.

D. Do It. Eq. (12-17), $\pi = \dfrac{RT}{v_{water}} \ln \left[\dfrac{VP_{water}}{VP_{solution}} \right]$

$$v_{water} = \frac{(MW)_w}{\rho_w} = \frac{18.016 \text{ g/gmole}}{0.996547 \text{ g/cc}} = 18.095 \text{ cc/gmole}$$

For 5 wt % solution at 30°C ($c_b = 0.05$),

$$\pi = \frac{\left[82.057 \, \dfrac{\text{cc atm}}{\text{gmole K}} \right] (303.16K)}{(18.095 \text{ cc/gmole})} \ln \left[\frac{31.824}{31.2} \right] = 27.2 \text{ atm}$$

Assuming linear dependence, Eq. (12-18b),

$$\pi = \frac{c}{0.5} (27.2) = 544.5c, \text{ or } a = 544.5$$

Part a. Ideal (R = 1). For pure water Eq. (12-20a) becomes

$$\frac{K_{solv}}{t_m} = \frac{J_{solv}}{\Delta p} = \frac{1500}{25} = 60 \text{ L/(m}^2 \text{ day atm)}$$

When M = 1, $\Delta p = 50 - 1 = 49$ atm, $\Delta\pi = 27.2$ atm ($\pi(c_p) = 0$). Note $\Delta\pi$ is the same everywhere since the membrane module is perfectly mixed.

$$J_{solv} = \frac{K_{solv}}{t_m} (\Delta p - \Delta\pi) = (60)(49 - 27.2) = 1306.6 \text{ L/m}^2 \text{ day}$$

When $M = 1.2$, $J_{solv} = \dfrac{K_{solv}}{t_m} [\Delta p - M \pi (c_b)]$

$J_{solv} = (60) [49 - (1.2) (27.2)] = 979.9 \text{ L/m}^2 \text{ day}$

Part b. Real Membrane. For $M = 1$ we observe $c_p = 0.005$. Rearranging Eq. (12-23a), we obtain

$$R = 1 - \frac{c_p}{c_b} = 1 - \frac{0.005}{0.05} = 0.9$$

For a linear dependence of osmotic pressure,

$$\pi (c_p) = (0.1) \pi (5\%) = 2.72 \text{ atm}$$

Equation (12-20a) can be written as,

$$J_{solv} = \frac{K_{solv}}{t_m} \{\Delta p - [\pi(c_b) - \pi(c_p)]\} \tag{12-20b}$$

This equation is valid everywhere since c_b and c_p are constants.

$$J_{solv} = 60 [49 - (27.2 - 2.72)] = 1469.9 \text{ L/m}^2 \text{ day}$$

Note that solvent flux of the real membrane is greater than that of the ideal membrane since $\Delta \pi$ is decreased.

Rearranging Eq. (12-24a) to solve for α,

$$\alpha = \frac{K_{solv}}{K_{solute}} = \frac{R}{(\Delta p - \Delta \pi) (1 - R)} \tag{12-24c}$$

Then, $\alpha = \dfrac{0.9}{(24.5) (0.1)} = 0.367$

$$\frac{K_{solute}}{t_m} = \frac{K_{solv}/t_m}{\alpha} = \frac{60}{0.367} = 163.32 \frac{L}{m^2 \text{ day}}$$

For M = 1.2 we need to solve Eqs. (12-22), (12-25) and (12-27) simultaneously. The resulting equation is

$$\frac{A\,K_{solv}}{t_m}\,c_p^2 + c_p\left[\frac{K_{solv}}{t_m}\left(\Delta p - M\,\pi\,(c_b)\right) + \frac{K_{solute}}{t_m}\right]$$

$$-\frac{K_{solute}}{t_m}\,M\,c_b = 0 \qquad\qquad (12\text{-}29)$$

where a is defined in Eq. (12-18b). Equation (12-29) is easily solved with the quadratic formula. The three constants for the quadratic formula are

$$\frac{a\,K_{solv}}{t_m} = (544.4)\,(60) = 32.669$$

and

$$\frac{K_{solv}}{t_m}\,(\Delta p - M\,\pi\,(c_b)) + \frac{K_{solute}}{t_m}$$

$$= 60\,[49 - (1.2)\,(27.2)] + 163.3 = 1143.2$$

and

$$-\frac{K_{solv}}{t_m}\,M\,c_b = -\,(163.32)\,(1.2)\,(0.05) = -\,9.8$$

From the quadratic formula,

$$c_p = \frac{-\,1143.2 \pm \sqrt{(1143.2)^2 - 4(32,669)\,(-\,9.8)}}{2\,(32,699)}$$

To have positive c_p must use + sign. $c_p = 0.00712$. Then from Eq. (12-27) and (12-15),

$$J_{solv} = 60\,\{49 - [(1.2)\,(27.2) - (0.00712)\,(544.5)]\} = 1212.5$$

$$J_{solute} = (163.3)\,[(1.2)\,(0.05) - 0.00712] = 8.64$$

E. Check. Can use Eq. (12-22) as one check. For Part b with M = 1.2 (the most difficult problem),

$8.64 = J_{solute} = c_p J_{solv} = (0.00712) (1212.5) = 8.63$ which is OK.

F. Generalize. There are several parts of this detailed example:

1. Note that the units on the gas constant R controls the units of π.

2. The value K_{solv}/t_m determined from data can be used under different conditions.

3. As M increases J_{solv} decreases.

4. Note that J_{solv} increased as R decreased since permeate osmotic pressure increased.

5. K_{solute}/t_m calculated from observed retention can be used under different conditions.

6. Calculation of c_p by simultaneous solution of mass balances when R < 1.0 and M > 1.0 using previously determined values of K_{solute}/t_m and K_{solv}/t_m, differed from the method used in Example 12-1 since different information was given.

7. If we do not have perfect mixing, c_b and c_p will both vary. Thus $\pi (c_b)$ and $\pi (c_p)$ vary which means the flux varies as we go down the membrane. Mass balances for other situations are illustrated in Section 13.3.

8. If the cut $\theta = F_p/F_{in}$ is specified, then the required feed concentration can be determined from the analogue to Eq. (12-8),

$$c_b = c_{out} = \frac{c_{in} - \theta c_p}{1 - \theta} \qquad (12\text{-}30)$$

9. This system was a continuous, steady state process. Batch operation is considered in Eqs. (12-43) to (12-46).

Determination of the polarization modulus M is important. When rejection is complete (R=1), a steady state, one-dimensional mass balance on the feed side of the membrane is (see Figure 12-4),

$$J_{solv}\,c + D\,\frac{dc}{dy} = 0 \qquad (12\text{-}31)$$

This equation is a statement that the movement of solute to the membrane by convection (the bulk flow through the membrane) is equal to the movement of solute away by diffusion. At the membrane wall (y=0) c equals c_w, and in the bulk fluid which starts at y=δ, c equals c_b. With constant diffusivity the solution to Eq. (12-31) is

$$M = \frac{c_w}{c_b} = \exp\left[\frac{J_{solv}\,\delta}{D}\right] \qquad (12\text{-}32a)$$

Since $D/\delta = k$, the mass transfer coefficient, this result is often written as

$$M = \frac{c_w}{c_b} = \exp\left[\frac{J_{solv}}{k}\right] \qquad (12\text{-}32b)$$

Although considerably over-simplified and difficult to use without a value for film thickness δ, or mass transfer coefficient k, these results do show that concentration polarization increases as:

1. Solvent flux increases. Thus highly permeable membranes have more of a problem with concentration polarization.

2. The boundary layer thickness δ increases. The boundary layer thickness can be decreased by decreasing the channel diameter or width or by promoting turbulence.

3. The diffusivity increases. This shows that large solutes will have worse concentration polarization.

More detailed theories are discussed in Chapter 13.

The effect of feed concentration on the productivity of an hollow fiber RO permeator was shown in Figure 12-12a (Caracciolo et al, 1977). This concentration effect is due to concentration polarization and the increased osmotic pressure at higher feed concentrations. Salt passage as a function of feed concentration and the recovery (which is the same as cut) is shown in Figure 12-12b (Caracciolo et al, 1977). As feed concentration or recovery increase, the salt passage increases. This would be expected, but the nonlinear increase illustrated is a surprise. This effect is due to the worsening of concentration polarization at increasing concentrations. Typical rejection coefficients for a variety of membranes are listed in Table 12-2 (Pusch and Walch, 1982). More detailed tables for a variety of inorganic and organic compounds are compiled by Eisenberg and Middlebrooks (1986).

The spiral wound and hollow fiber configurations are commonly used for RO. The common membrane polymers include cellulose acetate, polyamides (see Figure 12-3), and a composite membrane developed by FilmTec. The composite membrane is a crosslinked polyamide barrier layer supported by a microporous polysulfone coating on a polyester web. This complex membrane has high flux, high salt rejection, a pH range from 4 to 11, and a wide range of temperature stability. Other membranes are listed in Figure 12-3 and Table 12-2.

The skin of the RO membranes have pores which are several Angstroms or larger in diameter. These pores are larger than the hydrated ions, yet the ions are excluded. The separation is clearly not a sieving effect. The current physical model of the separation effect can be summarized as follows (Kesting, 1985). The water molecules are preferentially attracted to the hydrophilic membrane surface. An ordered water sheath of thickness t ($\sim$ 5Å) exists at the membrane surface and repels ions. This water sheath pours into pores. If the pore is less than 2t ($\sim$ 10 Å) in size the ordered water sheath will be continuous and ions will be excluded. In the occasional large pores (imperfections) with diameter > 2t, the ordered water sheath does not fill the pore. In the center of these pores ordinary water plus ions pass. The observed rejection coefficient is the sum of the almost pure water from the small pores and the contaminated water from the larger pores. These membranes are often called "solution-diffusion" membranes.

Table 12-2. Rejection coefficients and fluxes for a variety of RO membranes (Cadotte et al, 1988; Pusch and Walch, 1982). HF = hollow fiber, PF = plate and frame, SW = Spiral wound.

Membrane	Module	Manufacturer	R %	Flux L/m² day	Test Conditions
Cellulose-3 acetate	HF	Dow Chem	97	200	28 bar, 0.3% NaCl pH 6-8, 35°C
Cellulose-2.5 acetate	PF	DDS	≤ 99	≥400	40 bar, 1% NaCl pH 2-8, 30°C
Cellulose-2.5 acetate	SW	Millipore	90		14 bar, 0.1% NaCl pH 3-7, 30°C
Cellulose 2-acetate	HF	Toyobo	93		30 bar, 0.2% NaCl pH 3-7, 30°C
Cellulose acetate	Tube	UOP	97	450	40 bar, 0.5 % NaCl pH 3-7, 45°C
Cellulose-2.8 acetate	SW	UOP	≥ 99	400	70 bar, 3.5% NaCl pH 4-7.5, 35°C

Membrane	Config.	Manufacturer	Rejection (%)	Flux	Test conditions
Aromatic Polyamide (B9)	HF	DuPont	95	50	28 bar, 0.15% NaCl pH 4-11, 35°C
Aromatic Polyamide (B10)	HF	DuPont	98.5	40	56 bar, 3.5% NaCl pH 5-9, 35°C
Composite	PF	FilmTec	98	1800	40 bar, 1% NaCl ≤60°C
Composite, polyamide FT30	SW	Film Tech	99.5	20 gfd	1.4 MPa, dilute NaCl
Polyfuran, composite	SW	Osmonics	99	200	56 bar, pH 0.5-10.5 75°C
Composite	SW	Toray	99.7	700	400 bar, 0.25% NaCl pH 4-12, 40°C
Composite	SW	UOP	99.2	600	63 bar, 3.5% NaCl pH 2-12, 45°C
Composite, polyamide XP45 (Nanofilter)	SW	Film Tech	50 (NaCl) 97.5 ($MgSO_4$)	20 gfd	0.7 MPa, dilute
Composite, polyamide NF70 (Nanofilter)	SW	Film Tech	75 (NaCl) 97.5 ($MgSO_4$)	20 gfd	0.4 MPa, dilute

As shown in Figure 12-12a the required pressure depends on the feed concentration and also on the recovery of water. For brackish water (1500 mg/L dissolved solids) π is about 104 kPa (15psi) and a typical pressure range is from 2,760 to 3, 137 kPa (400 to 600 psig). For a typical seawater of 35,000 mg/L dissolved solids the osmotic pressure is about 2,415 kPa (350 psi). Since a 50% recovery will approximately double the osmotic pressure, operating pressures from 5,515 to 6895 kPa (800 to 1000 psig) are often used for seawater desalination (Applegate, 1984).

The effect of recovery on salt passage was illustrated in Figure 12-12b. Increasing the recovery decreases the average water flux since the average salt concentration on the high pressure side of the membrane is raised. This, in turn, increases the osmotic pressure and decreases the flux. Typical recoveries are about 33% for seawater and up to 90% for low salinity brackish water (Kesting, 1985). In under the sink units for treating tap water recoveries as low as 10% are used. These low recoveries decrease the purchase price of the unit, but raise the operating cost since more water is thrown away. However, the average consumer is much more aware of the initial purchase cost than the water costs. Calculating the effect of recovery or the product concentrations requires a knowledge of the flow geometry, the degree of concentration polarization, and the external mass balances. Details of the calculation procedures are in Chapter 13.

The reverse osmosis module needs a variety of supporting equipment to function properly (Applegate, 1984; Cheremisinoff and LaMendola, 1983; Eisenberg and Middlebrooks, 1986; Hwang and Kammermeyer, 1975; Porter, 1979; and Sourirajan, 1977). This is illustrated in Figure 12-13 where a water treatment plant is illustrated. The raw water must be stored to avoid temporary interruptions in supply. If required, chemicals will be added to adjust the pH, control biological growth, prevent calcium carbonate or other scaling, or aid in coagulation and settling. For very dirty waters a settling basin and/or a prefilter would be added to Figure 12-13. The water is then sent to a micron sized filter to remove particulates which could clog the membrane. Then a high pressure pump is used to boost the pressure. The pressure control valve is used for pressure control and the high pressure switch is for safety in case a valve is inadvertently closed or a pipe becomes clogged. A parallel-series arrangement of

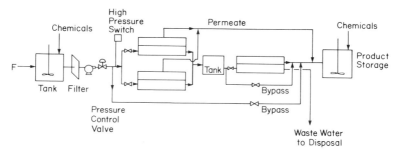

Figure 12-13.   Complete RO system showing auxiliary equipment.

permeators with bypass lines is shown in Figure 12-13. The bypass lines are used to mix in raw water if less pure water is required. The water which does not pass through the membranes is more concentrated in the dissolved solids. Usually, this stream is a waste stream which must be disposed of. The product water is sent to a storage tank where additional chemicals may be added. For example, if the water is for drinking chlorine or ozone will be added here. Chlorine is detrimental to the membranes and thus is added after the membranes unless it is required to stop biological growth. When treating highly fouling materials such as food products, a cleaning cycle must be added. This requires shut-down of the equipment, and it requires quite a bit of hardware in addition to that shown in Figure 12-13. Details of cleaning cycles and the chemicals used for cleaning are given by Eisenberg and Middlebrooks (1986). Unfortunately, this can greatly increase the costs.

Membranes have a finite lifetime which depends upon the operating conditions. Membrane replacement is usually treated as an operating cost. In addition, there is usually a long term flux decay caused by membrane compaction and fouling of the membrane. To take this into account the initial flux of the membrane is usually not used in the design calculations. Instead the flux after a few months of operation is used since the additional decay after this time is quite slow. Obviously, the membrane must be protected from chemical upsets since the membranes can be destroyed quite quickly.

There are, of course, other ways to purify water such as distillation, adsorption, ion exchange, and electrodialysis. The method used depends upon the economics of the particular case. The economics of RO are often favorable, and RO is used very extensively for treating brackish water, seawater, and tap water. One of the largest RO units is at Ras Abu Janjur, Bahrain, which produces 12.7 million gallons of potable water per day from brackish well water. The system consists of seven trains of hollow-fiber RO units with 2100 membrane modules per train. RO applications and economics are discussed by Belfort (1984), Cheremisinoff and LaMendola (1983), Applegate (1984), and Eisenberg and Middlebrooks (1986).

Reverse osmosis has also been used for separation of organics from water. Although this is not yet a common industrial separation, it may be important in particular cases. For example, dilute ε-caprolactam solutions are concentrated commercially using RO. If the organic recovered dissolves polymers or if the module needs to be steam sterilized, ceramic membranes can be used (Hsieh, 1988). Data is presented by Eisenberg and Middlebrooks (1986), Leeper (1986), and Sourirajan (1977).

Nanofiltration is a variant of reverse osmosis using membranes which pass small solutes but retain somewhat larger molecules such as sucrose. Nanofiltration membranes would typically have NaCl rejections from 20 to 70% and organic cutoffs in the 200 to 500 MW range. (Cadotte *et al*, 1988) This cutoff range corresponds to molecules with a diameter of approximately 10 Å which is one nanometer. These membranes are thus significantly looser than RO membranes but tighter than ultrafiltration membranes (minimum cutoff about 10,000 MW). The nanofiltration membranes operate at pressures in the range 0.4 MPa to 0.7 MPa which is from 1/4 to 1/2 a seawater RO membrane. Some results are given in Table 12-2. The rejection mechanism is the same as for RO, and the membranes can be thought of as loose RO membranes.

There are many applications where the ability to discriminate between salts and moderate molecular weight organics is useful. For instance, nanofiltration membranes can desalt whey or sugars. Nanofiltration membranes can also be made with 50% rejection of NaCl and 97.5% rejection of $MgSO_4$. These then are an alternative to water softening by ion exchange (see Section 9.5). Nanofiltration is a new development which can be expected to grow in the future.

Osmotic concentration can be considered a variant of osmosis. In osmotic concentration a dilute stream we wish to concentrate is separated from a concentrated salt solution by a reverse osmosis membrane such as cellulose acetate. Due to osmosis water migrates from the dilute stream to the concentrated salt stream. This concentrates the dilute stream and simultaneously dilutes the salt stream. The energy for this process comes from the energy required to evaporate water to reconcentrate the salt solution. If a waste brine stream (say from an RO plant) is available, than the energy required for concentration may be practically free.

12.5. ULTRAFILTRATION (UF)

Ultrafiltration (UF) is used for retaining larger solutes than in RO, but many of the operating characteristics are very similar to RO. The osmotic pressure in UF is invariably quite low since the molar concentration of the high molecular weight molecules separated by UF is quite low even when the weight concentrations are high. Because a large osmotic pressure does not have to be overcome, much lower operating pressures are used in UF than in RO. Typical operating pressures are in the range from 10 to 100 psig.

The membranes used in UF are usually asymmetric polymers used in one of the geometries shown in Figure 12-5. A variety of polymers such a cellulose acetate, aromatic polyamide, polysulfone, polyvinyl chloride, polyacrylonitrile and polycarbonate have been used to cast membranes (see Figure 12-3). Polysulfone has a wide temperature tolerance (to 93° C) and a wide pH range (0.5 to 13) and is probably the most commonly used membrane material (Applegate, 1984). The membranes are formed so that the dense skin is microscopically porous. Thus the separation mechanism can be considered (in a somewhat over-simplified form) to be sieving of the molecules. The membranes can be tailor made to fix the desired pore size distribution and thus provide for different molecular weight cutoffs. The molecular weight cutoff is loosely defined as the molecular weight below which species begin to pass through the membrane. The values for molecular weight cutoffs can range from 1000 to 80,000. Values for a variety of membranes are listed in Table 12-3. Molecular weight cutoffs should be employed with discretion since siev-

Table 12-3. Molecular weight cutoffs and fluxes of UF systems. (Pusch and Walch, 1982; and Warashina *et al.*, 1985). HF = hollow fiber, PF = plate and frame, SW = spiral wound

Membrane	Module	Manufacturer	MW	Flux L/m² day	Test Conditions
Cellulose 2-acetate	SW	Abcor	15,000	6000	3.5 bar, 50°C, pH 3-7.5
Polyvinylidene fluoride	SW	Abcor	10,000/20,000	7500	3.5 bar, 90°C, pH 2-9
Cellulose acetate	PF	DDS	6000 to 65,000	2-7000	5 bar, 50°C, pH 2-8
Polysulfone	PF	DDS	8000/20,000/ 65,000	1-7000	3 bar, 80°C, pH 0-14

675

Material	Type	Manufacturer			Conditions
Polysulfone	PF	Dorr-Oliver	10,000	10,000	2 bar, 70°C, pH 2-12
Polysulfone	SW	Millipore	80,000	2000	5 bar, 32°C, pH 3-11
Polysulfone	PF	Osmonics	1000/20,000	4000/12,000	3.5 bar, 93°C, pH 0.5-13
Cellulose acetate	Tube	Patterson Candy	1000-20,000	--	pH 3-6, 30–50°C
Co-polyacrylonitrile/ Methallyl sulfonate	PF	Rhone-Poulenc	20,000	7000	2 bar, 40°C, pH 1-10
Polyacrylonitrile	HF	Asahi Chem.	13,000	6380 to 19,100	3 kg/cm^2, 25C, pH 2-10
Polyacrylonitrile	HF	Asahi Chem.	6,000	14,900	3 kg/cm^2, 25C, pH 1-14

676

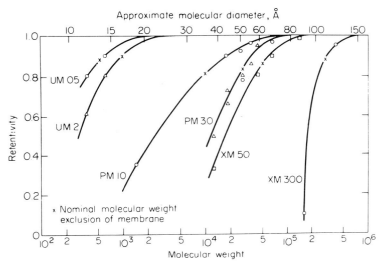

Figure 12-14.   Solute retention on Amicon Diaflo membranes (Porter, 1979).
Reprinted with permission from P.A. Schweitzer (Ed.), *Hand-book of Separation Techniques for Chemical Engineers* (1979).
Copyright 1979, McGraw-Hill.

ing depends on size and shape of the hydrated molecule, and molecular weight is only a rough guide to size and shape. In addition, there is considerable retention of molecules of lower molecular weight. Roughly, a sharp cut-off UF membrane will have $R = 0$ when the molecular weight is 1/2 the molecular weight which has $R = 0.9$. Diffuse cutoff membranes have a much broader range of fractionation. Typical retention data are shown in Figure 12-14 (Porter, 1979). A comparison of Tables 12-2 and 12-3 is interesting. Note that the UF membranes with their much larger pores have considerably larger fluxes at lower pressures than the RO membranes. Details of UF membranes are discussed by Blatt (1976), Cooper(1979), Kesting (1985), Lloyd (1985), Porter (1979), and Pusch and Walch (1982).

Concentration polarization, gel formation and fouling are extremely important in UF and need to be included in any detailed analysis. We will first look at the equations ignoring these effects, and then include them. Solvent flux without concentration polarization can be written as Eq. (12-10a or b).

For the large molecules separated by UF the molar concentration will be quite low even if the weight concentration is high. Thus, the osmotic pressure difference $\Delta\pi$ will be small and is usually ignored. The resulting solvent flux equation is,

$$J_{solv} = \frac{K_{solv}}{t_m} \Delta p \qquad (12\text{-}33)$$

For small and intermediate macromolecules (5000 or 100,000 daltons) it may be necessary to include the osmotic pressure term. This is discussed further in Chapter 13.

For sieve type membranes flow of both solvent and solute is in pores. Let R represent the fraction of solvent flux carried by pores which exclude the solute. Then 1-R of the solvent flux is in pores which do not exclude solute. With no concentration polarization the liquid passing through these pores will have a solute concentration c_b. This gives a solute flux of

$$J_{solute} = c_b(1 - R) J_{solv} \qquad (12\text{-}34)$$

In addition, Eq. (12-22) must remain valid since it represents a mass balance. Combining Eqs. (12-22), (12-33) and (12-34) and solving for R, we obtain Eq.(12-13). Thus in sieve type membranes the solute rejection can also be considered as the fraction of solvent flux in pores which reject solute molecules.

This analysis predicts that without concentration polarization the solvent flux is proportional to Δp and is independent of the feed concentration. In addition, the rejection coefficient should be constant. These results are a reasonable first approximation, but are drastically oversimplified. R is usually constant for very dilute systems, but may decrease for more concentrated systems. Some pores may pass solute molecules slowly so that the concentration in the pores is less than c_b, but the cut-off is not perfect.

Concentration polarization can cause an increase in solute concentration as shown in Figure 12-4, or it can cause a gel or cake layer to form. Assuming that there is no gel or cake layer formed, the solute flux equation becomes

$$J_{solute} = Mc_b (1 - R) J_{solv} \qquad (12\text{-}35)$$

678

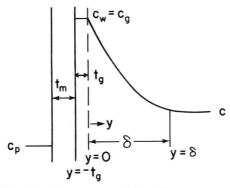

Figure 12-15.   Ultrafiltration system with gel layer at membrane wall.

where M is again the concentration polarization modulus, Eq. (12-26). Solving Eqs. (12-22) and (12-35) simultaneously, we obtain the apparent rejection coefficient R_{app},

$$R_{app} = 1 - \frac{c_P}{c_b} = 1 - M (1 - R) \qquad (12\text{-}36)$$

Unless R=1 (all pores completely reject solute), concentration polarization decreases the apparent rejection coefficient. When M=1, R_{app}=R. This non-gelling concentration polarization is predicted to have no effect on the solvent flux since osmotic pressure is negligible.

Unfortunately, many of the materials which the engineer desires to ultrafilter (paint pigments, foods, polymers, minerals, and so forth) form gels, cakes or slimes at the wall. This gel cake or slime can form at concentrations c_g below 1 wt% for polysaccharides to 50 vol% for suspensions of polymer lattices (Blatt et al, 1970). The concentration profile for UF with gel formation is shown in Figure 12-15. This gel layer acts as a porous solid which causes an additional resistance to flow. The solvent flux is now,

$$J_{solv} = \frac{\Delta p}{\dfrac{t_m}{K_{solv}} + \dfrac{t_g}{K_g}} \qquad (12\text{-}37)$$

where t_g is the thickness of the gel layer and K_g is the permeability of the gel layer. Since t_g can vary throughout a run, Eq. (12-37) is usually not useful for predictions. Often, the gel layer will have far more resistance to flow than the membrane and the gel will control the solvent flux. In these cases it does not matter what type of membrane is used as long as it retains the solute and causes a gel to form. The value of K_g can be estimated from the Carman-Kozeny equation (Blatt et al, 1970).

$$K_g = \frac{d_p^2 \, \varepsilon^3}{150 \, \mu \, (1 - \varepsilon)^2} \qquad (12\text{-}38)$$

Note that the gel permeability will be very sensitive to the particle diameter d_p in the gel layer. If $\varepsilon = 0.5$ and the viscosity is 1.0 cp, then $K_g = 3 \times 10^{-11}$ for one micron particles and $K_g = 2 \times 10^{-16}$ for 30 Angstrom particles. Thus a one micron layer of these gels with a pressure drop of 100 psi across the gel would have solvent fluxes of 200 and 0.0013 cm^3/cm^{2}sec, respectively. Obviously, a gel layer can have a major effect on the solvent flux.

A simplified steady state, one-dimensional mass balance is still given by Eq. (12-31). Now the concentration at the wall ($y = -t_g$) is $c_w = c_g$. The boundary conditions for the mass balance (see Figure 12-15) are at $y = 0$, $c = c_g$ and at $y = \delta$, $c = c_b$. The solution to this is

$$J_{solv} = \frac{D}{\delta} \ln \left[\frac{c_g}{c_b} \right] = k \ln \left[\frac{c_g}{c_b} \right] \qquad (12\text{-}37)$$

Since c_g and c_b are constants, the solvent flux is the variable. This is different from Eq. (12-32) where c_w was unknown. The solvent flux is *set* by the rate at which the solute can diffuse back from the gel layer to the bulk fluid. Increasing the pressure drop will cause a brief temporary increase in the solvent flux. However, during this period of increased flux transfer of solute to the gel layer is greater than the rate of transfer of solute back into the fluid. The gel layer must then become thicker. According to Eq. (12-37), J_{solv} will then decrease. This decrease in J_{solv} continues until the gel layer is thick enough so that the solvent flux has obtained the value predicted by Eq. (12-29). In other words, the engineer has no control over the flux rate except by increasing the diffusivity (increase temperature) or decreasing δ (stir or use thin channels). For high molecular weight polymers diffusivities are quite low and the solvent flux is low if gels form. The mass transfer coefficient k can be estimated for many flow geometries. This analysis is done in Chapter 13.

Example 12-3. Protein Ultrafiltration.

We wish to ultrafilter a 2 wt % aqueous solution of casein at 25°C. The casein gels with $c_g = 0.14$. We do two experiments as follows:

Experiment a: Run pure water and obtain $J_{solv} = 7000$ L/m^2 day with $\Delta p = 5$ atm.

Experiment b: Run casein solution at $\Delta p = 5$ atm and obtain $J_{solv} = 233$ L/m^{2}day, R = 1.

a. Calculate the mass transfer coefficient k and K_g/t_g for Experiment b.
b. If we increase Δp to 7 atm, determine the peak value of J_{solv}, the final value of J_{solv}, and the final value of K_g/t_g.

Solution

a. From the pure water data we can find K_{solv}/t_m from Eq. (12-33).

$$\frac{K_{solv}}{t_m} = \frac{J_{solv}}{\Delta p} = \frac{7000}{5} = 1400 \; \frac{L}{m^2 \; day \; atm}$$

From the casein data and Eq. (12-39),

$$k = \frac{J_{solv}}{\ln (c_g/c_b)} = \frac{233}{\ln (0.14/0.02)} = 119.74 \; \frac{L}{m^2 \; day}$$

Rearranging Eq. (12-37) and using the casein data,

$$\frac{t_g}{K_g} = \frac{\Delta p}{J_{solv}} - \frac{t_m}{K_{solv}} = \frac{5}{233} - \frac{1}{1400} = 0.0207$$

Thus, $K_g/t_g = 48.20 \, L/m^2$ day atm

b. If we increase Δp to 7 atm, we will have a momentary increase in water flux since t_g does not increase immediately. Using K_g/t_g found in part a and Eq. (12-37) we have,

$$J_{solv} = \frac{7}{\dfrac{1}{1400} + \dfrac{1}{48.2}} = 326.2 \, L/m^2 \text{ day}$$

After a short period of time, t_g increases and J_{solv} is given by Eq. (12-39). Since k, c_g and c_b are unchanged from part a, $J_{solv} = 233$. Solving for t_g/k_g

$$\frac{t_g}{K_g} = \frac{\Delta p}{J_{solv}} - \frac{t_m}{K_{solv}} = \frac{7}{233} - \frac{1}{1400} = 0.0293$$

and $K_g/t_g = 34.096$. Thus, t_g has increased by 40.8%.

Note that in both parts the resistance of the gel, t_g/K_g, is significantly greater than the membrane resistance, t_m/K_m. This is commonly the case when proteins are ultrafiltered.

Although simple and very appealing, there are significant problems with the gel layer model (Fane, 1986; Porter, 1979; Wijmans et al., 1984). The concentration c_g found by extrapolation may depend upon equipment geometry. The measured c_g may be too low and independent experiments show no gelling. In addition, c_g may be estimated as > 100% which is physically impossible. The mass balance, Eq. (12-31) does not include convection in the axial, x, direction and the boundary condition at $y = \delta$ is hypothetical. However, the model is useful for correlating data. Modifications of this model are discussed in Chapter 13.

The presence of a gel layer may have conflicting effects on the rejection of solutes. If the gel layer is very viscous, but remains fluid so that molecules diffuse in the layer, solute molecules will continue to pass through the membrane. Since $c_w > c_b$, the fluid passing through pores which do not reject solute will be concentrated. This will cause the apparent rejection coefficient to drop. This situation is similar to concentration polarization without a gel layer. The second case occurs when the gel layer has a solid-like nature and solute molecules are essentially immobile. Now the rejection coefficient can increase since the gel layer traps the solute molecules and very few of them can diffuse into the pores.

The formation of a gel layer also has a large effect on the separation of mixtures containing several solutes of widely different size. Suppose we wish to separate a low molecular weight compound from a very high molecular weight polymer. When run separately, the low molecular weight compound has R=0 while the polymer has R=1. What happens when the mixture is ultrafiltered? Our first guess is probably to use superposition and assume each molecule is unaffected by the presence of the other molecule. If no gel layer is formed, this assumption is probably close to true. Then the small molecules have R=0 and the polymer has R=1. The separation is easy. If a gel layer forms, the gel serves as a membrane which has different retention characteristics than the original membrane. The gel layer may retain the small molecules. If this happens both solutes may have retentions near 1.0 and separation will not be obtained. Thus gel layers change the fundamental nature of UF.

Once formed, the gel layer may not come off easily. In this case the membrane is said to be fouled. Fouling often occurs when the solute is adsorbed to the membrane or when charges on the membrane attract colloidal particles of opposite charge. The entire UF installation is often controlled by the presence of gel layers and fouling. Fouling can also occur from precipitation of salts, and is discussed in detail by Fane (1986) and Potts et al. (1981).

In non-fouling or moderate fouling applications hollow fiber and spiral wound configurations are commonly used. The hollow fibers have a 0.1 micron skin on the inside of the membrane. The fibers are from 500 to 1,100 microns inside diameter. Since pressures used in UF are much lower than in RO the membranes do not have to withstand very high pressures. Thus the high pressure liquid can be on the inside of the membrane. This has the advantage of reducing concentration polarization since velocities are higher and boundary layers thinner than for systems with the high pressure liquid on the outside of the fibers. The systems can be cleaned by washing with high velocity clean water or with chemical solutions. In many applications a dilute caustic wash is a very effective cleaning agent if the membrane can withstand the high pH. Hollow fiber membranes can also be cleaned by back-washing with a clean liquid. Back-washing forces liquid through the porous support and then through the skin. Any particles attached to the skin will tend to be washed off into the bulk fluid.

In highly fouling applications plate-and-frame and tubular membranes are often used. In food plants the membranes are cleaned daily and sometimes every few hours. Obviously, the cleaning cycle becomes very important in controlling costs. Biotechnology applications of UF with an emphasis on protein recovery are discussed by Belter *et al* (1988).

All of the cascade arrangements shown in Figure 12-8 can be used. When gel formation or fouling are severe, the cascade design as well as the module design are controlled by the concentration polarization. Designs which keep liquid velocities on the feed side of the membrane high are favored. These are the parallel-series and recycle cascades shown in Figures 12-8 c and d. In particular, the recycle system is often used since it is readily adaptable to the batch operation shown in Figure 12-8g which is required when cleaning must be frequent. Recycle systems are often cascaded in series to increase the recovery of the permeate or in parallel to increase capacity.

The batch system shown in Figure 12-8g is easily analyzed for simple cases. A mass balance on the entire system (tank + pipes + UF module) is

$$\frac{dV}{dt} = - A\, J_{solv} \qquad (12\text{-}40)$$

Where $V(t)$ is the volume of liquid in the tank + pipes + UF module. If osmotic pressure is negligible and no gel forms, J_{solv} is given by Eq. (12-33). Then

$$\frac{dV}{dt} = - \frac{A\, K_{solv}\, \Delta p}{t_m} \qquad (12\text{-}41)$$

The initial condition is $V = V_o$ for $t = 0$. Assuming that Δp is kept constant, we obtain the solution to Eq. (12-41).

$$V = V_o - \left[\frac{A \, K_{solv} \, \Delta p}{t_m} \right] t \qquad (12\text{-}42)$$

If a gel forms then J_{solv} is a constant given by Eq. (12-39). Now Eq. (12-40) becomes

$$\frac{dV}{dt} = -A \, k \, \ln(c_g/c_b) \qquad (12\text{-}43)$$

Since $R = 1$, the total moles of solute in the system, n, must remain constant.

$$n = c(t) \, V(t) = constant \qquad (12\text{-}44)$$

Then Eq. (12-43) becomes

$$\frac{dV}{dt} = - A \, k \, \ln (c_g \, V/n) \qquad (12\text{-}45)$$

The initial condition remains $V = V_o$ when $t = 0$. The solution to Eq. (12-45) is

$$\ln (\ln V) - \ln (\ln V_o) + \ln (V/V_o) + \frac{1}{(2)(2!)} \left[(\ln V)^2 - (\ln V_o)^2 \right]$$

$$+ \frac{1}{(3)(3!)} \left[(\ln V)^3 - (\ln V_o)^3 \right] + \cdots = -A \, kt \, \ln (c_g/n) \qquad (12\text{-}46)$$

which may be inconvenient to use since convergence may be slow.

If osmotic pressure is important, π is proportional to concentration, and no gel forms; then Eq. (12-27) should be used for J_{solv} with $\pi (c_p) = 0(c_p = 0$ since $R = 1$) (Belter et al, 1988). Assuming π is linear with respect to concentration, $\pi = ac$. Since $R = 1$, Eq. (12-44) remains valid. Then,

$$J_{solv} = \frac{K_{solv}}{t_m} \left[\Delta p - \frac{a \, Mn}{V} \right] \qquad (12\text{-}47)$$

Substituting Eq. (12-47) into Eq. (12-40), we obtain

$$\frac{dV}{dt} = -\frac{A\,K_{solv}\,\Delta p}{t_m}\left[1-\left[\frac{a\,Mn}{\Delta p}\right]\frac{1}{V}\right] \qquad (12\text{-}48)$$

with the initial condition $V = V_o$ when $t = 0$. The solution to Eq. (12-48) is (see Problem 12-C4),

$$V - V_o - \frac{a\,Mn}{\Delta p}\,\ln\left[\frac{V_o - \dfrac{a\,Mn}{\Delta p}}{V - \dfrac{a\,Mn}{\Delta p}}\right] = -\frac{A\,K_{solv}\,\Delta p}{t_m}\,t \qquad (12\text{-}49)$$

Note that when $a = 0$, Eq. (12-49) reduces to Eq. (12-42). Equation (12-49) is also valid for batch operation of RO when $R = 1$.

Ultrafiltration and reverse osmosis systems are often used together. For example, cheese whey is the left over liquid from making cheese. The whey is approximately 1% protein, 5% lactose (milk sugar), 1% salts, and the remainder is water. The whey has a very high Biological Oxygen Demand (BOD) and is expensive to dispose of properly. One processing route which utilizes all of the components of whey is shown in Figure 12-16. The protein is recovered by UF. This protein concentrate is quite valuable and can either be dried and sold or it can be added wet to cottage cheese or ice cream. The permeate from the UF system is sent to RO where the sugar and salts are concentrated by removing water. This is desirable since it makes both the downstream processing steps smaller and cheaper. The concentrated solution can then be fermented with yeast to produce a dilute ethanol solution. The ethanol is recovered by distillation or other separation scheme. The waste liquor containing about 3% salts is sent to evaporators to recover the salts which can be used as fertilizer. Note that the UF system is first. The UF system serves to protect the RO system from particulates and protein which can cause fouling and gel formation. Both UF and RO systems would be cleaned at least once a day.

Somewhat more complex combined UF and RO systems can be used for

686

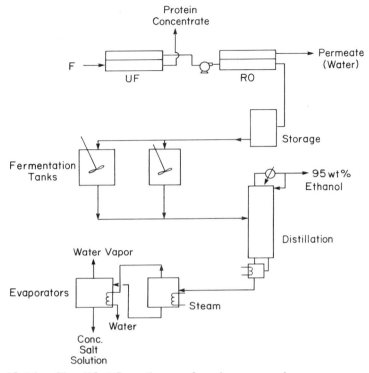

Figure 12-16. Simplified flow diagram for whey processing.

processing fruit juices (Stana, 1977). In concentration of fruit juices the processor wants to recover all of the pulp, the sugar, and the volatile flavor ingredients. The final product may be from 20 to 25% pulp and 20 to 25% sugars. This product is very viscous and has a very high osmotic pressure. (Open a can of frozen orange juice and let it melt. This is the desired final product.) A high recovery of sugar is desired; thus, the permeate leaving the RO system should be close to zero concentration. A 50 wt% solution of sugar has a very high osmotic pressure (see Table 12-1), and any leakage through the membrane will cause significant contamination of the waste stream. Thus a single RO module will be difficult to use and the membrane arrangement used in Figure 12-16 for whey processing is not a good scheme. Instead, the processing scheme shown in Figure 12-17 can be used (Stana, 1977). Note that

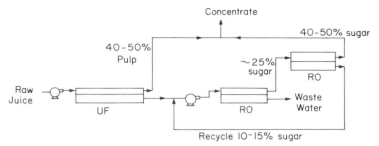

Figure 12-17.   Scheme for processing fruit juices. (Stana, 1977).

the UF system is again placed first to protect the RO systems. Since the UF membrane does not retain the sugar, the sugar concentration is the same in the permeate and the high pressure products. Thus, although π is significant, $\Delta\pi$ is approximately zero and the usual UF equations can be used. The first RO system produces the desired low concentration waste water, but the sugar solution is concentrated to only 25%. This keeps $\Delta\pi$ reasonable. The second RO system produces the desired sugar solution, but the permeate is a 10 to 15% solution which is recycled to the first RO system. This keeps $\Delta\pi$ modest in the second RO system also. The pulp and sugar are then mixed to produce the desired final product.

Other applications of UF include removal of colloidal matter in water treatment, pigment recovery in painting operations, concentration of oil emulsions, depyrogenating pharmaceutical process water, and recovery of dyes. Applegate (1984), Eykamp and Steen (1987), and Klinkowski (1978) discuss these applications.

12.6. DIALYSIS

Dialysis is a process where small molecules diffuse through a membrane because of a concentration driving force. Large molecules are excluded. The process differs from UF since the solute movement in dialysis is caused by diffusion while in UF the major flux is that of solvent caused by pressure gradients. In UF the small molecules are carried along with the solvent flux. In dialysis the flux of small molecules is independent of the solvent flux and may be in the opposite direction from the solvent flux. Dialysis also usually does not use asymmetric membranes, but instead uses homogeneous membranes without skins.

The major commercial use of dialysis is *hemodialysis* for removal of waste products such as urea and creatine from patients who have had kidney failure. This application is commonly known as the artificial kidney even though hemodialysis is not a good mimic of the way the kidney functions (Colton and Lowrie, 1981; Ward *et al*, 1985, Lysaght *et al*, 1986). Other commercial applications include the recovery of caustic in the manufacture of rayon, salt removal in pharmaceuticals manufacturing, and recovery of spent acid in the metal industry. Except in medical applications, the engineer is more likely to be involved with RO, UF, or electrodialysis than with dialysis. Both plate-and-frame and hollow fiber dialyzers are available (Lacey, 1979; Klein *et al*, 1987).

As small solutes pass through the microporous membrane, concentration gradients will develop on both sides of the membrane. This is illustrated in Figure 12-18. The flux of the permeable solutes through the membrane can be written as

$$J_{solute} = \frac{K_{solute}}{t_m} (c_{m,h} - c_{m,l}) \tag{12-50}$$

where K_{solute} is the permeability of the membrane to the nonexcluded solute. As shown in Figure 12-18, the concentration driving force is the difference in solute concentrations across the membrane. If both sides are very well mixed the membrane concentrations will be the same as the bulk concentrations. In most systems there will be a resistance to mass transfer on both sides of the membrane and concentration profiles will build up. When this occurs, the values of $c_{m,h}$ and $c_{m,l}$ will not be known. An overall driving force is more convenient. The usual mass transfer expression is (Hwang and Kammermeyer, 1975)

$$J_{solute} = k_{solute}^{T} (c_b - c_d)_{avg} \tag{12-51}$$

where c_b and c_d are the bulk fluid concentrations on the feed and dialysate sides, and k_{solute}^{T} is the total or overall mass transfer coefficient. If the solvent is

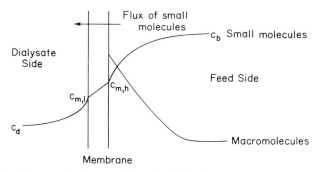

Figure 12-18.   Concentration gradients in dialysis.

stagnant, the overall mass transfer coefficient can be found from a sum of resistances.

$$\frac{1}{k_{solute}^T} = \frac{t_m}{K_{solute}} + \frac{1}{k_{solute}^I} + \frac{1}{k_{solute}^{II}} \qquad (12\text{-}52)$$

where k_{solute}^I and k_{solute}^{II} are the mass transfer coefficients on the feed and dialysate sides of the membrane. The individual mass transfer coefficients can be estimated from standard correlations such as those in Chapter 13. The three terms on the right hand side of Eq. (12-52) are often the same order of magnitude.

As illustrated in Figure 12-18 there can be concentration polarization of macromolecules if the solute flux is high enough. In some cases this may be severe enough to form a gel which can then interfere or stop the transfer of small molecules. The concentration polarization can be controlled by using thin channels or turbulence.

Solvent flux (see Eq. (12-27)) can be in either direction in Figure 12-18. If the pressures on both sides of the membrane are equal, the solvent will flow from the dialysate to the feed side because of osmosis. This osmotic flow can be drastically increased by the concentration polarization of macromolecules, and in turn will tend to reduce the concentration polarization. Unfortunately, the osmotic flow also decreases the flux of the small solutes since the convective flow is in the opposite direction to the solute diffusive flux. The solvent flow can be stopped or reversed by applying a positive pressure on the feed side of the membrane. Dialyzers are often operated with essentially no solvent flux, or with a small flux of solvent into the dialysate.

Any of the flow patterns shown in Figure 12-7 can be used in a dialyzer. Hemodialyzers are usually countercurrent. If the volumetric flow rates of liquids on the feed Q_F and dialysate sides Q_d and the overall mass transfer coefficient k^T can be assumed to be constant, a variety of steady-state flow case can be solved (Michaels, 1966). The correct average concentration difference in Eq. (12-51) is the logarithmic mean of the inlet and outlet concentration.

$$(c_b - c_d)_{lm} = \frac{(c_b - c_d)_1 - (c_b - c_d)_2}{\ln\dfrac{(c_b - c_d)_1}{(c_b - c_d)_2}} \tag{12-53}$$

where 1 and 2 are the two ends of the dialyses. For example, if countercurrent flow is used,

$$(c_b - c_d)_1 = c_{F,in} - c_{d,out} \tag{12-54a}$$

$$(c_b - c_d)_2 = c_{F,out} - c_{d,in} \tag{12-54b}$$

Solving Eqs. (12-51), (12-53) and (12-54) with the mass balance

$$N_A = Q_F(c_{F,in} - c_{F,out}) = Q_d(c_{d,out} - c_{d,in}) \tag{12-55}$$

where N_A is the amount transferred

$$N_A = J_A A \tag{12-56}$$

we can obtain the result for a counter-current dialyszer.

$$\frac{(c_{F,in} - c_{F,out})}{(c_{F,in} - c_{d,in})} = \frac{1 - \exp\left[\dfrac{k^T A}{Q_F}\left[1 - \dfrac{Q_F}{Q_d}\right]\right]}{\dfrac{Q_F}{Q_d} - \exp\left[\dfrac{k^T A}{Q_F}\left[1 - \dfrac{Q_F}{Q_d}\right]\right]} \tag{12-57}$$

In the derivation of Eq. (12-57) the volumetric flow rates Q_F and Q_d were assumed to be constant. At equilibrium, $c_{F,out} = c_{d,in}$. Thus the denominator on the LHS of Eq. (12-57) is the maximum possible concentration change in the feed stream while the numerator is the actual concentration change. The LHS of Eq. (12-57) is thus the fraction of maximum solute removal which is attained.

Results for other geometries are also easily obtained Michaels (1966). For parallel flow of feed and dialysate the result is,

$$\frac{c_{F,in} - c_{F,out}}{c_{F,in} - c_{d,in}} = \frac{1 - \exp\left[-\dfrac{k^T A}{Q_F}\left[1 + \dfrac{Q_F}{Q_D}\right]\right]}{1 + Q_F/Q_d} \qquad (12\text{-}58)$$

If the dialysate is completely mixed and the feed is in plug flow, the result is

$$\frac{c_{F,in} - c_{F,out}}{c_{F,in} - c_{d,in}} = \frac{1 - \exp\left[-\dfrac{k^T A}{Q_F}\right]}{1 - \dfrac{Q_F}{Q_d}\left[1 - \exp\left[-\dfrac{k^T A}{Q_F}\right]\right]} \qquad (12\text{-}59)$$

The counter-current system is superior. Dialysis is also used in batch processes (Klein *et al*, 1987).

Membranes used include cellulose, cellulose acetate, and polyacrylonitrile, but cellulose has been most common. For hemodialysis (dialysis of blood) isotropic cellulose hydrogels with a molecular weight cutoff of approximately 1000 are the most common membranes. The membranes are formed by the cuprammonium process and the membranes are homogeneous and do not have a skin. These membranes easily pass the low molecular weight waste products such as urea (MW=60) and creatinine (MW=113), but do not pass high molecular weight proteins which are desirable. In addition, the membranes will pass amino acids and salts which it is desirable to retain. This latter problem is solved by using a dialysate fluid which is a physiological electrolyte solution containing the appropriate concentrations of the salts. Since salt concentrations are the same on both sides of the membrane, there will be no transfer of the salts. In hemodialysis a positive pressure is applied to the feed (blood) side in order to remove some water (which can be considered the solvent). Equipment used in medical applications must satisfy a large number of constraints such as preventing blood clotting. Details of hemodialysis are discussed by Colton and Lowrie (1981), Lysaght et al (1986), and Ward et al (1985). Other membrane separations used in artificial organs are discussed by Lysaght et al (1986).

In the usual dialysis process exclusion of large solutes is based on steric effects. In *ion exchange dialysis* anion exchange membranes are used. The membranes are the same as those used in electrodialysis (see the next section). These membranes will exclude cations (ions with positive charge), but the exclusion of H^+ cations is poor (see Chapter 9 for a discussion of Ion Exchange). Thus, if a solution of acid and metal salts is on one side of the membrane and water or a dilute acid solution is on the other side of the membrane, the anions (ions of negative charge) readily transfer through the membrane. To keep electroneutrality cations must also transfer. Since the only cation which can transfer through the membrane is H^+, the acid is separated from the metal ion. This is illustrated in Figure 12-19a. Ion exchange dialysis is used commercially to recover metal ions in the plating industry. The systems use plate-and-frame arrangements similar to those used in electrodialysis except no current is required. Water and feed solutions are alternated in the different compartments. Other geometries could also be used.

Donnan dialysis is another variant using ion exchange membranes. The stack utilizes all cation or anion exchange membranes. For purposes of this explanation we will assume that all of the membranes are cation exchange membranes since our purpose is to concentrate a valuable cation. A dilute solution containing the valuable cation (for example Cu^{++}) is circulated in the odd-numbered compartments. In the even-numbered compartments a concentrated solution of cheap acid is circulated. One cell is illustrated in Figure 12-19b. The H^+ ions will transfer through the membranes due to the concentration driving force. To keep electroneutrality, either the anion must transfer through

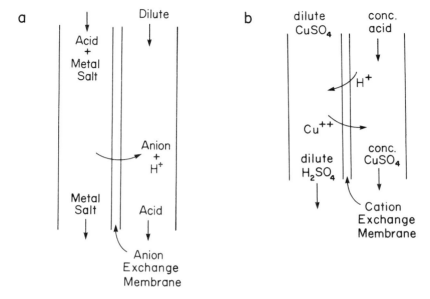

Figure 12-19.   Special dialysis systems. a. Ion exchange dialysis. b. Donnan dialysis.

the cation exchange membrane (which it cannot do because of Donnan exclusion), or Cu^{++} must transfer through the membrane in a direction opposite its concentration driving force. Thus the valuable cation (Cu^{++}) is concentrated at the price of diluting the acid. The copper can be concentrated from 30 ppm Cu SO_4 to as high as 4000 ppm $CuSO_4$. The cost of the separation is the dilution of the sulfuric acid.

12.7. ELECTRODIALYSIS (ED)

Electrodialysis is dialysis in the presence of an electrical field. The driving force for electrodialysis is the electrical potential difference. This driving force pushes cations through cation exchange membranes and anions through anion exchange membranes. The arrangement of membranes shown schematically in Figure 12-20 is used. Cation and anion exchange membranes are alternated. In

694

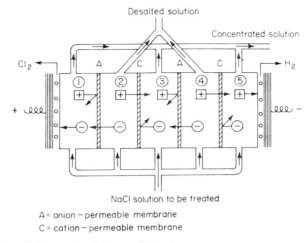

A = anion – permeable membrane
C = cation – permeable membrane

Figure 12-20.   Schematic of electrodialysis.

the presence of the electrical field the cations will migrate towards the cathode and anions towards the anode. The cations can pass through the cation exchange membranes but not through the anion exchange membranes. The anions can pass through the anion exchange membranes but not through the cation exchange membranes. Because of the alternation of the cation and anion exchange membranes the result is to concentrate ions in the odd numbered compartments and to dilute the ions in the even numbered compartments in Figure 12-20. In this way a desalted water and a concentrated brine are formed. In commercial systems from 100 to 600 unit cells (pairs of membranes) are in a stack. Reviews of electrodialysis are given by Applegate (1984), Hwang and Kammermeyer (1975), Klein et al (1985), Korngold (1984), Lacey (1979), Mintz (1963), Solt (1976), and Spiegler (1984).

Ion exchange membranes can be thought of as ion exchange resins which are formed as membranes. The same polymers used for ion exchange resins (see Chapter 9) are used for some of the commercially available ion exchange membranes. The most common cation exchange membrane has been a sulfonated polystyrene cross linked with divinylbenzene. The same basic polystyrene backbone is used for anion exchange with a $CH_2N^+(CH_3)_3$ group coupled to the benzene ring. Other membranes such as Nafion (Figure 12-3g) are used in special cases. Ion exchange membranes are discussed in detail elsewhere (Kesting, 1985; Flett, 1983; Klein et al, 1987; Korngold, 1984; Lacey, 1979; Pusch and Walch, 1982; Solt, 1976; Strathmann, 1985). Lists of suppliers and membrane properties are given by Korngold (1984), Spiegler (1984), and Strathmann (1985).

The usual reaction at the cathode is

$$2H_2O + 2e^- \longrightarrow H_2(g) + 2OH^- \tag{12-60a}$$

The OH^- formed must be neutralized in the cathode compartment. The cathode can be made from tantalum, niobuim, or titanium all of which must be coated with platinum. In the anode the usual reaction is

$$H_2O - 2e^- \longrightarrow \frac{1}{2} O_2(g) + 2H^+ \tag{12-60b}$$

while if Cl^- is present the reaction will be

$$2Cl^- - 2e^- \longrightarrow Cl_2(g) \tag{12-60c}$$

The anode can be made from the same materials as the cathode or from stainless steel. The anode and cathode compartments are separated from the stack by membranes. These compartments are vented to remove the gases formed.

Since the stack is in series, the current flow through each membrane and each compartment must be the same. The reason for using a large number of unit cells is to use this current many times and thus produce more desalted water. The current is carried by the ions. The fraction of current carried by an ionic species is the "transference number". This fraction can be different for the different ions since current is the product of the charge times the velocity times the number of ions transferred. Small ions such as H^+ will carry more current than large ions such as Cl^- since the H^+ have a higher velocity. In a solution such as KCl where the ions are approximately the same size and thus have the same velocity, the transference numbers will be approximately equal.

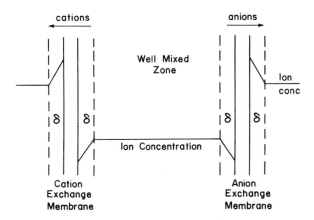

Figure 12-21.   Concentration polarization in electrodialysis.

In solution in the compartments both ions carry current. In the membranes one ion is excluded; thus, the other ion must carry all of the current. The transference number of the cation in the cation exchange membrane is essentially 1.0 while its transference number is essentially zero in the anion exchange membrane. Suppose that K^+ is carrying half the current in the compartment. Suddenly, in the cation exchange membrane K^+ must carry all of the current. This requires that more K^+ be transferred through the membrane than is transferred in solution. Referring to Figure 12-21, we see that the cations are diluted on the right hand side of the cation exchange membrane and concentrated on the left hand side of the membrane. Since concentration gradients have been developed, there will be diffusion of the cation towards the cation exchange membrane on the right hand side of this membrane (see Figure 12-21). This diffusion provides part of the cations needed to carry the current through the membrane. On the other side of the membrane the cations diffuse away from the membrane. Since electroneutrality must be satisfied, the total ion concentration will be diluted when the cation concentration is diluted and concentrated when the cation is concentrated. Exactly the same phenomena occurs at the anion exchange membrane where the anion transfers all of the current. This picture of concentration polarization is oversimplified since it does not include osmotic flow of water and other effects (Hwang and Kammermeyer, 1975).

Table 12-4. Basic electrical equations and units

$$V(\text{volts}) = I(\text{amps}) \, R(\text{ohms}) \qquad (12\text{-}61a)$$

$$I(\text{amps}) = Q(\text{charge in coloumbs}) \, /t(s) \qquad (12\text{-}61b)$$

$$E(\text{joules}) = V(\text{volts}) \, I(\text{amps}) \, t(s) \qquad (12\text{-}61c)$$

$$F = 96{,}500 \, \frac{\text{coloumb}}{\text{equivalent}} = 96{,}500 \, \frac{\text{amp sec}}{\text{equivalent}} \qquad (12\text{-}61d)$$

Concentration polarization has important ramifications for the operation of electrodialysis. If one increases the current density (current per area), then the rate of electrical transport also increases. This will require that the diffusive transport must also increase. This requires an increase in the concentration gradient and the ionic concentrations at the membrane surface will decrease. If these concentrations approach zero at the membrane, the ions will be unable to carry all the current. This point is called the *limiting current density*. The resistance at the membrane surfaces will be high and energy requirements will increase. At this point water will be ionized and H^+ and OH^- will transfer through the membranes to carry the current. This changes the pH in the compartments, and represents energy which is not used to separate the salts from the water. The changes in pH can cause precipitation of salts. The transfer of OH^- through the anion exchange membrane can cause dimensional changes in the membrane. Because of these adverse effects, operation is conducted at a current density below the limiting current density. This upper limit on the current density puts a lower limit on the area of membranes which must be used.

A brief review of electrical equations and units is given in Table 12-4. The energy consumption in electrodialysis can be calculated by combining Eqs. (12-61a) and (12-61c) for n cells.

$$E = I^2 nRt \qquad (12\text{-}62)$$

where E is the energy consumption in joules, I is the current in amps, n is the number of unit cells in the stack, R is the resistance per unit cell in ohms, and t is the time in second. The resistance in the dilute and concentrated parts of the cell differs. Thus, R is the average cell resistance. Alternately, we can calculate E from,

$$E = I^2 n \, t (R_{conc} + R_{dil})/2 \qquad (12\text{-}63)$$

if each chamber is completely mixed. The resistance is usually approximately inversely proportional to concentration,

$$R = b/c \qquad (12\text{-}64)$$

where b is a constant, and c is in equivalents/liter. After some algebraic manipulation, we obtain

$$E = \frac{I^2 nt \, R(c_F)}{\dfrac{2c_{dil}}{c_F} - \left[\dfrac{c_{dil}}{c_F}\right]^2} \qquad (12\text{-}65)$$

where $R(c_F)$ is the resistance per cell determined at the feed concentration. For example, if we recover a product water which is one half as concentrated as the feed this result is

$$E = \frac{4}{3} I^2 nt \, R(c_F)$$

The current requirements can be determined from the required concentration changes.

$$I = FQ \, (c_F - c_{dil})/\xi \qquad (12\text{-}66)$$

where F is Faraday's constant which is 96,500 coulombs/equivalent, Q is the volumetric flow rate of solution in liters/sec, and ξ is the current utilization. The concentration difference must be in gram equivalents per liter. The most important term in this equation is the current utilization ξ. The current utilization is directly related to the number of cells n in the stack and the efficiency of utilization of the current.

$$\xi = n\eta_s\eta_w\eta_m = n \, (\text{Elec. Eff.}) \qquad (12\text{-}67)$$

where n is the number of unit cells, η_s is the efficiency due to the semipermeability of the membrane (co-ions transfer through a membrane that they should be excluded from), η_w is the efficiency related to water transfer through the membrane, and η_m is the efficiency since some of the current invariably leaks through the manifold holding the membranes. All of the efficiencies are less than 1.0 and the overall electrical efficiency is often about 0.9. However, n often varies from 100 to 600. Thus, ξ will usually be significantly greater than 1.0. An important exception to this occurs as the feed concentration becomes high (3 to 5 mol/liter). As this happens η_s and hence Elec. Eff. approach zero since the coions are not strongly excluded from the membrane. At these high concentrations ξ becomes small and energy requirements become too large for electrodialysis to be economical.

The membrane area A for the cation and anion membrane can be estimated from

$$A = \frac{F n Q (c_F - c_{dil})}{i \xi} \qquad (12\text{-}68)$$

where i is the current density in amp/cm^2. The membrane area A is related to the area of each individual membrane A_m by

$$A = n A_m \qquad (12\text{-}69)$$

The area A_m is set by the dimensions of the plate-and-frame module which are standardized by the manufacturer. Substituting in

$$i = I/A_m \qquad (12\text{-}70)$$

plus Eqs. (12-67) and (12-69) into (12-68), we obtain

$$n = \frac{F Q (c_F - c_{dil})}{I \, \eta_s \, \eta_m \, \eta_w} \qquad (12\text{-}71)$$

Mintz (1963) presents a more detailed analysis.

The major commercial application of electrodialysis has been for desalting brackish water (1000 to 5000 mg/L of total dissolved salt) to produce potable water (less than 500 mg/L). ED is also used for producing salt from seawater in Japan, for desalting cheese whey, and for recovering metals from plating baths. In water treatment ED appears to be competitive with RO and ion exchange in the range from 1000 to 3000 mg/L TDS. Typical ED systems operate with current densities from 6 to 20 milliamp/cm^2. The cell would typically be 40 cm wide by 100 cm long and 0.1 cm thick (Mintz, 1963). The system would be designed for 50% demineralization. One major advantage of ED is that significantly less pretreatment is usually required than will be required for RO or ion exchange. The raw water does need to be filtered before the ED system, and the water may need to be treated chemically.

Many ED plants use *polarity reversal* to reduce scaling caused by precipitation of salts. Polarity reversal involves periodically switching the polarity of the electrodes so that the cathode becomes the anode and vice versa. This switches the direction of ion transfer. The purpose of this is to prevent scaling by causing precipitated salts to dissolve when the concentration drops after the direction of ion transfer is reversed. Unfortunately, when the polarity is reversed both streams will have a high salt concentration and must be sent to waste for a minute or two. In a commercial ED system using polarity reversal approximately 13% of the production is lost. Thus the polarity reversal system must be larger than a normal ED system. Since scaling can also be prevented by adding acid, the economics of polarity reversal depends upon acid costs. Since more than 500 of the 1000 commercial ED plants use polarity reversal, it appears to be economical in many cases (Applegate, 1984).

Example 12-4. Electrodialysis of Brackish Water

a. A laboratory electrodialysis unit is available to determine cell resistance and electrical efficiency for desalting a NaCl solution. The following experiment is done: Q = 30 L/min, n = 50, c_F = 20 g/L, c_{dil} = 0.8 g/L. We measure I = 21.5 amp and E = 60,670 joules in one minute. Determine the resistance per unit cell at c_F, and the electrical efficiency.

b. Assuming that R and electrical efficiency are unchanged for a commercial unit, design a system for $Q = 300$ L/min going from c_f = 2.0 g/L to c_{dil} = 0.49 g/L if A_m = 0.4 m^2 and i = 20 amp/m^2. Find I, n, and E in 1 minute.

Solution

a. Rearranging Eqs. (12-66) and (12-67),

$$(\text{Elec. Eff.}) = \frac{F \, Q \, (c_F - c_{dil})}{N \, I}$$

Since $MW_{NaCl} = 58.45$,

$$c_F - c_{dil} = (1.2 \,\frac{g}{L}) \left[\frac{1 \text{ equiv}}{58.45 \text{ g}} \right] = 0.0205 \, \frac{eq}{L}$$

$$(\text{Elec. Eff.}) = \frac{\left[96,500 \, \frac{\text{amp s}}{eq} \right] \left[30 \, \frac{L}{min} \right] \left[\frac{1min}{60 \text{ s}} \right] \left[0.0205 \, \frac{eq}{L} \right]}{(50) \, (21.5 \text{ amps})}$$

$$= 0.920$$

Assuming that cell resistance is inversely proportional to concentration Eq. (12-65) is valid. Rearranging,

$$R(c_F) = \frac{E}{t \, I^2 n} \left[\frac{2 \, c_{dil}}{c_F} - \left[\frac{c_{dil}}{c_f} \right]^2 \right]$$

$$R(c_F) = \frac{60,670 \text{ joules}}{(60 \text{ s}) \, (21.5 \text{ amp})^2 \, (50)} \left[\frac{2(0.8)}{2.0} - \left[\frac{0.8}{2.0} \right]^2 \right]$$

$$= 0.028 \text{ ohm/unit cell}$$

Note that the units work since

$$\text{joule} = (\text{volt})\,(\text{amp})\,(\text{s}) = (\text{amp})^2\,(\text{ohm})\,(\text{s})$$

b. We can use Eq. (12-70) to find I.

$$I = i\,A_m = \left[20\,\frac{\text{amp}}{\text{m}^2}\right](0.4\text{ m}^2) = 8\text{ amp}$$

Then from Eq. (12-71),

$$n = \frac{[96,500\,\frac{\text{amp sec}}{\text{eq}}]\left[300\,\frac{\text{L}}{\text{min}}\right]\left[\frac{1\text{ min}}{60\text{ sec}}\right]\left[\frac{2.0-0.49}{58.45}\,\frac{\text{eq}}{\text{L}}\right]}{(8\text{ amp})\,(0.92)}$$

where $\eta_s\,\eta_m\,\eta_n$ = elec. eff. = 0.92. n = 1693.6 or 1694.
From Eq. (12-65),

$$E = \frac{(8)^2\,(1694)\,(60)\,(0.028)}{\dfrac{2\,(0.49)}{2.0} - \left[\dfrac{0.49}{2.0}\right]^2} = 423,604\text{ joules}$$

Since there are 300 L/min, this is 1412 joules/L = 337.5 cal/L.

Notes: 1.)   One of the hardest parts of ED calculations is the use of unfamiliar units. Thus it is important to check units and refer to Table 12-4.

2.)   Equations (12-62) to (12-66) assume that electrode resistance is small compared to nR. If n is small, this may not be true. n = 50 is probably large enough.

3.)   If the cell design and size or spacer design are changed, R and Elec. Eff. may not be the same for laboratory and commercial units. Also, if the high concentrations are very different η_s may be different in the two units.

12.8. PERVAPORATION

Pervaporation is a membrane process where there is liquid on one side of the membrane and a vapor on the other side. The liquid diffuses through the membrane and vaporizes. This is illustrated in Figure 12-22. The partial pressure in the vapor phase is usually reduced by pulling a vacuum or using a sweep gas. Any of the modular geometries shown in Figure 12-5 could be used although the hollow fiber and spiral wound configurations are most likely. Unlike the other membrane processes discussed up to now, pervaporation is not currently a well established separation method. However, the method has considerable promise and commercial units are available (Sander and Soukup, 1988).

We usually want the least concentrated species to permeate preferentially through the membrane. This reduces the required membrane area and the load on the vacuum pump. For removal of trace organics rubbery polymers such as polyether block amide (PEBAX) are used. For removal of water from azeotropes such as the ethanol-water azeotrope either glassy polymers or ion exchange membranes are used.

Theoretically, pervaporation is the most complex membrane separation process. On the liquid side concentration polarization may be important particularly for the removal of trace organics from water. The membranes operate by a solution-diffusion mechanism. Since the polymer is highly swollen on the

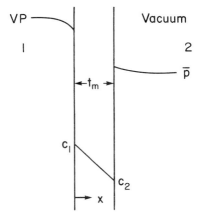

Figure 12-22.   Profiles for pervaporation.

704

liquid side and dry on the vapor side, the diffusivity varies markedly across the membrane. The evaporation at the vapor side may have a major effect on the observed selectivity. For the separation of trace organics from water, the relative volatility of the trace organic is often very high even though the boiling point of the organic is higher than water's boiling point. This occurs because these are very nonideal solutions with high activities. Finally, because of evaporation the process is nonisothermal. The temperature change affects solubility, diffusivity, and evaporation. Currently, a complete model including all these effects is not available.

Pervaporation must be analyzed by using a concentration dependent diffusivity. For the one dimensional system shown in Figure 12-22 the flux is

$$J_i = -D_i(c_1,c_2,..)\frac{dc_i}{dx} \qquad (12\text{-}72)$$

Since flux is proportional to dc_i/dx, the steady state form of Fick's second law becomes,

$$\frac{d}{dx}\left[D_i(c_1,c_2,..)\frac{dc_i}{dx}\right] = 0 \qquad (12\text{-}73)$$

Boundary conditions are

$$c_i = c_{i,1} \text{ at } x=0 \quad , \quad c_i = c_{i,2} \text{ at } x=t_m \qquad (12\text{-}74)$$

Concentration polarization on the liquid side may be important, and must be estimated to calculate $c_{i,1}$. To solve this set of equations a functional form for the diffusivity as a function of all solutes is required.

Unfortunately, solution of these coupled equations is very difficult and has only been done analytically for a pure fluid (Li and Long, 1969; Hwang and Kammermeyer, 1975). This has been done for an exponential dependence of diffusivity on concentration which is appropriate for polymer membranes.

$$D(c) = D_o \exp(ac) \qquad (12\text{-}75)$$

The parameters D_o and a are functions of temperature and the properties of the polymer.

If equilibrium follows a form of Henry's law, at the wall

$$c(\bar{p}) = S^*\bar{p} \tag{12-76}$$

where S^* is the Henry's law constant and is a form of solubility. Then the flux is

$$J = \frac{D_o}{a\,t_m}\,[\exp(aS^*\bar{p}_1) - \exp(aS^*\bar{p}_2)] \tag{12-77}$$

Note that Eq. (12-77) does not fit the standard form given in Eq. (12-1). If we force fit pervaporation into the form of Eq. (12-1) using $\Delta\bar{p}$ as the driving force, we obtain a "permeability" P of

$$P = \frac{J\,t_m}{\Delta\bar{p}} = \frac{D_o}{a\Delta\bar{p}}\,[\exp(aS^*\bar{p}_1) - \exp(aS^*\bar{p}_2)] \tag{12-78}$$

This result shows that the permeability is a function of the partial pressures, in addition to the diffusivity and the solubility. Since both solubilty and diffusivity usually increase as the temperature increases, the permeability and permeation rate increase with temperature increases. The selectivity between different species may decrease as temperature increases, although for commercial alcohol-water pervaporation there is little decrease in selectivity (Sander and Soukup, 1988).

For multicomponent systems the logical first attempt is to assume superposition. Then the partial pressures become

$$\bar{p}_1 = x_i(VP)_i \qquad \bar{p}_2 = y_ip \tag{12-79}$$

The flux and concentration profiles are assumed to be unchanged by the presence of the other diffusing components. Unfortunately, superposition is seldom valid. The presence of a second component affects the permeation rate of the

706

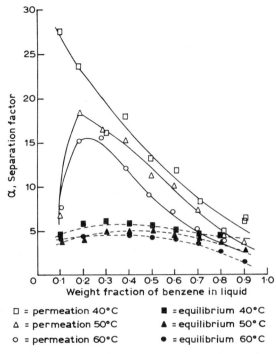

Figure 12-23.   Separation factors for separation of benzene and isopropyl alcohol mixtures through polyethylene by pervaporation. (Carter and Jagannadhaswamy, 1964). Reprinted with permission from *Symposium on The Less Common Means of Separation*, Institution of Chemical Engineers, London, 1984.

first component. Analysis becomes significantly more complicated and is beyond the scope of this book. The selectivity can be a complex function of concentration and temperature. This is illustrated in Figure 12-23 (Carter and Jagannadhaswamy, 1964). Note that selectivity can increase or decrease as mole fraction changes and as temperature increases depending on the system. The selectivity can be significantly higher than the vapor-liquid equilibrium selectivity.

If selectivity and flux are known from laboratory data, we can design the

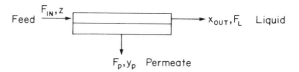

Figure 12-24.   One pass pervaporation system.

pervaporation system without knowing the details of the diffusion. Design does depend upon the details of the flow geometry. The simplest case, completely mixed liquid and vapor (Figure 12-7a), will be considered here. Hwang and Kammermeyer (1975) can be consulted for the analysis for other flow geometries.

A schematic of a pervaporation system is shown in Figure 12-24 for a binary separation. F_{in}, F_L and F_p are flow rates in moles/hr while z, x_{out} and y_p are mole fractions of the more permeable component. Defining the *cut* θ as $\theta = F_p/F_{in}$, the mass balances will be similar to Eqs. (12-5) to (12-7). The result is

$$x_{out} = \frac{z - \theta\, y_p}{1 - \theta} \qquad (12\text{-}80)$$

Since θ is usually determined based on energy balance considerations (see Eqs. (12-88) to (12-90b), Eq. (12-80) is one equation with two unknowns.

An additional equation can be obtained from selectivity data, α'_{AB}

$$\alpha'_{AB} = \frac{y_A/x_A}{y_B/x_B} = \frac{y_A\,(1 - y_A)}{x_A\,(1 - y_A)} \qquad (12\text{-}81)$$

Note that this definition is similar to the definition of relative volatility in vapor-liquid equilibrium although pervaporation is *not* an equilibrium system. Solving for y, we obtain

$$y = \frac{\alpha_{AB}\, x}{1 + \left[\alpha'_{AB} - 1\right] x} \qquad (12\text{-}82)$$

Equations (12-81) and (12-82) apply to local values at the same location of the membrane. For a perfectly mixed system

$$y_p = y \quad , \quad x_{out} = x \tag{12-83}$$

and Eq. (12-82) becomes

$$y_p = \frac{\alpha'_{AB} \, x_{out}}{1 + (\alpha'_{AB} - 1) \, x_{out}} \tag{12-84}$$

The global character of this expression for perfectly mixed systems greatly simplifies the remaining analysis.

Equations (12-80) and (12-84) can be combined. Upon clearing fractions this becomes

$$(\alpha'_{AB} - 1) \, \theta \, \alpha_p^2 - \left[(1 - \theta) + (\alpha'_{AB} - 1)z + \alpha'_{AB} \, \theta\right] y_p + \alpha'_{AB} \, z = 0 \tag{12-85}$$

This equation can obviously be solved for y_p with the quadratic formula (see Example 12-5). Equation (12-85) is linear in z and θ; thus, if y_p and θ are known

$$z = \frac{y_p \, (1 - \theta) - (\alpha'_{AB} - 1) \, \theta \, y_p^2 + \alpha_{AB} \, \theta \, y_p}{\alpha'_{AB} - (\alpha'_{AB} - 1) \, y_p} \tag{12-86}$$

or if y_p and z are known

$$\theta = \frac{\alpha'_{AB} \, z - (\alpha'_{AB} - 1) \, z \, y_p - y_p}{(\alpha'_{AB} - 1) \, (y_p - y_p^2)} \tag{12-87}$$

These equations are obviously valid and easy to use if α'_{AB} is constant. However, Figure 12-23 shows that α'_{AB} is a function of liquid mole fraction x. The equations are still valid, but must be used in a trial-and-error fashion. For example, if z and θ are given we can proceed as follows:

1. Guess $x_{out,guess}$

2. Determine α'_{AB} (x_{out}) from data.

3. Calculate y_p from the solution of Eq. (12-85).

4. Calculate $x_{out,calc}$ from Eq. (12-80).

5. Check: Is $x_{out,guess} = x_{out,calc}$? If not, return to step 1.

The value of the cut is often controlled by the energy balance. For the system shown in Figure 12-24 the energy balance is,

$$F_{in}c_{p,in}\left[T_{in}-T_{ref}\right] = F_{out}c_{p,L}\left[T_{out}-T_{ref}\right] + F_p\left[C_{p,v}\left[T_p-T_{ref}\right] + \lambda\right] \quad (12\text{-}88)$$

where λ is the latent heat of vaporization. With thermal equilibrium in a completely mixed system, $T_p = T_{out}$. Since the reference temperature is arbitrary, we can pick $T_{ref} = T_p = T_{out}$. Then, the energy balance simplifies to

$$F_{in}\,c_{p,in}\left[T_{in} - T_{out}\right] = F_p\,\lambda \quad (12\text{-}89)$$

which is

$$T_{in} - T_{out} = \frac{\theta\,\lambda}{c_{p,in}} \quad (12\text{-}90a)$$

or

$$\theta = \frac{\left[T_{in} - T_{out}\right]c_{p,in}}{\lambda} \quad (12\text{-}90b)$$

The high temperature, T_{in}, is limited by the stability of the membrane. The low temperature, $T_{out} = T_p$, is limited by the need to have a vapor on the permeate side. Thus, if T_p is decreased a very low pressure may be required. Since latent heats are significantly greater than specific heats, the amount of energy

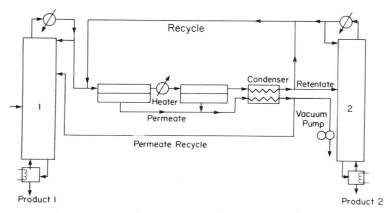

Figure 12-25.   Pervaporation system coupled with distillation.

required to vaporize the permeate will not be available in the feed unless the permeate rate is low. For removal of trace organics permeate rates will be low and sufficient energy is usually available in the feed. For breaking azeotropes conentrations are usually significantly higher and heat effects become important. A recycle stream and/or interstage heaters (see Figure 12-25) are used when necessary to provide sufficient sensible heat for the vaporization. Additional heat input into the pervaporation unit is provided by the hot distillate streams. The value of θ per pass is low, but θ_T for the entire unit shown in Figure 12-25 can be high. It is desireable to keep the temperature drop quite modest (5 to 10°C) since fluxes are significantly higher at higher temperatures (Sander and Soukup, 1988). Thus a large number of stages or high recycle rate is desirable. The use of these equations for a one-pass system is illustrated in Example 12-5. Recycle systems are left to Problem 12-C3.

What are the possible advantages of pervaporation as compared to other membrane processes? In pervaporation the driving force $\Delta \bar{p}$ can be increased by decreasing the downstream pressure by drawing a vacuum or using a sweep gas. In liquid permeation similar increases in the driving force usually require high upstream pressures. To use gas permeation the entire vapor stream must be vaporized instead of just the permeate as in pervaporation. If the feed is already vaporized, gas permeation will be a competing process. Pervaporation often has much larger selectivities but lower fluxes than RO. For trace oganics the high activity of the organic gives high relative volatilities and thus both high selectivities and high fluxes. In addition, pervaporation will not be limited by osmotic pressure.

Pervaporation has been extensively studied as a method of breaking azeotropes, and the method is now available commercially for the ethanol-water azeotrope (Sander and Soukup, 1988). Leeper (1986) has collected pervaporation data for separations of alcohols from water and from a variety of organics. Some of this data is shown in Table 12-5. It is useful to extract as much information as possible from this data. For example, the fluxes in Table 12-5 are considerably less than those in Tables 12-2 and 12-3 for RO and UF. Fluxes and selectivities in Table 12-5 vary significantly. In general, high selectivity membranes will have low fluxes and high flux membranes will have low selectivities. The cellophane data shows that additives can have a major effect on the selectivities. The acetone water data shows that downstream pressure has little effect as long as a vapor is present. Although not shown in Table 12-5, upstream pressure usually increases flux only slightly and has little effect on selectivity. Flux usually increases and selectivity usually decreases as temperature increases although there are exceptions (eg. the cellophane data). Leeper (1986) also presents RO data for the same separations. Reverse osmosis results show higher fluxes and lower selectivities.

In breaking azeotropes pervaporation will usually be coupled with distillation columns. One way of doing this is shown in Figure 12-25 (Goldblatt and Gooding, 1986; Leeper, 1986; Sander and Soukup, 1988). Two or more stages are used in series. The liquid is heated between the stages. Stages are shown operating under a vacuum since this technique is more common than using a sweep gas. Efficient permeate condensation is important since it greatly reduces the load on the vacuum pump. The vaccum pump normally represents the biggest energy cost. Refrigeration systems are used commercially to reduce the load on the vacuum pump (Sander and Soukup, 1988). The permeate recycle is required since permeate is unlikely to be pure. The method shown in Figure 12-25 could be used for separation of isopropyl alcohol and water. Optimization of the system shown in Figure 12-25 will be quite difficult.

Table 12-5. Pervaporation data (Leeper, 1986).

Separation Problem	Membrane	Conc. A in feed (wt%)	T, °F	p_2, mm Hg	Selectivity α_{AB}	Flux lb/ft^2/hr
Ethanol (B) from water (A)	Cellophane	50	77	-	0.94	0.21
	Cellophane	50	113	-	2.0	0.43
	Cellophane	50[1]	77	-	24.6	0.08
	Cellophane	50[2]	77	-	0.63	0.12
	Cellulose Acetate	50	68	0.1	2.0	0.22
	Polyvinylalcohol	10-50	104	0.1	220-75	-
	Polyvinylalcohol	50-90	104	0.1	–75	-
	Polyacrylonitrite	9-94	68	0.1	16-35	0.0001
	Polysulfone	50	68	0.1	332	0.001

713

	Polysulfone, Asymmetric	50	68	0.1	3.0	0.025
	Polysulfone, Composite	50	68	0.1	19.0	0.008
	Aromatic polyamide	4.5	90-130	0.5	0.59-0.36	1-2
	Aromatic polyamide	18.7	70-130	0.5	0.56-0.36	0.3-2
	Silicone rubber	8-12	86-140	-	0.14	0.02-0.05
	Silicone rubber	45-46	86-140	-	0.23-0.22	0.04-0.10
	Silicone rubber	81-87	86-140	-	0.67-0.71	0.04-0.16
n-Butanol(B)	Cellophane	10-24	140	20	10-15	0.2-0.4
from Water (A)	Cellulose 2.5 acetate	85	140	20	45	0.2
Acetone (A)	Polypropylene	45	230	10	2.5	0.094
from Water (B)	Polypropylene	45	230	49	2.8	0.094
	Polypropylene	45	230	488	2.8	0.092

(1) Includes 2 wt% sodium citrate. (2) Includes 2 wt% benzoic acid.

Distillation column 1 is used to approach the azeotrope concentration while column 2 is used to distill on the other side of the azeotrope. In some cases the retentate stream may be of high enough purity that the second distillation column is not required. This is the case for breaking the ethanol water azeotrope (Leeper, 1986; Sander and Soukup, 1988). The commercial ethanol water pervaporator uses a composite poly (vinyl alcohol) membrane which has a very high selectivity for water. The permeate recycle stream is still required for this simplified flowsheet. Of course, there are alternatives for separating the ethanol water azeotrope such as azeotropic distillation, extraction, adsorption, and gas permeation. The choice will depend on the economics of the particular case. Sander and Soukup (1988) state that capital costs were higher for pervaporation than the use of azeotropic distillation, but utility costs were about 1/3 those of azeotropic distillation.

Example 12-5. Pervaporation

We wish to remove water from n-butanol using a cellulose 2.5 acetate membrane. Feed 90 mole % n-butanol. Feed is at 60°C. Selectivity, $\alpha'_{WB} = 43$; Flux = 0.2 lb/ft^2 hr. Maximum permissible temperature drop is 30°C. Find the cut θ and the permeate and liquid mole fractions. If feed rate is 100 lb/hr, find the membrane area.

Data: $\lambda_B = 141.6$ cal/g, $\lambda_w = 9.72$ kcal/gmole
$c_{p,B}$ (45°C) = 0.625 cal/g°C, c_{pw} (45°C) = 1.0 cal/g°C
$MW_B = 74.12$, $MW_w = 18.016$

Solution

We can find the cut θ from Eq. (12-90b). First, we need consistent units.

$$\lambda_B = 141.6 \ \frac{cal}{g} \left[\frac{kcal}{1000 \ cal} \right] \frac{74.12 \ g}{gmole} = 10.5 \ kcal/gmole$$

For 90 mole % butanol, $\lambda = (0.1) 9.72 + (0.9) 10.5 = 10.4$.

Since liquid heat capacities are close to linear, c_p was estimated at

$$T_{avg} = \left[T_{in} + T_{out}\right]/2 = (60 + 30)/2 = 45°C$$

$$c_{p,B} = 0.625 \text{ cal/g°C} \left[\frac{cal}{1000 \text{ kcal}}\right] \left[\frac{74.12 \text{ g}}{gmole}\right] = 0.046 \frac{kcal}{gmole \text{ °C}}$$

$$c_{p,w} = 1.0 \text{ cal/g°c} \left[\frac{1}{1000}\right] \left[\frac{18.016}{1}\right] = 0.0180$$

Then, $c_{p,F} = (0.1)(0.0180) + (0.9)(0.046) = 0.0435$.
Eq. (12-83b) gives,

$$\theta = \frac{\left[T_{in} - T_{out}\right] c_{p,F}}{\lambda} = \frac{(30°C)\left[0.0435 \dfrac{kal}{gmole°C}\right]}{10.4 \text{ kcal/gmole}} = 0.125$$

Permeate mole fraction can be found by solving Eq. (12-85).

$$y_p = \frac{-b \pm \sqrt{b^2 - 4ac}}{2a}$$

where $a = (\alpha'_{WB} - 1)\,\theta = (43 - 1)(0.125) = 5.25$
$b = -[1 - \theta + (\alpha'_{WB} - 1)z + \alpha'_{WB}\,\theta\,] = -[0.875 + (42)(0.1) +$
$(43)(0.125)] = -10.45$
$c = \alpha'_{WB}z = (43)(0.1) = 4.3$

Note that $z = 0.1$ refers to water mole fraction since $\alpha' = \alpha'_{WB}$. Then y_p
is also water mole fraction.

$$y_p = \frac{10.45 \pm 4.35}{10.5} = 0.581 \text{ mole fraction water}$$

where the minus sign is used since $y_p < 1.0$.

716

From Eq. (12-80),

$$x_{w,out} = \frac{z - \theta\, y_p}{1 - \theta} = \frac{0.1 - (0.125)\,(0.581)}{(1 - 0.125)} = 0.031.$$

$$\text{Area} = \text{Feed Rate/Flux} = \frac{100 \text{ lb/hr}}{0.2 \text{ lb/hr ft}^2} = 500 \text{ ft}^2$$

Notes: 1. θ is small despite the significant temperature drop. Thus, recycle is often required.

2. y_p is increased significantly, but liquid product still contains 3% water. A cascade or recycle system is probably needed.

3. This separation can also be done by RO, distillation, adsorption and extraction. The choice will depend on economics.

4. In this example λ should be calculated at x_{out} and at the vacuum pressure. Both these corrections will be small.

There are two alternatives to pervaporation in addition to RO. One is to do gas permeation with the vapor stream. For reasons that are not completely understood, this method gives selectivities and fluxes which are significantly less than those observed for pervaporation. The second alternative is *perstraction* which is liquid permeation into a *carrier liquid* on the permeate side. Pervaporation has been more extensively studied than perstraction since recovery of permeate is normally easier from a vapor than from a liquid. In perstraction the permeate is usually recovered from the high boiling carrier liquid by distillation. Perstraction may be advantageous in some cases since a vacuum pump is not required.

12.9. LIQUID MEMBRANES

A liquid membrane has a layer of liquid which serves as the separation medium instead of the solid polymer used in the other membrane methods discussed

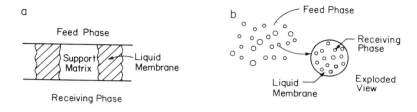

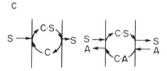

Figure 12-26. Liquid membrane systems. a. Supported liquid membranes. b. Emulsion liquid membranes. c. Facilitated transport.

previously. Two types of liquid membrane systems have been extensively studied. In *supported liquid membranes* the liquid is held in a porous matrix which serves to support the liquid (Danesi, 1984-85; Noble *et al*, 1986; Ward, 1970; Noble and Way, 1987; Way *et al*, 1982, 1985). The equipment and operating procedures for supported liquid membranes are very similar to those for the other membrane separations discussed in this chapter. In *emulsion liquid membranes* a double emulsion is formed with the receiving liquid encapsulated by an immiscible material which is also immiscible with the outer fluid (Cahn and Li, 1976; Li, 1971; Marr and Kopp, 1982; Noble *et al*, 1986; Way *et al*, 1982). The emulsion liquid membrane systems are operated in a manner very similar to liquid-liquid extraction. Liquid membrane systems have been an area of considerable research, but only waste water treatment and gas sensors for ion selective electrodes are commercial (Noble and Way, 1987). In the future these separation techniques may become important as commercial separation devices.

Supported liquid membranes are shown schematically in Figure 12-26a. The liquid membrane phase is held in a porous matrix which is usually a polymer. The liquid membrane itself must be chosen to be immiscible with both the feed phase and the receiving phase. The feed and receiving phases can be essentially the same liquid and in many cases will be an aqueous solution. The liquid membrane serves to separate the feed and receiving phases. In order to increase the capacity of the receiving phase, it will often contain a chemical which will react with the diffusing solute. The supported liquid membrane systems can use one of the geometries shown in Figure 12-5. One of the major problems with this type of liquid membrane is *bleeding* which is loss of the liquid membrane as it dissolves into the feed and receiving phases. Supported liquid membrane systems have apparently not been commercialized yet.

The emulsion liquid membrane system is shown schematically in Figure 12-26b. The system is a double emulsion with the receiving phase distributed within the liquid membrane drops which are dispersed within the feed phase. The emulsion type systems are fairly simple to make and have a very large surface area. Normal extraction equipment is used for the contacting. After the extraction, the liquid membrane usually must be broken to recover the solute. The receiving phase usually contains a chemical to react with the solute to increase the capacity. Emulsion type systems have been extensively designed and piloted for a variety of commercial processes such as copper recovery, phenol removal from waste water, and hydrocarbon separations.

Both types of liquid membrane systems can use *facilitated transport* (Cussler, 1971; Goddard, 1977; Noble et al, 1989). Facilitated transport is shown schematically in Figure 12-26c. A *carrier* contained within the liquid membrane reacts with the solute and then diffuses across the membrane. In the receiving phase the carrier-solute complex is broken and carrier diffuses into the receiving phase. The carrier then diffuses back across the membrane to pick up another "load". This mechanism is similar to the carrying of oxygen in blood by hemoglobin. In the second mechanism shown in Figure 12-26c a second molecule of A is back-transported across the membrane. The back-transported molecule supplies the energy for the process (Cussler, 1971). Examples of this process are using H^+ to supply energy to separate cations. Facilitated transport is of interest since it can provide much faster mass transfer rates with higher selectivities than the liquid membrane alone, and because facilitated transport appears to be important in transfer across cell membranes in living systems. In terms of a solution-diffusion membrane, facilitated transport involves increasing the solubility and/or the diffusion rate of the solute. Noble *et al* (1989) list a large number of systems which have been developed for facilitated transport. Note that these facilitated transport chemical systems can often be used to advantage in other separation processes such as absorption or extraction, and these alternatives may be cheaper than liquid membranes.

12.10. SUMMARY-OBJECTIVES

At the end of this chapter you should be able to meet the following objectives.

1. Explain and describe the following membrane separation processes: Gas permeation, reverse osmosis, ultrafiltration, dialysis, electrodialysis, pervaporation, and liquid membranes. Clearly delineate between the different processes.

2. Determine the flux for the different membrane separation techniques.

3. Describe concentration polarization, explain what can be done to reduce it, and estimate the effect of concentration polarization on flux and rejection coefficients.

4. Describe gelling and fouling, and estimate the effects on flux and rejection. Explain why flux is determined by back-diffusion when a gel layer exists.

5. Explain the effects of flow geometry qualitatively. Do this quantitatively for perfectly mixed systems.

REFERENCES

Applegate, L.E., "Membrane separation processes," *Chem. Eng., 91* (12) 164 (June 11, 1984).

Baker, R.W. and I. Blume, "Permselective membranes separate gases," *Chemtech, 16,* 232 (1986).

Beaver, E.R., P.V. Bhat, and D.S. Sarcia, "Integration of membranes with other air separations technologies," *AIChE Symp. Ser., 84* (261), 113 (1988).

Belfort, G. (Ed.), *Synthetic Membrane Processes. Fundamentals and Water Applications,* Academic Press, Orlando, FL, 1984.

Belter, P.A., E.L. Cussler, and W.-S. Hu, *Bioseparations. Downstream Processing for Biotechnology,* Wiley-Intersciences, 1988, Chapt. 9.

Blaisdell, C.T. and K. Kammermeyer, "Countercurrent and co-current gas separation," *Chem. Eng. Sci., 28,* 1249 (1973).

Blatt, W.F., A. Dravid, A.S. Michaels, and L. Nelson, "Solute polarizatio.` and cake formation in membrane ultrafiltration: Causes, consequences and coi trol techniques," in J.E. Flinn (Ed.), *Membrane Science and Technology,* Plenum Press, NY, 1970, 47-97.

Blatt, W.F., "Principles and practice of ultrafiltration," in P. Meares (Ed.), *Membrane Separation Processes,* Elsevier, Amsterdam, NY, 1976, Chapt. 3.

Cadotte, J., R. Forester, M. Kim, R. Petersen, and T. Stocker, "Nanofiltration membranes broaden the use of membrane separation technology," *Desalination, 70,* 77 (1988).

Cahn, R.P. and N.N. Li, "Hydrocarbon separation by liquid membrane processes," In P. Meares (Ed.), *Membrane Separation Processes,* Elsevier, Amsterdam, 1976, Chapt.9.

Caracciolo, V.P., N.W. Rosenblatt and V.J. Tomsic, "Du Pont's hollow fiber membranes," in S. Sourirajan (Ed.), *Reverse Osmosis and Synthetic Membranes,* Ottawa, Canada, National Research Council of Canada, 1977, Chapt. 16.

721

Carter, J.W. and B. Jagannadhaswamy, "Liquid separations using polymer films," *Proceedings Symposium on the Less Common Means of Separation*, Institution Chemical Engineers, London, 1964, 35-42.

Cheremisinoff, P.N. and A.R. LaMendola, "Industrial applications of reverse osmosis," in N.P. Cheremisinoff and D.S. Azbel (Eds.), *Liquid Filtration*, Ann Arbor Science, 1983, Chapt. 14.

Chern, R.T., W.J. Koros, H.B. Hopfenberg, and V.T. Stannett, "Material selection for membrane-based gas separations," in D.R. Lloyd (Ed.), *Materials Science of Synthetic Membranes*, Am. Chem. Soc., Washington, DC, 1985, Chapt. 2.

Colton, C.K. and E.G. Lowrie, "Hemodialysis: Physical principles and technical considerations," *The Kidney*, Vol. 2, 2nd ed., Philadelphia, W.B. Saunders Co. 1981, 2425-2489.

Cooper, A.R. (Ed.), *Ultrafiltration Membranes and Applications*, Plenum Press, NY, 1979.

Cussler, E.L., "Membranes which pump," *AIChE Journal, 17*, 1300 (1971).

Danesi, P.R., "Separation of metal species by supported liquid membranes, *Separ. Sci. Technol., 19*, 857 (1984-85).

Eisenberg, T.N. and E.J. Middlebrooks, *Reverse Osmosis Treatment of Drinking Water*, Butterworths, Boston, 1986.

Eykamp, W. and J. Steen, "Ultrafiltration and reverse osmosis," in R.W. Rousseau (Ed.), *Handbook of Separation Process Technology*, Wiley-Interscience, New York, 1987, Chapt. 18.

Fane, A.G., "Ultrafiltration: Factors influencing flux and rejection", in R.J. Wakeman (Ed.), *Progress in Filtration and Separation 4*, Elsevier, NY, 101-180 (1986).

722

Flett, D.S. (Ed.), *Ion Exchange Membranes*, Ellis Horwood Ltd., Chichester, England, 1983.

Finken, H., "Asymmetric membranes for gas separations," in D.R. Lloyd (Ed.), *Materials Science of Synthetic Membranes*, Amer. Chem. Soc., Washington, D.C., 1985, Chapt. 11.

Gienger, J.K. and R.J. Ray, "Membrane-based hybrid processes," *AIChE Symp. Ser., 84* (261), 168 (1988).

Goldblatt, M.E. and C.E. Gooding, "An engineering analysis of membrane-aided distillation", *AIChE Symposium Series, 82* (248) 51 (1986).

Goddard, J.D., "Further applications of carrier-mediated transport theory - A survey," *Chem. Eng. Sci., 32*, 795 (1977).

Henis, J. M.S. and M.K. Tripodi, "The developing technology of gas separating membranes," *Science, 220* (4592), 11 (April 1, 1983).

Hsieh, H.P., "Inorganic membranes," *AIChE Symp. Ser., 84* (261), 1 (1988).

Hwang, S.-T. and K. Kammermeyer, *Membranes in Separations*, Wiley, NY, 1975.

Kesting, R.E., *Synthetic Polymeric Membranes. A Structural Perspective*, 2nd ed., Wiley, NY, 1985.

Klein, E., R.A. Ward, and R.E. Lacey, "Membrane processes-Dialysis and electrodialysis", in R.W. Rousseau (Ed.), *Handbook of Separation Process Technology*, Wiley, New York, 1987, Chapt. 21.

Klinkowski, P.R., "Ultrafiltration: an emerging unit-operation," *Chem. Eng., 85* (11) 165 (May 8, 1978).

Korngold, E., "Electrodialysis - Membranes and mass transport", in G. Belfort

(Ed.), *Synthetic Membrane Processes. Fundamentals and Water Applications*, Academic Press, Orlando, FL 1984, Chapt. 6.

Koros, W.J. and R.T. Chern, "Separation of gaseous mixtures using polymer membranes," in R.W. Rousseau (Ed.), *Handbook of Separation Process Technology*, Wiley-Interscience, NEw York, 1987, Chapt. 20.

Kremen, S.S., "Membrane systems", in M.B. Chenoweth (Ed.), *Synthetic Membranes*, MMI Press, Midland, MI, 1986, 53-87.

Kremen, S.S., "Technology and engineering of ROGA spiral-wound reverse osmosis membrane modules," in S. Sourirajan (Ed.), *Reverse Osmosis and Synthetic Membranes*, Ottawa, Canada, National Research Council of Canada, 1977, Chapt. 17.

Lacey, R.E., "Dialysis and electrodialysis," in P.A. Schweitzer (Ed.), *Handbook of Separation Techniques for Chemical Engineers*, McGraw-Hill, NY, 1979, Section 1.14.

Leeper, S.A., "Membrane separation in the production of alcohol fuels by fermentation," in W.C. McGregor (Ed.), *Membrane Separations in Biotechnology*, Marcel Dekker, NY, 1986, Chapt. 8.

Li, N.N. and R.B. Long, "Permeation through plastic films," *AIChE Journal, 15*, 73 (1969).

Li, N.N., "Separation of hydrocarbons by liquid membrane permeation," *Ind. Eng. Chem. Process Des. Develop., 10,* 215 (1971).

Lloyd, D.R. (Ed.), *Materials Science of Synthetic Membranes*, Amer. Chem. Soc.," DC, 1985.

Lloyd, D.R. and T.B. Meluch, "Selection and evaluation of membrane materials for liquid separations," in D.R. Lloyd (Ed.), *Materials Science of Synthetic Membranes*, Amer. Chem. Soc., Washington, DC, 1985, Chapt. 3.

Loeb, S. and S. Sourirajan, "Seawater demineralization by means of an osmotic membrane," *Advan. Chem. Ser., 38*, 117 (1963).

Loeb, S. and S. Sourirajan, "Seawater demineralization by means of a semipermeable membrane," University of California at Los Angeles Engineering Report No. 60-60, 1960.

Lonsdale, H.K., "The growth of membranes technology," *J. Membrane Sci., 10*, 81 (1982).

Lysaght, M.J., D.R. Boggs, and M.H. Taimisto, "Membranes in artificial organs", in M.B. Chenoweth (Ed.), Synthetic Membranes, MMI Press, Midland, MI, 1986, 100-117.

Marr, R. and A. Kopp, "Liquid membrane technology - A survey of phenomena, mechanisms and models," *Internat. Chem. Eng., 22* (1), 44 (1982).

Michaels, A.S., "Operating parameters and performance criteria for hemodialyzers and other membrane-separation devices", *Trans. Amer. Artif. Intern. Organs, 12*, 387 (1966).

Mintz, M.S., "Electrodialysis, principles of process design," *Ind. Chem.,* 55(6) 18 (June 1963).

Noble, R.D., C.A. Koval, and J.J. Pellegrino, "Facilitated transport membrane systems," *Chem. Engr. Prog., 85* (3), 58 (March 1989).

Noble, R.D. and J.D. Way (Eds.), *Liquid Membranes, Theory and Applications,* ACS Symp. Ser., No. 347, ACS, Washington, D.C., 1987.

Noble, R.D., J.D. Way and A.L. Bunge, "Liquid membranes," in Y. Marcus (Ed.), *Ion Exchange and Solvent Extractions,* vol. 10, Marcel Dekker, NY.

Orofino, T.A., "Technology of hollow fiber reverse osmosis systems," in S.

Sourirajan (Ed.), *Reverse Osmosis and Synthetic Membranes*, Ottawa, Canada, National Research Council of Canada, 1977, Chapt. 15.

Porter, M.C., "Membrane filtration," in Schweitzer, P.A. (Ed.), *Handbook of Separation Techniques for Chemical Engineers*, McGraw-Hill, NY, 1979, Section 2.1.

Potts, D.E., R.C. Ahlert and S.S. Wang, "A critical review of fouling of reverse osmosis membranes," *Desalination, 36*, 235 (1981).

Pusch, W. and A. Walch, "Synthetic membranes-preparation, structure, and applications," *Angew Chem. Int. Ed. Engl., 21*, 660 (1982).

Reid, C.E., "Principles of reverse osmosis," in U. Merten (Ed.), *Desalination by Reverse Osmosis*, MIT Press, Cambridge, MA 1966, Chapt. 1.

Rogers, C.E., "Permeation of gases and vapours in polymers," in J. Comyn (Ed.), *Polymer Permeability*, Elsevier, London, 1985, Chapt. 2.

Sander, U. and P. Soukup, "Design and operation of a pervaporation plant for ethanol dehydration," *J. Memb. Sci., 36*, 463 (1988).

Schell, W.J., "Commercial applications for gas permeation membrane systems," *J. Memb. Sci., 22*, 217 (1985).

Solt, G.S., "Electrodialysis," in P. Meares (Ed.), *Membrane Separation Processes*, Elsevier, Amsterdam, NY, 1976, Chapt. 6.

Soltanieh, M. and W.N. Gill, "Review of reverse osmosis membranes and transport models," *Chem. Eng. Commun., 12*, 279 (1981).

Sourirajan, S. (Ed.), *Reverse Osmosis and Synthetic Membranes. Theory - Technology - Engineering*, National Research Council of Canada, Ottawa, Canada, 1977.

726

Spiegler, K.S., "Electrodialysis", in R.H. Perry and D. Green (Eds.), *Perry's Chemical Engineer's Handbook*, 6th ed., McGraw-Hill, N.Y., 1984, 17-37 to 17-47.

Spillman, R.W., "Economics of gas separation membranes", *Chem. Eng. Prog.*, *85*(1), 41 (Jan. 1989).

Stana, R.R., "Westinghouse membrane systems," in S. Sourirajan (Ed.), *Reverse Osmosis and Synthetic Membranes*, Ottawa, Canada, National Research Council of Canada, 1977, Chapt. 18.

Stannett, V.T., W.J. Koros, D.R. Paul, H.K. Lonsdale, and R.W. Baker, "Recent advances in membrane science and technology," *Adv. Polymer Sci.*, *32*, 69 (1979).

Stern, S.A., "New developments in membrane processes for gas separations", in M.B. Chenoweth (Ed.), *Synthetic Membranes*, MMI Press, Midland, MI, 1986, 1-37.

Stern, S.A. and H.L. Frisch, "The selective permeation of gases through polymers," *Ann. Rev. Mater. Sci.*, *11*, 523 (1981).

Stern, S.A., "The separation of gases by selective permeation," in P. Meares (Ed.), *Membrane Separation Processes*, Elsevier, NY, 1976, Chapt. 8.

Strathmann, H., "Membrane separation processes," *J. Memb. Sci.*, *9*, 121 (1981).

Strathmann, H., "Electrodialysis and its application in the chemical process industry," *Separ. Purific. Methods, 14*, 41 (1985).

Warashina, T., Y. Hashino and T. Kobayashi, "Hollow-fiber ultrafiltration," *Chem. Tech., 15*, 558 (1985).

Ward, R.A., P.W. Feldhoff and E. Klein, "Membrane materials for therapeutic applications," in D.R. Lloyd (Ed.), *Materials Science of Synthetic Membranes,* Amer. Chem. Soc., Washington, DC, 1985, Chapt. 5.

Ward, W.J., "Analytical and experimental studies of facilitated transport," *AIChE Journal, 16,* 405 (1970).

Way, J.D., R.D. Noble and B.R. Bateman, "Selection of supports for immobilized liquid membranes," in Lloyd, D.R. (Ed.), *Materials Science of Synthetic Membranes,* ACS, Washington, DC, 1985, Chapt. 6.

Way, J.D., R.D. Noble, T.M. Flynn and E.D. Sloan, "Liquid membrane transport: A survey," *J. Memb. Sci., 12,* 247 (1982).

Wijmans, J.G., S. Nakao, and C.A. Smolders, "Flux limitation in ultrafiltration: Osmotic pressure model and gel layer model," *J. Memb. Sci., 20,* 115 (1984).

HOMEWORK

A. *Discussion Problems*

A1. How does polymer structure affect selectivity?

A2. What are the advantages and disadvantages of each module shown in Figure 12-5?

A3. In pervaporation the permeate side is usually under a vacuum. Explain why. Would pulling a vacuum on the permeate side of a gas permeation system be useful? Explain why.

A4. In gas permeation too high a selectivity can be detrimental and may actually limit the removal of the permeating gas from the feed. Explain this phenomenon.

A5. How can RO and UF complement each other?

A6. Contrast concentration polarization without a gel to concentration polarization with a gel.

A7. Contrast how concentration polarization develops in RO and in ED.

A8. Figures 12-4 and 12-15 show no concentration polarization on the permeate side. Figures 12-18 and 12-21 show mass transfer on both sides of the membrane. Explain these differences.

A9. Why is ED more economical for separation of relatively dilute solutions than for concentrated solutions?

A10. Sketch a pervaporation system to break the ethanol-water azeotype when column 2 in Figure 12-25 is not required. Assume water is the preferred permeate. Why might a recycle stream be required for the permeator?

A11. Develop your key relations chart for this chapter.

B.   *Generation of Alternatives*

B1. The RM membrane is a clever and commercially successful solution to the problem of how to make essentially defect free gas permeation membranes. Brainstorm at least 5 other solutions to this problem.

C.   *Derivations*

C1. Show that Eq. (12-32a) is a solution to Eq. (12-31) and the appropriate boundary conditions.

C2. Show that Eq. (12-39) is a solution to Eq. (12-31) and the appropriate boundary conditions.

C3. A simple pervaporation unit with a recycle stream is shown below. Assume that the following variables are known: F_{new}, x_{new}, T_{new}, R, θ_T, T_R, $c_{p,in}$, $c_{p,new}$, $c_{p,R}$, α', λ, T_{out}. The module is perfectly mixed and operates at thermal equilibrium.

   a. Calculate θ

   b. Assuming θ is known, solve for y_p in terms of known variables.

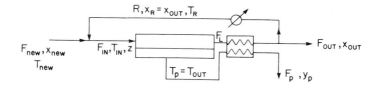

C4. Derive Eq. (12-49) from Eq. (12-48).

C5. Derive Eq. (12-46) from Eq. (12-45).

D. *Single-Answer Problems*

D1. Estimate the permeabilities for H_2 and CO of a RM membrane for gas permeation if both membranes are perfect. The top layer is 1μm silicone rubber. The second layer is polysulfone with a 1.2μm thin skin. Estimate $\alpha_{H_2,CO}$. Data are in the text. How will surface pores affect α?

D2. Data for a hollow fiber RO module from Dow Chemical is given in Table 12-2. Details of how the test were done are not complete.
a. If there was no concentration polarization, calculate K_{solv}/t_M for this system.
b. If $M = 2$ during the experiment, determine K_{solv}/t_M.
You can use the van't Hoff equation.

D3. An ultrafiltration membrane is first tested in a stirred cell where there is no concentration polarization. The experimental values obtained in the table are obtained. Then the same membrane is used in a spiral wound module where there is concentration polarization. Values listed are obtained. Assume membrane thickness and permeabilities are the same. Calculate the expected solvent flux and the concentration polarization modulus in the spiral wound membrane system. No gel layer forms.

	c_b(conc. solute)	c_p(conc. solute)	$J_{solv,}$ L/m^2 day	Δp, bars
Stirred Cell	10 g/L	0.25 g/L	7000	3.5
Spiral Wound	6 g/L	1.0 g/L		4.0

D4. Ultrafiltration of a dextran solution gives the following data

J, ml/cm^2 min	0.055	0.045	0.030	0.018
wt. frac dextran	0.01	0.02	0.05	0.10

Estimate the weight fraction at which dextran gels.

D5. A countercurrent dialyzer is using an experimental membrane to remove urea from an aqueous feed. The entering feed contains 10g/L urea and outlet should be 1g/liter. Feed rate is 1 L/min. Inlet dialysate is pure water and flow rate is 3 L/min.

   a. Determine the overall transfer rate N_A in g/min.

   b. Determine required value of k_T A.

   c. If A = 100 m^2 calculate k_T.

D6. We wish to desalinate 400 liters/min of a brackish water containing 1.5 g/L salt to 0.5 g/L salt in an ED system. The system has 200 cells. The efficiencies are estimated as: $\eta_s = 0.98$, $\eta_w = 0.99$, $\eta_M = 0.99$. The average resistance of each cell is 0.03 ohms. Determine,

   a. The current in amps and the voltage in volts.

   b. The energy required in cal/liter water.

   c. The power in kilowatts.

D7. An experimental RO cellulose-acetate membrane with an active layer 6 microns thick achieved a flux of 0.33 x 10^{-4} g/cm^2 sec for a 40 atmosphere pressure difference with 0.1 N NaCl in water (π=4.9 atm). What was the water permeability and list the units if:

   a1) $M = c_w/c_B = 1$ a2) $M = c_w/c_B = 3$

   b) This membrane had $R^0 = 0.96$. What was the salt permeability for

   b1) $M = c_w/c_B = 1$ b2) $M = c_w/c_B = 3$

D8. We are ultrafiltering a flexible chain polymer. In a stirred cell with no concentration polarization $R^0 = 0.996$ and $K_{solv}/t_m = 2000$ L/(m^2 day atm). In a hollow fiber system gelling occurs at $c_g = 80$ g/L. The gel layer appears to be completely mobile. In an experiment where a gel layer formed with $c_b = 26$ g/L and $\Delta p = 6$ atm we find $J_{solv} = 82.83$ L/m^2 day.

a. In the stirred cell find J_{solv} and J_{solute} if $\Delta p = 5$ atm and $c_b = 20$g/L.

b. In the hollow fiber system find J_{solv}, R_{app} and J_{solute} if $\Delta p = 5$ atm and $c_b = 20$g/L. Other conditions are the same as in previous experiment.

D9. In Example 12-1 we obtained $y_{out} = 0.0168$. Suppose we want $y_{out} = 0.010$. What value of θ is required? Other specifications are the same as in Example 12-1.

D10. A cellulose acetate membrane is separating a CO_2–N_2 mixture. The feed gas is 40 mole % N_2 and 60 mole % CO_2. The permeate pressure is 770 cm Hg while the feed pressure is 10,000 cm Hg. The effective membrane thickness is 1.5 μm. The membrane module can be assumed to be completely mixed on both sides. If the cut $\theta = F_p/F_{in} = 0.55$, determine y_{out} and y_p. Assume permeate is an ideal gas. Permeability data from Figure 12-9 gives $P_{N_2} \sim 0.3 \times 10^{-10}$ and $P_{CO_2} \sim 20 \times 10^{-10}$

D11. We are separating oxygen and nitrogen by gas permeation with a silicone rubber membrane. The membrane module is perfectly mixed. Inlet gas is 21 mole % O_2. We desire a permeate product which is 27 mole % O_2. Membrane has a selectivity $\alpha_{AB} = P_A/P_B = 2.1$. Pressure ratio is $p_L/p_H = 0.35$. Treat the gases as ideal gases. What cut θ must be used?

D12. Blood plasma proteins are known to gel at a concentration of $c_g = 0.2$ weight fraction. The proteins can be treated as particles approximately 30×10^{-10} meters diameter. With pure water the membrane has a flux of 2.5×10^{-5} m^3/m^2 sec at a transmembrane pressure drop of 68.96 kPa. At an operating pressure drop of 103.44 kPa with a plasma solution the flux is 0.416×10^{-5} m^3/m^2 sec. Assume the gel layer has a porosity of ε $= 0.5$.

    a)   What is the gel thickness at steady state?

    b)   If pressure is doubled, what is the gel thickness at steady state? Note: Watch your units on viscosity. Assume $\mu = \mu_{water}$ at 25°C.

D13.   We are separating oxygen and nitrogen with a composite membrane, $\alpha_{O_2-N_2} = P_{O_2}/P_{N_2} = 5.4$. We have set up a membrane cascade of perfectly mixed modulus to produce a final permeate product of $y_p = 0.95$ oxygen. In the last module $p_L/p_H = 0.25$ and $\theta = 0.60$. What must be the inlet mole fraction to this last module (feed contains only O_2 and N_2)?

F.   *Problems Requiring Other Resources*

F1.   Estimate the osmotic pressure of acetic acid, CH_3COOH, in a 25 wt % aqueous solution at 25°C.

    a. Use van't Hoff Eq.

    b. Use Eq. (12-17).

    c. Use Eq. (12-19).

Data is in Perry's and the *Handbook of Chemistry and Physics*.

F2.   (Derivation). It is unusual to have a ratio of gas constants in an equation such as in Eq. (12-19). Show in the derivation (see Reid, 1966) how this occurs. Note that Reid (1966) does not show this since he is not concerned with units.

Chapter 13

DETAILED THEORIES FOR MEMBRANE SEPARATIONS

The basic concepts, definitions, and theories for a variety of membrane separators were presented in Chapter 12. In order to cover the entire area of membrane separations while at the same time keeping that chapter a reasonable length some of the more involved analyses were not included. These more involved analyses will be discussed in this chapter. Chapter 12 is a prerequisite for this material.

The organization of this chapter is to divide the membrane separator into three parts. The first part (Sections 13.1, 13.2, and 13.5) is the transfer from the bulk fluid to the membrane wall. This part discusses concentration polarization, gel formation and fouling. The second part (Sections 13.3 and 13.4) considers the overall flow pattern in the membrane module such as those illustrated in Figure 12-6. The third part (Section 13.6) treats the transport of solvent and solute inside the membrane.

Concentration polarization was discussed in Chapter 12 and a simple theory was presented there. However, the equations were left in terms of the boundary layer thickness δ or the mass transfer coefficient k, and no mention was made of how to determine δ or k. The determination of k using correlations will be done in Section 13.1. The gel model for UF was also discussed in Chapter 12. A more complete analysis will be done in Section 13.2.

The bulk flow patterns in the membrane modules have a large effect on separation. In Chapter 12 fluid on both sides of the membrane was assumed to be perfectly mixed. In Section 13.3 perfectly mixed modules with concentration polarization are studied. Countercurrent flow is studied in Section 13.4.

The transfer phenomena *inside* the membrane was essentially ignored in

733

Chapter 12. In Section 13.6 an irreversible thermodynamics analysis of this transfer is developed. The solution-diffusion model for transfer inside of RO membranes and a frictional model appropriate for transfer inside of porous UF membranes will be presented.

13.1. APPROXIMATE ANALYSIS OF CONCENTRATION POLARIZATION

In this section a somewhat more detailed model of concentration polarization than that presented in Eqs. (12-25) to (12-32) will be developed. The analysis in this section uses mass transfer correlations to find k.

13.1.1. Basic Equations.

The usual picture of concentration polarization was shown in Figure 12-4. The solute mass balance was given by Eq. (12-31) when the rejection is 1.0 and c_p = 0. When the rejection is not 1.0, the mass balance can be written as:

$$J_{solv} \, c_p + J_{solv} \, c + D \, \frac{dc}{dy} = 0 \qquad (13-1)$$

where the first term represents solute which passes through the membrane. The boundary conditions are

$$c = c_w \quad \text{at} \quad y = 0 \qquad (13-2a)$$

$$c = c_b \quad \text{at} \quad y = \delta \qquad (13-2b)$$

Since $c_p = (1-R^\circ)c_w$, the solution to this set of equations is

$$M = \frac{c_w}{c_b} = \frac{\exp(J_{solv}\,\delta/D)}{R^\circ + (1-R^\circ)\exp(J_{solv}\,\delta/D)} \qquad (13-3a)$$

which reduces to Eq. (12-32a) when $R^o = 1.0$. In this result $R^o = 1 - c_p/c_w$ is the intrinsic rejection in the absence of concentration polarization.

To use this result we must be able to estimate δ. Since δ controls the boundary condition. This can be done by assuming that δ is the same as the δ for a semi-impermeable wall which has R=1. This is a reasonable estimate for low flux membranes since the solute flux through the membrane is much less than the solute flux parallel to the membrane. Then the mass transfer coefficient to the wall is

$$k = D/\delta \qquad (13\text{-}4)$$

This mass transfer coefficient k can be calculated from mass transfer correlations for different flow regimes. This is the subject of Section 13.1.2. Substituting Eq. (13-4) into (13-3a), we obtain

$$M = \frac{c_w}{c_b} = \frac{\exp(J_{solv}/k)}{R^o + (1 - R^o)\exp(J_{solv}/k)} \qquad (13\text{-}3b)$$

J_{solv} is given by Eq. (12-27). Note that Equations (12-27) and (13-3b) are valid at each point of the membrane since, in general, c_b, c_w, c_p, J_{solv}, and M vary throughout the membrane module. For a mixed system $c_b = c_{out}$ is constant and hence c_w, c_p, M, and J_{solv} are constant. When $R^o = 1$, simultaneous solution of Eqs. (12-27) and (13-3b) gives J_{solv} and M. If $R^o < 1$, we must simultaneously solve Eqs. (12-22), (12-25), (12-27) and (13-3b). For high flux membranes Eqs. (13-4) and (13-5) are both suspect.

Equations (13-3), (13-4) and the expressions for k are convenient to use when J_{solv} is constant and specified. If J_{solv} is unknown, these equations must be solved simultaneously with Eq. (12-27). Unfortunately, the polarization modulus M is required to calculate J_{solv} in Eq. (12-27) and J_{solv} is required to determine M in Eq. (13-3). Thus an iterative trial-and-error solution is often required. Fortunately, if $J_{solv}/k \ll 1.0$ an approximate solution can be developed (Rao and Sirkar, 1978). This solution is particularly simple for ideal semi-impermeable membranes where $R^o = 1$. Assume that the osmotic pressure is a linear function of concentration following Eq. (12-18b) which is reasonable for dilute solutions. When $J_{solv}/k \ll 1.0$, the exponential term in Eqs. (12-32a) and (13-3) can be expanded as

$$M = \frac{c_w}{c_b} = \exp\left(\frac{J_{solv}}{k}\right) \sim 1 + \frac{J_{solv}}{k} \tag{13-5}$$

where we have inserted $R^\circ = 1$. Setting $c_p = 0$ ($R^\circ = 1$) and $\pi(c_w) = ac_w$ in Eq. (12-27), we obtain

$$J_{solv} = \frac{K_{solv}}{t_m}(\Delta p - aMc_b) \tag{13-6}$$

Equations (13-5) and (13-6) can now be solved simultaneously for J_{solv}.

$$J_{solv} = \frac{\dfrac{K_{solv}}{t_m}(\Delta p - ac_b)}{1 + \dfrac{K_{solv}}{t_m}\dfrac{ac_b}{k}} \tag{13-7}$$

When using this equation, the assumption that $J_{solv}/k \ll 1.0$ should be checked. Equation (13-7) is useful when c_b is known. If c_b is not known, we need to include mass balances (see Section 13.3.2.).

If $R^\circ < 1$ and/or (J_{solv}/k) is not very small, the result from Eq. (13-7) can be used as the first guess for J_{solv}. Then Eq. (13-3b) can be solved for M. Now the solvent flux equation with $R^\circ < 1$, Eq. (12-27), can be solved simultaneously with Eqs. (12-22) and (12-25). This value of J_{solv} can be used in Eq. (13-3b) and the procedure can be continued until there is convergence.

Once M and J_{solv} have been determined the required membrane area and module length can be found. An external mass balance for the module is

$$J_{solv} A c_p + (F - J_{solv} A)c_{out} = F c_F \tag{13-8}$$

In this equation F is the volumetric feed rate to the module (e.g. liter/hr) and c_{out} is the concentrated product on the feed side of the membrane. Since c_{out} is usually given, Eq. (13-5) can be solved for A. For tubular or hollow fiber systems,

$$A = (\pi Ld)n \qquad (13-9)$$

where n is the number of tubes of diameter d and length L.

13.1.2. Mass Transfer Correlations

For turbulent flow the Nernst film theory can be used to estimate the value of k. Figure 12-4 can again be used. The boundary layer is assumed to contain all of the concentration gradient while the bulk flow is turbulent and well mixed. The mass transfer coefficient in turbulent flow can be written in terms of the Chilton-Colburn j factor.

$$k = u_b j_D Sc^{-2/3} \qquad (13-10a)$$

where $Sc = \mu/\rho D$ is the Schmidt number. In round tubes

$$j_D = f/2 \qquad (13-10b)$$

where f is the Fanning friction factor which in turbulent flow can be estimated from

$$f = 0.0791\, Re^{-1/4} \qquad (13-10c)$$

where $Re = du_b\rho/\mu$ is the Reynolds number. This allow estimation of k and δ. An alternate method is to use the standard correlation for mass transfer in round pipes in turbulent flow (Blatt et al., 1970; Porter, 1979).

$$k = 0.023\, \frac{D}{d}\, Re^{0.83}\, Sc^{1/3} \qquad (13-11)$$

Fully developed turbulent flow on tubes will certainly occur for Re > 20,000 and in UF devices appears to occur at Re = 2000 (Porter, 1979). These results can be substituted into Eq. (13-3) to estimate the concentration polarization modulus in turbulent flow. Note that concentration polarization in turbulent flow does not depend upon the distance down the tube. For turbulent flow between parallel sheets the same correlation can be used except the equivalent diameter of the channel d_{eq} should be used

$$d_{eq} = 4 \; \frac{\text{cross-sectional area}}{\text{wetted perimeter}} = 4 \; \frac{2hw}{2w + 2h} \qquad (13\text{-}12)$$

where $2h$ is the gap between the sheets and w is the width.

For turbulent flow in a stirred vessel (Blatt et al., 1970),

$$k = 0.0443 \; \frac{D}{d} \left[\frac{v}{D} \right]^{0.33} \left[\frac{\omega \, d^2}{v} \right]^{0.75} \qquad (13\text{-}13)$$

where d is the vessel diameter in cm, ω is the stirrer speed in radians/sec, v is the kinematic viscosity in cm^2/sec, and D is the diffusivity in cm^2/sec. This form is useful for laboratory stirred tanks, but the stirred tank configuration is unlikely to be used on a large scale. An example calculation is part of Example 13-2.

Turbulent flow can be important in tubular (Figure 12-5b), stirred tanks and plate-and-frame (Figure 12-5a) modules. Qualitatively, Eq. (13-3b) shows that M decreases if the mass transfer coefficient k increases. This can be achieved with high velocities u_b, high diffusivities, and low viscosities. Operating at high temperature increases D and decreases μ. Increasing J_{solv} *increases* concentration polarization. Thus high flux membranes have more concentration polarization.

For laminar flow conditions the average mass transfer coefficient can be estimated from (Blatt et al, 1970; Porter, 1979)

$$k = 0.816 \, [\gamma_w \; \frac{D^2}{L}]^{1/3} \qquad (13\text{-}14)$$

where γ_w is the fluid shear rate at the membrane surface and L is the length of the flow channel. The fluid shear rate in laminar flow in a round tube is

$$\gamma_w = \frac{4u_b}{R} \qquad (13\text{-}15)$$

and thus the average mass transfer coefficient in round tubes is

$$k = 1.295 \left[\frac{u_b D^2}{RL} \right]^{1/3} \tag{13-16}$$

For flow between parallel plates with a spacing of 2h

$$\gamma_w = \frac{3 u_b}{h} \tag{13-17}$$

and the mass transfer coefficient is

$$k = 1.177 \left[\frac{u_b D^2}{hL} \right]^{1/3} \tag{13-18}$$

These laminar flow correlations are used when the concentration polarization layer is thin, which holds when the axial distance is much less than the entrance length (see Example 13-2). These correlations be used when a gel does not form to estimate J_{solv} and M using Eqs. (13-3b) and (13-7), or when a gel forms (Section 13-2).

Unfortunately, these correlations do not cover many applications which are commercially significant. RO and gas permeation in hollow fibers usually have the feed on the outside. The appropriate mass transfer coefficient then depends on the flow on the shell side of the module. Spiral wound systems are not just parallel plates wound in a spiral; instead, the spacers are designed to promote mass transfer. For both these cases experimental data is required. Fortunately, the manufacturers have much of the required data.

Example 13-1. Concentration Polarization in Turbulent Flow

A 0.4 gmole/L NaCl solution in water is being purified by RO with a composite polymer membrane. The membrane has $J_{solv} = 750$ L/m^{2}day with pure water and $\Delta P = 70$ atm. With a 0.4 gmole/L solution, $R^\circ = 0.995$ when M = 1 and $\Delta P = 70$. An existing tubular module with 1 cm

id tubes is being used. The average fluid velocity u_b = 1300 cm/sec and ΔP = 50 atm. The cut θ = 0.10. Operation is at 18°C.
Find the average concentration polarization modulus $\overline{M}$, the average solvent flux $\overline{J}_{solv}$, c_{out}, and $\overline{c}_p$.
Data:
at 18°C: D_{NaCl} (0.4 gmoles/L) = 1.17×10^{-5} cm²/s
$\qquad\qquad D_{NaCl}$ (0.8 gmoles/L) = 1.19×10^{-5} cm²/s
(Sherwood et al. 1975, p. 37)

From Handbook Chemistry and Physics (p. D-175 of 48th Ed):
Freezing point depression: $T_f^* - T_f$ = 1.19°C for 0.346 gmole/L
$\qquad\qquad\qquad\qquad\qquad\quad$ = 1.49°C for 0.435 gmole/L
$\Delta H_{f,w}$ = 1436 cal/gmole, $T_{f,w}^*$ = 0°C = 273.16 K

For 2 wt% NaCl solutions: ρ = 1.01442 (10°C), ρ = 1.01112 (25°C)
$\qquad$ 4 wt% NaCl: $\qquad\quad$ ρ = 1.0292 (10°C), ρ = 1.0253 (25°C)
$\qquad\qquad\qquad\qquad$ (Perry and Green, 1984, p. 3-83)

Viscosities at 18°C: μ_w = 1.1 cp = 0.011 poise
$\qquad\qquad\qquad\quad$ μ (25 wt% NaCl) = 2.41 cp
(Perry and Green, 1984, p. 3-252)

Solution

A. *Define.* In problem statement.
B and C. *Explore and Plan.* In order to determine the mass transfer coefficient from the correlations we need the physical properties. Obviously, some interpolation will be needed. The osmotic pressure can be determined from the freezing point depression data with Eq. (12-19). If the flow is turbulent we will use Eq. (13-11) to find k. Since R is close to 1.0, we will first assume R = 1 and c_p = 0. Then from Eq. (12-30).

$c_{out} = c_{in}/(1-\theta) = 0.4/0.9 = 0.444$ gmoles/L.

The average $\overline{c}_b = (c_{in} + c_{out})/2 = 0.422$ gmoles/L. Assuming $\overline{J}_{solv}/k \ll 1$, we can determine $\overline{J}_{solv}$ from Eq. (13-7). Now $\overline{M}$ can be found from

Eq. (13-3b) and $\bar{R}$ and hence $\bar{c}_p$ from the solution to Eq. (12-29). We can then check that c_{out} is not changed significantly.

D. Do It. In a tube with turbulent flow, radial mixing is fairly uniform (high k), but axial mixing is incomplete. Thus c_b (and π) vary from c_{in} (π (c_{in})) to c_{out} (π (c_{out})). Average conditions are at $\bar{c}_b$. Thus, we will do all calculations at $\bar{c}_b = 0.422$ gmoles/L.

1. Calculate π. Eq. (12-19) is

$$\pi = \frac{(T_f^*-T_f) \, \Delta H_f \, T}{v_{solvent} \, T_f \, T_f^*} \left[\frac{R_{press}}{R_{energy}} \right]$$

$$= \frac{(1.45)\,(1436)\,(291.16)}{(18.05)\,(271.71)\,(273.16)} \left[\frac{82.057}{1.9872} \right] = 18.69 \text{ atm}$$

where $T_f^* - T_f$ is estimated at 0.422 gmole/L by linear interpolation

$$T_f^* - T_f = \frac{1.49-1.19}{0.435-0.346} (0.422-0.346) + 1.19 = 1.45°C$$

Then $T_f = T_f^* - 1.45 = 2.73.16 - 1.45 = 371.71$ K
$T = 18°C = 291.16$ K

The factor $\left[82.057 \dfrac{cc \, atm}{gmole \, K} \right] / \left[\dfrac{1.9872 \, cal}{gmole \, K} \right]$ converts two different values of the gas constant. The values R_{press} and R_{energy} depend on the units of ΔH_p, $v_{solvent}$, and the desired pressure units for π.

Since osmotic pressure data for NaCl is readily available (Perry and Green, 1984, p. 17-23), the purpose of this calculation is illustrative. Interpolating between concentrations and extrapolating to 18°C using the tabulated data, we find $\pi = 18.57$ which is a 0.6% difference. Assuming π is linear with concentration, a $= \pi/c = 18.69/0.422 = 44.29$ atm/gmole/L.

2. Calculate k.

A 0.422 gmole/L solution is about 2.4 wt% (same Table as Freezing point depression). Linearly interpolating, $\rho(10°C) \sim 1.0174$ and ρ $(25°C) \sim 1.0140$. Then doing *another* linear interpolation $\rho(18°C) \sim$ 1.0156 g/cc. [This is *not* the best way to estimate density, but since the differences are small it will not cause much error].

Viscosity of a mixture can be estimated from (Reid *et al*, 1977, p. 462)

$$\ln \mu_{mix} = x_1 \ln \mu_1 + x_2 \ln \mu_2$$

where the x_i are mole fractions. Here component 1 is pure water and component 2 is 25 wt% solution. From the same table which gives freezing point depression:

Water. 998.2 g/L = 55.4 gmoles/L
0.422 gmoles salt/L: has ~ 990.83g water/L = 55.0 gmole water/L
25 wt% has 5.086 mole NaCl/L and ~ 891.5 gwater/L = 49.48 gmoles/L of water.

Assuming volumes add, we need 0.422/5.086 = 0.083 fraction of 25 wt% and 0.917 fraction of pure water.

$$\ln \mu_{mix} = (0.917) \ln 0.011 + (0.083) \ln 0.024 = -4.445$$
$$\mu_{mix} = 0.0117 \text{ poise}$$

Then, $Sc = \mu/\rho D = 0.0117/(1.0156)(1.17 \times 10^{-5}) = 984.6$

$$Re = D \, u_b \, \rho/\mu = \frac{(1)(1300)(1.0156)}{0.0117} = 112,844$$
which is clearly tubulent.

From Eq. (13-11)

$$k = 0.023 \left[\frac{1.17 \times 10^{-5}}{1.0} \right] (112,844)^{0.83} (984.6)^{1/3} = 0.0418 \text{ cm/s}$$

3. Solvent flux.

From the pure water data:

$$\frac{K_{solv}}{t_m} = \frac{J_{solv}}{\Delta p} = \frac{750}{70} = 10.71 \text{ L/m}^2 \text{ day atm}$$

$$= 1.24 \times 10^{-5} \text{ cm/s atm}$$

Assuming $J_{solv}/k \ll 1.0$, we can use Eq. (13-7),

$$\overline{J}_{solv} = \frac{(1.24 \times 10^{-5})\,(50 - (44.29)\,(0.422))}{1 + \dfrac{(1.24 \times 10^{-5})\,(44.29)\,(0.422)}{0.0418}} = 0.000386 \text{ cm/s}$$

Which is 333.48 2/m²day

Check: $J_{solv}/k = 0.000386/0.0418 = 0.0092 \ll 1.0$.

4. Solute.

Now use actual $R° = 0.995$ in Eq. (13-3b)

$$\overline{M} = \frac{\exp (J_{solv}/k)}{R° + (1-R°)\exp (J_{solv}/k)} = \frac{\exp (0.0092)}{0.995 + 0.005 \exp (0.0092)} = 1.009$$

which is very modest due to the highly turbulent system.
The value of K_{solute}/t_m can be obtained from the salt rejection data with
$M = 1$. From Eq. (12-24C),

$$\alpha = \frac{K_{solv}}{K_{solute}} = \frac{R°}{(\Delta P - \Delta \pi)\,(1-R°)} = \frac{0.995}{(70 - (44.29)\,(0.4))\,(1 - 0.995)}$$

$$\alpha = 3.806$$

Then $\dfrac{K_{solute}}{t_m} = \dfrac{K_{solv}/t_m}{\alpha} = \dfrac{1.24 \times 10^{-5}}{3.806} = 3.25 \times 10^{-6} \text{ cm/s}.$

Now the solution to Eq. (12-29) gives $\bar{c}_p$. Constants for the quadratic formula are

$$\frac{a\,K_{solv}}{t_m} = (44.29)\,(1.24 \times 10^{-5}) = 0.000549$$

$$\frac{K_{solv}}{t_m}\,(\Delta p - M\,\pi\,(c_b)) + \frac{K_{solute}}{t_m}$$

$$= (1.24 \times 10^{-5})\,[50 - (1.009)\,(18.69)] + 3.26 \times 10^{-6} = 0.000389$$

$$\frac{K_{solute}}{t_m}\,M\,c_b = -(3.26 \times 10^{-6})\,(1.009)\,(0.422) = -1.387 \times 10^{-6}$$

From quadratic formula,

$$\bar{c}_p = \frac{-0.000389 \pm \sqrt{(0.000389)^2 - 4(0.000549)\,(-1.387 \times 10^{-6})}}{2\,(0.000549)}$$

Use the plus sign to obtain a positive value of $\bar{c}_p$.

$$\bar{c}_p = 0.0039 \text{ gmoles/L}$$

Note that, as expected, $\bar{c}_p$ is quite low. This is an average value of c_p since average values for c_b and π were used.

E. *Check.* The solute flux $J_{solute} = c_p\,\bar{J}_{solvent} = 1.515 \times 10^{-6}$ which is small compared to $J_{solvent}$. Thus ignoring this flux in Eq. (13-7) is reasonable. Recalculation of c_{out} using Eq. (12-30) gives

$$c_{out} = \frac{c_{in} - \theta\,c_p}{1 - \theta} = = \frac{0.4 - (0.1)\,(0.0092)}{0.9} = 0.443.$$

where $c_p = \bar{c}_p$ was used. This is essentially unchanged from our initial guess based on $c_p = 0$.

F. *Generalizations.* 1. In this example average values of $\overline{M}$, $\overline{J}_{solv}$, and $\overline{c}_p$ were found. Since concentration varies along the tube, an exact calculation requires an integration along the length of the tube. Usually, calculation of average conditions will be accurate enough for both turbulent and laminar flow.
2. Much of the effort in this example was involved with determining physical properties. This is often true.
3. Section 13.3.2 develops equations for completely mixed modules with concentration polarization.

13.2. GEL FORMATION AND FOULING

Gel formation was discussed in Chapter 12 following Eqs. (12-37) and (12-39). In this section more details of the calculation procedures will be given. The formation of a gel depends mainly upon the solute type and concentration although the membrane characteristics and hydrodynamics also affect gel formation (Blatt *et al,* 1970; Fane, 1986). Rigid chain, solvated macromolecules such as polysaccharides can gel at concentrations well below 1 wt %. Flexible chain, linear macromolecules often gel in the range of 2 to 5 wt%, while highly structured spheroidal macromolecules such as proteins and nucleic acids gel in the range from 10 to 30 wt %. Colloids can also form gels. Submicron pigments or minerals gel in the range from 5 to 25 vol % while polymer lattices require from 50 to 60 vol %.

For membranes with R=1, the solute mass balance was given in Eq. (12-31) and the solution was given in Eq. (12-39),

$$J_{solv} = k \ln \frac{c_g}{c_b} \qquad (12\text{-}39)$$

The mass transfer coefficient can be estimated from the mass transfer theories discussed in Section 13.1.2. Experimental UF data can be used to easily estimate k and c_g. If J_{solv} is determined at a series of bulk concentrations, c_b, a plot of J_{solv} versus $\ln c_b$ will have a slope of $-k$ and an intercept on the concentration axis of $\ln c_g$ (see Problem 12-D4). The resulting k and c_g values are then useful for correlating data. Changes in conditions such as velocity or temperature will change the mass transfer coefficient and can be correlated with Eqs. (13-11), (13-13), (13-16) or (13-18).

Should one employ a turbulent or a laminar flow system? For a given volumetric flow rate the mass transfer rate can be maximized by maximizing the shear rate. For tubular and plate-and-frame systems the flow can always be made turbulent by recycling liquid. This will give high k values but also results in high pressure drops along the length of the module. If the value of $k/\Delta p$ is found for both turbulent and laminar flow, one finds that this ratio is much larger for laminar flow. (See problem 13-C1). Thus, when energy costs are included in the calculation laminar flow is usually preferable. When UF is done in hollow fibers the feed flows inside the fibers, and flow almost has to be laminar. It is fortunate that laminar flow is desirable.

Although very appealing the gel formation theory often does not agree with experimental data (Fane, 1986; Le and Howell, 1984; Porter, 1979; Wijmans et al, 1984; Zydney and Colton, 1986). For instance, the model does not include any affect of the membrane, velocity, or feed concentration on c_g, but experimental results show such effects. Since c_g is usually much less than the solubility limit, it is difficult to determine fundamentally exactly what c_g is measuring. Solute-solute and solute-membrane interactions are important experimentally, but are not included in the model. Experiments with colloids show fluxes which can be one or two orders of magnitude greater than expected (Porter, 1979). (This is very helpful and helps explain why the earliest commercial applications of UF were for processing colloids, but it is a major problem for the theory.) Finally, the theory predicts a limiting flux which is independent of Δp while experiments often show a Δp dependence on the limiting flux.

Many attempts have been made to explain these problems. For example, in medium molecular weight applications the osmotic pressure can be important and should be included in the model (Fane, 1986; Wijmans et al, 1984). Unfortunately, models with osmotic pressure or with gels have very similar predictions and it is difficult to determine which is correct. For macromolecules > 100,000 daltons the osmotic pressure cannot have much influence.

Porter (1979) suggested that the colloid data can be explained by the *tubular pinch effect*. This is the tendency of small particles flowing in small tubes to migrate away from the tube walls. This effect will increase the mass transfer of particles away from the wall and will increase the solvent flux. Although this effect definitely exists, it does not appear to produce a large enough effect to completely explain the data (Le and Howell, 1984). Other explanations for high fluxes with particles are the particle diffusivity is much higher than Brownian diffusivity because it is caused by particle-particle interaction (Romero and Davis, 1988; Zydney and Colton, 1986). Other models which include variable diffusivity or cake aging or adsorption or leaky pores all seem to be able to explain only part of the phenomena. The mass balance, Eq. (12-31), does not include axial convection of solute and the boundary condition $c = C_b$ at $y = \delta$ is hypothetical. Shen and Probstein (1977) and Trettin and Doshi (1980) improved the model by including convection in the x direction (e.g. see Eq. (13-48)) and writing the boundary condition as $c = c_b$ at $y = \infty$. They also allowed for a concentration dependent diffusviity. Their results for the limiting flux agreed better with experimental data for protein UF than Eq. (12-39). At the current time gelling in UF must be considered only partially explained. Future research will eventually unravel the complexities involved. The simple gel formation model still serves as a simple physical picture and as an excellent method for correlating data.

Fouling can occur in both RO and UF although it is often worse in UF since dirtier streams are often processed. Fouling is a plugging or coating on (external) or in (internal) the membrane which is partially irreversible. That is, in normal operation the fouled membrane will stay fouled until a separate cleaning step is employed. After clean-up part or all of the original flux will be recovered. Fouling is complex because it can be caused by many different phenomena such as precipitation, adsorption, electrostatic attraction, biological growth, chemical reaction or polymerization.

In RO fouling can be classified as inorganic, particulate, or biological (Potts *et al*, 1981). Inorganic fouling occurs when compounds such as $CaCO_3$, $CaSO_4$, $MgCO_3$, and silica or iron precipitate out onto the membrane. Since the purpose of RO is to remove water and since the concentration of salts is highest at the membrane wall, it should not be surprising that precipitation can be a problem. The higher the water recovery the more likely precipitation is to be a problem. Fortunately, precipitation can often be controlled by adding sulfuric acid to adjust the pH in the range 4 to 6, and by adding compounds which bind calcium (e.g. Calgon). Fouling from particulates can be caused by particulates in the feed. This is relatively easy to control by prefiltering the feed. A more serious problem is the presence of both inorganic and organic colloids. Methods for solving these problems will be very specific for each case since the chemistry will differ from case to case. Some membranes such as cellulose acetate are susceptible to biological growth. This can be controlled by operating in the pH range from 4 to 6, removing dissolved oxygen, or chlorinating.

All of the above types of fouling can also occur in UF. In addition, since macromolecules are often ultrafiltered, polymer precipitates or gels may form which can be attached to the membrane by adsorption or electrostatic forces. The polymer may also react to form a cross-linked gel layer. Generally speaking, the higher the molecular weight of the solute the worse fouling will be. Modules should be designed to have no stagnant regions since fouling is invariably worse in these locations. Separate cleaning steps are often employed. These include pulsing clean water, back-flowing clean water through the membrane, mechanical cleaning with sponge balls or other methods, and chemical cleaning such as a caustic wash. Fouling may also be reduced by changing the membrane properties. For instance, electrostatic attraction can usually be reduced by giving the membrane a negative charge since fouling colloids are often negatively charged.

Flux decline in both RO and UF often follows an exponential decline and then levels off to a low asymptotic value.

$$J_{solv}(t) = (J_{init} - J_{asy}) \, t^m + J_{asy} \qquad (13\text{-}19)$$

where $J_{solv}(t)$, J_{init}, and J_{asy} are the fluxes at time t, initially and asymptotically. The time t is often measured in days, and $J_{solv}(\text{day } 1) = J_{init}$. The empirical constant m is negative. An m = −0.1 corresponds to about a 45% decline in flux in one year while an m = −0.03 corresponds to about a 16% flux decline in one year. If the membrane is chemically or mechanically cleaned, much of the original flux can be restored. The decline will then start again from this restored flux. Every time the membrane is cleaned some flux is permanently lost. Thus the membranes will have a finite life. This lifetime can vary from a few months to several years depending on the service conditions. Membrane replacement should be included as an operating cost. Membrane systems are usually designed with an average flux. For a parallel cascade membranes can be replace in a staggered pattern so that some membranes are always fresh and others are near the end of their useful life.

13.3. COMPLETELY MIXED SYSTEMS WITH CONCENTRATION POLARIZATION

In Chapter 12 the mass balances for completely mixed systems were considered. In this section we will first develop the external mass balances for reverse osmosis and ultrafiltration with concentration polarization. The possible occurrence of a gel will be included in Section 13.3.2.

13.3.1. Completely Mixed RO and UF With Concentration Polarization and No Gel Formation

In reverse osmosis and ultrafiltration concentration polarization must be included in the analysis. This will be done for a completely mixed flow case using the approximation developed by Rao and Sirkar (1978) in Eq. (13-5). In RO and UF rejection is quite high and it makes more sense to write equations in terms of rejections instead of selectivity as used in gas permeation. The development in this section will include osmotic pressure and is valid for RO and for UF when a gel does *not* form.

The balances will be done for the system shown schematically in Figure 13-1. The overall external mass balance is

$$F_{in} = F_{out} + F_P \tag{13-20}$$

while the external solute balance is

$$F_{in} c_{in} = F_{out} c_{out} + F_P c_P \tag{13-21}$$

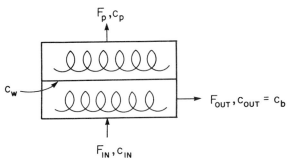

Figure 13-1.   Schematic of completely mixed RO or UF with concentration polarization.

The volumetric permeate flowrate can be determined from the flux as $F_P = JA$. For a perfectly mixed container $c_{out} = c_b$. Equations (13-20) and (13-21) can be solved to find c_{out}.

$$c_b = c_{out} = \frac{F_{in}c_{in} - F_P c_P}{F_{in} - F_P} = \frac{c_{in} - \theta c_p}{1-\theta} \tag{13-22}$$

which is Eq. (12-30). Note that these equations are essentially the same as Eqs. (12-5) to (12-8) since the external balances are unaffected by what happens inside the system. The permeate concentration is related to the wall concentration

$$c_P = c_w(1-R^\circ) \tag{13-23}$$

where R° is the intrinsic rejection which will be assumed to be constant. Combining Eqs. (13-23) and (13-22), we obtain

$$c_b = c_{out} = \frac{c_{in} - \theta\, c_w(1-R^\circ)}{1 - \theta} \tag{13-24}$$

The wall concentration can be removed from Eqs. (13-23) and (13-24) by substituting in Eq. (13-3b). The results are

$$c_P = \frac{c_b(1-R^\circ)\exp(J_{solv}/k)}{R^\circ + (1-R^\circ)\exp(J_{solv}/k)} \tag{13-25}$$

and, after some algebra,

$$c_b = \frac{c_{in}}{(1-\theta) + \dfrac{\theta(1-R^\circ)\exp(J_{solv}/k)}{R^\circ + (1-R^\circ)\exp(J_{solv}/k)}} \qquad (13\text{-}26)$$

Note that if $R^\circ = 1.0$, $c_P = 0$ and $c_{out} = c_{in}/(1-\theta)$. When $R^\circ = 1$, the flow patterns and solvent flux are unimportant for determining concentrations.

For $R^\circ < 1$ Eqs. (13-25) and (13-26) are very useful if J_{solv} is known. Unfortunately, J_{solv} is usually not known. The solvent flux must now be determined from the flux Eq. (12-27). We will assume that the osmotic pressure depends linearly on concentration so that Eq. (12-18b) is valid. Combining Eqs. (12-27), (12-18b) and (13-23), we have

$$J_{solv} = \frac{K_{solv}}{t_m}(\Delta p - aR^\circ c_w) \qquad (13\text{-}27)$$

The wall concentration can be removed using Eq. (13-3b), and this result can be solved simultaneously with Eq. (13-26). The equations are nonlinear and a closed form solution cannot be obtained. If the exponential term is approximated as in Eq. (13-5), an algebraic solution can be obtained. The wall concentration becomes

$$c_w = \frac{c_b(1+J_{solv}/k)}{R^\circ + (1-R^\circ)(1 + J_{solv}/k)} \qquad (13\text{-}28)$$

which gives

$$J_{solv} = \frac{K_{solv}}{t_m}\left[\Delta p - \frac{aR^\circ c_b(1 + J_{solv})/k}{R^\circ + (1-R^\circ)(1+J_{solv}/k)}\right] \qquad (13\text{-}29)$$

After some algebra the bulk concentration is

$$c_b = \frac{c_{in}}{1-\theta + \dfrac{\theta(1 + J_{solv}/k)(1-R^\circ)}{R^\circ + (1-R^\circ)(1 + J_{solv}/k)}} \qquad (13\text{-}30)$$

These two equations can now be solved simultaneously. After some manipulations the following quadratic equation results.

$$a' J_{solv}^2 + b' J_{solv} + c' = 0 \qquad (13\text{-}31)$$

where

$$a' = (1 - R^\circ)/k \qquad (13\text{-}32a)$$

$$b' = 1 - \theta R^\circ - \frac{K_{solv}}{t_m} \frac{(1 - R^\circ)}{k} \Delta p + \frac{K_{solv}}{t_m} \frac{c_{in} \, a}{k} R^\circ \qquad (13\text{-}32b)$$

$$c' = \frac{K_{solv}}{t_m} c_{in} \, aR^\circ - (1 - \theta R^\circ) \frac{K_{solv}}{t_m} \Delta p \qquad (13\text{-}32c)$$

After determining k from the appropriate mass transfer correlation, J_{solv} can be found from the quadratic formula.

$$J_{solv} = \frac{-b' \pm \sqrt{b'^2 - 4a'c'}}{2a'} \qquad (13\text{-}33)$$

Once J_{solv} is known, c_p and c_b can be calculated from Eqs. (13-25) and (13-26). If gel formation is possible, calculate c_w from Eq. (13-28). If $c_w < c_g$ a gel won't form and this solution is correct. If $c_w > c_g$, a gel forms and this solution is not correct (see Section 13.3.2). Also, this solution is based on $J_{solv}/k << 1$ and this restriction should be checked. If the assumption is invalid, we need to solve Eqs. (13-3b), (13-26) and (13-27) simultaneously. Equation (13-33) can be used for a first guess.

If $R^\circ = 1$ the solvent flux simplifies to

$$J_{solv} = \frac{(1-\theta)\dfrac{K_{solv}}{t_m}\Delta p - c_{in} \, a \dfrac{K_{solv}}{t_m}}{1 - \theta + \dfrac{c_{in} \, a \, K_{solv}}{k \, t_m}} \quad \text{for } R=1 \qquad (13\text{-}34)$$

It is interesting to compare this result to the solvent flux without concentration polarization and with $R°=1$. With no concentration polarization $c_w = c_b$ while $c_p = 0$. Solving Eqs. (12-18b), (13-6) and (13-24) simultaneously for these conditions we obtain,

$$J_{\text{solv w/o conc pol.}} = \frac{K_{\text{solv}}}{t_m}(\Delta p - \frac{ac_{in}}{1-\theta}) \quad \text{for } R°=1 \qquad (13\text{-}35)$$

Then the ratio of solvent fluxes with $R°=1$ is

$$\frac{J_{\text{solv w. conc pol.}}}{J_{\text{solv w/o conc. pol.}}} = \frac{1}{1 + \dfrac{c_{in} \, a \, K_{\text{solv}}}{k(1-\theta)t_m}} \quad \text{for } R° = 1 \qquad (13\text{-}36)$$

The flux without concentration polarization is always higher, and thus is an upper limit to the actual flux. As the mass transfer coefficient becomes very large the two solvent fluxes approach each other.

The flow pattern used in RO and UF is usually not completely mixed. However, stirred tanks and systems with a very large recycle (see Problem 13-D6) are often close to perfectly mixed. At higher concentrations π is usually not linearly dependent upon concentration. In addition, the pressure drop on the high pressure side decreases p_H and thus decreases Δp (Hwang and Kammermeyer, 1975). Complete design calculations are quite complex and require computer solutions. These design calculations are discussed by Harris et al (1976), and Sourirajan (1970,1977).

13.3.2. Completely Mixed UF with Gel Formation

If a gel forms, the analysis in Section 13.3.1 needs to be modified. Equations (13-23) and (13-24) become

$$c_p = c_g \, (1 - R°) \qquad (13\text{-}37)$$

$$c_b = c_{out} = \frac{c_{in} - \theta \, c_g \, (1 - R°)}{1 - \theta} \qquad (13\text{-}38)$$

where we assume that the solute is mobile in the gel and does not change R°. Since c_g is known, c_p and c_b can be calculated immediately.

When a gel is formed Eq. (13-3b) becomes

$$J_{solv} = k \ln \left[\frac{R^\circ\, c_g/c_b}{1 - (1 - R^\circ)\, c_g/c_b} \right] \qquad (13\text{-}39)$$

which reduces to Eq. (12-39) when $R^\circ = 1.0$. We can determine k from the appropriate correlation and then calculate J_{solv}. For laminar flow Eqs. (13-16) and (13-18) are convenient for first estimates of the average value of k.

If c_g is high, c_{in} is low, or θ is low, we may not know in advance if a gel will form. In this case, we can calculate c_w using the method in Section 13.3.1. A gel will form if $c_w > c_g$, and Eqs. (13-37) to (13-39) should be used. This procedure will be illustrated in Example 13-2.

Example 13-2. Concentration Polarization in Completely Mixed UF

A 10 cm diameter stirred tank with a mixer operating at 4000 rpm is being used to ultrafilter albumin. With pure water and $\Delta p = 5.0$ atm, the flux is 2500 L/m^2 day. $R^\circ = 0.992$. Operation of the stirred cell will be at 18°C with $\Delta p = 4.2$ atm.
Data: Albumin (Porter, 1979), $D = 6 \times 10^{-7}$ cm^2/s, $c_g = 0.45$ (wt. frac),
MW$_{albumin}$ = 70,000.
Water (Perry and Green, 1984): $\mu_w = 0.011$ poise, $\rho_w = 0.9986$ g/cm^3.
Assume $\nu = \mu/\rho$ is approximately constant.

Find c_p, c_b and J_{solv} for feed concentrations of 0.04 and 0.20 wt. frac. albumin if $\theta = 0.5$.

Solution

We will first assume a gel does not form and use Eqs. (13-32) and (13-33) to find J_{solv}. Then we will find c_b from Eq. (13-26) and c_w from

Eq. (13-28). If $c_w < c_g$, this solution is correct. If $c_w > c_g$ we need to use Eqs. (13-37) to (13-39). The mass transfer coefficient k for a stirred tank can be found from Eq. (13-13). To use this equation,

$$v = \mu/\rho_w = 0.011/0.9986 \text{ g/cm}^3 = 0.011 \text{ cm}^2/\text{s}$$

which we will (for now) assume to be constant.

$$\omega = 4000 \text{ rpm } \mid \frac{2\,\pi\,\text{radians}}{\text{revolution}} \mid \frac{1 \text{ min}}{60\text{s}} \mid = 418.8 \text{ radians/s}$$

Then from Eq. (13-13),

$$k = (0.0443) \left[\frac{6 \times 10^{-7}}{10} \right] \left[\frac{0.011}{6 \times 10^{-7}} \right]^{0.33} \left[\frac{(418.8)\,(10)^2}{0.011} \right]^{0.75}$$

$$= 0.00594 \text{ cm/s}$$

From the pure water flux we can find k_{solv}/t_m

$$\frac{k_{solv}}{t_m} = \frac{J_{solv}}{\Delta p} = \frac{2500}{5.0} = 500 \text{ L/m}^2\text{day atm} = 0.000578 \text{ cm/s atm}$$

To estimate a in Eq. (12-18b) we will use Eq. (12-18a). Since the solution will be approximately doubled in concentration, use $c = 8$ wt% albumin. Then for 1 liter have approximately: 960 g water = 53.3 gmoles water and 83.5 g albumin = 0.00119 gmoles albumin. Thus

$$\pi = \left[\frac{0.00119 \text{ gmole}}{\text{liter}} \right] \left[\frac{1 \text{ liter}}{1000 \text{ cc}} \right] \left[\frac{82.057 \text{ cc atm}}{\text{gmole k}} \right] (291.16 \text{ K})$$

$$= 0.0285 \text{ atm}$$

from Eq. (12-18a). We can use c_{in} as 0.08 wt. frac in Eq. (12-18b).

Then

$$a = \frac{\pi}{c} = \frac{0.0285 \text{ atm}}{0.08 \text{ wt frac}} = 0.356 \text{ atm/wt frac.}$$

Since $\pi/\Delta p = (0.0285/4.2) \times 100 = 0.68\%$, we can ignore osmotic pressure for the 4 wt% feed and set $a = 0$. Remember that the van't Hoff Eq. (12-18a) is highly unreliable; however, the basic conclusion that osmotic pressure can be ignored is probably valid.

Now, we can determine J_{solv} from Eq. (13-33), assuming $J_{solv}/k \ll 1$. From Eq. (13-32),

$$a' = (1-R^\circ)/k = 0.008/0.00594 = 1.347$$

$$b' = 1 - (0.5)(0.992) - (0.0005789)\left[\frac{0.008}{0.00594}\text{right})(4.2) + 0 = 0.5007\right.$$

$$c' = 0 - [1 - (0.5)(0.992)](0.000578)(4.2) = -0.001224$$

From Eq. (13-33)

$$J_{solv} = \frac{-0.5007 \pm \sqrt{(0.5007)^2 - (4)(1.347)(-0.001224)}}{(2)(1.347)}$$

$$= 0.00243 \text{ cm/s}$$

where the positive sign is used to make J_{solv} positive. To check the assumption calculate

$$J_{solv}/k = 0.00243/0.00594 = 0.409$$

There will be some error in the calculation (see Notes) and a second trial would be required for accurate results.

From Eq. (13-16) we find c_b

$$c_b = \frac{c_{in}}{0.5 + \dfrac{0.5\,(0.008)\exp(0.409)}{0.992 + (0.008)\exp(0.409)}} = 1.9763\,c_{in}$$

while from Eq. (13-38)

$$c_w = \frac{(1.9763)\, c_{in}\, (1.409)}{0.992 + (0.008)\, (1.409)} = 2.775\, c_{in}$$

and from Eq. (13-23)

$$c_p = c_w\, (1 - R^\circ) = (2.775\, c_{in})\, (0.008) = 0.0222\, c_{in}$$

Note that since osmotic pressure is negligible, c_{in} does not affect the calculation of J_{solv} and the other concentrations can be determined as functions of inlet concentration.

4 wt% feed: $c_b = 0.0791$, $c_w = 0.111 < c_g$, $c_p = 0.00089$

20 wt% feed: $c_w = 0.555 > c_g$

Thus, for the 20 wt% solution we need to use the solution when a gel forms. With a gel formed we use Eqs. (13-37) to (13-39).

$$c_p = (0.45)\, (0.008) = 0.0036$$

$$c_b = \frac{0.2 - (0.5)\, (0.45)\, (0.008)}{(0.5)} = 0.3964$$

$$J_{solv} = (0.00594)\, \ln\left[\frac{(0.992)\, (0.45)\, /\, (0.3964)}{1 - (0.008)\, (0.45)\, /\, (0.3964)}\right] = 0.00076 \text{ cm/s}$$

Notes:

A. There are several approximations involved in this solution.

   1. The worst approximation is $v = v_{water}$ in Eq. (13-13). The albumin solutions will be significantly more viscuous, v will

be higher, and k will be lower than predicted. We need viscosity data.

2. J_{solv}/k is really too large to use the approximation that $\exp(J_{solv}/k) = 1 + J_{solv}/k$, and $R \neq 1.0$. Using calculated $J_{solv}/k = 0.409$, $\exp(J_{solv}/k) = 1.505$ which is 6.8% greater than $1 + J_{solv}/k = 1.409$. Another trial should be done. For UF this approximation will often be suspect.

3. Ignoring osmotic pressure in reasonable for the 4 wt% feed. For the 20 wt% feed osmotic pressure is unimportant *because* a gel forms.

4. When the gel formed, we assumed R was unchanged. We need data to check this assumption. If the gel is rigid, R may become 1.0.

B.   The formation of the gel reduces J_{solv} by a factor of 3.

C.   Even with vigorous stirring $M = c_w/c_b = 2.775/1.9763 = 1.4$ which is significant.

13.4. COUNTERCURRENT GAS PERMEATION WITH NO CONCENTRATION POLARIZATION

The effect of flow patterns in gas permeators is discussed in great detail by Hwang and Kammermeyer (1975). We will follow their analysis for the countercurrent gas permeator shown schematically in Figure 13-2. Consider the

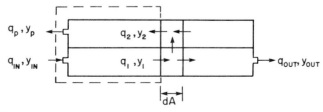

Figure 13-2.   Schematic of countercurrent gas permeator.

separation of a binary gas stream. The differential mass balances for components A and B are

$$-d(q_1 y_1) = -d(q_2 y_2) = \frac{\hat{\rho}_A P_A}{t_m}(y_1 p_H - p_L y_2)dA \qquad (13\text{-}40a)$$

$$-d\left[q_1(1-y_1)\right] = -d\left[q_2(1-y_2)\right] = \frac{\hat{\rho}_B P_B}{t_m}\left[(1-y_1)p_H - p_L(1-y_2)\right] \qquad (13\text{-}40b)$$

In these equations q_1 and q_2 are the flow rates in moles/hour on the feed and permeate sides of the membrane, and y_1 and y_2 are the mole fractions on the feed and permeate sides of the membrane, respectively. A is the membrane area. P_A and P_B are the permeabilities of the membrane. The second equation in each set comes from the flux Eq. (12-3). The molar density, $\hat{\rho}$, is required to convert the volumetric flux J_A to a molar flux. These two mass balances can be rearranged. Adding Eqs. (13-40a) and (13-40b) we obtain

$$\frac{dq_1}{dA} = \left\{y_1\, p_H - p_L y_2 + \frac{P_B \hat{\rho}_B}{P_A \hat{\rho}_A}\left[(1 - y_1)p_H - p_L(1-y_2)\right]\right\}\frac{P_A \hat{\rho}_A}{t_m} \qquad (13\text{-}41)$$

Rearranging Eq. (13-40b) we have a second equation.

$$q_1\frac{dy_1}{dA} = -\left[y_1 p_H - p_L\, y_2 + p_H y_1\frac{dq_1}{dA}\right]\frac{P_A \hat{\rho}_A}{t_m} \qquad (13\text{-}42)$$

A third equation is also required. This can be obtained from the overall and component mass balances for the mass balance envelope shown in Figure 13-2.

$$q_{in} - q_P + q_2 - q_1 = 0 \qquad (13\text{-}43a)$$

$$q_{in} y_{in} - q_P y_P + q_2 y_2 - q_1 y_1 = 0 \qquad (13\text{-}43b)$$

Removing the unknown flowrate q_2 and solving for y_2, we obtain

$$y_2 = \frac{q_P y_P + q_1 y_1 - q_{in} y_{in}}{q_P + q_1 - q_{in}} \tag{13-43c}$$

Equations (13-41), (13-42), and (13-43c) are solved simultaneously. The boundary conditions are:

$$y_1 = y_{out}, \quad y_2 = y_{2,0}, \quad q_1 = q_{out} \quad \text{at } A = A_{total} \tag{13-44a}$$

$$y_1 = y_{in}, \quad y_2 = y_P, \quad q_1 = q_{in} \quad \text{at } A = 0 \tag{13-44b}$$

In Eq. (13-44a) $y_{2,0}$ is the permeate mole fraction corresponding to y_{out}. This permeate mole fraction can be obtained by taking the ratio of flux Eq. (12-3) written for components A and B at the outlet. This result is

$$\frac{y_{2,0}}{1 - y_{2,0}} = \alpha_{AB} \frac{\hat{\rho}_A}{\hat{\rho}_B} \frac{y_{out} - \dfrac{p_L}{p_H} y_{2,0}}{1 - y_{out} - \dfrac{p_L}{p_H}(1 - y_{2,0})} \tag{13-44c}$$

Note that Eq. (13-44c) is essentially the same as Eq. (12-10) for a perfectly mixed system.

Obviously, a numerical solution of Eqs. (13-41), (13-42), and (13-43c) is required. This was done by Blaisdell and Kammermeyer (1973) for oxygen and nitrogen permeation through a silicone rubber membrane. Results are shown in Figure 13-3. The results in Figure 13-3 are the same for all flow configurations at $\theta = 0$. If we desire a concentrated oxygen product, operation should be at low cut (very little permeate product). If a concentrated nitrogen product is desired, a high θ with countercurrent flow should be used. The selectivity, $\alpha = 2.05$, used in these calculations is low. The best currently available oxygen membrane has a selectivity of about 7.5. This membrane is used for N_2 production. The countercurrent flow arrangement is best since the average driving force is highest while completely mixed is worst since the average driving force is lowest (see Problem 13-C4). Balances for flow arrangements

761

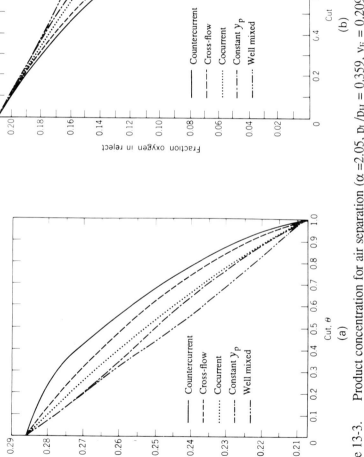

Figure 13-3. Product concentration for air separation ($\alpha = 2.05$, $p_L/p_H = 0.359$, $y_F = 0.209$). a. Permeate concentrations. b. Low pressure product concentrations. (Blaisdell and Kammermeyer, 1973). Reprinted with permission from *Chem. Eng. Sci.*, 28, 1249 (1973). Copyright 1973, Pergamon Press.

other than completely mixed and countercurrent are developed by Hwang and Kammermeyer (1975).

13.5. EXACT SOLUTION FOR CONCENTRATION POLARIZATION IN LAMINAR FLOW

In laminar flow both concentration and velocity boundary layers will form. Since diffifusivities are low, the concentration boundary layer will be thinner at the beginning of the tube. Both boundary layers become thicker as one progresses down the tube. If the tube is long enough (or the channel is thin enough) both boundary layers will eventualy fill the tube. Thus, one should expect two solutions for laminar flow: an entrance region solution and a fully developed far-downstream solution. The solutions have been generated for the case where the velocity profile is fully developed immediately, but the concentration profile is not. The solute was assumed to be completely rejected. Solutions for both parallel plates and round tubes are available (Sherwood et al, 1965.

The geometry for RO between two $parallel$ $sheets$ is shown in Figure 13-4a. For laminar flow the velocity must first be calculated from the following Navier-Stokes equations,

$$u \frac{\partial v}{\partial x} + v \frac{\partial v}{\partial y} = -\frac{1}{\rho} \frac{\partial p}{\partial y} + v \left[\frac{\partial^2 v}{\partial y^2} + \frac{\partial^2 v}{\partial x^2} \right] \qquad (13\text{-}45a)$$

$$u \frac{\partial u}{\partial x} + v \frac{\partial u}{\partial y} = -\frac{1}{\rho} \frac{\partial p}{\partial x} + v \left[\frac{\partial^2 u}{\partial y^2} + \frac{\partial^2 u}{\partial x^2} \right] \qquad (13\text{-}45b)$$

and the continuity equation

$$\frac{\partial u}{\partial x} + \frac{\partial v}{\partial y} = 0 \qquad (13\text{-}45c)$$

The boundary conditions are: a) no slip at the wall,

$$u = 0 \quad \text{at} \quad y = \pm h \qquad (13\text{-}46a)$$

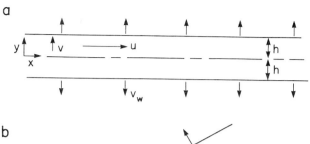

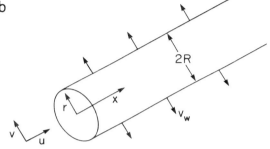

Figure 13-4.   Geometries for concentration polarization analysis. a. Parallel plates, b. Round tubes.

b) v equals solvent withdrawal rate at wall,

$$v = v_w \quad \text{at} \quad y = \pm h \qquad (13\text{-}46b)$$

and c) symmetry at the centerline.

$$v = \frac{\partial u}{\partial y} = 0 \quad \text{at} \quad y = 0 \qquad (13\text{-}46c)$$

The flow solution obtained by Berman (1953) is

$$\frac{u}{u_{in}} = \frac{3}{2}\left[1 - \frac{v_w\, x}{u_{in}\, h}\right](1 - y'^2)\left[1 - \frac{v_w\, h}{420\, v}\left[2 - 7\, y'^2 - 7\, y'^4\right]\right] \qquad (13\text{-}47a)$$

and

$$\frac{v}{v_w} = \frac{y'}{2}\,(3 - y'^2) - \frac{v_w y}{280\, v}\,(2 - 3y'^2 - y'^6) \qquad (13\text{-}47b)$$

where u_{in} is the average fluid velocity at the channel inlet, and $y' = y/h$. This solution reduces to the usual solution for laminar flow between flat plates when $v_w = 0$.

These solutions for velocity can be inserted in the steady state mass balance for solute. When rejection is perfect, $R = 1$, this balance is,

$$\frac{\partial}{\partial x}\left[uc - D\,\frac{\partial c}{\partial x}\right] + \frac{\partial}{\partial y}\left[vc - D\,\frac{\partial c}{\partial y}\right] = 0 \qquad (13\text{-}48)$$

The solute boundary conditions are: a) concentration equals c_{in} at inlet to RO system,

$$c = c_{in} \quad \text{at} \quad x = 0 \qquad (13\text{-}49a)$$

b) at the wall the flux of solute to the wall equals the backward difussion of salt

$$c\,v_w = D\,\frac{\partial c}{\partial y} \quad \text{at} \quad y = \pm\,h \qquad (13\text{-}49b)$$

and c) symmetry at the centerline.

$$\frac{\partial c}{\partial y} = 0 \quad \text{at} \quad y = 0 \qquad (13\text{-}49c)$$

The solution to Eqs. (13-47) to (13-49) is difficult; however, the equations can be simplified (Sherwood et al., 1965). For typical RO solvent fluxes, the terms divided by 420 v and 280 v in Eqs. (13-47) can be ignored. Also, since the axial concentration gradient will be small, the axial dispersion term, $-D\,\partial c/\partial x$, can be neglected in Eq. (13-48). The solution for the entire range of variables was obtained numerically by Sherwood et al. (1965), and is shown in Figure 13-5.

Sherwood and his coworkers also obtained asymptotic solutions for certain regions. The solutions are written in terms of the dimensionless variable

$$\xi = v_w^3\ hx/3\ u_{in}\ D^2 \qquad (13\text{-}50)$$

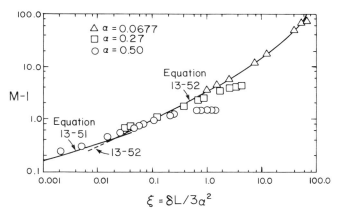

Figure 13-5.   Solutions for laminar flow between parallel plates (Sherwood *et al*, 1965). Reprinted with permission from *Ind. Eng. Chem. Fundam.*, 4, 113 (1965). Copyright 1965, Amer. Chem. Soc.

Very close to the inlet ($\xi << 1$),

$$M = 1 + 1.536(\xi)^{1/3} \tag{13-51}$$

For larger values of ξ the approximate solution for the entrance region is

$$M = 6 + \xi - 5\exp(-\sqrt{\xi/3}) \tag{13-52}$$

Very far downstream (large ξ) the boundary layer will completely fill the tube. Once this occurs M will be constant.

$$M = 1 + \frac{v_w^2 h^2}{3D^2} = \text{constant} \tag{13-53}$$

The locations of validity of these equations are shown in Figure 13-5.

To determine if the far downstream solution Eq. (13-53) or the entrance region solution Eq. (13-52) should be used, calculate M with both equations. The smaller M should be used. Very close to the channel entrance, $\xi << 1$, use the larger value of M calculated from Eqs. (13-51) and (13-52).

A similar but more complicated analysis can be done for laminar flow in *round tubes*. The geometry is shown in Figure 13-4b. The Navier-Stokes equations were solved by Yuan and Finkelstein (1956). Sherwood *et al.* (1965) used this velocity solution in the solute mass balance. The approximate solution for the entrance region for $v_w^3 \times R/(4\,u_{in}\,D^2) \leq 0.02$ is

$$M = \frac{c_w}{c_b} = 1.536\,(\frac{v_w^3 \times R}{4\,u_{in}\,D^2})^{1/3} + 1 \tag{13-54}$$

and for $v_w^3 \times R/(4\,u_{in}\,D^2) > 0.02$

$$M = \frac{v_w^3 \times R}{4\,u_{in}\,D^2} + 6 - 5\exp\left[-(\frac{v_w^3 \times R}{12\,u_{in}\,D^2})^{1/2}\right] \tag{13-55}$$

Note that the concentration polarization depends upon the axial distance x.

Far downstream the boundary layer will completely fill the tube. Once this occurs M will be constant. This far-downstream solution was obtained numerically and was presented in graphical form. This result is shown in Figure 13-6 (Sherwood, *et al*, 1965). To determine if the entrance region solutions, Eqs. (13-54) or (13-55), or the far-downstream solution (Figure 13-6) should be used, calculate M by both methods. The smaller M should be used.

If the average polarization modulus $\overline{M}$ is desired, this can be estimated by doing the calculation at x = L/2. If either the solvent velocity through the tube wall v_w or the solvent flux J_{solv} are given, the calculation of M(x) or $\overline{M}$ is straightforward for both geometries. However, if M, J_{solv} and v_w are unknown the problem is trial-and-error. This involves guessing M and then calculating J_{solv} from Eq. (12-27) or Eq. (13-6) if R=1. Then calculate M from the appropriate solution. If this M does not agree with the M used to calculate J_{solv}, the procedure is repeated.

Although usually quite accurate, these results for both turbulent and laminar flow are approximate for a variety of reasons. The no-slip boundary condition at the wall is not strictly true for a porous solid since there can be lateral fluid movement in the pores (Fane, 1986). Fluid properties ρ, μ and ν and

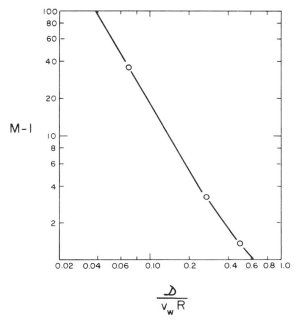

Figure 13-6. "Far-downstream" solution for round tubes. (Sherwood *et al*, 1965). Reprinted with permission from *Ind. Eng. Chem. Fundam.*, *4*, 113 (1965). Copyright 1965, Amer. Chem. Soc.

solute diffusivity vary if the polarization modulus M is large. Mass transfer coefficients are correlated for systems with impermeable walls, but will be increased by the flux through the walls. Since concentration polarization increases as the concentration boundary layer develops, the solvent flux and hence v_w usually decreases with increasing x. Including this variation is significantly more complex than the constant v_w case presented here (see Matthiasson and Sivik, 1980, for references).

Example 13-3. Concentration Polarization in Laminar Flow

Estimate the *average* concentration polarization modulus M for a dilute solution which is being concentrated in an RO system. The properties are $D = 5.2 \times 10^{-7}$ cm^2/sec, $\rho = 1.01$ g/cc, $\mu = 0.0095$ cm^2/sec, $c_L = 0.99$ gH$_2$O/ml (solvent concentration). The operation is inside round hollow fibers which are 0.01 cm in radius. Bulk velocity at the inlet is 3.2 cm/sec. Flux rate is 1.8×10^{-4} g/sec cm^2. The total length of each hollow fiber is 50 cm. Assume $R^o = 1.0$ and $\rho_{permeate} = 1.0$.

If the hollow fibers are increased to 500 cm long, estimate the average concentration polarization.

Solution

First, we need to check the Reynold's number.

$$R_e = \frac{D u_b}{\nu} = \frac{2R\, u_b}{\nu} = \frac{2(0.1)(3.2)}{(0.0095)} = 6.74$$

Flow is laminar. For average value of M use $x = L/2 = 25$ cm. Wall velocity,

$$v_w = \frac{\text{flux}}{\rho_w} = \frac{1.8 \times 10^{-4}}{1.00} = 1.80 \times 10^{-4} \text{ cm/s}$$

and parameter for abscissa of Figure 13-3 is

$$\frac{D}{v_w\, R} = \frac{5.2 \times 10^{-7}}{(1.8 \times 10^{-4})\,(0.01)} = 0.2888$$

Far downstream result from Figure 13-6, M-1 ~ 3.0 or M = 4. Also, need entrance region solution. Parameter value

$$\left[\frac{v_w^3\, x\, R}{4\, u_{in}\, D^2} \right] = \frac{(1.8 \times 10^{-4})^3\,(25)\,(0.01)}{(4)\,(3.2)\,(5.2 \times 10^{-7})^2} = 0.421$$

From Eq. (13-55),

$$M = 0.421 + 6 - 5 \exp\left[-\left[\frac{0.421}{3} \right]^{\frac{1}{2}} \right] = 2.98$$

Since entrance region result is smaller, use that value of M.

For L = 500, x = L/2 = 250 cm. Since abscissa in Figure 13-6 is unchanged, $M_{far\ downstream}$ = 4.0.

For entrance region

$$\frac{v_w^3 \times R}{4\ u_{in}\ D^2} = (0.421)\ \frac{250}{25} = 4.21$$

$$M = 4.21 + 6 - 5\ exp\ \left[-\left[\frac{4.21}{3} \right]^{\frac{1}{2}} \right] = 8.68$$

Since the far downstream solution is smaller, M = 4 when L = 500 cm.

Note that this method of calculating an average using x = L/2 is reasonable if all of the system is in the entrance region or most of the system is far downstream. The value of M calculated is always somewhat too large which makes this design approach conservative. A more accurate prediction can be made by calculating M at several points and then integrating numerically to find an average.

As a check on the solution for L = 50 we can use Eqs. (13-27) and (13-3b).

$$k = 1.295\ \left[\frac{u_b D^2}{R\ L} \right]^{1/3} = 1.295\ \left[\frac{(3.2)\ (5.2 \times 10^{-7})^2}{(0.01)\ (50)} \right]^{1/3} = 0.0001555\ cm/s$$

For $R^\circ = 1$, M = exp (J_{solv}/k)

$$J_{solv} = \frac{1.8 \times 10^{-4}\ g/s\ cm^2}{(1.00\ g/cm^3)} = 1.8 \times 10^{-4}\ cm/s$$

$$M = exp\ \left[\frac{1.8 \times 10^{-4}}{1.555 \times 10^{-4}} \right] = 3.18$$

$$\%\ Dif = \frac{3.18 - 2.98}{2.98} \times 100 = 6.7\%$$

Note that $\delta = D/k = 5.2 \times 10^{-7}/1.555 \times 10^{-4} = 3.34 \times 10^{-3}$ cm $<$ R. If we apply this correlation when L = 500,

$$k = 0.00007218, \quad M = 12.108$$

and $\delta = 0.0072$ which is close R = 0.01. This closeness of R and δ is a signal to not use this mass transfer correlation.

13.6. TRANSPORT INSIDE THE MEMBRANE

In this section two models for transport inside the membrane will be developed. The structure of irreversible thermodynamics will be used for these models and will be briefly presented first. Then the solution-diffusion model appropriate for RO membranes will be developed in a simplified form. Finally, a frictional model appropriate for UF membranes which have small pores will be discussed.

13.6.1. Basic Irreversible Thermodynamics

Irreversible thermodynamics has been extensively applied to study the transport inside the membrane (Hwang and Kammermeyer, 1975; Johnson et al, 1966; Lakshminarayanaiah, 1969; Merten, 1966; Soltanieh and Gill, 1981). The flux of species i through the membrane, J_i is

$$J_i = \text{Flux } i = L_{ii} \, (\text{Force on } i) + \sum L_{ij} \, (\text{Force on } j) \qquad (13\text{-}56)$$

Thus the flux of species i is proportional both to the force on that species and to the force on other species. This is usually written as

$$J_i = L_{ii} \, X_i + \sum_{j(j\neq 1)} L_{ij} \, X_j \qquad (13\text{-}57)$$

where X_i is the force on species i, L_{ii} is the phenomenological coefficient for the movement of species i caused by the force on that species, and L_{ij} is the phenomenological coefficient for the movement of species i caused by the force on another species j.

A thermodynamic analysis based on the continuous increase in entropy can be used to show that

$$L_{ii} L_{jj} - L_{ij}^2 \geq 0 \tag{13-58}$$

and

$$L_{ii} \geq 0 \tag{13-59}$$

Equation (13-59) states that a species will move in the direction of the force applied on it. Equation (13-58) requires that $L_{ij} = 0$ if $L_{ii} = 0$. Thus, if a component will not move through a membrane due to forces acting directly on the component then it will not pass through the membrane at all. Thermodynamically, L_{ij} can be either positive or negative since Eq. (13-58) only limits the absolute magnitude of the coupling coefficients L_{ij}. In practice all known L_{ij} are ≥ 0.

One other condition on the phenomenological coefficients is Onsager's reciprocal relationship.

$$L_{ij} = L_{ji} \tag{13-60}$$

This states that coupling of two species is the same regardless of which is experiencing the force and which flux we are considering. This relationship is based on microscopic reversibility.

The validity of these general statements concerning the phenomenological coefficients requires the appropriate choices of the forces X_i. Under isothermal conditions the forces are

$$X_i = - \text{grad } \mu_i + Y_i \tag{13-61}$$

where μ_i is the chemical potential of species i and Y_i is the external force on component i. The external force in ion exchange membranes is an electrical force. In porous membranes where separation is based on sieving the Y_i are frictional forces between the component and the membrane.

The chemical potential term can be expanded in terms of concentration gradients and pressure gradients.

$$\text{grad } \mu_i = \left[\frac{\partial \mu_i}{\partial c_i} \right]_{p,T} \text{grad } c_i + v_i \text{ grad } p \qquad (13\text{-}62)$$

where c_i is the concentration of species i in weight per volume and v_i is the partial molar volume of species i,

$$v_i = \left[\frac{\partial \mu_i}{\partial p} \right]_{T,N} \qquad (13\text{-}63)$$

where N is the number of molecules or particles. Equation (13-62) can be integrated for the solvent (which is usually called species 1).

$$\Delta \mu_1 = \int \left[\frac{\partial \mu_1}{\partial c_1} \right]_{p,T} dc_1 + \int v_1 dp = \int \left[\frac{\partial \mu_1}{\partial c_2} \right]_{p,T} dc_2 + \int v_1 dp \qquad (13\text{-}64)$$

Remembering that the osmotic pressure difference across a membrane is the pressure difference that exists when $\Delta \mu_1 = 0$, then Eq. (13-64) becomes

$$v_1 \Delta \pi = - \int \left[\frac{\partial \mu_1}{\partial c_2} \right]_{p,T} dc_2 \qquad (13\text{-}65)$$

Substituting this result into Eq. (13-64), we obtain

$$\Delta \mu_1 = v_1 (\Delta p - \Delta \pi) \qquad (13\text{-}66)$$

where we have assumed that v_1 is constant so that we could do the last integration in Eq. (13-64). Note that $\Delta \pi$ is from one membrane interface to the other. That is, from c'_m to c''_m in Figure 13-7.

It will be our purpose to first determine the appropriate terms for the external forces, to then arrange the equations in a form which allows experimental determination of the coefficients L_{ii} and L_{ij}, and finally to predict the phenomenological coefficients from other properties such as diffusivities and solubilities.

13.6.2. Solution-Diffusion Membranes (RO and Gas Permeation)

Assume that there is no coupling of fluxes ($L_{ij} = 0$), and that external forces are unimportant ($Y_i = 0$). This assumes that convective flow of water or carrier gas through pores or pinholes is negligible. This is appropriate for solution-diffusion membranes used in reverse osmosis and gas permeation. Combining Eqs. (13-57), (13-61), and (13-66), we obtain

$$J'_{solv} = J'_1 = - \frac{L_{11} \, v_1}{t_m} (\Delta p - \Delta \pi) \qquad (13\text{-}67)$$

where we have approximated grad μ_i as $\Delta\mu_i/t_m$. J' is the mass flux in units such as g/cm^2 s, and $J'_{solv} = J_{solv} \, \rho_{solv}$. This result agrees with Eq. (12-20a) if we relate

$$L_{11} = \frac{K_{solv} \, \rho_{solv}}{v_1} \qquad (13\text{-}68)$$

The minus sign in Eq. (13-67) comes in because the +x direction shown in Figure 13-7 is in the direction of osmotic flow for the irreversible thermodynamic argument. The solvent density appears because mass and volumetric fluxes are

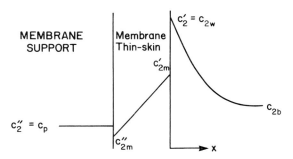

Figure 13-7.   Schematic of concentration profiles for RO membrane.

being compared. Since $\Delta\pi$ refers to the difference from concentration c'_m to c''_m, concentration polarization and solubilities are included. If π is proportional to concentration, Eq. (13-67) will have the same form as (12-27). Thus, after a lot of work we find that the solvent flux is given by the same equation we have been using all along. The advantage of the irreversible thermodynamics development is we can now relate the phenomenological coefficients and the fluxes to more fundamental quantities.

Assume that sorption and desorption at the membrane surface are rapid so that diffusion controls. Then L_{ii} can be related to the concentration within the membrane c_{im} and the mobility m_{im}.

$$L_{11} = c_{im}\, m_{im} \tag{13-69}$$

The mobility is the velocity per unit force on one mole of particles. In dilute solutions the mobility can be related to the diffusivity.

$$m_{im} = D_{1m}/RT \tag{13-70}$$

where R is the gas constant and D_{1m} is the solvent diffusivity within the membrane. Since the diffusivity and the solvent concentration are often approximately constant, L_{11} is often approximately constant. Now the solvent flux is

$$J'_{solv} = -\frac{c_{1m}\, D_{1m}\, v_1}{RT\, t_m}(\Delta p - \Delta\pi) \tag{13-71}$$

Remember that $\Delta\pi$ refers to the osmotic pressure difference across the membrane. The solvent permeability can be estimated by comparing Eqs. (13-71) to (13-67) and (13-68)

$$K_{solv} = \frac{c_{1m}\, D_{1m}\, v_1}{RT\, \rho_{solv}} \tag{13-72}$$

This allows estimation of permeabilities, and if permeability is determined experimentally it allows extrapolation to other conditions. This result also shows that K_{solv} will be approximately constant in dilute solutions where the solvent concentration and diffusivity are approximately constant. In concentrated solutions K_{solv} is not constant (Soltanieh and Gill, 1981).

The flux of solute (species 2) can also be estimated. In RO systems external forces and the coupling of fluxes can usually be ignored. Then combining Eqs. (13-57), (13-61) and (13-62) gives

$$J_2 = - L_{22} \left[\left[\frac{\partial \mu_2}{\partial c_2} \right]_{T,p} \frac{dc}{dx} + v_2 \frac{dp}{dx} \right] \qquad (13\text{-}73)$$

where J_2 is a mass flux which is the same as in Chapter 12. Since the last term is usually negligible, we obtain

$$J_2 = -L_{22} (\frac{\partial \mu_2}{\partial c_2})_{T,p} \frac{dc_2}{dx} \qquad (13\text{-}74)$$

The phenomenological coefficient L_{22} can again be related to the mobility and for dilute solutions to the diffusivity.

$$L_{22} = m_{2m}\, c_{2m} = \frac{D_{2m}}{RT}\, c_{2m} \qquad (13\text{-}75)$$

Since c_{2m} can change significantly in the membrane, L_{22} may not be constant. For dilute solutions

$$\left[\frac{\partial \mu_2}{\partial c_{2m}} \right]_{T,p} = \frac{RT}{c_{2m}} \qquad (13\text{-}76)$$

Combining Eqs. (13-74) to (13-76), we have

$$J_{solute} = J_2 = -\frac{D_{2m}}{t_m} \Delta c_{2m} \qquad (13\text{-}77)$$

where we have approximated dc_{2m}/dx as $\Delta c_{2m}/t_m$. In this equation Δc_{2m} is the concentration difference within the membrane. This is illustrated in Figure 13-7.

The relationship between the solute concentration in the membrane and in solution depends upon the solubility. We will assume that the membrane surfaces are in equilibrium with the solution and that the distribution coefficient is constant.

$$K_2 = \frac{c'_{2m}}{c_{2w}} = \frac{c''_{2m}}{c_p} \qquad (13\text{-}78)$$

Substituting this into Eq. (13-77), we have

$$J_{solute} = -\frac{D_{2m}K_2}{t_m}(c_{2w}-c_{2p}) = -\frac{D_{2m}K_2}{t_m}(M\,c_{2b} - c_p) \qquad (13\text{-}79)$$

This result agrees with Eq. (12-25) and shows that

$$L_{22} = D_{2m}K_2 \qquad (13\text{-}80)$$

Note that this result also agrees with Eq. (12-15) used for gas permeation which is also a solution-diffusion process.

It is interesting to use these results to study the change in salt concentration across a RO membrane. The salt concentration on the permeate side, $c_{2,p}$ can be calculated from

$$c_{2p}\left[\frac{\text{g salt}}{\text{cm}^3}\right] = \frac{J_2\left[\dfrac{\text{g salt}}{\text{cm}^2\,\text{s}}\right]}{J'_{solv}\left[\dfrac{\text{g water}}{\text{cm}^2\,\text{s}}\right]}\;c_{1p}\left[\frac{\text{g water}}{\text{cm}^3}\right] \qquad (13\text{-}81)$$

Then from Eqs. (13-71), (13-79) and (13-81), concentration ratio is

$$\frac{c_{2w}}{c_{2p}} = \frac{J'_1\,c_{2w}}{J_2\,c_{1p}} = \frac{c_{1m}\,D_{1m}\,v_1\,(\Delta p - \Delta\pi)\,c_{2w}}{D_{2m}\,K_2\,RT\,(c_{2w} - c_{2p})\,c_{1p}} \qquad (13\text{-}82)$$

Assuming that $c_{2w} \gg c_{2p}$ and defining $K_1 = c_{1m}/c_{1p}$ as the water distribution coefficient in the membrane, we obtain

$$\frac{c_{2w}}{c_{2p}} = \frac{D_{1m}\,K_1\,v_1}{D_{2m}\,K_2\,RT}\,(\Delta p - \Delta\pi) \qquad (13\text{-}83)$$

From Eq. (13-83) we can estimate the properties required to obtain a given concentration ratio. Note that the concentration ratio in RO membranes is proportional to $(\Delta p - \Delta \pi)$. More separation is achieved by increasing Δp.

Example 13-4. Water Desalination.

What membrane properties are required to desalinate sea water to potable water using RO?

Solution

A. *Define*. This problem is not well defined. Typical operating conditions are $\Delta p = 100$ atm with an average brine concentration of 5 wt %. Potable water is 500 ppm or 0.05 wt %. We wish to find the required value of $D_{1m} K_1 / D_{2m} K_2$.

B and C. *Explore and Plan*. We can use Eq. (13-83) to estimate the required properties. We will assume concentration polarization is negligible. The osmotic pressure of 5 wt % brine is about 37 atm while the osmotic pressure of 0.05 wt% is about 0.4 atm. The value of v_1/RT is

$$\frac{v_1}{RT} = \frac{18.095 \text{ cc/gmole}}{82.057 \left[\dfrac{\text{(cc atm)}}{\text{gmole K}} \right] (293.16 \text{ K})} \fallingdotseq 0.000752 \text{ atm}^{-1}$$

Solving Eq. (13-83)

$$\frac{D_{1m} K_1}{D_{2m} K_2} = \left[\frac{c_{2w}}{c_{2p}} \right] \left[\frac{RT}{v_1} \right] \frac{1}{(\Delta p - \Delta \pi)}$$

D. *Do It*. If concentration polarization is negligible,

$$\frac{c_{2w}}{c_{2p}} = \frac{c_{2b}}{c_{2p}} = 100$$

$$\Delta p - \Delta \pi = 100 - (37 - 0.4) = 63.4 \text{ atm}$$

and

$$\frac{D_{1m} K_1}{D_{2m} K_2} = 100 \left[\frac{1}{0.000752}\right] \left[\frac{1}{63.4}\right] = 2100$$

For typical RO membranes K_1 is slightly less than 1.0 and $D_{1m} = D_{\text{water in membrane}} \sim 2.5$ to 16×10^{-7} cm^2/s for high selectivity cellulose acetate. (Soltanieh and Gill, 1981). Thus, a typical required salt permeability is

$$D_{2m} K_2 = \frac{D_{1m} K_1}{2100} = 1.2 \text{ to } 7.6 \times 10^{-10} \text{ cm}^2/s$$

E. *Check.* These results agree with typical values of K_2 in cellulose acetate membranes from 0.017 to 0.039 and typical values of D_{1m} from 0.8 to 5×10^{-9} cm^2/s (Soltanieh and Gill, 1981).

F. *Generalization.* Obviously, these results can be changed for other operating conditions and other membranes. For less selective cellulose acetate membranes D_{1m} is higher. Values of diffusivities and distribution coefficients for a variety of membranes are tabulated by Soltanieh and Gill (1981). If concentration polarization is important, $\Delta\pi$ and $c_{2w} = M c_{2b}$ increase. Both these effects increase the value of $D_{1m} K_1 / D_{2m} K_2$. When RO is used to produce ultrapure water, $\Delta\pi$ is negligible and significantly higher values of $c_{2,w} / c_{2,p}$ can be obtained (see Problem 13-D8).

13.6.3. Frictional Model For Porous Membranes (UF)

In ultrafiltration separation appears to be based mainly on a sieving mechanism and not on solution and diffusion. The frictional model assumes that solvent flow through the membrane is mainly laminar convective flow. Thus the solvent flow can be estimated as Poiseuille flow. The solute flux depends upon the convective flow (that is coupled to the solvent flow), diffusion, and friction. In this model coupling between fluxes and external forces (friction) is important.

The solute flux is due to the sum of contributions from the convective flow and diffusion.

$$J_2 = c_{2m} u + J_{2dif} \tag{13-84}$$

where u is the center-of-mass velocity of the pore fluid. The term $c_{2m}u$ represents $-L_{21} d\mu_1/dx$. The diffusive flux can be written as $L_{22}X_2$. L_{22} can again be related to the mobility, and X_2 is the force from Eq. (13-61). Thus,

$$J_{2dif} = m_2 c_{2m} \left[- \left[\frac{\partial \mu_2}{\partial c_{2m}} \right]_{p,T} \frac{dc_{2m}}{dx} + Y_2 \right] \tag{13-85}$$

where Y_2 is the frictional force on the solute due to friction against the membrane. This external force can be related to the solute velocity within the pores as

$$Y_2 = -f_{23}u_2 = -\frac{f_{23} J_2}{c_{2m}} \tag{13-86}$$

where f_{23} is a friction factor between the solute (2) and the membrane (3). The mobility m_2 can also be related to a friction factor except now it is the friction between the solute and solvent.

$$m_2 = 1/f_{21} = D_{21} / RT \tag{13-87}$$

where (2) is solute and (1) is solvent. Combining these equations and solving for J_2, we obtain

$$J_2 = \frac{-c_{2m}}{(f_{21} + f_{23})} \left[\frac{\partial \mu_2}{\partial c_{2m}} \right]_{p,T} \frac{dc_{2m}}{dx} + \frac{f_{21} c_{2m}}{f_{21} + f_{23}} u \tag{13-88}$$

For dilute solutions Eq. (13-76) is valid and we have

$$J_2 = \frac{-RT}{f_{21} + f_{23}} \frac{dc_{2m}}{dx} + \frac{f_{21}}{f_{21}+f_{23}} c_{2m} u \tag{13-89}$$

As u approaches zero this gives us diffusion with a drag factor applied. The solute flux can also be related to the solvent flow as

$$J_2 = \varepsilon \, u \, c_{2p} \tag{13-90}$$

where ε is the porosity of the membrane and c_{2p} is the permeate concentration in the fluid. Assuming that the distribution coefficient given by Eq. (13-78) is constant for the porous membrane, Eqs. (13-89) and (13-90) can be combined and integrated to find c_2. The integration is from x=0 where $c'_{2m}=K_2c_{2w}$ to $x= - t_m\lambda$ where $c_{2m}''=K_2c_{2p}$. λ is the tortuosity which takes into account the fact that the pores are not straight, $\lambda > 1$. The result after some manipulation is

$$c_{2p} = \frac{f_{21} K_2 c_{2w} \exp (-u t_m \lambda \, f_{21}/RT)}{f_{21} K_2 - (f_{21} + f_{23}) \, \varepsilon + (f_{21} + f_{23}) \varepsilon \exp (-u t_m \, \lambda \, f_{21}/RT)} \tag{13-91}$$

which allows one to predict the permeate concentration once the solvent velocity is known. For high negative velocities Eq. (13-91) simplifies to,

$$c_{2p} = \frac{c_{2w} \, K_2 \, f_{21}}{(f_{23} + f_{21}) \, \varepsilon} \tag{13-92}$$

The solvent velocity due to Poiseuille flow in the pores without any friction would be,

$$\varepsilon \, u = -H \frac{dp}{dx} \sim -H \frac{\Delta p_m}{t_m \, \lambda} \tag{13-93}$$

where H is the hydrodynamic permeability of the membrane and Δp_m is the effective pressure driving force.

$$\Delta p_m = \Delta p - \Delta \pi' + \Delta \pi'' \tag{13-94}$$

The terms $\Delta \pi'$ and $\Delta \pi''$ are the osmotic pressure differences at the two membrane-liquid interfaces.

$$\Delta \pi' = \pi \left[\frac{c'_{2m}}{\varepsilon} \right] - \pi(c_{2w}) \tag{13-95a}$$

$$\Delta \pi'' = \pi \left[\frac{c''_{2m}}{\varepsilon} \right] - \pi(c_{2p}) \tag{13-95b}$$

The hydrodynamic permeability in Poiseuille flow can be estimated from

$$H = \frac{\varepsilon R_p^2}{8\mu} \qquad (13\text{-}96)$$

where R_p is the pore radius and μ is viscosity.

In addition to the pressure gradient there is a frictional force which must be added to the pressure gradient . Then,

$$u = -\frac{H}{\varepsilon} \left[\frac{dp}{dx} + Y_2 \frac{c_{2m}}{\varepsilon(MW)_2} \right] \qquad (13\text{-}97)$$

where Y_2 is the force per mole of pore fluid given by Eq. (13-86), and $c_{2m}/\varepsilon(MW)_2$ is the molar concentration of solute in the pore fluid. The product of these is the force per volume of the pore fluid. Combining Eqs. (13-86), (13-92), and (13-97), we obtain

$$u = -\frac{H}{\varepsilon} \left[\frac{\Delta p_m}{t_m \lambda} + \frac{f_{23} J_2}{\varepsilon(MW)_2} \right] \qquad (13\text{-}98)$$

The solute flux J_2 is given by Eq. (13-90). If this equation is substituted into Eq. (13-98) and the result is solved for u, we obtain

$$u = -\frac{H}{\varepsilon} \left[\frac{1}{1 + \dfrac{H f_{23}}{(MW)_2\, \varepsilon} c_{2p}} \right] \frac{\Delta p_m}{t_m\, \lambda} \qquad (13\text{-}99)$$

Note that u is negative because of the chosen direction for x. Solution of Eqs. (13-91) and (13-99) simultaneously allows prediction of the solvent velocity and the permeate concentration through the membrane. (See Problem 13-C3). In Eq. (13-91) c_{2w} is considered to be known since it can be calculated from the concentration polarization analysis. The solute flux can then be determined from Eq. (13-90). The solvent flux can be found from Eq. (13-81) which after substituting in Eq. (13-90), is

$$J'_{solv} = \varepsilon u\, c_{1p} \qquad (13\text{-}100)$$

This model appears to be a reasonable physical model for sieve type membranes with intrinsic rejections in the range $0 < R^{\circ} < 1$. The theory agrees qualitatively with experimental data. Unfortunately, predicting the necessary friction factors, f_{21} and f_{23}, and the tortuosity λ is difficult. Thus this model should probably be considered a qualitative model which helps to explain the transport processes inside sieving type membranes. It can serve as a guide to qualitatively predict or explain the effect of various variables and to help extrapolate data.

13.7. SUMMARY-OBJECTIVES

At the end of this chapter you should be able to meet the following objectives.

1. Predict the polarization modulus for both laminar and turbulent flow when no gel layer is formed using mass transfer correlations.

2. Predict the mass transfer coefficient and the solvent flux for UF when a gel forms. Determine whether or not a gel does form. Discuss the problems with the gel formation theory.

3. Explain the mass balances for a completely mixed RO systems with concentration polarization. Estimate the solvent flux for this system.

4. Explain the mass balances for countercurrent gas permeation and explain qualitatively why countercurrent operation is superior to other flow patterns.

5. Use the exact solutions for laminar flow to predict the concentration polarization modulus in tubes or between flat plates.

6. Discuss the application of irreversible thermodynamics to models of transport inside of membranes, and explain qualitatively both the solution-diffusion and the frictional models.

REFERENCES

Berman, A.S., "Laminar flow in channels with porous walls," *J. Appl. Phys.*, *24*, 1232 (1953).

Blaisdell, C.T. and K. Kammermeyer, "Countercurrent and co-current gas separation," *Chem. Eng. Sci.*, *28*, 1249 (1973).

Blatt, W.F., A. Dravid, A.S. Michaels, and L. Nelson, "Solute polarization and cake formation in membrane ultrafiltration: Causes, consequences and control techniques," in J.E. Flinn (Ed.), *Membrane Science and Technology*, Plenum Press, NY, 1970, 47-97.

Fane, A.G., "Ultrafiltration: Factors influencing flux and rejection," in R.J. Wakeman (Ed.) *Progress in Filtration and Separation 4*, Elsevier, NY, 101-180, 1986.

Harris, F.L., G.B. Humphreys and K.S. Spiegler, "Reverse osmosis (hyperfiltration) in water desalination," in P. Meares (Ed.) *Membrane Separation Processes*, Elsevier, Amsterdam, 1976, Chapt. 4.

Hwang, S.-T. and K. Kammermeyer, *Membranes in Separations*, Wiley, NY, 1975.

Johnson, J.S., L. Dresner and K.A. Kraus, "Hyperfiltration (Reverse Osmosis)," in K.S. Spiegler (Ed.), *Principles of Desalination*, Academic Press, NY, 1966, 345-439.

Lakshminarayanaiah, N. *Transport Phenomena in Membranes*, Academic Press, NY 1969.

Le, M.S. and J.A. Howell, "Alternative model for ultrafiltration," *Chem. Eng. Res. Des.*, *62*, 373 (1984).

Matthiasson, E. and B. Sivik, "Concentration polarization and fouling", *Desalination*, *35*, 59 (1980).

784

Merten, U. "Transport properties of osmotic membranes," in U. Merten (Ed.), *Desalination by Reverse Osmosis*, MIT Press, Cambridge, MA, 1966, 15-54.

Porter, M.C., "Membrane filtration," in Schweitzer, P.A. (Ed.), *Handbook of Separation Techniques for Chemical Engineers*, McGraw-Hill, NY, 1979, Section 2.1.

Potts, D.E., R.C. Ahlert and S.S. Wang, "A critical review of fouling of reverse osmosis membranes," *Desalination, 36*, 235 (1981).

Rao, G. and K.K. Sirkar, "Explicit flux expressions in tubular reverse osmosis desalination," *Desalination, 27*, 99 (1978).

Romero, C.A. and R.H. Davis, "Global model of crossflow microfiltration based on hydrodynamic particle diffusion," *J. Membrane Sci., 39*, 157 (1988).

Shen, J.J.S. and R.F. Probstein, "On the prediction of limiting flux in laminar ultrafiltration of macromolecular solutions," *Ind. Eng. Chem. Fundam., 16*, 459 (1977).

Sherwood, T.K., P.L.T. Brian, R.E. Fisher and L. Dresner, "Salt concentration at phase boundaries in desalination by reverse osmosis," *Ind. Eng. Chem. Fundam., 4*, 113 (1965).

Soltanieh, M. and W.N. Gill, "Review of reverse osmosis membranes and transport models," *Chem. Eng. Commun., 12*, 279 (1981).

Sourirajan, S., *Reverse Osmosis*, Logos Press, London 1970.

Sourirajan, S. (Ed.), *Reverse Osmosis and Synthetic Membranes. Theory - Technology - Engineering*, National Research Council of Canada, Ottawa, Canada, 1977.

Trettin, D.R. and M.R. Doshi, "Limiting flux in ultrafiltratio of macromolecular solutions," *Chem. Eng. Commun., 4*, 507 (1980).

Wijmans, J.G., S. Nakao, and C.A. Smolders, "Flux limitation in ultrafiltration: Osmotic pressure model and gel layer model," *J. Memb. Sci., 20,* 115 (1984).

Yuan, S.W. and A.B. Finkelstein, "Laminar pipe flow with injection and suction through a porous wall," *Transactions ASME, 78,* 719 (1956).

Zydney, A.L. and C.K. Colton, "A concentration polarization model for the filtrate flux in cross-flow microfiltration of particulate suspensions," *Chem. Eng. Commun., 47,* 1 (1986).

HOMEWORK

A.   *Discussion Problems*

A1.   UF systems will almost always show concentration polarization. Under what conditions would you expect this to lead to gel formation? When would fouling be likely?

A2.   Why are there multiple solutions for concentration polarization in laminar flow?

A3.   Theoretical analyses of turbulent flow are much more complicated than laminar flow analysis. However, the concentration polarization analysis for turbulent flow is simpler than the exact analysis for laminar flow. Explain this paradox.

A4.   Qualitatively, why is a countercurrent flow pattern superior to completely mixed?

A5.   How can you determine if the solution obtained with Eqs. (13-3b) and (13-16) or (13-18) is reasonable?

A6.　On one page develop your key relations chart for this chapter. This will be a challenge because you will have room for only the more important equations.

C.　*Derivations*

C1.　Derive the ratio of $k/\Delta p$ for both laminar and turbulent flow. Compare these results.

C2.　Derive Eq. (12-57) for a countercurrent dialyzer.

C3.　If a constant $b < < 1$, then $\exp (b) \sim 1+b$. Using this approximation, simplify Eq. (13-91) when $(- u \, t_m \lambda f_{21}/RT) < <1$. Then solve Eqs. (13-91) and (13-99) simultaneously to determine c_{2p}. Note $u < 0$. Note that this assumption of small b will often not be valid.

C4.　Prove that the lowest driving force for a countercurrent gas permeation module equals the driving force for a completely mixed module.

D.　*Single-Answer Problems*

D1.　We are doing an ultrafiltration experiment with a high molecular weight solute in water. The bulk concentration is 0.005 weight fraction. The osmotic pressure can be ignored. A 1.5 cm id tubular membrane is used. Feed to each tube is 100 ml/sec. The membrane has a pure water flux of 10.5×10^{-4} g/sec cm^2 at a pressure of 38 atmospheres. The inherent rejection coefficient (M=1) for the membrane is $R^{\circ} = 0.972$. Under the conditions of this experiment (M > 1) the measured rejection coefficient is $R = 0.85$. Estimate the solute diffusivity.
Data: $\rho = 1.0$ g/cm^3, $\mu = 0.0105$ poise, no gel is formed.

D2.　We are ultrafiltering a dextran solution in a laminar thin-channel system. The channel consists of two flat plates 0.1 cm apart. Fluid flows at 3.0 cm/min and is recycled through a 20 cm length of the channel. The dextran is known to gel at ~30 wt %. The solvent flux is measured as a function of dextran concentration. Kinematic viscosity $v = 8.96$ cm^2/s. For the data given in problem 12-D4 estimate the dextran diffusivity.

D3. We wish to ultrafilter a 2 wt % aqueous solution of casein at 25°C. The c_g for casein is approximately 14 wt %. The channel is to be 25 cm long and is a rectangular slit 0.025 cm deep. The bulk velocity is 50 cm/sec. The pressure drop across the membrane is 40 psi and casein diffusivity is approximately 10^{-7} cm^2/sec.

a. Predict the water flux at steady state.

b. If $R^\circ = 0.99$ (without concentration polarization) and assuming that the casein is mobile in the gel, estimate R when a gel layer forms.

D4. Estimate the average concentration polarization modulus for a 4 wt% NaCl solution. $D = 1.61 \times 10^{-6}$ cm^2/sec. $\rho_b = 1.025$ g/cc, Sc = 560, $c_L = 0.987$ gH$_2$O/ml. Operation is in round tubes 0.05 cm in radius, 50 cm long, and with a bulk velocity at the inlet of 2.0 cm/sec. Flux rate is 3×10^{-4} g/sec cm^2. Use the exact solution for laminar flow.

D5. We wish to do a reverse osmosis experiment on a 0.98 % salt solution. The osmotic pressure is 6.958 atmospheres and $\pi = bc$ is valid. Operation is at 45 atmospheres. For pure distilled water a flux of 8.5×10^{-4} g/sec cm^2 is observed. Salt retention without concentration polarization is 0.998. Tubular membranes 2 cm in diameter are used. Each tube is 80 cm long. Feed to each tube is 1.0 g/sec. Including concentration polarization find the average water flux.
Physical properties: $D = 1.6 \times 10^{-6}$ cm^2/sec, $\rho = 1.01$ g/cc, Sc = 560, $c_L = 0.99$g H$_2$O/ml (solvent concentration)

D6. We are ultrafiltering a polymer in a hollow fiber system. The hollow fibers are 100 cm long and 0.1 cm id. The polymer gels at $c_g = 0.015$ wt frac. Inlet velocity $u_{in} = 3.5$ cm/s and $c_{in} = 0.001$ wt frac. Flux rate before gelling occurs is 3.2×10^{-4} cm^3/cm^{2}s. $R^\circ = 1.0$.
a. Estimate the distance down the tube at which the polymer starts to gel (± 0.1 cm).

b. What is the flux after gelling occurs?

DATA: $\rho = 1.01$ g/cc (assume constant)

$\mu = 0.03$ poise (assume constant)

$D = 5 \times 10^{-7}$ cm^2/s

D7. An experimental gas permeation system with flat plates is being tested. Rejection, $R^\circ = 0.96$. The flow path is 100 cm long and the plates are 0.02 cm apart. The high pressure side is at ten atmospheres and the low pressure side is at one atmosphere. The total gas flux through the membrane is $J = 1.0 \times 10^{-3} \dfrac{cc\ (STP)}{cm^2\ s}$. The inlet gas velocity is 100 cm/s. Operation is at 25°C and the system is an ideal gas. Find the average concentration polarization modulus.

DATA: Average MW on high pressure side = 40

$D = 0.42$ cm^3/s

$\mu = 1.4 \times 10^{-4}$ poise

D8. We wish to use a cellulose acetate membrane to purify tap water for an electronics plant. The tap water contains 120 ppm TDS (total dissolved salts) and we wish a product which is 1 ppm or less. $\Delta p = 110$ atm.

a. Can we do this with existing membranes?

b. If we can do it, what cut θ should be used if the RO module is perfectly mixed? Set $c_p = 1$ ppm

c. Predict J'_{solv} and J_{solute} if $t_m = 1.2 \times 10^{-4}$ cm for part b.

d. If $M = 2.0$, set $c_p = 1$ ppm and find θ, J'_{solv} and J_{solute}.

DATA: Operate at 18°C. Assume properties of water (see Example 13-1). Use p. 17-23 in Perry and Green (1984) to estimate π. Assume salts can be treated as if they are NaCl. $K_2 = 0.025$, $D_{2m} = 2.5 \times 10^{-9}$ cm^3/s, $D_w = 1.0 \times 10^{-6}$ cm^2/s, $K_1 = 0.98$.

Ignore concentration polarization in parts a, b, and c.

D9. Merten (1966) reports values for transfer of sucrose through a cellophane membrane at 25°C. At infinite dilution, $\varepsilon = 0.67$ and

$$\frac{K_2 f_{21}}{(f_{21} + f_{23})\, \varepsilon} = 0.65 \quad , \quad \frac{t_m\, \lambda\, f_{21}}{RT} = 6 \times 10^3 \text{ s/cm} \quad ,$$

$$D_{21} = \frac{RT}{f_{21}} = 5 \times 10^{-6} \text{ cm}^2/\text{s}$$

If $-u\varepsilon = 0.9 \times 10^{-4}$ cm/s at $\Delta p_m = 1$ atm, determine:

a. c_{2p}/c_{2w}

b. R_p

Note: Watch your units.

Part IV
SELECTION AND SEQUENCING

NOMENCLATURE CHAPTER 14

A_i	linear equilibrium constant for adsorption
B_c	bottoms flow rate of melted crystals
$C_{P,B}$	heat capacity bulk adsorbent
$C_{p,sorb}$	heat capacity sorbate
D	distillate rate
k_i'	capacity factor in chromatography Eq. (7-32a)
K_{solv}	membrane permeability
L	column length, m
L_{MTZ}	length of mass transfer zone, m
M	concentration polarization modulus
N_{ads}	rate adsorbate product
p	pressure
P	permeate rate
q_{avg}	average adsorbed phase loading
q_{sat}	adsorbate loading at saturation
Q	heat supplied or removed
Q_c , Q_M	heat for condenser and melter
Q_R	heat for reboiler
Q_{reg}	heat required for regeneration
R	gas constant
R_D	L/D, external reflux ratio
R_M	external reflux ratio for melter
t_m	membrane thickness

T	temperature, K
T_o	surroundings temperature, K
T_c	cold (refrigeration) temperature
T_{RG}	temperature regeneration gas is supplied at
T_s	steam temperature
T_{sm}	supply temperature for melter
W_{eq}	equivalent work
W_{min}	minimum reversible work
W_{rev}	reversible work
W_{RO}	equivalent work for RO
$x_{i,j}$	mole fraction component i in phase j
y_i	mole fraction in vapor

Greek

α_{ij}	separation factor, Eq. (14-1)
γ_i	activity coefficient
ΔH_{ads}	heat of adsorption
ε_p	power cycle efficiency
ε_R	Carnot cycle efficiency for refrigeration
λ	latent heat of vaporization
λ_f	latent heat of freezing
ξ	factor defined in Eq. (14-21)
π	osmotic pressure
ψ	factor for excess regeneration gas

Chapter 14

SELECTION AND SEQUENCING OF SEPARATIONS

Throughout this book we have been discussing mainly known results - we now move into the unknown area of selection and sequencing of separations. This is an area which has been extensively studied for distillation and to a lesser extent for extractive and azeotropic distillation - all equilibrium staged processes. Very little research has been done for the rate controlled separations which are the subject of this book. In this chapter we will discuss what has been done, and extend by analogy the results obtained for equilibrium staged processes to rate controlled processes. The results obtained are logical, but are not proven; thus, they should be used carefully.

We will first consider the general characteristics of separation problems. Then, an overview of separation methods will be presented. The purpose of this overview is to aid in the selection of separation methods which will work. Energy criteria for evaluating separation processes will be presented. After a brief introduction to the strategy of process design and synthesis, heuristics (rules of thumb) for developing separation schemes will be discussed. Evolutionary methods which are used to improve the initial sequences will be briefly introduced. Finally, needed research will be outlined.

14.1. GENERAL CHARACTERISTICS OF THE SEPARATION PROBLEM

There are so many possible types of separation problems that it is hard to be specific about your immediate problem which becomes *the* separation problem.

However, there are a few abstract ideas which are useful in looking at the separation problem.

1. Invariably, there are several (n) components present and the initial problem is multicomponent. Often only one or two of these components are valuable.

2. Most real problems will require several methods in series. Often, one or more separation methods capable of separating most or all of the components are readily available. There is a strong temptation to immediately use these methods. Resist this temptation.

3. The separation can be split into n - 1 binary pairs. These binary pairs are not unique since they depend upon the physical properties used by different separation methods (see Section 14.2). For any given set of n - 1 binary pairs there will be one separation which is most difficult. This most difficult separation may be different for different choices of separation methods.

4. If we know how to do all of the separations then the problem becomes one of choosing the appropriate set of separation methods. If we do not know how to do all of the separations, then the initial problem is to find some set of separation methods which will do the separation. The next problem is determining the optimum set of separation methods.

5. The appropriate separation method depends upon where you are in the life cycle of the product. If you are racing to be first on the market and the product can demand a high price, then the series of separation processes which can be put on stream fastest has a definite edge. For more mature products the cost of the separation methods becomes much more important and different separation processes may be optimum.

6. The scale of operation is also important. A process which is economic on a small scale may not be economic on a large

scale and vice versa. For example, cyrogenic distillation of air is currently the most economic air separation method at very large scale, but either adsorption or membrane processes or more economic at small scale.

7. The concentration of the feed stream affects the separation costs. The effect of the naturally occuring concentration on

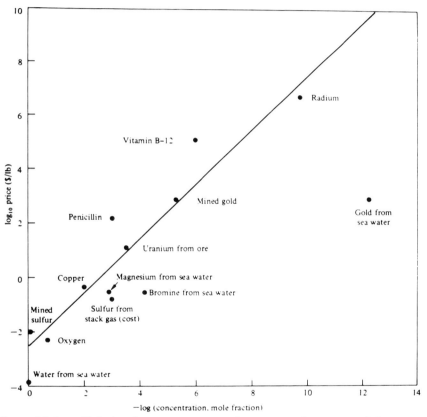

Figure 14-1.   Relation between pure product cost and raw material concentration (Sherwood *et al*, 1975). Reprinted with permission from T.K. Sherwood, R.L. Pigford and C.R. Wilke, *Mass Transfer*, McGraw-Hill, 1975. Copyright 1975, McGraw-Hill.

798

price is illustrated in Figure 14-1 (Sherwood et al, 1975). In general, products which are dilute cost more to separate. Gold is an interesting example of this. Gold can be recovered from sea water, but this is not currently economic since mined gold is more concentrated and hence is cheaper.

8. Every industry has its favorite separation methods. Since these methods are known to work within that industry, there is a stong predisposition to use those methods.

9. The criteria used to select a separation method for research and development (either academic or industrial) are different than the criteria used to select separation methods to solve a problem. The focus of this chapter is on solving separation problems. Bravo et al (1986) and Fair (1987) discuss the results of a study to evaluate separation processes as candidates for further research with respect to significant energy savings.

14.2 OVERVIEW OF SEPARATION METHODS

The purpose of this section is to provide an overview of separation methods and a very preliminary guide on methods of selecting separation methods which will work.

There are a variety of ways to classify separation methods. One approach is shown in Figure 14-2. This book has been concerned with *diffusional* separation processes where the separation is at a molecular level. *Mechanical* separation processes involve the separation of bulk phases. Real problems will often require both mechanical and diffusional separation methods. The mechanical separation processes are covered in detail elsewhere (Evans, 1980; Jacobs and Penney, 1987; Ludwig, 1979; Perry and Green, 1984; Schweitzer, 1979).

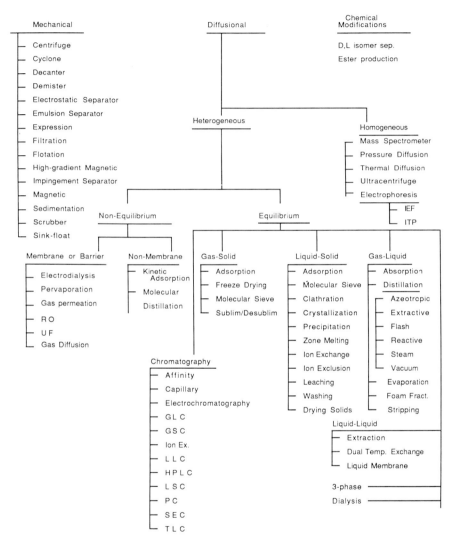

Figure 14-2.   Classification of separations.

The third major category, *chemical modification*, involves doing a reaction which simplifies the separation. In the production of esters and MTBE in distillation columns the reaction and the separation are done simultaneously. In D, L amino acid separations one of the isomers first reacts to form an ester, and then the remaining isomer in the acid form is easily separated from the ester.

The diffusional separation processes can be further subdivided into *homogeneous* (one phase present) and *heterogeneous* (two or more phases present). Electrophoretic processes (Chapter 11) are considered to be homogeneous since the actual separation occurs in a single phase-the addition of a second phase as a anticonvective medium is optional. The heterogeneous separation processes have been further subdivided into equilibrium and nonequilibrium separations. Nonequilibrium processes without a membrane or barrier present are relatively rare. Kinetic adsorption was discussed in Chapters 6 and 8. The nonequilibrium processes with a membrane include all the membrane processes discussed in Chapters 12 and 13. The equilibrium processes have been subdivided based on the phases present except for chromatography which is listed separately. I have included chromatography as an equilibrium process since the major reasons for separation in these methods are equilibrium differences even though the column may never be at equilibrium. The equilibrium processes also include crystallization methods (Chapters 2 to 5), adsorption and ion exchange (Chapters 6 to 10), and the equilibrium staged processes such as distillation, extraction and absorption which are covered in many other books. The most commonly used diffusional separations are the equilibrium processes.

Figure 14-2 has over 70 separation methods listed, and it does not include all methods. In addition most methods have many variants which are not listed, and many methods can be done with a variety of solvents, adsorbents, additives, or membranes. The result of all these variations is there are literally thousands of separation methods available if one includes all the variations. The engineer's job is to select methods which will solve the problem economically.

There are many other approaches to classifying separation methods which may be useful in selecting the appropriate methods. Since separations are based on physical property differences, a classification based on the physical property differences can be very useful. One way of doing this is shown in Table 14-1 where the sizes of species being separated is also indicated. Some separations are listed more than once in Table 14-1 since different property differences can be used. For example, absorption can be due to vapor pressure differences (physical absorption) or due to reversible or irreversible chemical reaction.

The separations listed in Table 14-1 are also marked as to whether they use an *energy* (E) or *mass* (M) separating agent. Separations using an energy separating agent use heat (e.g. crystallization) or pumping energy (e.g. gas permeation) to effect the separation. Separations using a mass separating agent add an additional species such as a solvent or purge gas to the mixture to be separated. Note that the insoluble membrane, adsorbent or packing material is not considered to be a mass separating agent. However, the solvent or carrier gas in chromatography and the purge gas or displacer in adsorption is a mass separating agent. The disadvantage of adding a mass separating agent is that usually the mass separating agent has to be removed before the product can be used. Thus, a separation scheme using an energy separation agent is usually required in addition to the mass separating agent processes. Separations such as precipitation or adsorption can use either an energy or a mass separating agent depending on how they are operated. Separations such as electrochromatography use both energy and mass separating agents. Gradient chromatography systems have two or more mass separating agents.

The separation factor obtainable with the different separations listed in Figure 14-2 and Table 14-1 is a very important first indication of the feasiblity of a given separation method. For equilibrium processes the inherent separation factor is defined as (King, 1980)

$$\alpha_{ij} = \frac{x_{i,1} / x_{j,1}}{x_{i,2} / x_{j,2}} \qquad (14\text{-}1)$$

where $x_{i,1}$ is the mole fraction of component i in phase 1. Phases 1 and 2 are assumed to be in equilibrium. For distillation $\alpha_{i,j}$ is the relative volatility. For

Table 14-1. Property Differences for Separations
(King, 1980; Null, 1987; Rudd *et al.*, 1973)

Property Differences	Molecules	Macromolecule	Particles
	GLC(M)		
	flash dist. (E)		
vapor	distillation (E)		
pressure	absorption (M)		
(rel. volatility)	sublimation/desublimation (E)		
	stripping (M)		
	evaporation (E)		
	high vacuum distillation (E)		
rel. volatity	azeotropic dist. (M+E)		
+ chem. interact	extractive dist. (M+E)		
	reactive dist (M+E)		
distribution	extraction (M)		
2 liquids	liquid membranes (M)		
	← two-aqueous phase extraction (M) →		
	-LLC(M)-		

melting point — crystallization (E)
zone melting (E)

solubility — crystallization
absorption/stripping (M)
leaching (M)
precipitation (E or M)

solubility + diffusivity — gas permeation (E)
reverse osmosis (E)
pervaporation (E)
liquid membrane (M)

size & shape — molecular sieves (M)
← size exclusion chromatography (M)   → filtration/demister
clathration (M)   centrifuge (filtering)
← ultrafiltration (M)   → microfiltration (M)

Property Differences	Molecules	Macromolecule	Particles
electric	← ion exchange (M)	→	
charge	← ion exchange chromatography (M)	→	
	ion exclusion (M)		
electric charge	← electrodialysis (E)	→	
& mobility	← electrophoresis (E)	→	
	← isotachophoresis (E)	→	
electric mobility	← immunoelectrophoresis (M+E)	→	
& chem. rxn	← affinity electrophoresis (M+E)	→	
surface	GSC (M)		
adsorption	← TLC (M)	→	
	← LC (M)	→	
	adsorption (M or E)		
	← foam fractionation (M)	→	
adsorption and shape	molecular sieves (M)		
adsorption & charge	← paper chromatography (M)	→	

adsorption & diffusivity	carbon sieves (M)
hydrophobic interaction	← hydrophobic chromatography (M)
rate of evaporation	molecular distillation (E)
diffusivity	gas diffusion (M + E)
electric mobility & size	← electrochromatography (M + E) (w. SEC)
electric mobility & adsorption	← electrochromatography (M) (w. adsorption)
reversible chem. rxn	absorption/stripping (M)
	liquid membrane (M)
	extraction (M)
	dual-temperature exchange (M)
	← affinity chromatography (M)
irreversible chem. rxn	absorption (M)

Property Differences	Molecules	Macromolecule	Particles
density & size		ultracentrifuge (E)	settling centrifuge (sedimentation) cyclone sink-float decanter
magnetic		high gradient mag. separation	magnetic separator
surface wettability			floatation
electrical conductivity			electrostatic separator
thermal diffusivity	thermal diffusion (E)		
isoelectric point	← isolectric focusing (M+E)	→	
molecular wt.	← SDS electrophoresis (M+E)	→	

linear adsorption or chromatographic systems $\alpha_{i,j}$ is the ratio of equilibrium constants.

$$\alpha_{ij} = \frac{A_i}{A_j} = \frac{k_i'}{k_j'} \qquad (14\text{-}2)$$

For eutectic crystallization systems in the concentration range where a pure species is in equilibrium with the eutectic the inherent separation factor is infinite.

For non-equilibrium processes the inherent separation factor can always be determined experimentally. The inherent separation factor is again defined by Eq. (14-1), but $x_{i,1}$ is now the mole fraction of species i in product 1, and the two product streams are not in equilibrium with each other. In certain cases where simplifying assumptions can be made $\alpha_{i,j}$ can be estimated. For example, for reverse osmosis irreversible thermodynamics arguments were used in Chapter 13 to estimate the change in salt concentration across a membrane. If Eq. (13-83) is combined with Eq. (14-1) and we assume that the water distribution coefficient $K_w = K_1$ is the same on both sides of the membrane, we obtain

$$\alpha_{w,s} = \frac{c_{w,p} / c_{w,waste}}{c_{s,p} / c_{s,waste}} = \frac{D_{w,m} K_w v_w (\Delta p - \Delta \pi)}{D_{s,m} K_s RT} \qquad (14\text{-}3)$$

where terms are defined in Chapter 13.

The value of the separation factor required before the separation method is of interest depends on several factors. The ease of multistaging is very important. In this context multistaging means that the separation acheived can be multiplied many times and the separation agent can be reused. A packed bed chromatograph and a packed bed distillation column are both multistage systems even though no physical stages are present. Equilibrium processes such as distillation, adsorption and chromatography can easily be operated with many stages, and the separation agent can be reused many times with low additional capital investment. Thus the separation acheived with a low separation factor can easily be multiplied many times in an economical fashion. Other equilibrium processes such as crystallization can be staged, but the staging is not nearly as convenient. Membrane processes can be staged (operated in series), but the low pressure product needs to be repressurized after each stage and a new module is needed. Thus staging is not easy. The easier staging, the lower the inherent separation factor can be. As a rough guide the ease of staging is

$$\text{adsorption, chromatography} > \text{distillation} > \text{crystallization} > \text{membrane} \quad (14\text{-}4)$$

In addition to ease of staging we prefer energy separation processes compared to mass separation agent processes since an additional separation is not automatically required. This choice favors distillation, crystallization and membrane processes.

Ultimately, the choice of separation method usually depends upon economics (occassionally government regulations control the choice). Energy use is important and the low energy use of the membrane processes is one of their most appealing features; however, energy is not the only important factor. Keller (1982) and Ho and Keller (1987) show that for distillation the per year cost of capital is equal or greater than the energy cost. This is significant since distillation is normally considered to be a low capital, high energy process. Thus, capital costs must be included. Energy criteria for selecting separation processes are discussed in more detail in Section 14.3. Since capital costs are important, simple systems are favored. This favors distillation, absorption, and membranes. Very complex processes such as displacement adsorption and electrophoresis tend to be used only when necessary. Some rough guidelines for chosing processes are given in Section 14.5.

Distillation keeps appearing in the list of possible alternatives. Distillation is an energy separating agent process which is easy to stage and simple to construct. The design principles are well understood and many companies will bid to design and build distillation systems. Distillation has good economy of scale and can be operated in very large sizes. Two pure products can be recovered, and the principles for sequencing columns have been extensively

809

studied. Although energy use may be high, the energy is usually supplied by low pressure steam which is often very cheap. The net result is that if distillation can be used it should be considered as one of the alternatives. Guidelines for when distillation cannot be used are discussed in Section 14.5.

Example 14-1. Generation of Possible Separation Processes

Generate possible separations to separate ethanol from water.

Solution

A. Define. This problem was purposely ill-defined. The choice of separation process will depend upon:

  a. The purpose of the separation. Do we want pure ethanol or the azeotrope, or is it a pollution control problem?

  b. The feed concentration.

  c. The scale of operation.

  d. Presence of other components.

To further define the problem assume a fermentation process is used to produce approximately an 8 wt% ethanol in water mixture. We want a water waste stream which can be discarded and pure (99.9%) ethanol. Both small and large plants should be considered. For now, the trace contaminants such as glycerol will be ignored.

B. and C. Explore and Plan. There are obviously a variety of ways to proceed. For this example we will consider the physical property differences listed in Table 14-1 to develop possible separation methods.

D. **Do It.** We will list the physical property and the separation methods that result.

1. *Relative Volatility:* Vapor-liquid equilibrium data is readily available (e.g. Seader, 1984; Wankat, 1988). At low concentrations the relative volatility is quite high (~ 12); however, there is an azeotrope at 0.894 mole fraction ethanol at 1 atm pressure. Thus *distillation* can produce pure water and the azeotrope, and is a commercial method. The azeotrope contains less water as the pressure is decreased (Seader, 1984). At 70 mm Hg the azeotrope disappears. Thus *distillation* at 70 mm Hg could be used, but does not appear to be economically feasible (Black, 1980).

2. Relative volatility and chemical interaction. *Azeotropic distillation* is commonly used to break the azeotrope. A hydrocarbon entrainer such as pentane or benzene can be used to form a heterogeneous, ternary azeotrope overhead (e.g., Black, 1980; Seader, 1984; Wankat, 1988). Extractive distillation can also be used (Black, 1980), but unlike azeotropic distillation is not a commercial process.

3. Distribution between two liquids. Equilibrium data is available in several sources such as Leeper and Wankat (1982); and Roddy (1981). Liquid-liquid extraction can be used to either extract the ethanol from the azeotrope (Leeper and Wankat, 1982) or extract ethanol from the feed. The first may be economical while the second does not appear to be economically feasible.

4. Melting point. Data is available in the *Handbook of Chemistry and Physics* and *Lange's Handbook of Chemistry*. Addition of ethanol to water causes a significant freezing point depression (-51.3°C at 71.9 wt% ethanol). Freezing can be used for removing water at low ethanol concentrations although a countercurrent wash column (see Chapter 5) will

be needed. This method might be useful for breaking the azeotrope, but more data is needed.

5 Solubility and diffusivity. Membranes can be fabricated which preferentially pass either water or ethanol. Some data was given in Chapter 12. Reverse osmosis can be used to preconcentrate a dilute feed, but by itself cannot produce pure ethanol. Pervaporation units are available commercially for breaking the azeotrope (see Chapter 12).

6. Surface adsorption. Adsorbents will show preference for either ethanol or water. Activated carbon preferentially adsorbs ethanol and is used for ethanol recovery from air while activated alumina, corn grits, starches and molecular sieves prefer water. Cornmeal is used commercially for breaking the azeotrope (Ladisch, et al., 1984). Operation is in the vapor phase.

7. Adsorption and shape. 3A molecular sieves exclude ethanol and adsorb water (Garg and Ausikaitis, 1983). This method is used commercially for breaking the azeotrope operating with a vapor.

8. Rate of evaporation. Water will evaporate more rapidly and thus molecular distillation could be used, but will be very expensive.

9. Chromatography. Both GLC and LLC work with a variety of packings and are used for analysis. They are likely to be expensive, but could be considered for breaking the azeotrope.

E. Check. Data can be checked from other sources, but this is probably not necessary for an initial list like this.

F. Generalization. This list is not inclusive. It certainly does not include all possible solvents, entrainers and adsorbents. A detailed literature search will generate additional information. This list does show that there are a variety of possibilities several of which compete commerically. Also, use of an organized list such as Table 14-1 is a good method to generate possible separation schemes.

14.3. ENERGY CRITERIA

Energy requirements for separation processes are discussed in many sources (Ho and Keller, 1987; Keller, 1982; King, 1980; Null, 1980; Robinson and Gilliland, 1950). In this section we will first discuss minimum work requirements for separations, and then compare the equivalent work required for some separation processes. Before starting, we will reiterate that energy use is only one of the criteria used in selecting a separation process.

14.3.1. Minimum Work

The minimum reversible work required for the complete separation of a mixture of ideal gases is (Keller, 1982)

$$W_{min,T} = RT \sum_{i=1}^{c} \left[y_{i,F} \ln \left[p_p / y_{i,F} \, p_F \right] \right] \qquad (14\text{-}5)$$

If the feed, p_F, and product, p_p, pressures are equal this result simplifies to

$$W_{min,T,p} = -RT \sum_{i=1}^{c} (y_{i,F} \ln y_{i,F}) \qquad (14\text{-}6)$$

For the separation of a mixture of nonideal liquids the result is

$$W_{min,T,p} = -RT \sum_{i=1}^{c} \left[x_{i,F} \ln (\gamma_i \, x_{i,F}) \right] \qquad (14\text{-}7)$$

These results are easily derived by postulating a reversible process. One way of doing this is to postulate the existence of perfect semipermeable membranes which will pass one component but none of the other components

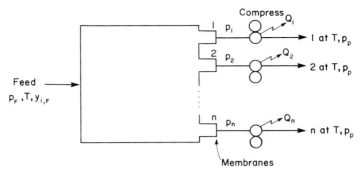

Figure 14-3.   Reversible membrane separation process for calculating minimum work.

(Keller, 1982). This process is illustrated in Figure 14-3. After passing through the membranes, the gases are completely pure but are at reduced pressures.

$$p_i = y_{i,F} \, p_F \qquad (14-8)$$

Each of these gas streams is compressed isothermally to the product pressure p_p. For an ideal gas the reversible work required to isothermally compress one mole from $p_{initial}$ to p_{final} is

$$W_{rev} = RT \ln (p_{final} \, / \, p_{initial}) \qquad (14-9)$$

Since $p_{final} = p_p$ and $p_{i,initial} = p_i$ in Eq. (14-8), the reversible work for one gas is

$$W_{rev,i} = RT \ln (p_p \, / \, y_{i,F} \, p_F) \qquad (14-10)$$

The total reversible (and hence minimum) work for the separation is the sum of $W_{rev,i}$ for all components. The result is Eq. (14-5). More detailed developments which include partial separation and nonisothermal operation are given by King (1980).

The minimum work required for any separation is easily determined. This is illustrated in Example 14-2.

Example 14-2. Minimum Work of Separation

We wish to separate a liquid mixture of ethylbenzene and styrene at 110°C. Determine $W_{min,T,p}$ for mole fractions ethylbenzene of 0, 10, 20, ..., 100 in the feed.

Solution

Since the liquid can be assumed to be ideal, $\gamma_i = 1$. Then Eq. (14-7) becomes

$$W_{min,T,p} = -RT \left[x_E \ln x_E + (1-x_E) \ln (1-x_E) \right] \qquad (14\text{-}11)$$

for this ideal binary mixture. For this problem,

R = 1.9872 cal/gmole K, T = 383.16 K.

As an example, for a 0.1 mole fraction ethylbenzene feed

$W_{min,T,p}(0.10) = -(1.9872)(383.16)[0.1 \ln 0.1 + 0.9 \ln 0.9]$

$= 247.52$ cal/gmole feed

The remaining results are similiar and are listed in the Table.

$x_{E,F}$	$W_{min,T,p}$ (cal/gmole feed)	$W_{min,prod}$ (cal/gmole EB prod)
0	0	--
0.1	247.52	2475.2
0.2	381.01	1905.1
0.3	465.12	1550.4
0.4	512.44	1281.1
0.5	527.77	1055.5
0.6	512.44	854.1
0.7	465.12	664.5
0.8	381.01	476.3
0.9	247.52	275.0
1.0	0	0

Note that the minimum work required to separate a 0.0 and a 1.0 mole fraction feed are both zero since these feeds are already pure. The minimum work required for separation per mole of feed is symmetric around a feed mole fraction of 0.5. For nonideal liquids this will not be true. The third column in the table is of considerable interest since it shows the minimum energy required per mole of ethylbenzene product. As expected, this value decreases as the feed becomes more concentrated in ethylbenzene.

The energy requirements calculated in Example 14-2 seem quite reasonable. The minimum work of separation is easily calculated and gives a simple first approach to compare the difficulty of different separations. Unfortunately, the fractional efficiency (W_{min}/W_{actual}) of most separation processes ranges from a few percent to about twenty percent (Keller, 1982). Since distillation is a benchmark process which other processes are compared to, it is interesting to look at the maximum efficiency of distillation processes. This is shown in Figure 14-4 (Ho and Keller, 1987) for a simple distillation column producing two pure products at minimum reflux. Actual columns must operate above the minimum reflux ratio and the real efficiency will be 5 to 20% lower than the values shown in Figure 14-4 (Ho and Keller, 1987).

Further research is required on the minimum energy requirements for some of the more complex processes. In addition, research is required on how the minimum energy requirements can be incorporated into a search for the best separation method for a given problem.

14.3.2. Equivalent Work Requirements

Equations (14-5) to (14-11) determine the minimum mechanical work requirement. Many separations use heat instead of mechanical work as the energy source. In order to compare different processes we will calculate the *equivalent work* which is the work which could have been obtained by a reversible heat engine. This equivalent work can be calculated from (Null, 1980)

$$W_{eq} = Q \left[\frac{T - T_o}{T} \right] \varepsilon_p \qquad (14-12)$$

816

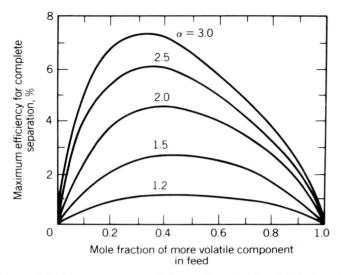

Figure 14-4.   Maximum energy efficiency for simple distillation (Ho and Keller, 1987). Reprinted with permission from Y.A. Liu, H.A. McGee and W.R. Epperly (Eds.), *Recent Developments in Chemical Process and Plant Design*, Wiley-Interscience, 1987. Copyright 1987, Wiley-Interscience.

where Q is the heat supplied at absolute temperature T and the surroundings are at T_o. The efficiency ε_p is the power cycle efficiency compared to a Carnot cycle. From this definition of equivalent work Null (1980) derives approximate equations for the energy requirements of several commercial separation processes. The following development is based on Null's (1980) development.

Consider first a simple *distillation* column with one feed, a condenser, and a reboiler. The approximate energy requirements are

$$Q_R = |Q_c| = D \lambda (R_D + 1) \qquad (14\text{-}13)$$

where Q_R and Q_c are the reboiler and condenser heat loads, respectively; D is the distillate product rate; λ is the latent heat of vaporization of the distillate product; and $R_D = L/D$ is the external reflux ratio. Combining Eqs. (14-12) and

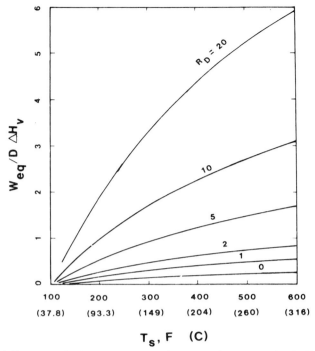

Figure 14-5.   Equivalent work requirement for normal distillation. T_o = 37.8°C (Null, 1980). Reprinted with permission from *Chem. Eng. Prog.*, *76*(8), 42 (1980). Copyright 1980, American Institute of Chemical Engineers.

(14-13), we can determine the equivalent work required for simple distillation.

$$W_{eq,dist} = D \lambda (R_D + 1) \varepsilon_p \frac{(T_s - T_o)}{T_s} \qquad (14\text{-}14)$$

where T_s is the temperature of the steam used to supply the heat. Note that T_s > $T_{reboiler}$ since some temperature difference is necessary for heat transfer. T_o is the temperature of the cooling water used. The predicted equivalent work values normalized by $D\lambda$ are given in Figure 14-5 (Null, 1980). Null (1980) also presents results for somewhat more complicated distillation columns.

Although the relative volatility does not appear explicitly in Eq. (14-14) or Figure 14-5, α is an important parameter in determining W_{eq} since α controls the required external reflux ratio. The value of W_{eq} for distillation can now be compared to the results for other processes.

Melt crystallization is analogous to distillation with the solid crystals taking the place of the liquid in distillation, and the melt taking the place of the vapor. Processes were shown in Figures 5-4, 5-5, and 5-6. Consider the center feed system shown in Figure 5-5. In the melter the approximate amount of energy required to melt all the crystals is

$$Q_M = B_c \, (R_M + 1) \, \lambda_f \qquad (14\text{-}15)$$

where B_c is the bottoms product of melted crystals, λ_f is the latent heat of freezing, and R_M is the external reflux ratio for the melter. If the heat is supplied to the melter at temperature T_{sM} where $T_{sM} > T_M$, then the equivalent work for the heated end of the crystallizer is

$$W_{eq,M} = B_c \, \varepsilon_p \, (R_M + 1) \, \lambda_f \, \frac{(T_{sM} - T_o)}{T_{sM}} \qquad (14\text{-}16)$$

where T_o is the ambient temperature of the surroundings. At the cooled end of the crystallizer approximately the same amount of heat is removed. Usually, refrigeration will be required to form the crystals for reflux. The refrigeration is required at temperature T_c. Then the equivalent work for cooling is

$$W_{eq,cool} = B_c \, (R_M + 1) \, \lambda_f \, \frac{(T_o - T_c)}{T_o \, \varepsilon_R} \qquad (14\text{-}17)$$

where ε_R is the Carnot cycle efficiency of the refrigeration system. The total equivalent work for the melt crystallization process is the sum of Eqs. (14-16) and (14-17).

$$W_{eq,cry} = B_c \, (R_M + 1) \, \lambda_f \left[\frac{\varepsilon_p(T_{sM} - T_o)}{T_{sM}} + \frac{(T_o - T_c)}{T_o \, \varepsilon_R} \right] \qquad (14\text{-}18)$$

Based on energy considerations only, we can now compare crystallization to simple distillation by comparing the equivalent work terms from Eqs. (14-18) and (14-14). Crystallization will be preferred on an energy basis if $W_{eq,cry} < W_{eq,dist}$ which occurs if

$$R_D > (R_M+1) \frac{\lambda_f}{\lambda} \frac{B_c}{D} \left[\left[\frac{T_{sM}-T_o}{T_s-T_o} \right] \frac{T_s}{T_{sM}} + \frac{1}{\varepsilon_p \varepsilon_R} \left[\frac{T_o-T_c}{T_s-T_o} \right] \left[\frac{T_s}{T_o} \right] \right] - 1 \quad (14-19)$$

Null (1980) shows some step-by-step simplifications. If $B_c = D$ (same amount of product), $T_s = T_{sM}$ (normally $T_s > T_{sM}$), and cooling can be done with normal cooling water ($T_c = T_o$), then Eq. (14-19) becomes

$$R_D > (R_M + 1) (\lambda_f / \lambda) - 1 \quad (14-20)$$

Since latent heats of freezing are typically about 1/5 of the latent heat of vaporization, Eqs. (14-19) and (14-20) often show an energy advantage for crystallization. However, Fair (1987) notes, "The specific energy advantages of crystallization have not been a factor in its selection for commercial use." These results do show the potential of crystallization particularly if energy costs escalate.

Temperature swing adsorption of gases is another process which is amenable to this type of analysis. Assuming that the column is adiabatic and that the energy required to heat the column itself is small, we obtain a simplified energy balance for the energy required for regeneration.

$$Q_{reg} = \left[C_{p,sorb} + C_{p,B} / q_{avg}) (T_{reg} - T_{ads}) + \Delta H_{ads} \right] \psi N_{ads} = \xi N_{ads} \quad (14-21)$$

where $C_{p,sorb}$ and $C_{p,B}$ are the heat capacities of the sorbate and the bulk adsorbent in kJ/kgmole K and kJ/kg adsorbent K, respectively, and q_{avg} is the average adsorbed phase loading at the end of the feed step. For a symmetric mass transfer zone,

$$q_{avg} = q_{sat} (L - 0.5 L_{MTZ}) / L \quad (14-22)$$

ψ in Eq. (14-21) is a factor to account for the use of excess regeneration gas, T_{ads} is the average bed temperature at the end of the feed step, T_{reg} is the average temperature of the bed after the regeneration step, ΔH_{ads} is the heat of adsorption in kJ/kgmole, N_{ads} is the average rate the adsorbate product is produced in kgmole/hr. Then ξ is the total regeneration heat required per kg mole adsorbed.

Combining Eqs. (14-12) and (14-21), we obtain the equivalent work required

$$W_{eq,ads} = \xi \, N_{ads} \, \varepsilon_p \, (T_{RG} - T_o) \, / \, T_{RG} \tag{14-23}$$

where T_{RG} is the supply temperature of the regeneration gas, $T_{RG} > T_{reg}$. This result can be compared to Eq. (14-14) for distillation. Adsorption uses less equivalent work when

$$R_D > \left[\frac{N_{ads}}{D} \right] \left[\frac{\xi}{\lambda} \right] \left[\frac{T_s}{T_{RG}} \right] \left[\frac{T_{RG} - T_o}{T_s - T_o} \right] - 1 \tag{14-24}$$

Usually, $\Delta H_{ads} > \lambda$, and hence $\xi/\lambda >> 1$. Adsorption typically adsorbs the least volatile component. Thus, N_{ads}/D corresponds to B/D if either adsorption or distillation can do a separation. Adsorption will be favored if B/D is small which means that a small amount of nonvolatile material is to be removed. Adsorption is also favored if distillation is difficult and a large reflux ratio is required. Null's (1980) numerical results are shown in Figure 14-6.

Reverse osmosis directly uses mechanical energy and the work required is easily calculated. The mechanical work required is the volumetric flow rate times the pressure increase. Although the entire feed stream is pressurized, part of the mechanical work can be recovered from the high pressure waste stream. Only the permeate product is completely degraded. Assuming that the permeate pressure and feed pressures (before pressurizing) are the same, we obtain

$$W_{RO} = P \, \Delta p \tag{14-25}$$

where P is the volumetric flow rate of permeate product and Δp is the pressure

821

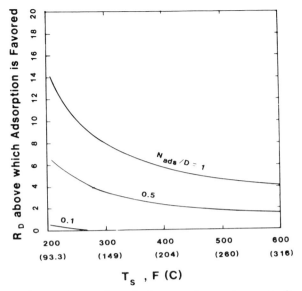

Figure 14-6.   Comparison of equivalent work requirements for temperature
swing adsorption with regeneration at 316°C versus simple distillation (Null, 1980). Reprinted with permission from *Chem.
Eng. Prog.*, *76*(8), 42 (1980). Copyright 1980, American Institute of Chemical Engineers.

drop across the membrane. We have also assumed that the efficiency of energy
recovery from the high pressure waste stream is 100%. Obviously, Δp must be
greater than the osmotic pressure difference. From Eq. (12-27) Δp can be
related to the volumetric solvent flux $J_{solv} = P/A$ and the osmotic pressure
difference

$$\Delta p = \frac{P/A}{K_{solv} / t_m} + M \pi (c_b) - \pi (c_p) \tag{14-26}$$

where π is the osmotic pressure, A is the membrane area, and M is the concentration polarization modulus. Combining these equations, we obtain

$$W_{RO} = P \left[\frac{J/A}{K_{solv} / t_m} + M \pi (c_b) - \pi (c_p) \right] \tag{14-27}$$

The work required is inversely proportional to the permeability of the membrane which is a rate constant. Thus, the work requirements depend upon the membrane rate properties in addition to physical properties. This differs from previous results obtained for equilibrium processes where rate properties do not enter into the equivalent work expressions. Note that one must be careful with units in Eqs. (14-25) and (14-17). In SI units W_{RO} will be in J/S.

With reasonable values for fluxes and permeabilities the work calculated from Eqs. (14-25) or (14-27) is very low when compared to the equilibrium processes which involve a phase change (note that there is no latent heat term in these equations). Thus, from an energy point of view reverse osmosis and the other membrane separations are very appealing. However, RO is not a complete separation process since the reject stream is a concentrated solute in solvent, and cannot be pure solute. The concentration of the reject stream is limited by the osmotic pressure which increases rapidly at high concentrations. If a complete separation of solute and solvent is required then RO can be advantageously coupled with another separation method in a *hybrid* process.

Further research is required to determine the equivalent work requirements for more complex separation processes. Also, methods for using the equivalent work results to aid in the selection of the appropriate separation process are needed.

14.4. STRATEGY OF PROCESS DESIGN AND SYNTHESIS

The appropriate strategy to use for process design and synthesis has been extensively studied recently (Douglas, 1988; Rudd et al, 1973; Westerberg, 1982). We will follow Westerberg (1982) and present some guidelines without examples. Detailed examples are given in these references, and in Blumberg (1988) for liquid-liquid extraction.

Westerberg (1982) presents five guidelines for attacking design problems.

1. Evolve from simple to complex calculations.

   Use approximate calculation methods initially. So many changes will be made in the design that the use of complex and time-consuming detailed calculation methods is unecessary. Douglas (1988) discusses short-cut calculation methods for equilibrium staged processes. Detailed calculation methods should be used in the later stages of design.

2. Quickly develop a complete feasible solution.

This is a *depth first* approach and requires that one avoid backtracking to improve the design of subproblems. The first feasible design should be considered to be a learning experience. It shows where the easy and where the difficult steps are. It may even show that the entire project probably cannot be done economically with existing technology. It serves as a guide for later backtracking to improve steps. Douglas (1988) considers this step in detail.

3. Develop approximate criteria for screening among alternatives.

It is not possible to determine if one has a good design until one has a design. It is also impossible to evaluate the criteria which will be used to assess the design without a completed design. To avoid this dilemma one should use aproximate criteria and heuristics (see Section 14.5.) to obtain an initial design.

4. Alternate between global and detailed solutions.

A global approach is needed to keep the overall goal of the design in mind. This goal is then partitioned into subgoals which are further subdivided into additional subgoals until one obtains subgoals which can be designed without further partitioning. This is known as a *top-down* approach. Once the lowest level subgoals have been identified, detailed design using approximate, short-cut methods is done. Initially, the purpose of this design is to find those subgoals which preclude obtaining an economic solution. This is called a *bottom-up* approach. If any impossible subgoals are found one returns to the global design and makes appropriate changes. Some sort of strategy such as heuristics or an evolutionary approach (see Section 14.6.) should be used for generating the next global design.

5. When trying to prove that concepts will not work, use optimistic conditions. Most initial design concepts will not work. During the screening process the designer's job is to prove things will not work or cannot be economic. This type of comparison is convincing only when optimistic guesses are made (e.g. make the optimistic guesses that there is no entrainment in a crystallization process or that there is no concentration polarization in a membrane separation). If one were conservative in making the guesses, the failure of the design might be due to the guess and one does not have a clear reason for rejecting the design.

14.5 HEURISTICS

Heuristics are rules of thumb which allow us to make preliminary choices in complicated situations without doing a large number of detailed calculations. The use of heuristics for general selection of separation processes has been considered by Douglas (1988), Hendry *et al* (1973), Keller (1982), Kelly (1987), King (1980), Liu (1987), Nishida *et al* (1981), and Rudd *et al* (1973) among others. The heuristics have been most highly developed for distillation. Some work on heuristics has been done for modifications of distillation such as azeotropic and extractive distillation, and for absorption and extraction. Only the heuristics for sequencing distillation systems have been rigorously tested. The other heuristics appear to be valid, and have received some modest testing.

One problem with heuristics is that different heuristics often conflict with each other. Then the proper choice of heuristic is unclear. All of the heuristics should be preceeded with the words, " If all things are equal ..." Liu (1987) has rank ordered heuristics for distillation and modified distillation systems.

In this section a large number of possible heuristics for the selection and sequencing of separations will be listed and the reasoning for the heuristic will be explained. These heuristics were developed either by generalizing the heuristics developed for the equilibrium staged separations or from comments in the literature. Except for the distillation heuristics, these heuristics have not been rigorously tested and should always be checked with calculations.

14.5.1. G. General and Flowsheet Heuristics

1G. Always generate more than one alternative separation method or sequence.
Although not usually explicitly stated, this idea is inherent in the ideas of process synthesis and good problem solving practice.

2G. In developing a flow sheet select the separation schemes first before adjusting temperatures or flow rates.
This heuristic is stated by Rudd et al (1973) and Kelly (1987). Compared to temperature and flow rate adjustment separations are much more expensive and require more energy. Thus, the separation problems should receive priority.

3G. Reduce the separation load by splitting streams, blending or mixing as appropriate.
This heuristic applies to the development of flow sheets and was stated by Rudd et al (1973) and Kelly (1987).

4G. Favor schemes which give the smallest product set.
This heuristic states that components which will eventually be in the same product should not be separated. This heuristic was listed by Kelly (1987), King (1980), Liu (1987), Nath and Motard (1981) and Thompson and King (1972) and others. Nath and Motard (1981) consider this the primary heuristic while Liu (1987) ranks it third. If extended to chromatography it implies that components which will be lumped together as a waste stream should not be separated.

5G. Do not produce purer products than required.
This can be considered as a corollary of heuristic 4G.

6G. Do not remix partially separated streams.
If components are ultimately to be separated, any partial separation should be retained since remixing is an increase in entropy. Although not explicitly stated elsewhere, this heuristic is a generalization of common practices such as the use of two-feed distillation columns, "super-loading" in adsorption columns, and segregated recycle in chromatography.

7G. Consider using the standard separation methods of the industry.

These methods may not be optimum, but they will probably give a working base case. This heuristic is often standard operating procedure, but should always be used in conjuction with heuristic #1G.

8G. Favor separation methods which are known within the company.

The separation methods which the company is familiar with will require the least design and development time. These methods will also be easiest to sell to management. Heuristic #1G should not be forgotten when applying this heuristic.

9G. For new products look for separations which can be put on stream quickly. With new products the company which gets to the market first often captures a large proportion of the market. Thus, separation schemes which will take a long time to develop are not favored for the first plant. Known separation processes will be favored (See heuristics 7G and 8G).

10G. Consider hybrid plants when one separation method by itself is not ideal for a given separation problem.

Hybrid plants use two or more separations for the same problem. An example would be concentrating a stream by reverse osmosis before doing evaporation even though evaporation by itself could do the separation. Hybrid plants can utilize the strength of a separation in the concentration range where it is best, and avoid weaknesses.

14.5.2. D. Design Heuristics

1D. Favor separations using energy separation agents.

These separations do not add anything to the mixture to be separated. This heuristic is explicitly stated by Liu (1987) and is first in his ordered list. This heuristic leads to heuristic 1S (favor distillation).

2D. If a mass separating agent is used remove it early and do not use a mass separating agent to recover a mass separating agent.

This heuristic is commonly stated (Kelly, 1987; Liu, 1987; Nath and Motard, 1981; Rudd et al, 1973). It probably does not strictly apply when solutes must be dissolved in a solvent so that they can be processed. Rudd et al (1973) also suggest considering the use of a chemical already present in the process even if it is not optimum based on its properties alone.

3D. Prefer processes with only one and not two mass separating agents.
The use of an additional mass separating agent such as a gradient in chromatography makes the downstream recovery more difficult. However, Mazsaroff and Regnier (1986) note that gradients are required for elution of macromolecules when separation is due to surface forces.

4D. Avoid excursions in temperature and pressure.
Both very high and very low temperatures should be avoided, but when necessary go high not low (Kelly, 1987; King 1980; Liu, 1987; Rudd et al, 1973). This implies that vacuum distillation and distillation with refrigeration are less likely to be economical. It also favors PSA over VSA. This heuristic also shows a preference for liquid chromatography instead of gas chromatography since LC operates at lower temperatures. Both pervaporation (which uses a vacuum) and low temperature crystallization are contraindicated.

5D. Do the cheapest separation next.
This heuristic was developed by Thompson and King (1972) and is also used by Douglas (1988). The reasoning is that every separation method used reduces the volume of material to be processed; thus the more expensive separations will process less material and will cost less. Although the use of this heuristic alone may not give optimum flowsheets, it does appear to generate reasonably good flowsheets quickly. However, this heuristic was tested only with distillation type separations. Heuristics 7S and 8S for adsorption and chromatography follow this heuristic.

6D. Avoid solids and if they are present remove them early.
Solids cause processing problems. Separations involving solids (e.g. adsorption and chromatography) are difficult to operate as countercurrent processes.

7D. When a solid material needs to be processed consider putting the sample into solution and removing insolubles to be a separation step.

This heuristic is explicitly stated for chromatography by McDonald and Bidlingmeyer (1987), but can be extended to any process such as extraction, crystallization, or adsorption where solids are first dissolved.

8D. Consider side withdrawals for sloppy splits.

Sloppy splits are problems where the product does not have to be of high purity. This heuristic was developed by Tedder and Rudd (1978) for distillation, but can be extended to other separations. For example, a side withdrawal for column switching of chromatography (see Figure 7-16) is roughly analogous to a side withdrawal in distillation. Side withdrawals would be relatively easy to use in fractional extraction or crystallization. A single cascade with a side withdrawal will be quite inexpensive when the side withdrawal can produce the desired purity.

14.5.3. C. Component and Composition Heuristics

1C. Remove corrosive, hazardous, and unstable compounds early.

This heuristic is commonly stated (Douglas, 1988; Kelly, 1987; Liu, 1987; Rudd *et al*, 1973). Corrosive materials often require expensive materials of construction, and overall cost can be reduced by removing these components early. Hazardous materials may require special conditions and also cost more to process. Unstable compounds decompose less if they are removed early. In particular, reactive monomers and proteases should be removed early.

2C. Do the difficult separations last.

The difficult separations will require the longest column. It usually makes sense to do these separations with no other compounds present unless these other components change the equilibrium and make the separation easier. This heuristic has been commonly presented for both equilibrium stage separations (Douglas, 1988; Kelly, 1987; Liu, 1987; Rudd *et al*, 1973) and for chromatography (Guiochon and Colin, 1986; McDonald and Bidlingmeyer, 1987; Wankat, 1986). Nath and Motard (1981) state that the "easiest separation should be done first", which is essentially the inverse.

3C. Do high recovery and high purity separations last.
This heuristic is closely related to heuristic 2C and is based on the same reasoning.

4C. Remove most plentiful component next.
This heuristic was developed for distillation (Douglas,1988; Kelly, 1987; Liu, 1987; Rudd *et al*, 1973) but is probably applicable to other separations as well. Use of this heuristic reduces the load on downstream processes.

5C. If component compositions are similiar, favor 50/50 splits or equal size parts.
This was also derived for distillation and serves to balance the distillation column (Douglas, 1988; Kelly, 1987; Liu, 1987; Rudd *et al*, 1973). Its use for other separations is not clear.

6C. In organic systems remove water early.
In organic systems water often causes significant problems due to immiscibility (in distillation), freezing out (in crystallization), or strong adsorption (in adsorption). Thus, removing the water early even though it may be only a trace component is often good practice.

14.5.4. S. Separation Specific Heuristics

1S. Favor distillation unless $\alpha < \alpha_{critical}$.
This heuristic is commonly stated, but the value of $\alpha_{critical}$ varies. Null (1987) uses $\alpha_{critical} = 1.05$, Nath and Motard (1981) and Douglas (1988) use $\alpha_{critical} = 1.10$, for comparison with adsorption Ruthven (1984) uses $\alpha_{critical} = 1.25$ while Keller (1982) uses a range from 1.2 to 1.5.

2S. In distillation remove products as distillates.
This heuristic is commonly stated (Douglas, 1988; Kelly, 1987; Rudd *et al*, 1973). The reason is that most degradation products have high boiling points and will appear in the bottoms. Thus, distillate products are more likely to be pure. This heuristic can be extended to other separations (see Problem 14-A11).

3S. If the product is sold as a solid the last purification step should probably be crystallization.
Crystallization can be used both to produce crystals with the desired size distribution and as a final polishing step.

4S. Start considering adsorption instead of distillation when have:

   a. $\alpha < 1.2$ to 1.5.

   b. An azeotrope forms.

   c. light gases

   d. α_{ads} is very high

   e. feed is dilute (< 10 to 25% of product). This is particularly important if the product is the heavier component.

   f. product is thermally unstable

   g. there are two sets of compounds with boiling point overlap. Note that extraction is also commonly used in this case.
This set of heuristics is from Keller (1982).

5S. Consider temperature swing adsorption if adsorbate concentration in the feed is < 5 mole%.
Keller (1982) notes that energy costs in TSA can be very high and they increase as the adsorbate concentration in the feed increases.

6S. Consider displacement adsorption only when $\alpha_{ads} > 2$ and $\alpha_{dist} < 1.2$ to 1.3.
Keller (1982) notes that displacement adsorption processes are quite complex, and the process should be considered as a last resort.

7S. In adsorption and chromatography consider methods with cheap packings first.
This heuristic is related to heuristic 5D. For adsorption this heuristic favors activated carbon. For chromatography it favors plain silica, activated alumina, or ion exchange chromatography systems.

8S. In adsorption and chromatography use expensive packings last.
This is common practice particularly with HPLC and affinity chromatography where the packing can be very expensive. Using the expensive packing last means that the solution is cleaner and is less likely to foul the packing.

9S. Chromatography is expensive - use it only when necessary.
This heuristic is stated by McDonald and Bidlingmeyer (1987).

10S. In large scale liquid chromatography always optimize the solvent stationary phase system.
McDonald and Bidlingmeyer (1987) note that the selectivity α is the most important parameter, and increasing α by optimization is well worth the effort. However, Kopaciewicz and Regnier (1983) note that solvents need to be compatible for chromatography columns in series or an extra separation will be required between columns. Solvent selection is also very important in absorption (Keller, 1982), azeotropic and extractive distillation (Van Winkle, 1967; Wankat, 1988), and extraction (Blumberg, 1988; King, 1981).

11S. Consider large-scale gas-liquid chromatography instead of distillation if $\alpha < 1.10$. If $\alpha > 1.2$ prefer distillation or vacuum distillation.
This heuristic was stated by Bonmati et al (1984). However, note that liquid chromatography will also be a competing process and LC has been more successful for large-scale applications.

12S. Do ultrafiltration or microfiltration before reverse osmosis.
This heuristic is implied by many process flow sheets. The reasons are that UF and microfiltration are better able to handle feeds containing particulates, and they have has higher fluxes. Thus the UF or microfiltration system will protect the RO system and will decrease the volume which has to be processed by the RO system.

13S. Consider RO for preconcentration of dilute aqueous streams in a hybrid process.
This is one of the classical uses of hybrid processes and is often done with RO followed by evaporation.

14S. If hydrogen or carbon dioxide need to be purified, consider gas permeation.

With currently available membranes these two gases have the highest permeabilities, and these applications have now been widely commercialized.

As was noted at the beginning of this section many of these heuristics have not been rigorously tested. In addition, an ordering of these heuristics for nondistillation applications is needed. This implies that considerable research is needed. In the meantime the heuristics must be used with caution.

Example 14-3. Use of Heuristics

Use heuristics to generate preliminary separation flowsheets for Example 14-1.

Solution

Following heuristic 1G, we will generate several sequences. Heuristics 2G to 6G, 8G and 9G are not applicable. Heuristic 8G suggests:

Distillation to produce waste water and azeotrope (also supported by 1D, 1S and 2S).

Adsorption or azeotropic distillation for breaking the azeotrope.

Heuristics 9G and 13S suggest preconcentrating feed with RO.

Heuristic 2D suggests removing mass separating agent early. This can easily be done in the azeotropic distillation since the azeotrope is heterogeneous.

Heuristics 3D and 6S suggest adsorption should be either temperature or pressure swing.

Heuristics 5D and 2C lead to distillation first, followed by breaking the azeotrope.

Heuristics 7D, 8D, 1C and 3C are not applicable.

Heuristic 4C suggests removing water first.

Heuristic 2S is satisfied by distillation taking the azeotrope as overhead, but is not satisfied by the usual azeotropic distillation.

Heuristic 5S suggests TSA may have high energy costs for breaking the azeotrope. An alternative such as PSA should be considered.

Heuristic 9S probably rules out chromatography.

Heuristic 12S would be applicable if solids were present in the feed.

The net result are the flow sheets shown in Figure 14-7. Figure 14-7a is a fairly standard distillation column followed by azeotropic distillation. Reverse osmosis is optional as a preconcentrator (Note: because of the unusual shape of the VLE curve this preconcentration has little effect on the reflux ratio R_D. Then according to Eq. (14-13) Q_R is not changed much by preconcentration. Although suggested by the heuristics RO is probably not useful for ethanol-water and is not shown on the other flow sheets. Preconcentration by RO can be useful for other systems.) Figure 14-7b uses distillation followed by liquid phase adsorption. This requires a drain step, evaporation of liquid, and then thermal regeneration. Since energy requirements will be quite high the vapor phase adsorption alternative shown in Figure 14-7c should be considered. The adsorption can be done as TSA or PSA. TSA is done commercially, but from heuristic 5S we should also consider PSA. This will require operating the distillation column under pressure. This may be advantageous since a smaller diameter distillation column can be used although equilibrium is less favorable.

Other known processes can be substituted for breaking the azeotropes. Examples are extraction and pervaporation. Heuristic 4D suggests pervaporation may not be advantageous; however, since it is commercially available it should be considered.

The heuristics give several reasonable flowsheets. Generation of a final flowsheet will require further economic comparisons. Note that in plants there are also solids and trace components to be removed.

834

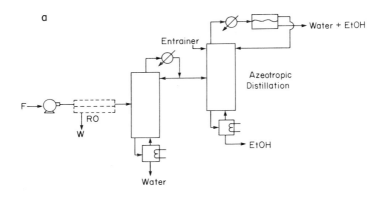

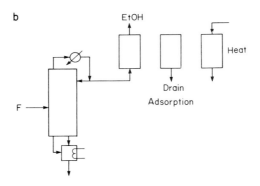

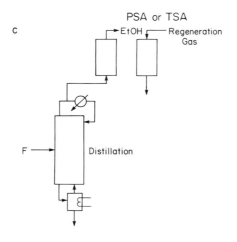

14.6. EVOLUTIONARY METHODS

Evolutionary methods are used to systematically modify an existing flowsheet to improve it. Although evolutionary methods do not guarentee that the optimum flowsheet will be generated, they are excellent insurance against catastrophic failure. Evolutionary methods are discussed by Liu (1987), Nath and Motard (1981), Nishida et al (1981), Seader and Westerberg (1977), and Stephanopoulos and Westerberg (1977) among others.

To use an evolutionary method one must first generate an initial sequence. The initial flowsheet is important. The better this flowsheet is, the easier it will be to apply evolutionary methods and find a result close to the optimum. Generation of the initial flowsheet is usually done using heuristics (Liu, 1987; Nath and Motard, 1981; Nishida et al, 1981; and Seader and Westerberg, 1977). This is one reason that heuristics have a prominent place in this chapter. An alternative to using heuristics is to use the solution to a similiar problem solved in the past. Conversion of flowsheets for similar liquid-liquid extraction problems is discussed by Blumberg (1988).

The second step is to develop the evolutionary rules. Local evolutionary methods look only at separation problems which are neighbors (Liu, 1987; Seader and Westerberg, 1977; Stephanopoulos and Westerberg, 1976). The local methods have the advantage of reducing the number of calculations which have to be done, but at the price of limiting the search field. The two evolutionary rules used for the local evolutionary method are (Seader and Westerberg, 1977):

1. Interchange the relative position of two neighboring subproblems.

2. Substitute an alternate separation method.

Figure 14-7.   Possible flowsheets for Example 14-3. a. Distillation followed by azeotropic distillation with optional RO. b. Distillation followed by liquid phase adsorption. c. Distillation followed by vapor phase adsorption (TSA or PSA).

Application of the rules requires a strategy. The strategy developed by Seader and Westerberg (1977) consisted of the following:

1. Generate each possible neighbor using the two rules. This will result in a lot of possibilities.

2. Keep a neighbor as a candidate if the heuristic used to choose the original separation did not clearly discriminate between the two choices, or if a competing heuristic would have selected the neighbor.

3. Evaluate the neighboring flowsheets until a locally "best" flowsheet is found.

4. Consider neighbors which are plausible, but were not included in strategy item 2.

It should be evident that this method can involve a lot of work. Thus, one needs to use short-cut estimation methods in the evaluation of flowsheets.

A global evolutionary method was developed by Nath and Motard (1981) and was used by Liu (1987). Unfortunately, this development included only distillation and extractive distillation; however, the method can probably be expanded to include other separation processes. Nath and Motard (1981) used heuristics in the following order:

1 (4G). Favor the smallest product set.
2 (1S). Favor distillation.
3 (Inverse of 2C). Easiest separation first.
4 (2D). Do not use a mass separating agent to recover a mass separating agent.
5. (1S). Separations with $\alpha < \alpha_{min}$ are unacceptable.
6 (4D). Set operating pressure close to ambient.
7. Use user set split fractions.
8. Use $L/D = 1.3 \ (L/D)_{min}$.

These heuristics are used in the order listed to generate the initial flowsheet. The following evolutionary rules are then applied:

1. Challenge Heuristic 1 (smallest product set).
To obtain the smallest product set one may have to use a mass separating agent. Relaxing heuristic 1 may result in a flowsheet without the mass separating agent, and this may be a better flowsheet.

2. Challenge neighboring separations if the difficulty of separation is about equal or if refrigeration is required for condensation of distillate.
Nath and Motard (1981) define a Coefficient of Difficulty of Separation to aid in the application of this rule.

3. Challenge heuristic 2 (favor distillation).
This rule allows one to consider mass separating agent processes.

4. Examine neighbors to see if removal of a mass separating agent should be delayed.
Heuristic rule 3 (easiest separation) will almost always force the removal of the mass separating agent next. If the mass separating agent can be used in more than one separation it is advantageous to leave it in the process longer.

5. Challenge heuristic 3 (easiest separation) if the following separation is much more difficult than the one being looked at.
Removing a component may make the next separation very difficult because of composition effects on the equilibrium parameters.

Liu (1987) notes that rules 1, 3, and 4 may be very valuable in developing less expensive designs.

These evolutionary rules can be applied in a variety of ways. The strategy chosen by Nath and Motard (1981) makes this a global method. Evolutionary rule 1 is done first. Then rules 2 to 5 are treated equally. When a change proves to be advantageous, the downstream process is eliminated and regenerated. All parts of the process are checked with rules 2 to 5. Nath and Motard (1981) give examples, but they include only distillation and extractive distillation.

The evolutionary approach or some other systematic approach to improving flowsheets are very useful in developing better flowsheets. Unfortunately, the evolutionary approaches need to be developed and validated for separations other than distillation and extractive distillation. This requires more research.

14.7. SUMMARY - OBJECTIVES

At the end of this chapter you should be able to meet the following objectives.

1. Discuss the type of separation problems which occur.

2. Develop tables of properties to compare separation alternatives for a given problem.

3. Use energy considerations to compare separation alternatives.

4. Discuss and use different strategies for developing flowsheets.

5. Use heuristics to develop an initial flowsheet. Discuss the rationale for each heuristic.

6. Discuss and use evolutionary methods.

7. List and discuss the areas which need further research in selecting a separation method.

REFERENCES

Bonmati, R., G. Chapelet-Letourneax, and G. Guiochon, "Gas chromatography: A new industrial process of separation. Application to essential oils", *Separ. Sci. Technol., 19*, 113 (1984).

Black, C., "Distillation modelling of ethanol recovery and dehydration processes for ethanol and gasohol," *Chem. Eng. Prog.*, *76* (9), 78 (1980).

Blumberg, R., *Liquid-Liquid Extraction*, Academic Press, London, 1988.

Bravo, J.L., J.R. Fair, J.L. Humphrey, C.L. Martin, A.E. Seibert and S. Joshi, *Fluid Mixture Separation Technologies for Cost Reduction and Process Improvement*, Noyes Publications, Park Ridge, N.J., 1986.

Douglas, J.M., *Conceputal Design of Chemical Processes*, McGraw-Hill, New York, 1988.

Evans, F.L., Jr., *Equipment Design Handbook for Refineries and Chemical Plants*, 2nd ed., Gulf Pub. Co., Houston, TX, 1980.

Fair, J.R., "Energy-efficient separation process design", in Y.A. Liu, H.A. McGee and W.R. Epperly (Eds.), *Recent Developments in Chemical Process and Plant Design*, Wiley-Interscience, New York, 1987, Chapt. 3.

Garg, D.R. and J.P. Ausikaitis, "Molecular sieve dehydration cycle for high water content streams," *Chem. Eng. Prog.*, *79* (4) 60 (1983).

Guiochon, G. and H. Colin, "Theoretical concepts and optimization in preparative scale liquid chromatography", *Chromatography Forum*, *21*, (Sept.-Oct., 1986).

Hendry, J.E., D.F. Rudd, and J.D. Seader, "Synthesis in the design of chemical processes," *AIChE Journal*, *19*, 1 (1973).

Ho, F.-G. and G.E. Keller, II, "Process integration", in Y.A. Liu, H.A. McGee, and W.R. Epperly (Eds.), *Recent Developments in Chemical Process and Plant Design*, Wiley-Interscience, New York, 1987, Chapt. 4.

Jacobs, L.J., Jr., and W.R. Penney, "Phase Segregation", in R.W. Rousseau

(Ed.), *Handbook of Separation Process Technology*, Wiley-Interscience, New York, 1987, Chapt. 3.

Keller, G.E., II, *Adsorption, Gas Absorption, and Liquid-Liquid Extraction: Selecting a Process and Conserving Energy*, Manual 9 in *Industrial Energy-Conservation*, The MIT Press, Cambridge, MA, 1982.

Kelly, R.M., "General Processing Considerations," in R.W. Rousseau (Ed.), *Handbook of Separation Process Technology*, Wiley-Interscience, New York, 1987, Chapt. 4.

King, C.J., *Separation Processes*, 2nd ed., McGraw-Hill, New York, 1980.

Kopaciewicz, W. and F.E. Regnier, "A system for coupled multiple-column separation of proteins", *Anal. Biochem. 129*, 472 (1983).

Ladisch, M.R., M. Voloch, J. Hong, P. Bienkowski and G.T. Tsao "Commercial adsorber for dehydrating ethanol vapors," *Ind. Eng. Chem. Process Des. Develop., 23*, 437 (1984).

Leeper, S. and P.C. Wankat, "Gasohol production by extraction of ethanol from water using gasoline as solvent," *Ind. Eng. Chem. Process Des. Develop., 21*, 331 (1982).

Liu, Y.A., "Process Synthesis: Some simple and practical developments," in Y.A. Liu, H.A. McGee, Jr., W.R. Epperly (Eds.), *Recent Developments in Chemical Process and Plant Design*, Wiley-Interscience, New York, 1987, Chapt.6.

Ludwig, E.E., *Applied Process Design for Chemical and Petrochemical Plants*, 2nd ed., Gulk Pub. Co., Houston, TX, 1979.

Mazsaroff, I. and F.E. Regnier, "An economic analysis of performance in preparative chromatography of proteins", *J. Liqd. Chromatogr. 9*, 2563 (1986).

McDonald, P.D. and B.A. Bidlingmeyer, "Strategies for successful preparative liquid chromatography," in B.A. Bidlingmeyer (Ed.), *Preparative Liquid Chromatography*, Elsevier, Amsterdam, 1987.

Nath, R. and R.L. Mothard, "Evolutionary synthesis of separation processes", *AIChE Journal, 27*, 578 (1981).

Nishida, N., G. Stephanopoulos and A.W. Westerberg, "A review of process synthesis," *AIChE Journal, 27*, 321 (1981).

Null, H.R., "Energy economy in separation processes," *Chem. Engr. Prog., 76* (8), 42 (Aug. 1980).

Null, H.R. "Selection of a separation process," in R.W. Rousseau (Ed.)., *Handbook of Separation Process Technology*, Wiley-Interscience, New York, 1987, Chapt. 22.

Perry, R.H. and D.W. Green (Eds.), *Chemical Engineers' Handbook*, 6th ed., McGraw-Hill, New York, 1984.

Robinson, C.S. and E.R. Gilliland, *Elements of Fractional Distillation*, 4th ed., McGraw-Hill, New York, 1950.

Roddy, J.W., "Distribution of ethanol-water mixtures to organic liquids," *Ind. Eng. Chem. Process Des. Develop., 20*, 104 (1981).

Rudd, D.F., G.J. Powers, and J.J. Siirola, *Process Synthesis*, Prentice-Hall, Englewood Cliffs, N.J., 1973.

Ruthven, D.M., *Principles of Adsorption and Adsorption Processes*, Wiley, New York, 1984.

Schweitzer, P.A. (Ed.), *Handbook of Separation Techniques for Chemical Engineers*, McGraw-Hill, New York, 1979.

Seader, J.D., "Distillation," in R.H. Perry and D.W. Green (Eds.), *Perry's Chemical Engineers' Handbook*, 6th ed., McGraw-Hill, New York, 1984, Section 13.

Seader, J.D. and A.W. Westerberg, "A combined heuristic and evolutionary strategy for synthesis of simple separation sequences", *AIChE Journal, 23*, 951 (1977).

Sherwood, T.K., R.L. Pigford and C.R. Wilke, *Mass Transfer*, McGraw-Hill, New York, 1975, Chapt. 1.

Stephanopoulos, G. and A.W. Westerberg, "Studies in process synthesis - II", *Chem. Eng. Sci., 31*, 195 (1976).

Tedder, D.W. and D.F. Rudd, "Parametric studies in industrial distillation. Part I. Design Comparisons", *AIChE Journal, 24*, 303 (1978).

Thompson, R.W. and C.J. King, "Systematic synthesis of separation schemes," *AIChE Journal, 18*, 941, (1972).

Van Winkle, M., *Distillation*, McGraw-Hill, New York, 1967.

Wankat, P.C., *Large-Scale Adsorption and Chromatography*, CRC Press, Boca Raton, FL, 1986.

Wankat, P.C. *Equilibrium-Staged Separations*, Elsevier, New York, 1988.

Westerberg, A.W., "Design research. Both theory and strategy", *Chem. Eng. Educ., 16*, 12 (1982) and *16*, 62 (1982).

HOMEWORK

A. *Discussion Problems*

A1.Define the following terms

    a. Minimum work

b. Equivalent work

c. Heuristic

d. Evolutionary method

e. Local evolution

f. Global evolution

g. Separation factor

h. Diffusional separations

i. Mechanical separations

j. Hybrid process

k. Neighbor

j. Top-down/Bottom-up

A2. When one is developing new separation processes, distillation is often considered "the enemy". Explain why.

A3. Heuristics can be misleading. For example, heuristic 4D could be misleading when high pressure gas streams are processed. Explain why one probably wants to do the separation at high pressure.

A4. Based on an equivalent work analysis crystallization is a very attractive separation process. Why isn't crystallization used more often?

A5. Explain the differences and similarities between local and global evolution.

A6. Expand on the idea of using flowsheets for similar problems to generate an initial flowsheet. How similar must the problems be? What are some sources of flowsheets?

A7. On Figure 14-1 "Water from sea water", vitamin B-12, and "gold from sea water" all fall off the empirical straight line. Hypothesize why each of these three is different.

844

A8.Why is adsorption favored compared to distillation when a small amount of nonvolatile material is to be removed?

A9.List and discuss the areas requiring additional research.

A10. What are "optimistic conditions" for comparison of the following separation processes?

    a. zone melting

    b. UF

    c. ED

    d. LC for protein purification

A11. Extend heuristic 2S to the following separations:

    a. crystallization

    b. adsorption

    c. membrane separations

A12. Westerberg (1982) suggests that theories evolve from simple to complex. Explain how one can do this for

    a. Chromatography

    b. Reverse osmosis

    c. Solution crystallization

A13. Compare depth-first with breadth-first approaches. Why should both depth and breadth be included? List and discuss the areas requiring additional research.

A14. Develop your key relations chart for this chapter.

B. *Generation of Alternatives*

B1.Hybrid processs allow the designer to stretch his/her imagination. Membrane processes in particular seem to be very useful in hybrid processes. Develop two novel hybrid processes involving membranes.

B2. Suppose you work for a company whose business is selling processes. Brainstorm and then pare down a list of separations which should be explored further by R&D. Explain your final list of 5 items.

B3. Generate possible separations to recover acetic acid from a dilute aqueous solution.

B4. Use heuristics to generate preliminary separation flowsheets for Problem 14-B3.

C. *Derivations*

C1. Develop a local evolutionary process which uses Nath and Motard's (1981) evolutionary rules.

C2. Derive Eq. (14-19).

C3. Derive Eq. (14-14).

C4. Many of the heuristics in this chapter were developed from material in previous chapters. Generate two additional S heuristics based on information in previous chapters.

D. *Problems*

D1. We wish to separate a gas mixture of ethylbenzene and styrene at $110°C$. Determine $W_{min,T}$ for mole fractions of ethylbenzene of 0,10,20,...,100 in the feed. Ratio $p_p/p_F = 1.5$.

D2. Determine the equivalent work requirement for a melt crystallization system purifying p-xylene from a mixture of para and meta xylenes. The feed is 40 mole % p-xylene, crystal product is 99.9 mole % p-xylene. Operation of the crystallizer is very slightly above the eutectic temperature (221 K).

Assume the melt product is essentially at the eutectic composition (13 mole % p-xylene). Pressure is 101.3 kPa. Determine the ideal equivalent work ($\varepsilon_P = \varepsilon_R = 1$) for melt crystallization if a 10°C approach temperature is used in the melter and the crystallizer. The ambient temperature T_o is 18°C. Melter reflux ratio $R_M = 0.5$. Use a feed rate of 100 kg/hr as a basis.

Xylene Data (King, 1980, p. 740): MW = 106.16, λ_p = 340 kJ/kg, λ_M = 343 kJ/kg, $T_{boiling,p}$ = 411.8 K., $T_{boiling,m}$ = 412.6 K, $T_{f,M}$ = 225.4 K, $T_{f,p}$ = 286.6 K,

(Perry and Green, 1984, p. 3-123) $\lambda_{f,M}$ = 26.045 cal/g, $\lambda_{f,p}$ = 38.526 cal/g

D3. Find the equivalent work in cal/(kg product) required for the RO system in Example 12-2b for M = 1.2. Watch your units. Use a water density of 1 kg/liter.

F. *Problems Requiring Other Resources*

F1. Different chromatographic methods used for protein purification have different solvent requirements. Read Kopaciewicz and Regnier (1983) and develop heuristics for sequencing chromatography columns for protein purification.

F2. Extend Nath and Motard's (1981) "Coefficient of Difficulty of Separation" to center-feed melt crystallization of solid solutions.

APPENDIX. ANSWERS TO SELECTED PROBLEMS

Chapter 2

2-D1. $CuSO_4 \cdot 5\,H_2O$, $a = -1610$, $b = 1.727$

2-D3.   a. $Na_2\,CO_3 \cdot 7\,H_2O(45.9\ kg)$, $Na_2\,CO_3 \cdot H_2O(40.4\ kg)$ and
        eutectic (13.6 kg)
        b. $Na_2CO_3 \cdot 7\,H_2O$ (65.0 kg) , $Na_2CO_3 \cdot H_2O$ (35.0 kg)
        30,500 KJ

2-D5.   Add water. 66.8 kg KNO_3 ,   Point $b = 0.28\ KNO_3$

2-D7. $F(b(0)) = 116.97$ kg/hr , $F(b(30)) = 188.08$ kg/hr.
        $W_{in,1} = 16.11$ kg/hr   , $W_{in,2} = 9.96$ kg/hr.
        $F_{hydrate} = 81.07$ kg/hr

2-D11. 3.503 M

Chapter 3

3-D2.   Linear. 30°C proportionality $= 7.514 \times 10^{-10}$
                  70°C proportionality $= 6.334 \times 10^{-9}$

3-D3.   a. $B^\circ = 41.75$ #/cm$^3 \cdot$ s , b. $B^\circ \approx 0$

Chapter 4

4-D1.   65 mesh, M = 21.9
        48 mesh, M = 58.6
        35 mesh, M = 134.1
        28 mesh, M = 254.4
        20 mesh, M = 385

4-D5a. $\overline{G} = 0.0041$ cm/hr , $n^\circ = 1.61 \times 10^8$ #/cm $\cdot$ L

4-D6.   G = 0.0821 mm/hr

4-D9. $M_T = 0.28$ gm/cm^3, $L_D = 0.31$ mm

4-E1. $G = 6.068 \times 10^{-7}$ m/s
          Median size 0.9016 mm.

Chapter 5

5-D2.   a. $y_{tot} = 0.00178$
          b. $y_{Prod} = 0.00102$

5-D3. $k_i = 0.4525$, $e = 0.1243$

5-D5. $L = 239.1$ cm

5-D7.   b. $x = 0.0024$

Chapter 6

6-D2. $c = 0.02$ until $t = 24.6$ min then $c = 0.50$ until $t = 25.5$ min. At this
          point get a diffuse wave.
$c = 0.34$	at	$t = 28.0$ min
$c = 0.10$	at	$t = 42.0$ min
$c = 0.02$	at	$t = 92.2$ min

6-D4.   a. $t_G = 4.71$ min, $t_F = 6.19$ min
          b. $t_{feed} = 1.48$ min
               $t_{next} = 2.96$ min (1.48 min waiting period)

6-D6. $\alpha_{EP} = 7.36$

6-D8.   b. $t_{out} = 14.12$ min based on data
               $t_{out} = 13.46$ min based on Langmuir fit.

Chapter 7

7-D1.   a. $u_N = 0.0115$, $u_A = 0.00853$, $u_p = 0.0062$ m/min
          b. $L = 0.66$ m
          c.   wait 49.1 minutes after end of pulse

7-D2. $A_B = 4.25$

7-D3. $x = 1 - X(L,t) + X(L, t - t_1)$

7-D5. $c/c_F = 0.5$ at 74.29 minutes

7-D7.   a. $R = 0.317$
          b. $L = 799$ cm

7-D11. $d_p = 5.97$ μm

7-D13. $t_{sh} = 10.15$ min, $c = 0.0052$

7-D14. $H_{col} = 0.0651$ cm, $\sigma_{ec}^2 = 0.266$ cm^2

Chapter 8

8-D1.   a. $L = 42.71$ cm, $t_{br} = 36.9$ min
          b. $L = 56.94$ cm, $t_{br} = 36.9$ min

8-D3. $v_{super} = 0.0116$ cm/s

8-D4. $d_{p,new} = 0.639$ mm , $D_{new}/D_{old} = 1.166$

8-D7.   a. $L = 268.4$ cm
          b. $c_{methane} = 0.0036$ gmole/L

8-D8.   frac bed util col B = 0.82
          For 90% util, $L = 119.1$ cm, $t_{br} = 900$ min.

Chapter 9

9-D3.   From 0 to 3 minutes, $c_T = 0.1$, $x_{Ni} = 0.2$.
          From 3 to 6.10 min, $c_T = 5.1$, $x_{Ni} = 0.78$
          After 6.10 min, $c_T = 5.1$, $x_{Ni} = 0.2$

9-D5.   a. $L_{MTZ} = 8.13$ cm

9-D6.   In bands $y_{Na} = 1$ and $y_{NH4} = 1$.
              $t_{Na,band} = 4$ min, $t_{NH4,band} = 6$ min

Chapter 10

10-D1. $N = 4$ stages

10-D3.   88% of protein is recovered.

10-D5. $V_R/V_S = 11.93$

10-D7. $h = 23.4$ cm. $c_{out} = 1.095$ mg/ml

Chapter 11

11-D1. $\zeta = 19.265$ mV

11-D2. $\mu = 7.907 \times 10^{-6}$ cm^2/sV
$D = 3.07 \times 10^{-8}$ cm^2/s

11-D4.   a. $w_y = 0.485$ cm , $w_z = 2.40$ cm

11-D6. $\mu = 5.12 \times 10^{-4}$ cm^2/sV

11-D7.   a. $E = 16.39$ V/cm
b. $\sigma_A = 1.0935$ cm , $w_A = 4.375$ cm
c. $\sigma_A = 0.495$ cm , $w_A = 1.98$ cm

11-D8.   a. $\Delta pI = 0.018$ pH units
b. $pI = 5.53$

Chapter 12

12-D1. $\alpha_{H2,CO2} = 39.3$

12-D3. $J_{solv} = 8000$ L/m^2 day, $M = 6.67$

12-D4. $c_g = 0.314$

12-D6.   a. $I = 57.27$ amp , $V = 343$ volts
b. $E = 705.5$ cal/L
c.   Power = 19.68 kilowatts

12-D9. $\theta = 0.160$

12-D10. $y_p = 0.889$, $y_{out} = 0.247$

12-D12.   a. $t_g = 6.98 \times 10^{-5}$ cm
b. $t_g = 1.48 \times 10^{-4}$ cm

Chapter 13

13-D1. $D = 3.09 \times 10^{-8}$ cm^2/s

13-D4. M = 5.23

13-D6. a. Gelling starts at 18.93 cm
 b. $J = 3.2 \times 10^{-4}$ cm/s

13-D7. M ≈ 1.0

13-D9. a. $c_{2p}/c_{2w} = 0.771$
 b. $R_p = 5.6 \times 10^{-7}$ cm

Chapter 14

14-D1. $y_{EF} = 0$, $W_{min} = 308.7$ cal/gmole feed
 $y_{EF} = 0.1$, $W_{min} = 556.25$ cal/gmole feed

14-D2. $W_{eq,cry} = 5.27$ Kcal/kg feed

Breakthrough, 306, 311, 366-370,
Bromine, 797
Butane adsorption, 223
Butanol, 413, 713-716
Butyric acid, 416

C
C term, 327-329
Calcium acetate, 21,24
Calcium carbonate, 747
Calcium sulfate, 747
Canister systems, 414, 435-437, 446
Capacity, 369, 456-458
Capillary chromatography, 291, 799
Capillary condensation, 223, 415
Capillary electrophoresis,
    See Electrophoresis, capillary
Caprolactam, 672
Carbon adsorption systems,
    See Activated carbon and
    Carbon molecular sieves
Carbon dioxide, 226, 293, 367, 408,
    643, 646-651, 831
Carbon monoxide, 649-651
Carbon molecular sieves, 225, 804
Carbon tetrachloride, 223, 418
Carman-Kozeny equation, 385, 679
Carrier ampholytes, See Ampholytes
Carriers, 649
Cascades, membrane,
    See Membrane, cascades
Casein, 680-681, 787
Cations, 452, 461
Cellophane membrane, 711-713, 789

Cellulose, 634-635, 691
Cellulose acetate membrane, 570, 633,
    635, 638, 643, 646-648, 650,
    667-668, 673-675, 691, 712-716,
    748, 778
Center feed columns, 178, 183
Centrifuge, 151, 799, 803
Cesium chloride, 585
Channeling, 219, 489
Characteristic temperature, 408
Charcoal, 230
Chemical modification, 799-800
Chem-Seps process,
    See Higgins process
Chlorine, 416, 419-420, 671
Chlorobenzene, 418
Chloroform, 418
Chromatofocusing, See focusing,
Chromatography, See also specific
    topics, 4-6, 217, 288-364, 807-808,
    810, 825, 827-828, 830-831
    analytical, 288-296, 306, 316
    large-scale, 306, 320, 330-331, 336,
        341-347
    linear, 297, 306-334
    nonlinear, 298-306
    resolution, 319-320
    scaling, 389
    solute movement theory, 296-305,
        395-400
    theories, 296-335, 347
Chung and Wen correlation, 312
Citric acid, 25, 87, 91
Classification, See Separations,
    classification

PAGE, *See* Electrophoresis,
  polyacrylamide gel
Paper chromatography, 295, 605, 799,
  804
Paper electrophoresis, *See*
  Electrophoresis, paper
Parex, 177
Partial melting, 171-176, 184-186, 200
Pb(NO₃)₂, *See* Lead nitrate
Peak maximum, 313, 317, 326
Peak width, 318-319
Peclet number, 310-312, 317
Penicillin, 797
Pentane, 394-395, 433
Permeability, gas, 631, 643-644, 646,
  652, 776
Permeability, liquid, 657-665, 679,
  680-681, 688, 705, 774-775
Permittivity free space, 551
Perstraction, 716
Pervaporation 703-716, 728-729, 799,
  803, 810, 827, 833
pH effects, 69-70, 286-287, 289
pH gradient, 286-287, 336, 338-339
pH marker, 553, 598
Pharmaceuticals, 342
Phase equilibria, *See* Equilibrium data
Phenanthrene, 39
Phenol, 39, 40, 162, 420, 433-434, 718
Phenomenological coefficients,
  770-771, 773-776, 779
Phillips process, 176-177
Philpot-Harwell device, 585-587
pI, *See* Isoelectric point
Plasma proteins, *See* Blood proteins

Plate-and-frame, 637-638, 640,
  668-669, 674-675, 683, 688, 692,
  694, 699-700, 738, 746, 762-765
Plate generation, 573
Plate height, *See* HETP
Plate theories, *See* Staged theory
Plateau, 394-395
Point fines trap, 132
Poiseuille flow, 780-781
Poisson distribution, 315
Poisson-Boltzmann distribution, 556
Polarity, chemical, 336-337
Polarity reversal, 700
Polarization, *See*
  Concentration polarization
Polarization Modulus, 661-666,
  677-678, 734-736, 765-770
Polishing, 481-482
Polyacrylamide gel electrophoresis,
  See Electrophoresis,
  polyacrylamide gel
Polyacrylic acid, 456-459
Polyacrylonitrile, 634, 673, 675, 691,
  712
Polyamide, 634, 638, 667, 669, 673,
  713
Polycarbonate, 633, 673
Polyether block amide (PEBAX), 703
Polyfuran, 669
Polymeric adsorbent, 227-228, 433
Polymeric resin, 433, 455-459
Polymorphism, 81
Polynucleotide, 550, 552-553
Polypropylene, 713
Polysaccharide, 678, 745